HOW NOT TO DIE

Also by
MICHAEL GREGER, M.D., FACLM

The How Not to Die Cookbook
How Not to Diet
The How Not to Diet Cookbook
How to Survive a Pandemic
How Not to Age
The How Not to Age Cookbook

HOW NOT TO DIE

REVISED AND UPDATED

DISCOVER THE FOODS
SCIENTIFICALLY PROVEN TO PREVENT
AND REVERSE DISEASE

Michael Greger, M.D., FACLM
with Gene Stone

First revised edition published 2025 by Flatiron Books

First published in the UK 2025 by Bluebird
an imprint of Pan Macmillan
The Smithson, 6 Briset Street, London EC1M 5NR
EU representative: Macmillan Publishers Ireland Ltd, 1st Floor,
The Liffey Trust Centre, 117–126 Sheriff Street Upper,
Dublin 1 D01YC43
Associated companies throughout the world

ISBN 978-1-0350-6018-4

Copyright © Michael Greger with Gene Stone 2015, 2025

This book contains the opinions and ideas of its author. It is intended to provide helpful general information on the subjects that it addresses. It is not in any way a substitute for the advice of the reader's own physician(s) or other medical professionals based on the reader's own individual conditions, symptoms, or concerns. If the reader needs personal medical, health, dietary, exercise, or other assistance or advice, the reader should consult a competent physician and/or other qualified health care professionals. The author and publisher specifically disclaim all responsibility for injury, damage, or loss that the reader may incur as a direct or indirect consequence of following any directions or suggestions given in the book or participating in any programs described in the book. The reader is advised not to undertake, cease, or modify any treatments, diets, or health procedures without consulting a professional. Failure to adhere to this recommendation may result in adverse health impacts, for which the author and publisher accept no responsibility.

The rights of Michael Greger and Gene Stone to be identified as the
authors of this work have been asserted in accordance
with the Copyright, Designs and Patents Act 1988.

Figures and illustrations by Caroline Garriott, Kat Farrell, and Vance Lehmkuhl

Designed by Steven Seighman

All rights reserved. No part of this publication may be reproduced,
stored in a retrieval system, or transmitted, in any form, or by any means
(including, without limitation, electronic, mechanical, photocopying, recording
or otherwise) without the prior written permission of the publisher.

Pan Macmillan does not have any control over, or any responsibility for,
any author or third-party websites (including, without limitation, URLs,
emails and QR codes) referred to in or on this book.

1 3 5 7 9 8 6 4 2

A CIP catalogue record for this book is available from the British Library.

Printed and bound in the UK using 100% Renewable Electricity by CPI Group (UK) Ltd

This book is sold subject to the condition that it shall not, by way of
trade or otherwise, be lent, hired out, or otherwise circulated without
the publisher's prior consent in any form of binding or cover other than
that in which it is published and without a similar condition including this
condition being imposed on the subsequent purchaser. The publisher does not
authorize the use or reproduction of any part of this book in any manner
for the purpose of training artificial intelligence technologies or systems.
The publisher expressly reserves this book from the Text and Data Mining
exception in accordance with Article 4(3) of the European Union
Digital Single Market Directive 2019/790.

Visit **www.panmacmillan.com/bluebird** to read more about
all our books and to buy them.

To my grandma Frances Greger

Contents

AUTHOR'S NOTE — IX
PREFACE — XIII
INTRODUCTION — 1

PART 1

1. How Not to Die from Heart Disease — 19
2. How Not to Die from Lung Diseases — 35
3. How Not to Die from Brain Diseases — 53
4. How Not to Die from Infections — 76
5. How Not to Die from High Blood Pressure — 102
6. How Not to Die from Digestive Cancers — 125
7. How Not to Die from Diabetes — 144
8. How Not to Die from Liver Diseases — 170
9. How Not to Die from Blood Cancers — 183
10. How Not to Die from Kidney Disease — 195
11. How Not to Die from Suicidal Depression — 212
12. How Not to Die from Breast Cancer — 227
13. How Not to Die from Parkinson's Disease — 252
14. How Not to Die from Prostate Cancer — 268
15. How Not to Die from Iatrogenic Causes — 285

PART 2

Introduction	305
Dr. Greger's Daily Dozen	323
Beans	327
Berries	340
Other Fruits	348
Cruciferous Vegetables	359
Greens	366
Other Vegetables	377
Flaxseeds	394
Nuts and Seeds	398
Herbs and Spices	407
Whole Grains	431
Beverages	442
Exercise	456
Conclusion	465
Acknowledgments	471
Appendix: Supplements	473
Appendix: Cooking Legumes	479
Appendix: Cooking Whole Grains	483
Notes	487
Index	635

Author's Note

I didn't want to write *How Not to Die*.

When a book agent approached me with the offer, my first thoughts were: *All my work is available for free online, so why would anyone buy a book?* I was already reaching millions through NutritionFacts.org, the nonprofit organization I had started years before. *Do people even read books anymore?* I knew it would take at least a year to write it. Who has the time?

But he kept coming back with higher and higher offers from the publisher. I knew I wouldn't personally accept any money from a book. There is too much corrupting commercial influence in the wellness world. I didn't want to be another author profiting off book sales (or gadgets or supplements). Whenever I see a purported health or wellness "expert" hawking this or that, I'm left wondering whether they actually care about the health of me and my family or if they're just pushing sales to enrich themselves.

There were charities I wanted to support, though. Think how many lives I could help and maybe even save! (Charity evaluators like GiveWell estimate that $3,000 spent on targeted malaria prevention, for example, could save a life in Nigeria.[1]) Eventually, the book advance offer got so high, reaching a level that donating all of it would do more good in the world than anything else I could imagine doing, that I couldn't say no. So I didn't. I said yes, and I'm so glad I did.

How Not to Die became an instant *New York Times* bestseller and went on to sell more than a million copies. It's been translated into more than thirty languages. (I don't know if I could even *name* thirty languages!) Beyond all the money that got distributed to effective charities was the impact the book was having on readers' lives around the world. Every day the stories would pour in. Though there are fleeting moments when I regret publicly posting my personal cell phone number and email address, I was joyfully overwhelmed to hear about all the life and health transformations.

I had always had warm receptions at my speaking events, but there was a palpable shift after *How Not to Die* came out. People would wait in book-signing lines for hours to tearfully share how much my work had meant to their family. I realized just how intimate the connection can be between writer and reader. By the time we first met, they had already spent days—maybe weeks—curling up with me on the couch. It can be such a powerful bond. This book's reach allowed me to serve and help in a way I had never been able to before. I knew then that I'd be writing books for the rest of my life.

My professional trajectory isn't the only thing that's shifted over the past decade. The COVID crisis helped lay bare the limitations of our "pill for every ill" sickcare system, which focuses on managing the consequences of chronic disease rather than treating the underlying cause to potentially reverse it—or prevent it in the first place.[2] Approximately 80 percent of protracted disease and premature death may be attributable to choices each one of us makes on a day-to-day basis, yet for too long this lifestyle lever has been largely ignored by mainstream medicine.[3] But that's changing.

I am honored that more than twenty years ago I became a founding member of the American College of Lifestyle Medicine (ACLM), a professional society dedicated to using diet and lifestyle interventions to treat the roots of many of the chronic diseases that plague humanity. Lifestyle medicine has grown from humble beginnings to become one of the fastest-growing medical specialties.[4] Now with more than ten thousand clinician members, ACLM is more than just a professional association; it is a galvanizing force for change. Most medical schools now have student-run lifestyle medicine groups, and hundreds of residency programs for budding doctors have incorporated a lifestyle medicine curriculum. Thousands of physicians in the United States alone have now become board certified in lifestyle medicine.[5] (I am so proud to have been in the first cohort.) A global network of national lifestyle medicine associations has sprung up, dedicated to the use of daily healthy habits to prevent, treat, and cure chronic disease.[6] What started as fringe has become more and more mainstream.

Look what happened in New York City. Consistent with its namesake, the Big Apple became a leader in food policy innovation. All eleven NYC public hospitals started offering plant-based meals *by default*. Healthy food in a *hospital*? What a concept! Patient meal satisfaction exceeds 90 percent, and the hospital saves money in a win-win that should be replicated throughout the country and around the world.[7] Lifestyle medicine clinics were started in all five New York City boroughs.[8] Its schools have Meatless Mondays and Plant-Powered Fridays,[9] and under enhanced food standards, sugary drinks were removed from vending machines and processed meat eliminated from the city's schools, hospitals, prisons, homeless shelters, and older adult centers.[10,11] If the country's largest city can institute sweeping food reform, why can't other cities follow suit?

I'm thrilled to present this tenth-anniversary edition of *How Not to Die*. The needle hasn't moved as much as I'd hoped in the last decade. We're still eating ourselves into early graves, but there has been much progress. Lifestyle medicine is marching along, gaining support and supporters, and there have been significant, even wildly exciting, advances in treating diseases like Alzheimer's. The good news is that we have tremendous power over our health destiny and longevity. Indeed, the vast majority of premature death and disability is preventable with a healthy enough diet and lifestyle.

If this is your first time reading *How Not to Die*, I hope you find it inspiring, illuminating, and empowering. If you're reading this updated tenth-anniversary edition, I hope you find more hope in what our day-to-day choices can do to help us live longer and healthier lives.

I look back at the "More Doctors Smoke Camels" type of ads that ran in medical journals up through the 1950s.[12] We had already had decades of science linking smoking with lung cancer,[13] but it was ignored because smoking was mainstream. Smoking was normal. Even most doctors smoked.[14] The average per capita cigarette consumption was four thousand cigs a year, meaning the average American smoked half a pack a day.[15] Despite all the evidence to the contrary, the American Medical Association was reassuring everyone that smoking *in moderation* was okay.[16] There was a disconnect between the science and public policy. It took more than twenty-five years and seven thousand studies before the first U.S. Surgeon General report against smoking came out in the 1960s.[17] You'd think that maybe after the first *six thousand* studies we could have been given a heads-up?

In 2017, our diet overtook tobacco use as the leading lifestyle risk factor for death in the United States. In 2021, diet-related deaths were poised to overtake tobacco-related deaths globally as well. Cigarettes still kill hundreds of thousands of Americans every year, but so does the American diet.[18] The medical establishment went from defending the tobacco industry to eventually leading the way in the fight against smoking.[19] Medical momentum is slowly gathering against our new leading killer, but we don't have to wait. Until the system changes, we can take personal responsibility for our own health and that of our loved ones. We can't wait until society catches up to the science again, because it's a matter of life and death.

In health,

March 1, 2025

Preface

It all started with my grandmother.

I was only a kid when the doctors sent her home in a wheelchair to die. Diagnosed with end-stage heart disease, she had already had so many bypass operations that the surgeons essentially ran out of plumbing—the scarring from each open-heart surgery had made the next more difficult until they finally ran out of options. My grandma was confined to a wheelchair with crushing chest pain, and her doctors told her there was nothing else they could do. Her life was over at age sixty-five.

I think what sparks many kids to want to become doctors when they grow up is watching a beloved relative become ill or even die. But for me, it was watching my grandma get better.

Soon after she was discharged from the hospital to spend her last days at home, a segment aired on *60 Minutes* about Nathan Pritikin, an early lifestyle medicine pioneer who had been gaining a reputation for reversing terminal heart disease. He had just opened a new center in California, and my grandmother, in desperation, somehow made the cross-country trek to become one of its first patients. This was a live-in program where everyone was placed on a plant-based diet and then started on a graded exercise regimen. They wheeled my grandmother in, and she walked out.

I'll never forget that.

She was even featured in Pritikin's biography *Pritikin: The Man Who Healed America's Heart*. My grandma was described as one of the "death's door people":

Frances Greger, from North Miami, Florida, arrived in Santa Barbara at one of Pritikin's early sessions in a wheelchair. Mrs. Greger had heart disease, angina, and claudication; her condition was so bad she could no longer walk without great pain in her chest and legs. Within three weeks, though, she was not only out of her wheelchair but was walking ten miles a day.[20]

When I was a kid, that was all that mattered: I got to play with Grandma again. But over the years, I grew to understand the significance of what had happened. At that time, the medical profession didn't even think it was possible to reverse heart disease. Drugs were given to try to slow its progression, and surgery was performed to circumvent clogged arteries to try to relieve symptoms, but the disease was expected to get worse and worse until you died. Now, however, we know that as soon as we stop eating an artery-clogging diet, our bodies can start healing themselves, in many cases opening up arteries without drugs or surgery.

My grandma was given her medical death sentence at age sixty-five. Thanks to a healthy diet and lifestyle, she was able to enjoy another thirty-one years on this earth with her six grandchildren. The woman who was once told by doctors she only had weeks to live didn't die until she was ninety-six. Her near-miraculous recovery not only inspired one of those grandkids to pursue a career in medicine but granted her enough healthy years to see him graduate from medical school.

By the time I became a doctor, giants like Dean Ornish, M.D., president and founder of the nonprofit Preventive Medicine Research Institute, had already proven beyond a shadow of a doubt what Pritikin had shown to be true. Using the latest high-tech advances—cardiac PET scans,[21] quantitative coronary arteriography,[22] and radionuclide ventriculography[23]—Dr. Ornish and his colleagues showed that the lowest-tech approach—diet and lifestyle—can undeniably reverse the progression of heart disease, our leading killer.

Their studies were published in some of the most prestigious medical journals in the world. Yet medical practice hardly changed. Why? Why were doctors still prescribing drugs and using Roto-Rooter-type procedures to just treat the symptoms of heart disease and try to forestall what they chose to believe was the inevitable—an early death?

This was my wake-up call. I opened my eyes to the depressing fact that there are other forces at work in medicine besides science. The U.S. health care system largely runs on a fee-for-service model in which doctors get paid for the pills and procedures they prescribe, rewarding quantity over quality. We may not get reimbursed for time spent counseling our patients about the benefits of healthy eating. If doctors were instead paid for performance, there would be a financial incentive to treat the lifestyle causes of disease. Until the model of reimbursement changes, I don't expect great changes in medical care or medical education.[24]

Only a quarter of U.S. medical schools appear to offer a single dedicated course on nutrition.[25] During my first interview for medical school, at Cornell University, I remember the interviewer emphatically stating, "Nutrition is superfluous to human health." And he was a pediatrician! I knew I was in for a long road ahead. Come to think of it, I think the only medical professional who ever asked me about a family member's diet was our veterinarian.

I was honored to be accepted by nineteen medical schools. I chose Tufts because it boasted the most nutrition training—twenty-one hours' worth, although this was still less than 1 percent of the curriculum.

During my medical training, I was offered countless steak dinners and fancy perks by Big Pharma representatives, but not once did I get a call from Big Broccoli. There is a reason we hear about the latest drugs on television: Huge corporate budgets drive their promotion. The same reason we'll probably never see a commercial for sweet potatoes is the same reason breakthroughs on the power of foods to affect our health and longevity may never make it to the public: There's little profit motive.

In medical school, even with our paltry twenty-one hours of nutrition training, there was no mention of using diet to treat chronic disease, let alone reverse it. I was only aware of this body of work because of my family's personal story.

The question that haunted me during training was this: *If the potential cure to our number one killer could get lost down the rabbit hole, what else might be buried in the medical literature?* I made it my life's mission to find out.

Most of my years in Boston were spent scouring the dusty stacks in the basement of Harvard's Countway Library of Medicine. I started practicing medicine, but no matter how many patients I saw in the clinic every day, even when I was able to change the lives of entire families at a time, I knew it was just a drop in the bucket, so I went on the road.

With the help of the American Medical Student Association, I set out with the goal of speaking at every medical school in the country every two years to influence an entire generation of new doctors. I didn't want another doctor to graduate without this tool—the power of food—in their toolbox. If my grandma didn't have to die from heart disease, perhaps no one's grandparent did.

There were periods where I was giving forty talks a month. I'd roll into town to give a breakfast talk at a Rotary Club, deliver a presentation at the medical school over lunch, then speak to a community group in the evening. I was living out of my car, one key on my keychain. I ended up giving more than a thousand presentations around the world.

Not surprisingly, life on the road was not sustainable. I lost a marriage over it. With more speaking requests than I could accept, I started putting all my annual research findings into a DVD series, *Latest in Clinical Nutrition*. Every penny I received from selling those DVDs went directly to charity, as does the money I get from my speaking engagements and book sales to this day, including the book you're reading now.

As corrupting an influence as money is in medicine, it appears to me to be even worse in the field of nutrition, where it seems everyone has their own brand of snake-oil supplement or wonder gadget. Dogmas are entrenched and data too often cherry-picked to support preconceived notions.

True, I have biases of my own to rein in. Although my original motivation was health, over the years, I've grown into quite the animal lover. Three dogs run our household, and I spent much of my early professional life proudly serving The Humane Society of the United States as the charity's public health director. So, like many people, I care about the welfare of the animals we eat, but first and foremost, I am a physician. My primary duty has always been to care for people, to accurately provide the best available balance of evidence.

In the clinic, I could reach hundreds, and on the road, thousands. But this life-or-death information needed to reach millions. Enter Jesse Rasch, a Canadian philanthropist who shared my vision of making evidence-based nutrition freely accessible and available to all. The foundation he and his wife, Julie, set up put all my work online. NutritionFacts.org was born. Today, I can reach more people while working from home in my jammies than I ever could when I was traveling the world.

Now a self-sustaining nonprofit organization itself, NutritionFacts.org has thousands of bite-sized videos on nearly every conceivable nutrition topic, and I post new videos (captioned in many languages, so follow our YouTube channel) and articles every week. Everything on the website is free for all, for all time. There are no ads, no corporate sponsorships. It's just a labor of love, a tribute to my grandmother.

When I started this work more than a decade ago, I thought the answer was to train the trainers, educate the profession. But with the democratization of information, doctors no longer hold a monopoly as gatekeepers of knowledge about health. When it comes to safe, simple lifestyle prescriptions, I've realized it may be more effective to empower individuals directly. In a national survey of doctor office visits, only about one in five smokers were told to quit.[26] Just as we don't have to wait for our physician to tell us to stop smoking, we don't have to wait to start eating healthier. Together, we can show my medical colleagues the true power of healthy living.

Last year alone, there were more than a quarter million papers published in the medical literature on nutrition, nearly a thousand articles a day. Thankfully, I now have a whole team of researchers, a wonderful staff, and an army of volunteers who help me dig through the mountains of new information. This book is not just another platform through which I can present my findings but a long-awaited opportunity to share practical advice about how to put this life-changing, life-*saving* science into practice in our daily lives.

I think my grandma would be proud.

Introduction

PREVENTING, ARRESTING, AND REVERSING THE PROGRESSION OF OUR LEADING KILLERS

There may be no such thing as dying from old age. From a study of more than forty-two thousand consecutive autopsies, centenarians—those who live past one hundred—were found to have succumbed to diseases in 100 percent of the cases examined. Though most were perceived, even by their physicians, to have been healthy just prior to death, not one "died of old age."[27] Until recently, advanced age had been considered to be a disease itself,[28] but people don't die as a consequence of maturing. They die from disease, most commonly heart attacks.[29]

Most deaths in the United States are preventable, and most are related to what we eat.[30] Our diet is one of the top causes of premature death and disability in the world.[31] Surely, diet must also be a top subject taught in medical schools, right?

Sadly, it's not. According to the most recent national survey, only a quarter of medical schools offer a *single* course in nutrition, down from 37 percent forty years ago.[32] While most of the public reportedly considers doctors to be "very credible" sources of nutrition information,[33] six out of seven graduating doctors surveyed felt that physicians were inadequately trained to counsel patients about their diets.[34] One study found that people off the street sometimes know more about basic nutrition than their doctors, concluding "physicians should be more knowledgeable about nutrition than their patients, but these results suggest that this is not necessarily true."[35]

To remedy this situation, a bill was introduced in the California State Legislature to mandate physicians get at least twelve hours of nutrition training any time over the next four years. It might surprise you to learn that the California Medical Association came out strongly *opposed* to the bill, as did other mainstream medical groups, including the California Academy of Family Physicians.[36] The bill was amended from a mandatory minimum of twelve hours over four years down to seven hours and then doctored, one might say, down to zero. No nutrition training at all.

The California medical board does have one subject requirement: twelve hours on pain management and end-of-life care for the terminally ill.[37] This disparity between prevention and mere mitigation of suffering could be a metaphor for modern medicine. A doctor a day may keep the apples away.

Back in 1903, Thomas Edison predicted that the "doctor of the future will give no medicine, but will instruct his patient in the care of [the] human frame in diet and in the cause and prevention of diseases."[38] Sadly, all it takes is a few minutes watching pharmaceutical ads on television imploring viewers to "ask your doctor" about this or that drug to know that Edison's prediction hasn't come to light. A study of thousands of patient visits found that the average length of time primary-care doctors spend talking about nutrition is about ten seconds.[39]

But this is the twenty-first century. Can't we eat whatever we want and simply take meds when we begin having health problems? For too many patients and even my physician colleagues, this seems to be the prevailing mindset. Global spending for prescription drugs surpasses $1 trillion annually, with the United States accounting for about 45 percent of this market, nearly as much as the rest of the world combined.[40] Why do we spend so much on pills? Many people assume that our manner of death is preprogrammed into our genes. High blood pressure by fifty-five, heart attacks at sixty, maybe cancer at seventy, and so on. . . . But for most of the leading causes of death, the science shows that our genes often account for only 10 to 20 percent of risk at most.[41] For instance, as you'll see in this book, the rates of killers like heart disease and major cancers differ up to a hundredfold among various populations around the globe. But when people move from low- to high-risk countries, their disease rates almost always change to those of the new environment.[42] New diet, new diseases. So, while a sixty-year-old American man living in San Francisco has about a 5 percent chance of having a heart attack within five years, should he move to Japan and start eating and living like the

Japanese, his five-year risk would drop to only 1 percent. Japanese Americans in their forties can have the same heart attack risk as Japanese in their sixties. Switching to an American lifestyle in effect aged their hearts a full twenty years.[43]

The Mayo Clinic estimates that nearly 70 percent of Americans take at least one prescription drug.[44] Yet despite the fact that more people in the United States are on medication than aren't, not to mention the steady influx of ever newer and more expensive drugs on the market, we aren't living much longer than others. In terms of life expectancy, the United States was only around twenty-seven or twenty-eight out of the thirty-four top free-market democracies. That was in 2010, down from ranking twentieth in 1990. People in Slovenia live longer than we do.[45]

More recently, U.S. life expectancy dipped to forty-third in the world and is expected to drop to sixty-fourth by 2040,[46] despite our spending trillions on health care a year, more than any other country.[47] The problem is that those trillions in health care spending are not addressing the root causes of disease, disability, and death. The leading risk factors for death in the United States are related to what we eat.[48] It's the food. The standard American diet is just to die for. Literally.

Thanks in large part to the obesity epidemic, we may now be raising the first American generation to live shorter lives than their parents.[49] Longevity gains faltered, then, in 2015, started to reverse.[50] And that was before COVID-19 knocked two years off the U.S. life expectancy, a decline not experienced since 1943, the deadliest year for Americans during World War II.[51]

And we aren't just living shorter lives, but sicker ones. A twenty-year-old in 1998 could expect to live about fifty-eight more years, while a twenty-year-old in 2006 could look forward to fifty-nine more years. However, the twenty-year-old from the 1990s might live ten of those years with chronic disease, whereas now it's more like thirteen diseased years. So it feels like one step forward, three steps back. Researchers also note that we're living two fewer *functional* years—that is, for two years, we're no longer able to perform basic life activities, such as walking a quarter of a mile, standing or sitting for two hours without having to lie down, or standing without special equipment.[52]

Students of public health learn that there are three levels of preventive medicine. The first is primary prevention, as in trying to prevent people at risk for heart disease from suffering their first heart attack. An example of this level of preventive medicine would be your doctor prescribing you a statin drug for high cholesterol. Secondary prevention takes place when you already have the disease and are trying to prevent it from becoming worse, like having a second heart attack. To do this, your doctor may add an aspirin or other drugs to your regimen. At the third level of preventive medicine, the focus is on helping people manage long-term health problems, so your doctor, for example, might prescribe a cardiac rehabilitation program that aims to prevent further physical deterioration and pain.[53] In 2000, a fourth level was proposed. What could this new "quaternary" prevention be? Reduce the complications from all the drugs and surgery from the first three levels.[54] But people seem to forget about a fifth concept, termed *primordial prevention*, that was first introduced by the World Health Organization back in 1978. Decades later, it's finally being embraced by the American Heart Association.[55]

Primordial prevention was conceived as a strategy to prevent whole societies from experiencing epidemics of chronic-disease risk factors. This means not just preventing chronic disease but preventing the risk factors that lead to chronic disease.[56] For example, instead of trying to prevent someone with high cholesterol from suffering a heart attack, why not help prevent them from getting high cholesterol (which leads to the heart attack) in the first place?

With this in mind, the American Heart Association came up with "The Simple 7" factors that can lead to a healthier life: not smoking, not being overweight, being "very active" (defined as the equivalent of walking at least twenty-two minutes a day), eating healthier (for example, lots of fruits and vegetables), having below-average cholesterol, having normal blood pressure, and having normal blood sugar levels.[57] The American Heart Association's goal was to reduce heart-disease deaths by 20 percent over the next decade.[58] If more than 90 percent of heart attacks may be avoided with lifestyle changes,[59] why so modest an aim? Even 25 percent was "deemed unrealistic."[60] The American Heart Association's pessimism may have something to do with the frightening reality of the average American diet.

An analysis of the health behaviors of thirty-five thousand adults across the United States was published in the American Heart Association's premiere journal. Most of the participants didn't smoke, about half reached their weekly exercise goals, and about a third of the population got a pass in each of the other categories—except diet. Their diets were scored on a scale from zero to five to see if they met a bare minimum of healthy eating behaviors, such as hitting recommended targets for fruit, vegetable, and whole-grain consumption or drinking fewer than three cans of fizzy drink a week. How many reached four out of five on their Healthy Eating Score? About 1 percent.[61] Maybe if the American Heart Association achieves its goal of an "aggressive"[62] 20 percent improvement, we'll get up to 1.2 percent.

Medical anthropologists have identified several major eras of human disease, starting with the Age of Pestilence and Famine, which largely ended with the Industrial Revolution, and the stage we're in now, the Age of Degenerative and Man-Made Diseases.[63] This shift is reflected in the changing causes of death over the last century. In 1900 in the United States, the top three killers were infectious diseases: pneumonia, tuberculosis, and diarrheal disease.[64] Now the fatal diseases are largely related to our lifestyle: cardiovascular disease, cancer, and chronic lung disease.[65] Is this simply because antibiotics have enabled us to live long enough to suffer from degenerative diseases? No. The emergence of these epidemics of chronic disease was accompanied by dramatic shifts in dietary patterns. This is best exemplified by what's been happening to disease rates among people in the developing world over the last few decades as they've rapidly Westernized their diets.

In 1990 around the world, most years of healthy life were lost to undernutrition, such as diarrheal diseases in malnourished children, but now the greatest disease burden is attributed to high blood pressure, a disease of overnutrition.[66] The pandemic of chronic disease has been ascribed in part to the near-universal shift toward a diet dominated by animal-sourced and processed foods—in other words, more meat, dairy, eggs, oils, fizzy drinks, sugar, and refined grains.[67] China is perhaps the best-studied example. There, a transition away from the country's traditional, plant-based diet was accompanied by a sharp rise in diet-related chronic diseases, such as obesity, diabetes, cardiovascular diseases, and cancer.[68]

Why do we suspect these changes in diet and disease are related? After all, rapidly industrializing societies undergo multitudes of changes. How are scientists able to parse out the effects of specific foods? To isolate the effects of different dietary components, researchers can follow the diets and diseases of large groups of defined individuals over time. Take meat, for example. To see what effect an increase in meat consumption might have on disease rates, researchers studied lapsed vegetarians. People who once ate vegetarian diets but then started to eat meat at least once a week experienced a 146 percent increase in odds of heart disease, a 152 percent increase in stroke, a 166 percent increase in diabetes, and a 231 percent increase in odds for weight gain. During the twelve years after the transition from vegetarian to omnivore, meat-eating was associated with a decrease of 3.6 years in life expectancy.[69]

Even vegetarians can suffer high rates of chronic disease, though, if they eat a lot of processed foods. Take India, for example. This country's rates of diabetes, heart disease, obesity, and stroke have increased far faster than might have been expected given its relatively small increase in per capita meat consumption. This has been blamed on the decreasing "whole plant food content of their diet," including a shift from brown rice to white and the substitution of other refined carbohydrates, packaged snacks, and fast-food products for India's traditional staples of lentils, fruits, vegetables, whole grains, nuts, and seeds.[70] In general, the dividing line between health-promoting and disease-promoting foods may be less plant- versus animal-sourced foods and more whole plant foods versus most everything else.

To this end, a dietary quality index was developed that simply reflects the percentage of calories people derive from nutrient-rich, unprocessed plant foods[71] on a scale of zero to one hundred. The higher people score, the more body fat they may lose over time[72] and the lower their risk may be of abdominal obesity,[73] high blood pressure,[74] high cholesterol, and high triglycerides.[75] Comparing the diets of 100 women with breast cancer to 175 healthy women, researchers concluded that scoring higher on the whole plant food diet index (greater than about thirty compared to less than about eighteen) may reduce the odds of breast cancer more than 90 percent.[76]

Sadly, most Americans hardly make it past a score of ten. The standard American diet rates eleven out of one hundred. According to estimates from the U.S. Department of Agriculture, 32 percent of our calories comes from animal foods, 57 percent comes from processed plant foods, and only 11 percent comes from whole grains, beans, fruits, vegetables, and nuts.[77] That means on a scale of one to ten, the American diet would rate about a one.

We eat almost as if the future doesn't matter. And, indeed, there are actually data to back that up. A study entitled "Death Row Nutrition: Curious Conclusions of Last Meals" analyzed the last meal requests of hundreds of individuals executed in the United States during a five-year period. It turns out that the nutritional content didn't differ much from what Americans normally eat.[78] If we continue to eat as though we're having our last meals, eventually they will be.

What percentage of Americans hit all the American Heart Association's "Simple 7" recommendations? Of 1,933 men and women surveyed, most met two or three, but hardly any managed to meet all seven simple health components. In fact, just a single individual hit all seven recommendations.[79] One person out of nearly two thousand. As a recent past president of the American Heart Association responded, "That should give all of us pause."[80]

The truth is that adhering to just four simple healthy lifestyle factors can have a strong impact on the prevention of chronic diseases: not smoking, not being obese, getting half an hour of exercise a day, and eating more healthfully—defined as consuming more fruits, veggies, and whole grains and less meat. Those four factors alone were found to account for 78 percent of chronic disease risk. If you start from scratch and manage to tick off all four, you may be able to eliminate more than 90 percent of your risk of developing diabetes, more than 80 percent of your risk of having a heart attack, cut in half your risk of having a stroke, and reduce your overall cancer risk by more than one-third.[81] For some cancers, like our number two cancer killer, colon cancer, up to 71 percent of cases appear to be preventable through a similar portfolio of simple diet and lifestyle changes.[82]

Maybe it's time we stop blaming genetics and focus on the more than 70 percent that is directly under our control.[83] We have the power.

Does all this healthy living also translate into a longer life? The Centers for Disease Control and Prevention (CDC) followed approximately eight thousand Americans aged twenty years or older for about six years. They found that three cardinal lifestyle behaviors exerted an enormous impact on mortality: People can substantially reduce their risk for early death by not smoking, consuming a healthier diet, and engaging in sufficient physical activity. And the CDC's definitions were pretty laid-back: By not smoking, the CDC just meant not *currently* smoking. A "healthy diet" was defined merely as being in the top 40 percent in terms of complying with the weak federal dietary guidelines, and "physically active" meant averaging about twenty-one minutes or more a day of at least moderate exercise. People who managed at least *one* of the three had a 40 percent lower risk of dying within that six-year period. Those who hit two out of three seemed to cut their chances of dying by more than half, and those who scored all three behaviors appeared to slash their chances of dying in that time by 82 percent.[84]

Of course, people sometimes fib about how well they eat. How accurate can these findings really be if they're based on people's self-reporting? A similar study on health behaviors and survival didn't just take people's own word for how healthfully they were eating; the researchers measured how much vitamin C participants had in their bloodstreams. The level of vitamin C in the blood was considered a "good biomarker of plant food intake" and hence was used as a proxy for a healthy diet. The conclusions held up. The drop in mortality risk among those with healthier habits was equivalent to being fourteen years younger.[85] It's like turning back the clock fourteen years—not with a drug or a DeLorean but just by eating and living more healthfully.

Let's talk a little more about aging. In each of our cells, we have forty-six strands of DNA coiled into chromosomes. At the tip of each chromosome, there's a tiny cap called a *telomere*, which keeps our DNA from unraveling and fraying. Think of telomeres as the plastic tips on the ends of shoelaces. Every time our cells divide, however, a bit of that cap is lost. And when the telomere is completely gone, our cells can die.[86] Though this is an oversimplification,[87] telomeres have been thought of as our life "fuse": They can start shortening as soon as we're born, and when they're gone, we're gone. In fact, forensic scientists can take DNA from a bloodstain and roughly estimate how old the person was based on how long their telomeres are.[88]

Sounds like fodder for a great scene in *CSI*, but is there anything we can do to slow the rate at which our fuses burn? The thought is that if we can slow down this ticking cellular clock, we may be able to slow down the aging process and live longer.[89] So what would we have to do if we wanted to prevent this telomere cap from burning away? Well, smoking cigarettes is associated with triple the rate of telomere loss,[90] so the first step is simple: Stop smoking. But the food we eat every day may also have an impact on how fast we lose our telomeres. The consumption of fruits,[91] vegetables,[92] and other antioxidant-rich foods[93] has been associated with longer protective telomeres. In contrast, the consumption of refined grains,[94] fizzy drinks,[95] meat (including fish),[96] and dairy[97] has been linked to shortened telomeres. What if we ate a diet composed of whole plant foods and stayed away from processed foods and animal foods? Could cellular aging be slowed?

The answer lies in an enzyme found in Methuselah. That's the name given to a bristlecone pine tree growing in the White Mountains of California that happens to be the oldest recorded living being, nearing its 5,000th birthday. It was already hundreds of years old before construction of the pyramids in

Egypt began. There's an enzyme in the roots of bristlecone pines that appears to peak a few thousand years into their lifespan, and it actually rebuilds telomeres.[98] Scientists named it *telomerase*. Once they knew what to look for, researchers discovered the enzyme was present in human cells too. The question then became, *How can we boost the activity of this age-defying enzyme?*

Seeking answers, the pioneering researcher Dr. Dean Ornish teamed up with Dr. Elizabeth Blackburn, who was awarded the Nobel Prize in Medicine for her discovery of telomerase. In a study funded in part by the U.S. Department of Defense, they found that three months of whole food, plant-based nutrition and other healthy changes could significantly boost telomerase activity, the first intervention ever shown to do so.[99] The study was published in one of the most prestigious medical journals in the world. The accompanying editorial concluded that this landmark study "should encourage people to adopt a healthy lifestyle in order to avoid or combat cancer and age-related diseases."[100]

So were Drs. Ornish and Blackburn able to successfully slow down aging with a healthy diet and lifestyle? A five-year follow-up study measured the lengths of the participants' telomeres. Those in the control group did not change their lifestyles, and their telomeres predictably shrank with age. But for the healthy-living group, not only did their telomeres shrink less, they *grew*. Five years later, their telomeres were even longer on average than when they started, suggesting a healthy lifestyle can boost telomerase enzyme activity and *reverse* this aspect of cellular aging.[101]

Subsequent research has shown that the telomere lengthening wasn't just because the healthy-living group was exercising more or losing weight. In fact, weight loss through caloric restriction and an even more vigorous exercise program failed to improve telomere length, so it appears that the active ingredient is the quality, not quantity, of the food eaten. As long as people were eating the same diet, it didn't appear to matter how small their portions were, how much weight they lost, or even how hard they exercised; after a year, they saw no benefit.[102] In contrast, individuals on the plant-based diet exercised only half as much, enjoyed the same amount of weight loss after just three months,[103] and achieved significant telomere protection.[104] In other words, it wasn't the weight loss and it wasn't the exercise that reversed cell aging—it was the food.

In my book *How Not to Age*, I document the effects a healthy diet can have on the other ten aging pathways,[105] helping to explain why those who eat more plant-based appear to age slower.[106] To demonstrate cause and effect, hundreds of individuals were randomized either to a diet centered around healthy plant foods, exercise, or neither. Though, sadly, physical activity alone failed to slow the aging process, those in the plant-based dietary intervention group experienced a significant slowing of biological aging. In the study featured in the Netflix documentary *You Are What You Eat* that randomized identical twins to a healthier omnivorous diet or a plant-based one, not only did the plant-based diet slow telomere loss but researchers found a significant slowing in three other measures of biological aging, "aligning with anti-aging effects of plant-based diets," and this was achieved within just eight weeks.[107]

Some people have expressed concern that boosting telomerase activity could theoretically increase cancer risk, since tumors have been known to hijack the telomerase enzyme and use it to ensure their own immortality.[108] But as we'll see in chapter 14, Dr. Ornish and his colleagues have used the same diet and lifestyle changes to halt and apparently *reverse* the progression of cancer in certain circumstances. We will also see how the same diet can reverse the progression of heart disease.

What about our other leading killers? It turns out a more plant-based diet may help prevent, treat, or reverse *every single one* of our fifteen leading causes of death. In this book, I'll go through this list, with a chapter on each.

Certainly there are prescription medications that can help with some of these conditions. For example, we can take statin drugs for our cholesterol to lower risk of heart attacks, inject insulin for diabetes, and pop a slew of diuretics and other blood pressure medications for hypertension. But there is only one unifying diet that may help prevent, arrest, or even reverse the progression of each of these killers. Unlike with medications, there isn't one kind of diet for optimal liver function and a different way of eating to improve our kidneys. A heart-healthy diet is a brain-healthy diet is a lung-healthy diet. The diet that helps prevent cancer just so happens to be the *same* diet that may help prevent type 2 diabetes and every other cause of death on the top-fifteen list. Unlike drugs—which only target specific functions, can have dangerous side effects, and may only treat the symptoms of disease—a healthy diet can benefit all organ systems at once, has *good* side effects, and can treat the underlying cause of illness.

That one unifying diet that's been found to best prevent and treat many of these chronic diseases is a whole food, plant-based diet, defined as an eating pattern that encourages the consumption of unrefined plant foods and dis-

MORTALITY IN THE UNITED STATES

	Annual Deaths
1. Coronary heart disease[109]	383,000
2. Lung diseases (lung cancer,[110] COPD, and asthma[111])	277,000
3. Brain diseases (stroke[112] and Alzheimer's[113])	274,000
4. You'll be surprised! (see chapter 15)	~250,000
5. Infections (respiratory and blood[114,115])	133,000
6. High blood pressure[116]	120,000
7. Digestive cancers (colorectal, pancreatic, and esophageal)[117]	117,000
8. Diabetes[118]	95,000
9. Liver diseases (cirrhosis, fatty liver,[119] and cancer[120])	81,000
10. Blood cancers (leukemia, lymphoma, and myeloma)[121]	56,000
11. Kidney disease[122]	55,000
12. Suicide[123]	49,000
13. Breast cancer[124,125]	43,000
14. Parkinson's disease[126]	40,000
15. Prostate cancer[127]	33,000

courages meats, dairy products, eggs, and processed foods.[128] In this book, I don't advocate for a vegetarian diet or a vegan diet. I advocate for an evidence-based diet, and the best available balance of science suggests that the more whole plant foods we eat, the better—both to reap their nutritional benefits and to displace less healthful options.

Most doctor visits are for lifestyle-based diseases, which means they're preventable diseases.[129] As physicians, my colleagues and I were trained not to address the root cause but rather the consequences by giving a lifetime's worth of medications to treat risk factors like high blood pressure, blood sugar, and cholesterol. This approach has been compared to mopping up the floor around an overflowing sink instead of simply turning off the faucet.[130] Drug companies are more than happy to sell us a new roll of paper towels every day for the rest of our lives while the water continues to spill. As Dr. Walter Willett, the former chair of nutrition at Harvard University's School of Public Health, put it: "The inherent problem is that most pharmacologic strategies do not address the underlying causes of ill health in Western countries, which are not drug deficiencies."[131]

Treating the cause is not only safer and cheaper, but it can work better. So why don't more of my medical colleagues do it? Not only were they not trained how to do so, but doctors don't get paid to do it. No one profits from lifestyle medicine—other than the patient—so it's not a major part of medical training or practice.[132] That's just how the current system works. The medical system is set up to financially reward prescribing pills and procedures, not produce. After Dr. Ornish proved that the progression of heart disease could be reversed without drugs or surgery, he thought that his studies would have a meaningful effect on the practice of mainstream medicine. After all, he effectively found a potential cure for our number one killer! But he was mistaken—not about his critically important findings regarding diet and disease reversal but about how much influence the business of medicine has on the practice of medicine. In his words, Dr. Ornish "realized reimbursement is a much more powerful determinant of medical practice than research."[133]

Though there are vested interests, such as the processed food and pharmaceutical industries, which fight hard to maintain the status quo, there is one corporate sector that actually benefits from keeping people healthy—namely, the insurance industry. Kaiser Permanente, the largest managed-care organization in the United States, published a nutritional update for doctors in its official medical journal, informing its nearly fifteen thousand physicians that healthy eating may be "best achieved with a plant-based diet, which we define as a regimen that encourages whole, plant-based foods and discourages meats, dairy products, and eggs as well as all refined and processed foods."[134]

"Too often, physicians ignore the potential benefits of good nutrition and quickly prescribe medications instead of giving patients a chance to correct their disease through healthy eating and active living. . . . Physicians should consider recommending a plant-based diet to all their patients, especially those with high blood pressure, diabetes, cardiovascular disease, or obesity."[135] Physicians should give their patients a chance to first correct their disease themselves with plant-based nutrition.

The major downside Kaiser Permanente's nutritional update describes is that this diet may work a little too well. If people begin eating plant-based diets while still taking medications, their blood pressure or blood sugar could drop so low that physicians may need to adjust medications or eliminate them altogether. Ironically, the "side effect" of the diet may be not having to take drugs anymore. The article ends with a familiar refrain: Further research is needed. In this case, though, "Further research is needed to find ways to make plant-based diets the new normal. . . ."[136]

We're a long way off from Thomas Edison's 1903 prediction, but it is my hope that this book can help you understand that most of our leading causes of death and disability are more preventable than inevitable. The primary reason diseases tend to run in families may be that *diets* tend to run in families.

For most of our leading killers, nongenetic factors like diet can account for at least 80 or 90 percent of cases. As I noted before, this is based on the fact that the rates of cardiovascular disease and major cancers differ fivefold to a hundredfold around the world. Migration studies show this is not just genetics. As I mentioned, when people move from low- to high-risk areas, their disease risk nearly always shoots up to match the new setting.[137] As well, dramatic changes in disease rates within a single generation highlight the primacy of external factors. Colon cancer mortality in Japan in the 1950s, for instance, was less than one-fifth that of the United States (including Americans of Japanese ancestry).[138] But now colon cancer rates in Japan are as bad as they are in the United States, a rise that has been attributed in part to the fivefold increase in meat consumption.[139]

Research has shown us that identical twins separated at birth will get different diseases based on how they live their lives. An American Heart Association–funded study comparing the lifestyles and arteries of nearly five hundred twins found that diet and lifestyle factors clearly trumped genes.[140] Even among identical twins who have the exact same genes, one could die early of a heart attack and the other could live a long, healthy life with clean arteries depending on what they ate and how they lived. Even if *both* our parents died with heart disease, we should be able to eat our way to a healthy heart. Our family history does not have to become our personal destiny.

Just because we may be born with bad genes doesn't mean we can't effectively turn them off. As you'll see in the breast cancer and Alzheimer's disease chapters, even if we're born with high-risk genes, we have tremendous control over our medical destiny. Epigenetics is a hot new field of study that deals with this control of gene activity. Skin cells look and function a lot differently from bone cells, brain cells, or heart cells, but each of our cells has the same complement of DNA. What makes them act differently is that they each have different genes turned on or off. That's the power of epigenetics. Same DNA, but different results.

Let me give you an example of how striking this effect can be. Consider the humble honeybee. Queen bees and worker bees are genetically identical, yet queens may live for three years and lay up to two thousand eggs a day, while worker bees may live only for three weeks and are functionally sterile.[141] How can this be if there is no difference between them genetically? There is another difference: their diets. When the hive's queen is dying, a larva is picked by nurse bees to be fed a secreted substance called royal jelly. (The workers just get mostly a mixture of honey and pollen adorably named beebread.)[142] When the chosen larva eats this jelly, the enzyme that had been silencing the expression of royal genes is turned off and a new queen is born.[143] The queen bee has the exact same genes as any of the worker bees, but simply because of what she ate, different genes are expressed, resulting in dramatic alterations to her life and lifespan. A fiftyfold increase in longevity, thanks to epigenetics.

Cancer cells can use epigenetics against us by silencing tumor-suppressor genes that could otherwise stop cancer in its tracks. So even if we're born with good genes, cancer can sometimes find a way to turn them off. A number of chemotherapy drugs have been developed to restore our bodies' natural defenses, but their use has been limited due to their high toxicity.[144] There are, however, a number of compounds distributed widely throughout the plant kingdom—including beans, greens, and berries—that appear to have the same effect naturally.[145] For example, dripping green tea on colon, esophageal, or prostate cancer cells has been shown to reactivate genes that had been silenced by the cancers.[146] This hasn't just been demonstrated in a petri dish. Three hours after eating 68 grams of broccoli sprouts, the enzyme that cancers use to help silence our defenses is suppressed in our bloodstream[147] to an extent equal to or greater than the chemotherapy agent specifically designed for that purpose[148] and without the toxic side effects.[149]

What if we ate a diet chock-full of plant foods? In the Gene Expression Modulation by Intervention with Nutrition and Lifestyle (GEMINAL) study, Dr. Ornish and colleagues took biopsies from men with prostate cancer before and after three months of intensive lifestyle changes that included a whole food, plant-based diet. Without any chemotherapy or radiation, beneficial changes were noted in gene expression for five hundred different genes. Within just a few months, the expression of disease-preventing genes was boosted, and oncogenes that promote breast and prostate cancers were suppressed.[150] Whatever genes we may have inherited from our parents, what we eat can affect how those genes affect our health. The power is mainly in our hands and on our plates.

This book is divided into two parts: the *why* and the *how*. In Part 1—the *why* to eat healthfully section—I will explore the role diet can play in the prevention, treatment, and reversal of the progression of the fifteen leading causes of death in the United States. I'll then take a closer look at more practical aspects in the *how* to eat healthfully section presented in Part 2. For example, we'll see in Part 1 *why* beans and greens are among the healthiest foods on earth. Then, in Part 2, we'll take a look at *how* best to eat them and explore such issues as how many greens to eat every day and whether they're best cooked, canned, fresh, or frozen. We'll see in Part 1 why it's important to eat at least nine servings of fruits and vegetables daily; then Part 2 will help us decide whether to buy organic or conventional produce. I'll try to answer all the common questions I regularly receive and offer real-world tips for grocery shopping and meal planning to make it as easy as possible to best feed yourself and your family.

Besides writing more books, I intend to keep lecturing at medical schools and speaking at hospitals and conferences for as long as I can. I'm going to keep trying to reignite the spark that led my colleagues into the healing profession in the first place: to help people get better. There are tools missing from too many doctors' medical toolboxes, powerful interventions that can make many of our patients well again instead of merely slowing their decline. I'll keep working on trying to change the system, but you, the reader, don't have to wait. You can start now by following the recommendations within the following chapters. Eating more healthfully is easier than you think, it's inexpensive, and it might just save your life.

PART 1

1

How Not to Die from Heart Disease

On December 30, 2019, Dr. Li Wenliang, an ophthalmologist at Central Hospital of Wuhan in the Hubei province of China, messaged his fellow physicians, alerting them to the appearance of a concerning cluster of pneumonia cases. In response, he was summoned to the public security bureau and reprimanded for "spreading rumors" and "making false statements that disturbed the public order." Thirty-nine days later, after becoming infected with the very virus he had tried to warn his colleagues about, he was dead at age thirty-three.[151] By that time, the disease had already spread to dozens of countries.[152] His initial message read "7 SARS cases confirmed at Hua'nan Seafood Market."[153] SARS stands for *severe acute respiratory syndrome*, which, seventeen years earlier, had been the first deadly global outbreak known to be triggered by a coronavirus. (Sadly, the doctor who first alerted the world to that epidemic, Carlo Urbani, also succumbed to the disease.[154]) Coronaviruses are named for their crown-like appearance under an electron microscope—from the Latin *corona* for "crown," as in coronation—due to a fringe of protein spikes that radiate from the surface.[155]

The COVID-19 pandemic, as we came to know it, became front-page news all day, every day, around the world. Much of humankind retreated—isolating, masking, sanitizing, social distancing—as scientists scrambled to find solutions. Within two years, about fifteen million lives would be lost in one of the deadliest pandemics on record.[156]

Globally, we came together to battle this threat, however imperfectly, and emerged beleaguered yet ultimately triumphant. But what about another epidemic—another global pandemic—that has been taking millions of lives every single year?[157] It kills more Americans every few years than have all our past wars combined.[158] It can be stopped not in a laboratory but right in our supermarkets, kitchens, and dining rooms. As far as weapons go, we don't need vaccines or safety protocols. A simple fork will do.

This epidemic is already present on such a massive scale and so preventable. Why aren't we doing more about it?

The killer I'm talking about is coronary heart disease, and it's affecting nearly everyone raised on the standard American diet.[159]

Our Top Killer

America's number one killer is fatty deposits in the walls of our arteries called *atherosclerotic plaque*. For most Americans raised on a conventional diet, plaque accumulates inside the coronary arteries—the blood vessels that crown the heart (hence "coronary") and supply it with oxygen-rich blood. This buildup of plaque, known as *atherosclerosis*, from the Greek words *athere* (gruel) and *sklerosis* (hardening), is the hardening of the arteries by pockets of cholesterol-rich gunk that builds up within the inner linings of the blood vessels. This process occurs over decades, slowly bulging into the space inside the arteries, narrowing the path for blood to flow. The restriction of blood circulation to the heart muscle can lead to chest pain and pressure, known as *angina*, when people try to exert themselves. If the plaque ruptures, a blood clot can form within the artery. This sudden blockage of blood flow can cause a heart attack, damaging or even killing part of the heart.

When you think about heart disease, you may think of friends or loved ones who suffered for years with chest pain and shortness of breath before they finally succumbed. However, for the majority of Americans who die suddenly from heart disease, the very first symptom may be their last.[160] It's called "sudden cardiac death." This is when death occurs within an hour of symptom onset. In other words, we may not even realize we're at risk until it's too late. We could be feeling perfectly fine one moment, and then an hour later, we're gone forever. That's why it's critical to prevent heart disease in the first place, before we even necessarily know we have it. An ounce of prevention is worth much more than a pound of cure, because there is no cure for dead.

When I used to work in the hospital, my patients sometimes asked me, "Isn't heart disease just a consequence of getting old?" I can see why this is a common misconception. After all, our heart pumps literally billions of times during the average lifespan. Does our ticker just conk out after a while? No.

A large body of evidence shows there were once enormous swaths of the world where the epidemic of coronary heart disease simply didn't exist. For instance, in the famous China-Cornell-Oxford Project (known as the China Study), researchers investigated the eating habits and incidence of chronic disease among hundreds of thousands of rural Chinese. In Guizhou province, for example, a region comprising half a million people, over the course of three years, not a single death could be attributed to coronary artery disease among men under the age of sixty-five.[161]

During the 1930s and 1940s, Western-trained doctors working throughout an extensive network of missionary hospitals in sub-Saharan Africa noticed that many of the chronic diseases laying waste to populations in the so-called developed world were largely absent across most of the continent. In Uganda, a country of millions in eastern Africa, coronary heart disease was described as "almost non-existent."[162]

But were the peoples of these nations simply dying early of other diseases, never living long enough to develop heart disease? No. Doctors compared autopsies of Ugandans to autopsies of Americans who had died at the same age. Researchers found that out of 632 people autopsied in Saint Louis, Missouri, there had been 136 heart attacks. But in 632 age-matched Ugandans? One. A single heart attack. The Ugandans experienced more than one hundred times fewer heart attacks than the Americans. The doctors were so blown away that they examined another 800 deaths in Uganda. Out of more than 1,400 Ugandans autopsied, researchers found just that one body with a small, healed lesion of the heart, meaning the attack wasn't even fatal. Then and now, in the industrialized world, heart disease is a leading killer. In central Africa, heart disease was so rare it killed fewer than one in a thousand.[163]

Immigration studies show that this resistance to heart disease is not just something in the Africans' genes. We know that when people move from low-risk to high-risk areas, their disease rates skyrocket as they adopt the diet and lifestyle habits of their new homes.[164] The extraordinarily low rates of heart disease in rural China and Africa have been attributed to the extraordinarily low cholesterol levels among these populations. Though their diets are very different, they share commonalities: They are both centered on plant-derived foods, such as grains and vegetables. By eating so much fiber and so little animal fat, the total cholesterol levels of Chinese and African people studied averaged under 3.88 mmol/L,[165,166] similar to people who eat contemporary plant-based diets.[167]

What does all of this mean? Heart disease may be a choice.

If you looked at the teeth of people who lived more than ten thousand years before the invention of the toothbrush, you'd notice they had almost no cavities.[168] They never flossed a day in their lives, yet no cavities. That's because candy bars hadn't been invented yet. The reason people get cavities now is that the pleasure they derive from sugary treats may outweigh the cost and discomfort of the dentist's chair. I certainly enjoy the occasional indulgence. (I'm lucky to have a good dental plan!) But what if instead of the dental plaque on our teeth, we're talking about the atherosclerotic plaque building up in our arteries? Then we're not just talking about scraping tartar anymore. We're talking about life and death.

Heart disease is the number one reason we and most of our loved ones will die. Of course, it's up to each of us to make our own decisions as to what to eat and how to live, but shouldn't we try to make these choices consciously by educating ourselves about the predictable consequences of our actions? Just as we could avoid sugary foods that rot our teeth, we can avoid trans fats, saturated fats, and cholesterol-laden foods that clog up our arteries.

Let's take a look at the progression of coronary heart disease throughout life and learn how simple dietary choices at any stage may prevent, stop, and even reverse the progression of heart disease before it's too late.

Is Fish Oil Just Snake Oil?

Thanks in part to the American Heart Association's recommendation that individuals at high risk for heart disease should ask their physicians about omega-3 fish oil supplementation,[169] fish oil pills have grown into a multibillion-dollar industry. We now consume more than one hundred thousand tons of fish oil every year.[170]

But what does the science say? Are the purported benefits of fish oil supplementation for the prevention and treatment of heart disease just a fish tale? A systematic review and meta-analysis published in the *Journal of the American Medical Association* looked at all the best randomized clinical trials evaluating the effects of omega-3 fats on lifespan, cardiac death, sudden death, heart attack, and stroke. These included studies not only on fish oil supplements but also studies on the effects of advising people to eat more oily fish. What did they find? Overall, the researchers found no protective benefit for overall mortality, heart disease mortality, sudden cardiac death, heart attack, or stroke.[171]

What about individuals who had already had a heart attack and were trying to prevent another? Still no benefit was found.[172]

Where did we even get this idea that the omega-3 fats in fish and fish oil supplements are good for us? There was a notion that some indigenous people of the Arctic* were protected from heart disease, but that appears to be a complete myth.[173] Some early studies, however, looked promising. For example, the famous DART trial from the 1980s involving two thousand men found that those advised to eat fatty fish had a 29 percent reduction in mortality.[174] That's impressive, so it's no wonder the study got a lot of attention. But people seem to have forgotten about the sequel, the DART-2 trial, which found the exact opposite. Run by the same team of researchers, the DART-2 trial was an even bigger study—three thousand men—but this time, participants who had been advised to eat oily fish and particularly those who were supplied with fish oil capsules had a *higher* risk of cardiac death.[175,176]

After putting all the studies together, the meta-analysis concluded that there was no longer justification for the use of omega-3s in everyday clinical practice.[177] The latest gold-standard review of the evidence concluded that fish oil supplementation or advice to eat fish has "little or no effect on deaths and cardiovascular events . . ."[178] What should doctors do when their patients follow the American Heart Association's advice and inquire about fish oil supplements? As the director of Lipids and Metabolism at Mount Sinai's cardiovascular institute put it: "Given this and other negative meta-analyses, our job [as doctors] should be to stop highly marketed fish oil supplementation to all our patients . . ."[179]

---

* The study refers to "Eskimos" and was conducted at a time when that term was the norm, though, today, it is offensive to many communities.

Heart Disease Starts in Childhood

In 1953, a study published in the *Journal of the American Medical Association* radically changed our understanding of the development of heart disease. Researchers conducted a series of three hundred autopsies on American casualties of the Korean War, with an average age of around twenty-two. Shockingly, 77 percent of soldiers already had visible evidence of coronary atherosclerosis. Some even had arteries that were blocked off 90 percent or more.[180] The study "dramatically showed that atherosclerotic changes appear in the coronary arteries years and decades before the age at which coronary heart disease (CHD) becomes a clinically recognized problem."[181]

Later studies of accidental death victims between the ages of three and twenty-six found that fatty streaks—the first stage of atherosclerosis—were found in nearly all American children by age ten.[182] By the time we reach our twenties and thirties, these fatty streaks can turn into full-blown plaques like those seen in the young American GIs of the Korean War. And by the time we're forty or fifty, they can start killing us off.

So, if anyone reading this is over the age of *ten*, the question isn't whether you want to eat healthier to help *prevent* heart disease but whether you want to try to *reverse* the progression of heart disease you very likely already have.

Just how early do these fatty streaks start to appear? Atherosclerosis may develop even before birth. Italian researchers looked inside arteries taken from miscarriages and premature newborns who died shortly after birth. It turns out that the arteries of fetuses whose mothers had high LDL cholesterol levels were more likely to contain arterial lesions.[183] This finding suggests that atherosclerosis may not just start as a nutritional disease of childhood but one during pregnancy.

It's become commonplace for pregnant women to avoid smoking and drinking alcohol. It's also never too early to start eating healthier for the next generation.

According to William C. Roberts, the longtime editor in chief of *The American Journal of Cardiology*, the only critical risk factor for atherosclerotic plaque buildup is cholesterol, specifically elevated LDL cholesterol in our blood.[184] LDL is called "bad" cholesterol because it's the vehicle by which cholesterol is deposited into our arteries. Autopsies of thousands of young accident victims have shown that the level of cholesterol in the blood was closely correlated with the amount of atherosclerosis in the arteries.[185] To drastically reduce LDL cholesterol levels, we need to drastically reduce our intake of three things: trans fat, which comes from processed foods and naturally from meat and dairy; saturated fat, found mainly in animal products and junk foods; and, to a lesser extent, dietary cholesterol, found exclusively in animal-derived foods, especially eggs.[186]

Notice a pattern here? The three boosters of bad cholesterol—the number one risk factor for our number one killer—all stem from eating processed foods and animal products. This likely explains why populations living on traditional diets revolving around whole plant foods have largely remained free from the epidemic of heart disease.

It's the Cholesterol, Stupid!

Dr. Roberts wasn't only the editor in chief of *The American Journal of Cardiology* for forty years; he was Chief of Pathology at the National Institutes of Health before heading up the Baylor Heart and Vascular Institute. He authored more than a thousand scientific publications and wrote more than a dozen textbooks on cardiology.

In his editorial "It's the Cholesterol, Stupid!," Dr. Roberts argued that there is only one true risk factor for coronary heart disease: cholesterol.[187] You could be an obese, cigarette-smoking couch potato with diabetes and *still* not develop atherosclerosis, he argues, as long as the cholesterol level in your blood is low enough.

The optimal LDL cholesterol level is probably 1.29 to 1.81 mmol/L, and apparently, the lower, the better. That's where we start out at birth, that's the level seen in populations largely free of heart disease, and that's the level at which the progression of atherosclerosis appears to stop in cholesterol-lowering trials.[188] An LDL around 1.81 mmol/L corresponds to a total cholesterol reading of about 3.88, the level below which no deaths from coronary heart disease were reported in the famous Framingham Heart Study, a generations-long project to identify risk factors for heart disease.[189] The population target should therefore be a total cholesterol level under 3.88 mmol/L. "If such a goal was created," Dr. Roberts wrote, "the great scourge of the Western world would be essentially eliminated."[190]

The average cholesterol for people living in the United States is much higher than 3.88 mmol/L; it hovers around 5.17 mmol/L. If your blood test results came back with a total cholesterol of 5.17 mmol/L, your physician might reassure you that your cholesterol is normal. But in a society where it's normal to die of heart disease, having a "normal" cholesterol level is probably not a good thing.

To become virtually heart-attack proof, you need to get your LDL cholesterol at least under 1.81 mmol/L. Dr. Roberts noted that there are only two ways to achieve this for our population: to put more than a hundred million Americans on a lifetime of medications or to recommend they all eat a diet centered around whole plant foods.[191]

So: drugs or diet. All health plans cover cholesterol-lowering statin drugs, so why change your diet if you can simply pop a pill every day for the rest of your life? Unfortunately, as we'll see in chapter 15, these drugs don't work nearly as well as most people think, and they can cause undesirable side effects.

Want Fries with That Lipitor?

The cholesterol-lowering statin drug Lipitor has become the best-selling drug of all time, generating more than $140 billion in global sales.[192] This class of drugs garnered so much enthusiasm in the medical community that some U.S. health authorities facetiously proposed they be added to the public water supply like fluoride.[193] One cardiology journal even offered the tongue-in-cheek suggestion for fast-food restaurants to offer "McStatin" condiments along with ketchup packets to help neutralize the effects of unhealthy dietary choices.[194]

For those at high risk for heart disease who are unwilling or unable to bring down their cholesterol levels naturally with dietary changes, the benefits of statins outweigh the risks. These drugs do have side effects, though, such as the potential for liver injury or muscle damage. The reason some doctors routinely order regular blood tests for patients on these drugs is to monitor for liver toxicity. We can also test the blood for the presence of muscle breakdown products, but biopsies reveal that people on statins can show evidence of muscle damage even if their blood work is normal and they exhibit no symptoms of muscle soreness or weakness.[195] The decline in muscular strength and performance sometimes associated with these drugs may not be such a big deal for younger individuals, but they can place seniors at increased risk for falls and injury.[196]

Other concerns have also been raised. In 2012, the U.S. Food and Drug Administration announced newly mandated safety labeling on statin drugs to warn doctors and patients about their potential for brain-related side effects, such as memory loss and confusion. Statin drugs appeared to increase the risk of developing diabetes, as well.[197] The primary killer is heart disease, not diabetes, so the benefits of statins may still outweigh the risks, but why accept any risk at all if we can lower our cholesterol naturally?

Plant-based diets have been shown to lower cholesterol just as effectively as first-generation statin drugs, but without the risks.[198] In fact, the "side effects" of healthy eating tend to be good—*less* cancer and diabetes risk and *protection* of the liver and brain, as we'll explore throughout the rest of this book.

Are Statins Right for You?

The number one take-home message from the latest cholesterol clinical practice guidelines from the American Heart Association and the American College of Cardiology is to have a lifelong heart-healthy lifestyle. If, however, you have a history of cardiovascular disease, cholesterol-lowering medications are considered nonnegotiable. But what about *primary prevention*, meaning preventing that first heart attack or stroke? If you have an LDL cholesterol of 4.91 mmol/L or more, go directly to statins. That's a case of "Don't pass Go, and don't collect $200." Similarly, if you're between forty and seventy-five years of age and you have diabetes, then even an LDL of 1.81 mmol/L gets you a statin recommendation. But if you don't yet have known cardiovascular disease or diabetes *and* if your LDL is between 1.81 and 4.91, then statins are generally recommended if your risk of having a cardiovascular event (like a heart attack or stroke) over the next ten years is 7.5 percent or higher.[199]

My favorite online risk calculator is u-prevent.com. It's free and endorsed by the European Society of Cardiology. Not only does it give you a ten-year risk estimate and a lifetime risk estimate, but it estimates how long you may have before the event.[200] And, best of all, you can then toggle various treatment options to see what may happen to your risk if you adopt certain lifestyle changes, such as stopping smoking, increasing your step count, or starting a statin.

Under the current guidelines, if your ten-year risk is below 5 percent, then you should just stick to diet, exercise, and smoking cessation to further lower your numbers, unless there are extenuating circumstances. If your ten-year risk hits 20 percent or higher, though, the recommendation is to add a statin drug on top of lifestyle modification. Between 5 and 7.5

percent, the tendency is to adhere to lifestyle interventions unless you have risk-enhancing factors, and between 7.5 and 20 percent, most lean toward adding drugs. Risk-enhancing factors your doctor should take into account when helping you make the decision include a family history of heart disease or stroke, a really high LDL cholesterol (≥ 4.14 mmol/L), metabolic syndrome, chronic kidney or inflammatory conditions, and persistently high triglycerides (≥ 4.53 mmol/L), C-reactive protein (≥ 2.0 mg/L), or Lp(a) (≥ 107.5 nmol/L).[201]

If you're still not sure if you should take statins, the American Heart Association and American College of Cardiology guidelines suggest considering getting a coronary artery calcium score,[202] though the U.S. Preventive Services Task Force has said explicitly that the current evidence is insufficient to conclude that the benefits of the test outweigh the harms (even though the radiation exposure is relatively low these days).[203]

Heart Disease Is Reversible

It's never too early to start eating healthfully, but is it ever too late? Such lifestyle medicine pioneers as Nathan Pritikin, Dean Ornish, and Caldwell Esselstyn Jr. took patients with advanced heart disease and put them on the kind of plant-based diet followed by Asian and African populations who didn't suffer from epidemic heart disease. Their hope was that a healthy enough diet would stop the disease process and keep it from progressing further.

Instead, something miraculous happened.

Their patients' heart disease started to reverse. These patients were getting *better*. As soon as they stopped eating an artery-clogging diet, their bodies were able to start dissolving away some of the plaque that had built up. Arteries began opening up without drugs or surgery, even in some cases of patients with severe triple-vessel heart disease. This suggests their bodies wanted to heal all along but were just never given the chance.[204]

Let me share with you what has been called the "best kept secret in medicine": Given the right conditions, the body heals itself.[205]

If we whack our shin really hard on a coffee table, it can get red, swollen, and painful. But our shin will heal naturally if we just stand back and let our body work its magic. But what if we kept whacking it in the same place three times a day—say, at breakfast, lunch, and dinner? It would never heal.

We could go to our doctor and complain that our shin hurts. "No problem," they might say, whipping out a pad and writing a prescription for painkillers. We'd go back home, still whacking our shin three times a day, but the pain pills would make it feel *so* much better. Thank heavens for modern medicine! That's what happens when people take nitroglycerin for chest pain. Medicine can offer tremendous relief, but it's not doing anything to treat the underlying cause.

Our body wants to regain its health if we let it. But if we keep reinjuring ourself three times a day, we interrupt the healing process. Consider smoking and lung cancer risk: One of the most amazing things I learned in medical school was that within about fifteen years of stopping smoking, lung-cancer risk approaches that of a lifelong nonsmoker.[206] Our lungs can clear out all that tar buildup and, eventually, it's almost as if we never smoked at all.

Our body wants to be healthy. Every night of our smoking life, as we fall asleep, that healing process is restarted until . . . *bam!*—we light up that first cigarette the next morning. Just as we can reinjure our lungs with every puff, we can reinjure our arteries with every bite. We could choose moderation and hit ourselves with a *smaller* hammer, but why beat ourselves up at all? Instead, we can choose to stop redamaging ourself, get out of our own way, and let our body's natural healing process bring us back toward health.

Endotoxins Crippling Our Arteries

Unhealthy diets don't just affect the structure of our arteries; an unhealthy diet can also affect their functioning. Our arteries are not merely inert pipes through which blood flows. They are dynamic, living organs. We've known for nearly three decades that a single fast-food meal—Sausage and Egg McMuffins were used in the original study—can stiffen our arteries within hours, cutting in half their ability to relax normally.[207] And just as this inflammatory state starts to calm down five or six hours later, it's lunchtime. We may once again whack our arteries with another load of harmful food, leaving many of us stuck in a danger zone of chronic, low-grade inflammation. Unhealthy meals don't just cause internal damage decades down the road but right here and now, within hours of going into our mouth.

Originally, researchers blamed the animal fat or animal protein, but attention has recently shifted to bacterial toxins known as *endotoxins*. Certain foods, such as meats, appear to harbor bacteria that, dead or alive, can trigger inflammation, even when the food is fully cooked. Endotoxins are not destroyed by cooking temperatures, stomach acid, or digestive enzymes, so after a meal of animal products, these endotoxins may end up in our intestines. They are then thought to be ferried by saturated fat across the gut wall into our bloodstream, where they can trigger the inflammatory reaction in our arteries.[208]

This may help explain the remarkable speed at which cardiac patients can experience relief when placed on a diet composed primarily of plant foods, including fruits, vegetables, whole grains, and beans. Dr. Ornish reported a 91 percent reduction in angina attacks within just a few weeks in patients placed on a plant-based program.[209] This rapid resolution in chest pain occurred well before their bodies could have cleared the plaque from their arteries, suggesting plant-based diets don't just help clean out arteries but also improve their day-to-day function. In contrast, control-group patients who were instead told to follow the advice of their doctors had a 186 percent *increase* in angina attacks.[210] It's no surprise their conditions worsened, given that they continued to eat the same diet that crippled their arteries in the first place.

We've known about the dramatic power of dietary changes for decades. For example, there was a paper entitled "Angina and Vegan Diet" published in the *American Heart Journal* back in 1977. Vegan diets are exclusively plant-based, avoiding meat, dairy, and eggs. Doctors described cases like that of Mr. F. W. (initials are often used to protect patient confidentiality), a sixty-five-year-old man with angina so severe he had to stop every nine or ten steps. He couldn't even make it to the mailbox. He was started on a vegan diet, and his pain improved within days. Within months, he was reportedly climbing mountains with no pain at all.[211]

Not ready to start eating healthier? Well, there is a new class of anti-angina drugs, such as ranolazine (sold as Ranexa). A drug company executive suggested its product be used for people not "able to comply with the substantial dietary changes required to achieve a vegan diet."[212] The medication hit the market at more than $2,000 a year, but the side effects are relatively minor, and it does work . . . technically speaking. At the highest dose, Ranexa was able to prolong exercise duration by *33.5 seconds*.[213] It does not look like those choosing the drug route will be climbing mountains anytime soon.

Brazil Nuts for Cholesterol Control?

Can a single serving of Brazil nuts bring down cholesterol levels faster than statin drugs and keep them down even a month after eating them that one time?

It was one of the wildest findings I'd ever seen. Researchers from—where else?—Brazil gave ten men and women a single meal containing one to eight Brazil nuts. Amazingly, compared to the control group who ate no nuts at all, just a single serving of four Brazil nuts almost immediately improved cholesterol levels. The "bad" LDL cholesterol levels were a staggering half a point lower just nine hours after eating the Brazil nuts.[214] Even drugs don't work nearly that fast.[215]

Here's the truly astonishing part: The researchers went back thirty days later and measured the study participants' cholesterol again. Even a month after ingesting a single serving of Brazil nuts, their cholesterol levels were still down.

Normally, when a study comes out in the medical literature showing some too-good-to-be-true result like this, doctors wait to see the results replicated before they change their clinical practice and begin recommending something new to their patients, particularly when the study is conducted with only ten subjects, and especially when the findings seem too incredible to believe. But when the intervention is cheap, easy, harmless, and healthy—we're talking just four Brazil nuts per month—then, in my opinion, the burden of proof is somewhat reversed. I think the reasonable default position is to do it until proven otherwise.

More is not better, however. Brazil nuts are so high in the mineral selenium that eating four every *day* may actually bump us up against the tolerable daily limit for selenium. Nevertheless, this is not something we have to worry about if we're only eating four Brazil nuts once a month.

Follow the Money

Research showing that the progression of coronary heart disease can be reversed with a plant-based diet—with or without other healthy lifestyle changes—has been published for decades in some of the most prestigious medical journals in the world. Why hasn't this news translated into public policy yet?

In 1977, the U.S. Senate Committee on Nutrition and Human Needs tried to do just that. Known as the McGovern Committee, they released *Dietary Goals for the United States*, a report advising Americans to cut down on animal-based foods and increase their consumption of plant-based foods. As a founding member of Harvard University's nutrition department recalls, "The meat, milk and egg producers were very upset."[216] That's an understatement. Under industry pressure, not only was the goal to "decrease meat consumption" removed from the report but the entire Senate nutrition committee was disbanded. Several prominent senators reputedly lost their election bids as a result of supporting the report.[217]

In more recent years, it's been uncovered that many members of the U.S. Dietary Guidelines Advisory Committee have had financial ties to everything from candy bar companies to entities like McDonald's Council on Healthy Lifestyles and Coca-Cola's Beverage Institute for Health and Wellness. One committee member even served as "brand girl" for cake-mix maker Duncan Hines and then as the official Crisco "brand girl" before going on to help write the official *Dietary Guidelines for Americans*.[218]

As one commentator noted in the *Food and Drug Law Journal*, historically, the Dietary Guidelines Advisory Committee reports contained:

> [n]o discussion at all of the scientific research on the health consequences of eating meat. If the Committee actually discussed this research, it would be unable to justify its recommendation to eat meat, as the research would show that meat increases the risks of chronic diseases, contrary to the purposes of the Guidelines. Thus, by simply ignoring that research, the Committee is able to reach a conclusion that would otherwise look improper.[219]

And what about the medical profession? Why haven't my colleagues fully embraced this research demonstrating the power of good nutrition? Sadly, the history of medicine holds many examples of the medical establishment rejecting sound science when it goes against the prevailing conventional wisdom. There's even a name for it: the "Tomato Effect." The term was coined in the *Journal of the American Medical Association* in reference to the fact that tomatoes were once considered poisonous and were shunned for centuries in North America, despite overwhelming evidence to the contrary.[220]

It's bad enough that most medical schools don't even require a single course on nutrition,[221] but it's even worse when mainstream medical organizations actively lobby *against* increased nutrition education for physicians.[222] When the American Academy of Family Physicians (AAFP) was called out on their proud new corporate relationship with Coca-Cola to support patient education on healthy eating, an executive vice president of the academy tried to quell protests by explaining that this alliance was not without precedent. After all, it had had relationships with PepsiCo and McDonald's for some time.[223] Before that, it had financial ties to cigarette maker Philip Morris.[224]

This argument didn't seem to placate the critics, so the AAFP executive quoted them the policy statement of the American Dietetic Association (ADA) that "[t]here are no good or bad foods, just good or bad diets." No bad foods? Really? The tobacco industry used to broadcast a similar theme: Smoking per se wasn't bad, only "excess" smoking.[225] Sound familiar? Everything in moderation.

The ADA, which produces a series of nutrition fact sheets with guidelines on maintaining a healthy diet, also has its own corporate ties. Who writes these fact sheets? Food industry sources pay the ADA $20,000 per fact sheet to explicitly take part in the drafting process. So we can learn about eggs from the American Egg Board and about the benefits of chewing gum from the Wrigley Science Institute.[226]

In 2012, the American Dietetic Association changed its name to the Academy of Nutrition and Dietetics but didn't appear to change its policies. It continues to take millions of dollars every year from processed junk food, meat, dairy, fizzy drink, and candy bar companies. In return, the academy lets them offer official educational seminars to teach dietitians what to say to their clients.[227] When you hear the title "registered dietitian," this is the group they are registered through. Thankfully, a movement within the dietitian community, exemplified by the formation of the organization Dietitians for Professional Integrity, started to buck this trend.

What about individual doctors, though? Why aren't all my colleagues telling their patients to lay off the KFC? Insufficient time during office visits is a common excuse physicians cite, but the top reason given by doctors for not counseling patients with high cholesterol to eat more healthfully is that they think patients may "fear privations related to dietary advice."[228] In other words, doctors perceive that patients would feel deprived of all the junk they've been eating. Can you imagine a doctor saying, "I'd like to tell my patients to stop smoking, but I know how much they love it"?

Neal Barnard, M.D., president of the Physicians Committee for Responsible Medicine, wrote a compelling editorial in the American Medical Association's journal of ethics, describing how doctors went from being bystanders—or even enablers—of smoking to leading the fight against tobacco. Doctors realized they were more effective at counseling patients to quit smoking if they no longer had tobacco stains on their own fingers.

Today, Dr. Barnard says, "Plant-based diets are the nutritional equivalent of quitting smoking."[229]

2

How Not to Die from Lung Diseases

The worst death I ever witnessed was that of a man dying of lung cancer. I was interning at a public health hospital in Boston. Evidently, people dying behind bars looks bad for prison statistics, so terminally ill prisoners were shipped to my hospital for their final days, even if there was little we could do for them.

It was summer, and the hospital's prison ward had no air-conditioning, at least for the inmates. We doctors could retreat to the chilled confines of the nursing station, but the inmates, handcuffed to their beds, just lay prostrate in the heat on that top floor of the tall brick building. When they were shuffled down the hall in front of us, ankles chained together, they left a trail of sweat.

The night the man died, I was on a thirty-six-hour shift. We worked 117-hour workweeks back then. It's amazing we didn't kill more people ourselves. Overnight, there were only two of us—myself and a moonlighting doctor who preferred to sleep for his $1,000 paycheck. So most of the time I was on my own to cover hundreds of patients, some of the sickest of the sick. It was on one of those nights that, staggering through a sleep-deprived haze, I got the call.

Up until then, all the deaths I had seen were those in which the patient was either dead on arrival or had died during cardiac "codes," when we try desperately, and nearly always unsuccessfully, to resuscitate.

This man was different.

He was wide-eyed, gasping for air, his cuffed hands clawing at the bed. The cancer was filling his lungs with fluid. He was being drowned by lung cancer.

While he thrashed desperately, pleading, my mind was in medical mode, all protocols and procedures, but nothing much could be done. The man needed morphine, but that was held on the other side of the ward, and I'd never get to it in time, let alone back to him. I was not popular on the prison floor. I had once reported a guard for beating a sick inmate and was rewarded with death threats. There was no way they'd let me through the gates fast enough. I begged a nurse to try to get some, but she didn't make it back in time.

The man's coughing turned to gurgling. "Everything's going to be okay," I said. Immediately I thought, *What a stupid thing to say to someone choking to death.* Just another lie in probably a long line of condescension from other authority figures throughout his life. Helpless, I turned from doctor back to human being. I took his hand in my own, which he then gripped with all his might, tugging me toward his tear-streaked, panic-stricken face. "I'm here," I said. "I'm right here." Our gaze remained locked as he suffocated right in front of me. It felt like watching someone being tortured to death.

Take a deep breath. Now imagine what it would feel like if you weren't able to breathe. We all need to take care of our lungs.

America's number two killer, lung disease, claims the lives of nearly 300,000 people each year. And like our number one domestic killer, heart disease, it's largely preventable. Lung disease can come in many forms, but the three types that kill the most people are lung cancer, chronic obstructive pulmonary disease (COPD), and asthma.

Lung cancer is our number one cancer killer. Most of the 130,000 lung cancer deaths[230] every year are the direct result of smoking. However, a healthy diet may help mitigate the DNA-damaging effects of tobacco smoke, as well as perhaps help prevent lung cancer from spreading.

COPD kills approximately 140,000 people annually,[231] either from damage to the walls of tiny air sacs in the lungs (emphysema) or inflamed and thickened airways plugged with thick mucus (chronic bronchitis). Although there is no cure for the permanent lung scarring that COPD causes, a diet rich in fruits and vegetables may help slow the progression of the disease and improve lung function for its thirteen million sufferers.

Finally, asthma, which claims more than 3,000 lives each year, is one of the most common chronic diseases among children,[232] yet it may be largely preventable with a healthier diet. Research suggests a few extra daily servings of fruits and vegetables can reduce both the number of cases of asthma during childhood and the number of asthma attacks among people with the disease.

LUNG CANCER

Lung cancer is diagnosed about 210,000 times each year in the United States[233] and causes more deaths annually than the next two cancers—colorectal and breast—combined.[234] At any given moment, more than 600,000 Americans are living under lung cancer's dark shadow.[235] Unlike with heart disease, which has yet to be fully acknowledged as the direct result of an artery-clogging diet, there is widespread recognition that tobacco is by far the most common cause of lung cancer. According to the American Lung Association, smoking tobacco contributes to up to 90 percent of all lung cancer deaths. Men who smoke are twenty-three times more likely and women thirteen times more likely to develop lung cancer than nonsmokers. And smokers aren't just harming themselves; thousands of deaths each year have been attributed to secondhand smoke. Nonsmokers have a 20 to 30 percent higher risk of developing lung cancer if they're regularly exposed to cigarette smoke.[236]

Those warning labels on cigarette packs are everywhere now, but for a long time, the link between smoking and lung cancer was suppressed by powerful interest groups—much as the relationship between certain foods and other leading killers is suppressed today. For example, in the 1980s, Philip Morris, the nation's leading cigarette manufacturer, launched the notorious Whitecoat Project. The corporation hired doctors to publish ghostwritten studies purporting to negate links between secondhand smoke and lung disease. These papers cherry-picked various scientific reports to conceal and distort the damning evidence of the dangers of secondhand smoke. This whitewashing, coupled with the tobacco industry's clever marketing campaigns, including cartoonlike ads, helped hook generations of Americans onto its products.[237]

If, despite all the evidence and warnings, you're currently a smoker, the most important step you can take is to stop. Now. Please. The benefits of quitting are immediate. According to the American Cancer Society, just twenty minutes after quitting, your heart rate and blood pressure drop. Within a few weeks, your blood circulation and lung function improve. Within a few months, the sweeper cells that help clean the lungs, remove mucus, and reduce the risk of infection start to regrow. And within a year of quitting, your smoking-related risk of coronary heart disease becomes half that of current smokers.[238] As we saw in chapter 1, the human body possesses a miraculous ability to heal itself as long as we don't keep reinjuring it. Simple dietary changes may help to roll back the damage wrought by the carcinogens in tobacco smoke.

Does Marijuana Cause Lung Cancer?

There are at least thirty-three carcinogens[239] in marijuana smoke, including polycyclic aromatic hydrocarbons,[240] combustion by-products blamed in part for the link between cancer and grilled meat.[241] The levels flowing through the bodies of those who smoke marijuana were found to be similar to what flows through the bodies of cigarette smokers, which is surprising, since most tobacco users typically inhale much more smoke into their lungs over the course of a day than do those exclusively smoking cannabis.[242] So, on a puff-by-puff basis, is marijuana smoke really that much worse?

Compared to unfiltered cigarette smoke, cannabis smoke does seem to contain more benzopyrene and benzanthracene, which are polycyclic aromatic hydrocarbon procarcinogens.[243] However, cannabis users may just inhale more deeply and then hold in the smoke longer, resulting in the deposition of four times more tar in the lungs.[244] What about bubbling the smoke through water, like in a bong? That method does little to reduce the risks of tar buildup.[245]

The tar in marijuana smoke may have similar tumor-promoting effects to cigarette smoke—in mice.[246] But what about in people? Longtime marijuana users do have more cancers—more lung cancer, oral cancer, and voice box cancer—but it seems that's only because they also tend to be more likely to smoke tobacco too. After cigarettes were taken out of the equation, no increased cancer risk was found.[247]

The same holds for head and neck cancers. One study found increased risk, but five studies reported no association, and one study even found decreased risk.[248] Regular use of marijuana can cause chronic bronchitis in some smokers due to airway injury, but no evidence has been found of long-term emphysema-like lung damage. And, despite the carcinogenic components in marijuana smoke, there is no apparent increased risk of lung cancer either. Evidence is mixed, however, regarding the risk of heavy, long-term use.[249]

In terms of smoke exposure, smoking a joint every single day for ten years may only translate to six months of pack-a-day cigarette smoking. In most studies on tobacco smoke and lung cancer, six months in a lifetime might even classify you as a "never smoker."[250] It may take a couple of years of cigarette smoking to significantly bump up lung cancer risk, so that would be like smoking a joint every day of your adult life. This may help explain the lack of a lung cancer link with casual marijuana use.[251]

Load Up on Broccoli

First, it's important to understand the toxic effects of cigarettes on the lungs. Tobacco smoke contains chemicals that weaken the body's immune system, making it more susceptible to disease and handicapping its ability to destroy cancer cells. At the same time, tobacco smoke can damage cell DNA, increasing the chance for cancer cells to form and flourish in the first place.[252]

To test the power of dietary interventions to prevent DNA damage, scientists often study chronic smokers. Researchers rounded up a group of longtime smokers and asked them to consume thirty-eight times more broccoli than the average American—in other words, a single stalk a day. Compared to broccoli-avoiding smokers, the broccoli-eating smokers suffered 41 percent fewer DNA mutations in their bloodstream over ten days. Is that just because the broccoli boosted the activity of the detoxifying enzymes in their livers, which helped clear carcinogens before they even made it to the smokers' cells? No, even when DNA was extracted from the subjects' bodies and exposed to a known DNA-damaging chemical, the genetic material from the broccoli eaters showed significantly less damage, suggesting that eating vegetables like broccoli may make us more resilient at a subcellular level.[253]

Now, don't think this means that eating a stalk of broccoli before smoking a pack of Marlboro Reds is going to completely erase the cancer-causing effects of cigarette smoke. It won't. But as you're trying to quit, such vegetables as broccoli, cabbage, and cauliflower may help prevent further damage.

The benefits of broccoli-family (cruciferous) vegetables may not stop there. While breast cancer is the most common internal cancer among American women, lung cancer is actually their number one cancer killer. About 85 percent of women with breast cancer are still alive five years after diagnosis, but the numbers are reversed when it comes to lung cancer: 85 percent of women die within five years of a lung cancer diagnosis. Ninety percent of those deaths are due to metastasis, the spread of the cancer to other parts of the body.[254]

Certain compounds in broccoli may have the potential to suppress this metastatic spread. In a 2010 study, scientists laid down a layer of human lung cancer cells in a petri dish and cleared a swath down the middle. Within twenty-four hours, the cancer cells had crept back together, and within thirty hours, they had completely closed the gap. But when the scientists dripped some cruciferous-vegetable compounds onto the cancer cells, the cancer creep was stunted.[255]

Whether or not eating broccoli will help prolong survival in cancer patients has yet to be tested in clinical trials, but a cohort study found that lung cancer patients eating more whole plant foods in general have a 34 percent lower risk of dying in the subsequent few years.[256] We don't have to keep waiting for further research, though. The nice thing about healthy dietary interventions is that since they have no downsides, they can be added to whatever other treatments one chooses.

Smoking vs. Kale

Researchers have found that kale—that dark green leafy vegetable dubbed the "queen of greens"—might help control cholesterol levels. Thirty study participants with high cholesterol consumed three to four shots of kale juice each day for three months. That's like eating 13.5 kilos' worth of kale, or the amount the average American consumes in about a century. So what happened? Did they turn green and start to photosynthesize?

No. What the kale did do was substantially lower their "bad" LDL cholesterol.[257] By the end of the study, the antioxidant activity in the blood of most participants had shot up. But curiously, the antioxidant activity in a minority remained flat. Sure enough, these were the smokers. The free radicals created by the cigarettes were thought to have actively depleted the body of antioxidants. When your smoking habit erases the antioxidant-boosting effects of eight hundred cups of kale, you know it's time to quit.

Carcinogen-Blocking Effects of Turmeric

The Indian spice turmeric, which gives curry powder its characteristic golden color, may also help prevent some of the DNA damage caused by smoking. Since 1987, the National Cancer Institute has tested more than a thousand different compounds for *chemopreventive* (cancer-preventing) activity. Only a few dozen have made it to clinical trials, but among the most promising is curcumin, the bright-yellow pigment in turmeric.[258]

Chemopreventive agents can be classified into different subgroups based on which stage of cancer development they help fight: Carcinogen blockers and antioxidants help prevent the initial triggering DNA mutation, and antiproliferatives work by keeping tumors from growing and spreading. Curcumin is special in that it appears to belong to both groups, meaning it may potentially help prevent and arrest cancer cell growth.[259]

Researchers have investigated the effects of curcumin on the DNA-mutating ability of various carcinogens and found that curcumin was indeed an effective antimutagen against several common cancer-causing substances.[260] But these experiments were done in vitro, meaning effectively in a laboratory test tube. After all, it wouldn't be ethical to expose humans to carcinogens to observe whether they got cancer. However, someone got the bright idea of finding a group of people who already, of their own accord, had carcinogens coursing through their veins. Smokers!

One way to measure the level of DNA-mutating chemicals in peoples' bodies is dripping their urine on bacteria growing in a petri dish. Bacteria, like all life on Earth, share DNA as a common genetic language. Unsurprisingly, scientists who tried this experiment found that the urine from nonsmokers caused far fewer DNA mutations—after all, they had a lot fewer carcinogens flowing through their systems. But when the smokers were given turmeric, the DNA-mutation rate dropped by up to 38 percent.[261] They weren't given curcumin pills; they merely got less than a teaspoon a day of just the regular turmeric spice you'd find at the supermarket. Of course, turmeric can't completely mitigate the effects of smoking. Even after the study participants ate turmeric for a month, the DNA-damaging ability of the smokers' urine still exceeded that of the nonsmokers'. But smokers who make turmeric a staple of their diets may help lessen some of the damage.

The anticancer effects of curcumin extend beyond its ability to potentially prevent DNA mutations. It also appears to help regulate programmed cell death. Our cells are preprogrammed to die naturally to make way for fresh cells through a process known as *apoptosis* (from the Greek *ptosis*, "falling," and *apo*, "away from"). In a sense, our bodies are rebuilding themselves every few months[262] with the building materials we provide through our diets. Some cells, however, overstay their welcome—namely, cancer cells. By somehow disabling their own suicide mechanism, they don't die when they're supposed to. Because they continue to thrive and divide, cancer cells can eventually form tumors and potentially spread throughout the body.

So how does curcumin affect this process? It appears to have the ability to reprogram the self-destruct mechanism back into cancer cells. All cells contain so-called death receptors that trigger the self-destruction sequence, but cancer cells can disable their own death receptors. Curcumin, however, appears able to reactivate them.[263] Curcumin can also directly kill cancer cells by activating "execution enzymes" called *caspases*. They are present inside cancer cells and can destroy them from within by chopping up their proteins.[264] Unlike most chemotherapy drugs, against which cancer cells can develop resistance over time, curcumin affects several mechanisms of cell death simultaneously, making it potentially harder for cancer cells to avoid destruction.[265]

Curcumin has been found to be effective against a variety of other cancer cells in vitro, including those of the breast, brain, blood, colon, kidney, liver, lungs, and skin. For reasons not fully understood, curcumin seems to leave noncancerous cells alone.[266] Unfortunately, turmeric has yet to be tested in clinical trials for the prevention or treatment of lung cancer, but with no downsides at culinary doses, I'd suggest trying to find ways to incorporate the spice into your diet. I offer a number of suggestions in Part 2.

Dietary Secondhand Smoke

Though the majority of lung cancer is attributed to smoking, approximately a quarter of all cases occur in people who've never smoked.[267] Although some of these cases are due to secondhand smoke, another contributing cause may be another potentially carcinogenic plume: fumes from frying.

When fat is heated to frying temperatures, whether it be animal fat, such as lard, or plant fat, such as vegetable oil, toxic volatile chemicals with mutagenic properties (those able to cause genetic mutations) are released into the air.[268] This happens even before the "smoke point" temperature is reached.[269] If you do fry at home, good ventilation in the kitchen may reduce lung cancer risk.[270]

Cancer risk may also depend on what's being fried. A study of women in China found that smokers who stir-fried meat every day had nearly three times the odds of lung cancer compared to smokers who stir-fried foods other than meat on a daily basis.[271] This is thought to be because of a group of carcinogens called heterocyclic amines that are formed when muscle tissue is subjected to high temperatures. (We'll talk more about these in chapter 12.)

The effects of meat fumes can be hard to separate from the effects of eating the meat itself, but a recent study on pregnant women and barbecuing attempted to tease them out. When meat is grilled, polycyclic aromatic hydrocarbons (PAHs) are also produced, one of the probable carcinogens in cigarette smoke. The researchers discovered that not only was the ingestion of grilled meat in the third trimester associated with smaller birth weights, mothers merely exposed to the fumes tended to give birth to babies with a birth weight deficit. Exposure to the fumes was also associated with a smaller head size, an indicator of brain volume.[272] Air pollution studies suggest prenatal exposure to polycyclic aromatic hydrocarbons may then translate into adverse effects on children's future cognitive development (as manifested by a significantly lower IQ).[273]

Even just living next to a restaurant may pose a health hazard. Scientists estimated the lifetime cancer risk among those residing near the exhaust outlets at Chinese restaurants, American restaurants, and barbecue joints. While exposure to fumes from all three types of restaurants resulted in exposure to unsafe levels of PAHs, the Chinese restaurants proved to be the worst. This is thought to be due to the amount of fish being cooked,[274] as the fumes from pan-fried fish have been found to contain high levels of PAHs capable of damaging the DNA of human lung cells.[275] Given the excess cancer risk, the researchers concluded that it wouldn't be safe to live near the exhaust of a Chinese restaurant for more than a day or two a month.[276]

What about that enticing aroma of sizzling bacon? The fumes produced by frying bacon contain a class of carcinogens called *nitrosamines*.[277] Although all meat may release potentially carcinogenic fumes, processed meat like bacon may be the worst: A study from the University of California, Davis, found that bacon fumes cause about four times more DNA mutations than the fumes from beef patties fried at similar temperatures.[278]

What about tempeh bacon? Tempeh is a fermented soya bean product used to make a variety of meat alternatives. Researchers compared the DNA-mutating effects of the fumes from frying bacon and beef to tempeh. The bacon and burger fumes were mutagenic, but the tempeh fumes were not. Nevertheless, it's still not a good idea to eat fried foods. Though no DNA changes were detected after exposure to tempeh smoke, the fried tempeh itself did cause some DNA mutations (though 45 times fewer than the beef and 346 times fewer than the bacon). The researchers proposed that these findings might account for the higher incidence of respiratory diseases and lung cancer among cooks and lower incidence overall among vegetarians.[279]

If you do need to be around frying bacon or eggs, it would be safer to limit your exposure by using a backyard grill. Studies show that the number of particles deposited into the lungs increases by a factor of ten when frying indoors versus outdoors.[280]

CHRONIC OBSTRUCTIVE PULMONARY DISEASE

Chronic obstructive pulmonary disease (COPD), such as emphysema and chronic bronchitis, is a condition that makes it difficult to breathe and gets worse and worse over time. In addition to shortness of breath, COPD can cause severe coughing, excess mucus production, wheezing, and chest tightness. The disease affects more than fourteen million Americans.[281]

Smoking is far and away the leading cause of COPD, but other factors can contribute, such as prolonged exposure to air pollution. Unfortunately, there is no cure for COPD, but there is some good news: A healthy diet may help to prevent COPD and help keep it from getting worse.

Data going back fifty years show that a high intake of fruits and vegetables is positively associated with good lung function.[282] Just one extra serving of fruit each day may translate into a 24 percent lower risk of dying from COPD.[283] On the other hand, a twin pair of studies from Columbia and Harvard Universities found that consumption of cured meats—like bacon, ham, hot dogs, sausage, and salami—may increase the risk of COPD.[284,285] It's thought to be due to the nitrite preservatives in meat, which may mimic the lung-damaging properties of the nitrite by-products of cigarette smoke.[286]

What if you already have the disease? Can the same foods that appear to help prevent COPD be used to treat it? We didn't know until a landmark study was published in 2010. More than a hundred COPD patients were randomized into two groups—half were instructed to boost their fruit and vegetable consumption, while the others remained on their normal diet. Over the next three years, the standard-diet subjects became progressively worse, as expected. In contrast, the disease progression was halted in the group consuming more fruits and veggies. Not only did their lung function not get worse, it actually *improved* a little. The researchers suggested this could be due to a combination of the antioxidant and anti-inflammatory effects of the fruits and vegetables, along with a potential reduction in the consumption of meat, which is thought to act as a pro-oxidant.[287]

Regardless of the mechanism, a diet with more whole plant foods may help prevent and arrest the progression of this leading killer. In the large Harvard cohort studies, which followed the diets and diseases of more than 200,000 doctors, nurses, and other health professionals for decades, those eating more healthy plant foods had a 46 percent lower risk of developing COPD. The researchers concluded: "These findings provide further evidence for consuming a diet that emphasizes healthful plant foods to optimize lung health."[288]

Combatting Air Pollution with Food

Outdoor air pollution may be the ninth leading cause of death and disability in the world, responsible for millions of deaths from lung cancer, emphysema, heart disease, stroke, and respiratory infection.[289,290] In the United States, living in a polluted city was associated with 16, 27, and 28 percent increases in total, cardiovascular, and lung cancer deaths, respectively, compared to living in a city with cleaner air.[291] As well, living in a city with polluted air may lead to up to a 75 percent increase in the risk of a heart attack.[292] The risk of dying in a traffic jam is two and a half times greater in a polluted city. No one wants to be living in a traffic jam, but it's better than dying in one.

In addition to causing deaths, air pollution is also the cause of a number of health problems. It may not only exacerbate asthma but also increase the risk of developing asthma in the first place.[293] These pollutants may trigger liver disease[294] and even increase the risk of diabetes.[295] They can be harmful to health even when pollutant levels are within legal established limits.[296] So, what can we do about it?

We need better vehicle inspections, efficient public transport, bus lanes, bicycle lanes, and even urban tolls to help clean up the air, but such measures might inconvenience the population "and, therefore, might not be politically acceptable."[297] Until then, what can we do to protect ourselves?

Our body naturally has detoxifying enzymes, not only in our liver but also lining our airways. Studies show that people born with less effective detox enzymes have an exaggerated allergic response to diesel exhaust, suggesting that these enzymes actively combat the inflammation caused by pollutants in the air.[298] A significant part of the population has these substandard forms of the enzyme, but, either way, what can we do to boost the activity of whichever detoxification enzymes we do have?

In chapter 12, I'll talk about how broccoli can dramatically boost the activity of the detox enzymes in our liver, but what about our lungs? Smoking cigarettes is so inflammatory that we can have elevated C-reactive protein (CRP) levels for up to thirty years after quitting,[299] and that inflammation can start almost immediately after we start smoking, so it's critical to never start in the first place.[300] If you do, though, you can cut your level of the inflammation biomarker CRP nearly in half after just ten days of eating a lot of broccoli. Broccoli appears to cut inflammation in nonsmokers as well,[301] which may explain in part why consuming broccoli even just one to two times per week was associated with a 32 to 43 percent lower risk of dying prematurely.[302]

What about air pollution? We know that the cruciferous compound sulforaphane "is the most potent known inducer"[303] of our detox enzymes, so most of the research has been on its ability to fight cancer. But, for the first time, researchers tried to see if it could combat the pro-inflammatory impact of pollutants, such as diesel exhaust. They put some human lung lining cells in a petri dish, and the number of detox enzymes produced after dripping on some broccoli goodness skyrocketed. Interesting, but we don't inhale broccoli or snort it. We eat it. Can it still get into our lungs and help? Yes. After study participants consumed broccoli sprouts for two days, researchers took some cells out of their noses and found up to a hundred times more detox enzyme expression compared to eating a non-cruciferous vegetable, alfalfa sprouts.[304] If only we could squirt some diesel exhaust up people's noses. That's just what some UCLA researchers did, at an amount equal to daily rush hour exposure on a Los Angeles freeway. Within six hours, the number of inflammatory cells in their noses shot up and continued to rise. But in the group who had been getting a broccoli sprout extract, the inflammation went down and stayed down.[305]

> What about detoxifying air pollutants throughout the rest of our body? We didn't know, until a study in China found that eating broccoli sprouts enables people to detoxify 60 percent more benzene from their bodies. "The key finding . . . was the observed rapid and highly durable elevation of the detoxification of . . . a known human carcinogen." Now, this was using broccoli sprouts, which are highly concentrated, equivalent to about 900 grams of broccoli a day, so we don't know how well more modest doses would work. But if they do, eating broccoli could "provide a frugal means to attenuate . . . the long-term health risks [of air pollution]."[306]

ASTHMA

Asthma is an inflammatory disease characterized by recurring attacks of narrowed, swollen airways, causing shortness of breath, wheezing, and coughing. Asthma can start at any age, but it usually emerges during childhood. One of the most common chronic diseases in kids, asthma's prevalence has been increasing year after year.[307] In the United States, twenty-five million people suffer from asthma, and about five million of them are children.[308]

A groundbreaking study recently demonstrated that the rates of asthma vary dramatically around the world. The *International Study of Asthma and Allergies in Childhood* followed more than a million children in nearly one hundred countries, making it the most comprehensive survey ever undertaken of this disease. The study found a twentyfold to sixtyfold difference in the prevalence of asthma, allergies, and eczema.[309] Why does the prevalence of rhinoconjunctivitis (itchy eyes and runny nose) range from 1 percent of children in parts of India, for instance, to as much as 45 percent elsewhere?[310] While such factors as air pollution and smoking rates may play a role, the most significant associations were not with what was going into their lungs but what was going into their stomachs.[311]

Adolescents living in areas where more starchy foods, grains, vegetables, and nuts were consumed were significantly less likely to exhibit chronic symptoms of wheezing, allergic rhinoconjunctivitis, and allergic eczema.[312] Boys and girls eating two or more servings of vegetables a day appear to have only half the odds of suffering from allergic asthma.[313] In general, the prevalence of asthma and respiratory symptoms reportedly appears to be lower among populations eating more foods of plant origin.[314]

On the other hand, foods of animal origin have been associated with increased asthma risk. A study of more than one hundred thousand adults in India found that those who consumed meat daily, or even occasionally, were significantly more likely to suffer from asthma than those who excluded meat and eggs from their diets altogether.[315] Eggs (along with fizzy drinks) have also been associated with asthma attacks in children, as well as respiratory symptoms, such as wheezing, shortness of breath, and exercise-induced coughing.[316] Removing eggs and dairy from the diet has been shown to improve asthmatic children's lung function in as few as eight weeks.[317]

The mechanism by which diet affects airway inflammation may lie with the thin coating of fluid that forms the interface between our respiratory-tract lining and the outside air. Using the antioxidants obtained from the fruits and vegetables we eat, this fluid acts as our first line of defense against the free radicals that contribute to asthmatic airway hypersensitivity, contraction, and mucus production.[318] Oxidation by-products can be measured in exhaled breath and are significantly lowered by shifting toward a more plant-based diet.[319]

If those with asthma eat fewer fruits and vegetables, does their lung function decline? Researchers out of Australia tried removing these plant foods from asthma patients' diets to see what would happen. Within two weeks, their asthma symptoms grew significantly worse. Interestingly, the low-fruit, low-vegetable diet used in the study—a restriction to no more than one serving of fruits and two servings of vegetables per day—is typical of Western diets. In other words, the diet they used experimentally to impair people's lung function and worsen their asthma was effectively the standard American diet.[320]

The Side Effects of Burning Incense

Frankincense and myrrh date back thousands of years before the three wise men, and their burning as incense may have had a hygienic function. When put to the test, incense fumes were able to kill off some bacteria and mold in the air,[321] but they may also carry health risks.

Although the adverse health effects of secondhand tobacco smoke are well recognized, the impact of burning incense in the home has received less attention. However, burning incense has been found to generate around four times the particulate matter as cigarettes,[322] helping to explain why home incense use has been linked to adverse health effects, particularly on the heart and lungs, including childhood asthma.[323]

In addition to little ash particles that can settle in the lungs, there are harmful compounds in the smoke, including carbon monoxide, sulfur dioxide, carcinogenic polycyclic aromatic hydrocarbons, benzene, and formaldehyde.[324] The World Health Organization guideline for indoor formaldehyde is about 80 parts per billion, but even with a window open during the hour or so incense burns, formaldehyde levels could exceed the safety limit.[325] What does this all mean in terms of disease outcomes?

A study of thousands of children in Hong Kong followed over time found that exposure to household incense burning was associated with impaired lung function, reduced lung function growth, and increased risks of respiratory diseases and symptoms.[326] Daily exposure is also associated with impaired lung function in adolescents.[327]

What about the heart? Long-term exposure to incense burning in the home environment was associated with an increased risk of cardiovascular mortality. Approximately 8 percent of heart disease deaths and 12 percent of stroke deaths could potentially be attributed to incense use, though, in the study, researchers looked at long-term exposure equivalent to incense burning at home on a daily basis for at least twenty years.[328]

What about cancer? Temple workers exposed to incense day in and day out were found to have evidence of significantly more DNA damage, including DNA strand breaks.[329] Does this translate into greater cancer risk? One unsolved mystery has been why nonsmoking Asian women have such high lung cancer rates. Might it be incense? Probably not, since the association between incense use and lung cancer remains inconclusive,[330] though incense use appears to be linked to cancers of the upper respiratory tract,[331] as well as brain tumors among children whose mothers used incense during pregnancy.[332]

Even without tumors, a study of 15,000 infants found that household incense burning was associated with a delay in brain development milestones, such as when they started to walk.[333] On the other side of the life cycle, incense exposure among older adults was associated with reduced cognitive performance and adverse structural changes in the brain. The

> researchers concluded that this calls for safer practices, such as avoiding burning incense indoors.[334]
>
> Despite being a recognized health hazard by the medical community, burning incense remains in widespread use.[335] At the very least, we may want to avoid burning incense in the home when susceptible individuals are present, such as the very young, the very old, or people with a family history of allergy or preexisting cardiovascular or respiratory disease.[336]

What about improving asthma by adding fruits and vegetables? Researchers repeated the experiment, but this time increased fruit and vegetable consumption to seven servings a day. This simple act of adding a few more fruits and vegetables to their daily diet ended up successfully cutting the study participants' exacerbation rate in half.[337] That's the power of eating healthfully.

If it's the antioxidants, why not just take an antioxidant supplement? After all, popping a pill is easier than eating an apple. The reason is simple: Supplements don't appear to work. Studies have repeatedly shown that antioxidant supplements have no beneficial effects on respiratory or allergic diseases, underscoring the importance of eating whole foods rather than trying to take isolated components or extracts in pill form.[338] For example, the Harvard Nurses' Health Study found that women who obtained high levels of vitamin E from a nut-rich diet appeared to have nearly half the risk of asthma of those who didn't, but those who took vitamin E supplements saw no benefit at all.[339]

Who do you think did better? A group of asthma patients who ate seven servings a day of fruits and vegetables, or a group who ate three daily servings plus fifteen "serving equivalents" in pill form? Sure enough, the pills didn't seem to help at all. Improvements in lung function and asthma control were evident only after subjects increased their *actual* fruit and vegetable intake, strongly suggesting that consuming whole foods is paramount.[340]

If adding a few daily servings of fruits and vegetables can have such a significant effect, what if asthma sufferers were put on a diet composed entirely of plant foods? Researchers in Sweden decided to test a strictly plant-based diet on a group of people with severe asthma who weren't getting better despite the best medical therapies—thirty-five patients with long-established, physician-verified asthma, twenty of whom had been admitted to hospitals for acute attacks during the previous two years. One patient had received emergency intravenous infusions a total of twenty-three times, another reported he'd been hospitalized more than a hundred times, and one person had even suffered a cardiac arrest after an attack and had to be revived and placed on a ventilator.[341]

Of the twenty-four patients who adhered to the plant-based diet, 70 percent improved after four months, and 90 percent improved within one year. And these were all people who had experienced no improvement in their conditions at all in the year prior to switching to a plant-based diet.[342]

Within just one year of eating more healthfully, all but two patients were able to drop their dose of asthma medication or get off their steroids and other drugs completely. Objective measures like lung function and physical working capacity improved; meanwhile, subjectively, some patients said their improvement was so considerable that they felt "they had a new life."[343]

There was no control group, so the placebo effect may have accounted for some of the improvement, but, again, what's nice about a healthier diet is there are only good side effects. In addition to improvements in their asthma control, the study participants lost an average of eighteen pounds, and their cholesterol and blood pressures got better. From a risk-benefit standpoint, then, it's definitely worth giving a plant-based diet a try. A 2024 systematic review concluded: "The most successful diets for asthma patients seem to be those in which the consumption of fruit, vegetables, and high-fiber foods is increased. . . ."[344]

The most lethal lung diseases vary widely in presentation and prognosis. As noted, smoking is far and away the leading cause of lung cancer and COPD, but diseases like asthma typically develop during childhood and can be associated with a range of contributing factors, such as low birth weight and frequent respiratory infections. While quitting smoking remains the most effective way to ward off the worst kinds of lung disease, we can also help the body bolster its defenses by eating a diet rich in protective plant foods. The same kind of diet that appears to help severe asthmatics may also help prevent all three diseases from occurring in the first place.

If you're one of the millions of Americans who already suffer from lung disease, quitting smoking and changing your diet can still make a difference. It's never too late to start living and eating more healthfully. The restorative powers of the human body are remarkable, but our body needs our help. By including foods that contain cancer-fighting compounds and loading up on antioxidant-rich fruits and veggies, we may be able to strengthen our respiratory defenses and breathe easier.

In my clinical practice, whenever I felt I was under too much time pressure to address a patient's smoking or bad dietary habits, I would stop and think back to the hideous death of that man in Boston. No one deserves to die like that. I'd like to think no one has to.

How Not to Die from Brain Diseases

My mom's father died of a stroke, and her mother died of Alzheimer's disease.

As a kid, I loved going to see my grandma in Long Island. We lived out west, so I got to fly on a plane—sometimes all by myself! She was the perfect—and perfectly doting—grandmother. She'd want to take me to toy stores, but, geeky me, I just wanted to go to the library. When we'd get back to the house, my arms filled with borrowed books, she'd let me sit way back on her big couch—shoes off, of course—and read and draw pictures. Then she'd bring me blueberry muffins she made with a big mechanical mixer that took up half the kitchen counter.

Later in life, my grandma started to lose her mind. By then, I was in medical school, but my newfound knowledge was useless. She had turned. My previously sweet and stately grandmother? Now she threw things at people. She cursed. Her caretaker showed me the teeth marks on her arm where my once kind, loving grandma had bitten her.

That's the horror of brain disease. Unlike a problem with our foot or our back or even another vital organ, brain disease can attack our *self*.

The two most serious brain diseases are stroke, which kills 160,000 Americans each year,[345] and Alzheimer's disease, which kills 114,000.[346] Most strokes can be thought of as "brain attacks"—like heart attacks, but the rupturing plaques in our arteries cut off blood flow to parts of the brain rather than to parts of the heart. Alzheimer's is more like a mind attack.

Alzheimer's disease is one of the most physically and emotionally burdensome diseases, for both sufferers and caregivers. Unlike stroke, which can kill instantly and without any warning, Alzheimer's involves a slower, more subtle decline over months or years. Instead of cholesterol-filled plaques in our arteries, plaques made of a substance called *amyloid* develop in the brain tissue itself, associated with the loss of memory and, eventually, loss of life.

While the pathology of stroke and Alzheimer's are different, one key factor unites them: Mounting evidence suggests that a healthy diet may help prevent them both.

STROKE

In about 90 percent of strokes,[347] blood flow to part of the brain gets cut off, depriving it of oxygen and killing off the part that was fed by the now-clogged artery. That's called an *ischemic stroke* (from the Latin *ischaemia*, meaning "stopping blood"). A small minority of strokes are *hemorrhagic strokes*, which are caused by bleeding into the brain when a blood vessel bursts. The damage wrought by a stroke depends on which area of the brain was deprived of oxygen (or where bleeding occurred) and how long the deprivation lasts. People who experience a brief stroke might only need to contend with arm or leg weakness, while those who suffer a major stroke can develop paralysis, lose the ability to speak, or, as is too often the case, die.

Sometimes the blood clot lasts only a moment—not long enough to notice but still long enough to kill off a tiny portion of our brain. These so-called silent strokes can multiply and slowly reduce cognitive function until full-blown dementia develops.[348] The goal is to reduce the risk of both the massive strokes that can kill us instantly and the ministrokes that maim us over the course of years. Just as with heart disease, a healthy diet can reduce stroke risk by reducing cholesterol and blood pressure while improving blood flow and antioxidant capacity.

Fiber! Fiber! Fiber!

In addition to its well-known effects on bowel health, high fiber intake appears to reduce the risk of cancers of the colon[349] and breast,[350] diabetes,[351] heart disease,[352] obesity,[353] and premature death in general.[354] A number of studies now show that high fiber intake may also help ward off stroke.[355] Unfortunately, only 6 percent of Americans meet the minimum daily recommendation for fiber.[356]

This means about 94 percent of Americans eat fiber-deficient diets. Fiber is naturally concentrated in only one place: whole plant foods. Processed foods have less, and animal-derived foods have no fiber at all. Animals have bones to hold them up; plants have fiber.

It apparently doesn't take much fiber to cut stroke risk. Increasing fiber intake by just seven grams a day may be associated with a 7 percent risk reduction.[357] Different strokes for different folks—depending, evidently, on how much fiber they ate. An additional seven grams of fiber is easy to add to our diet; it's the equivalent of a bowl of oatmeal with berries or a serving of baked beans.*

How does fiber protect the brain? We're not exactly sure. We do know that fiber helps control our cholesterol[358] and blood sugar levels,[359] which can help reduce the amount of artery-clogging plaque in our brain's blood vessels. High-fiber diets may also lower blood pressure,[360] which reduces the risk of brain bleeds. But scientists don't have to know the exact mechanism before we act on this knowledge. As the biblical passage goes: "A man scatters seed on the ground . . . the seed sprouts and grows, though he does not know how." Had the farmer from scripture postponed his sowing until he understood the biology of seed germination, he wouldn't have survived for very long. So why not go ahead and reap the benefits of eating fiber by eating more unprocessed plant foods?

It's never too early to start eating healthier. Though stroke is considered an older person's disease—only about 2 percent of stroke deaths occur before the age of forty-five[361]—the risk factors may begin accumulating in childhood. In a remarkable study, hundreds of children were followed for a period of twenty-four years, from junior high school to adulthood. Researchers found that low fiber intake early on was associated with stiffening of the arteries leading up to the brain—a key risk factor for stroke. By the time these adolescents were only fourteen, clear differences in arterial health were found for those consuming different amounts of fiber-containing foods in their daily diets.[362]

Again, it did not appear to take much. One more apple, an extra 45 grams of broccoli, or just two tablespoons of beans a day during childhood may

---

* Anytime a nutrient claim is made, it is from the U.S. Department of Agriculture's Food-Data Central database, hosted by the National Agricultural Library at https://fdc.nal.usda.gov/.

translate into a meaningful effect on artery health later in life.[363] If we *really* want to be proactive, the best available science[364] suggests we can minimize stroke risk by eating a minimum of 25 grams a day of soluble fiber (fiber that dissolves in water, typically found in beans, oats, nuts, and berries) *and* 47 daily grams of insoluble fiber (fiber that does not dissolve in water, found primarily in whole grains, such as brown rice and whole wheat). Granted, we'd have to eat an extraordinarily healthy diet to attain this level of fiber intake, far beyond what is arbitrarily determined as adequate by most health authorities.[365] Rather than patronizing us with what they think is "achievable"[366] by the masses, though, I wish these authorities would just tell us what the science says and let us make up our own mind.

Potassium

Take a plant, any plant, and burn it to ash. Throw that ash in a pot of water, boil it, skim off the ashes, and eventually you'll be left with a white residue known as *potash* ("pot ash"). Potash has been used for millennia for making everything from soap and glass to fertilizer and bleach. It wasn't until 1807 that an English chemist figured out that this "vegetable alkali" contained an undiscovered element, which he called *pot-ash-ium*—that is, potassium.

I mention this simply to emphasize the primary source of potassium in our diet—namely, plants. Every cell in our body requires potassium to function, and we need to get it from our diet. For much of human history, we ate so many plants that we got upward of 10,000 mg of potassium every day.[367] Nowadays, less than *2 percent* of Americans even reach half that.[368]

The major reason is simple: We don't eat enough unprocessed plant foods.[369] What does potassium have to do with stroke? A review of all the best studies on the relationship between potassium and our top-two killers, heart disease and stroke, determined that a 1,640 mg increase per day in potassium intake was associated with a 21 percent reduction in stroke risk.[370] That may not be enough to bring the average American's potassium levels to where they should be, but it's still enough to substantially reduce the risk of stroke. Imagine how much lower our risk would be if we doubled or tripled our intake of whole plant foods.

Bananas, although they've been marketed for their potassium content, aren't actually particularly rich in the mineral. According to the U.S. Department of Agriculture database, bananas don't even make the list of the top one thousand foods with the highest levels of potassium; in fact, they come in at number 1,611, right after Reese's Pieces.[371]

What are some of the truly potassium-rich foods? The healthiest common whole food sources are probably greens, beans, and sweet potatoes.[372]

Citrus

Good news for all you orange lovers: Citrus fruit intake has been associated with reduced stroke risk—even more so than apples.[373] Say I can't compare them? I just did! The key may lie with a citrus phytonutrient called *hesperidin*, which appears to increase blood flow throughout the body, including the brain. Using a machine known as a doppler fluximeter, scientists can measure blood flow through the skin using a laser beam. If we hook people up to this machine and give them a solution containing the amount of hesperidin found in 500 ml of orange juice, blood pressure decreases and overall blood flow increases. When study participants drank straight orange juice instead of the hesperidin solution, their blood flow was even better. In other words, the stroke-reducing effects of oranges extend beyond just the hesperidin.[374] When it comes to food, the whole is often greater than the sum of its parts.

The positive effects of citrus fruits on blood flow don't require a machine to measure them. In one study, scientists recruited women who suffered from sensitivity to cold weather due to poor blood flow—women with chronically cold hands, feet, and toes—and placed them in a highly air-conditioned room. The women in the experimental group drank a solution containing actual citrus phytonutrients, while another (control) group drank a placebo (an artificially flavored orange drink). The placebo drinkers got colder and colder. Because of decreased blood flow, the temperature of their fingertips dropped nearly 9°F during the course of the study. The fingertips of the women who drank real citrus, meanwhile, cooled less than half as fast, because their blood flow remained steadier. (The researchers also had both groups of women plunge their hands into icy water and saw the citrus drinkers recover about 50 percent faster than those in the control group.)[375]

So eating a few oranges before snowboarding may help keep our fingers and toes from getting as chilly. But while warm digits are nice, the reduced stroke risk associated with higher citrus intake is even nicer.

Optimal Sleep Duration and Stroke

Lack of sleep, or even too much of it, is associated with increased stroke risk.[376] But how much sleep may be too little? How much too much?

Scientists in Japan were the first to take a major stab at this question. They followed nearly 100,000 middle-aged men and women for fourteen years. Compared with people who slept an average of seven hours per night, subjects who got four hours of sleep or less, or ten hours or more, had roughly a 50 percent greater likelihood of dying from a stroke.[377]

A recent study of 150,000 Americans was able to examine the issue more thoroughly. Higher stroke rates were found among individuals sleeping six hours or less, or nine hours or more. Those at lowest risk got around seven or eight hours of sleep a night.[378] Large studies in Europe,[379] China,[380] and elsewhere[381] have confirmed that seven or eight hours appears to be associated with the lowest risk. We're not sure if the relationship is cause and effect, but until we know more, why not aim for that range? Sleep well!

Antioxidants and Stroke

Awarded the National Medal of Science, the highest honor for scientific achievement in this country, revered biochemist Earl Stadtman was quoted as saying, "Aging is a disease. The human lifespan simply reflects the level of free radical damage that accumulates in cells. When enough damage accumulates, cells can't survive properly anymore and they just give up."[382]

First proposed in 1972,[383] this concept—now called the *mitochondrial theory of aging*—suggests that free radical damage to our cells' power source, known as *mitochondria*, leads to a loss of cellular energy and function over time. This process may be a little like charging your smartphone battery over and over—each time, its capacity gets less and less.

But what exactly are free radicals, and what can we do about them?

Here's my best attempt to simplify the quantum biology of oxidative phosphorylation: Plants get their energy from the sun. Through a process called *photosynthesis*, the chlorophyll in their leaves harnesses the sun's energy and transfers it to tiny building blocks of matter called *electrons*.

The plant starts out with low-energy electrons and, using the energy of the sun, charges them up into high-energy electrons. In this way, plants store the sun's energy. When we then eat the plant (or the animals who ate the plant), these electrons (in the form of carbohydrates, protein, and fat) are delivered to all our cells. Then our mitochondria take the plant's power-packed electrons and use them as an energy source—that is, as fuel—and slowly release their energy. Mind you, this process has to occur in a precise, tightly controlled manner, because these electrons are packed with energy and are therefore volatile, like petrol.

In fact, petrol, petroleum, oil, and charcoal aren't called fossil fuels for nothing. The tanks of our vehicles are filled with mostly prehistoric plant matter that stored the energy of the sun that shone millions of years ago as high-energy electrons.

And just as it would be dangerous to toss a match into a can of petrol and release all its energy at once, our body has to be cautious. That's why our cells take these same high-energy electrons from the plants we eat and release their energy in a controlled manner, like a gas stove—just a little at a time until the energy is used up. Our body then passes these used-up electrons to an all-important molecule you may have heard of: oxygen. In fact, the way poisons like cyanide kill us is by preventing our body from giving up these spent electrons to oxygen.[384]

Fortunately, oxygen loves electrons, although maybe a little too much. While our body is taking its sweet time, slowly releasing the electrons' energy, oxygen is waiting impatiently at the end of the line, eager to get a high-energy electron. Our body says, "Hold on. We've got to do this slowly, so wait your turn and let it cool off first. We'll give you your electron, but only after we've removed the energy so it's safe."

But the oxygen molecule may spy a stray high-energy electron and pounce on it. Our body isn't perfect; it can't keep an eye on oxygen all the time. About 1 to 2 percent[385] of all high-energy electrons that pass through our cells leak out where oxygen can grab them.

When oxygen gets its hands on a high-energy electron, it basically turns into the Hulk, changing from lowly oxygen into what's called *superoxide*, a type of free radical. A free radical is what it sounds like—a molecule that can be unstable, out of control, and violently reactive. The superoxide is just pumped up with energy and can start smashing around the cell, knocking stuff down and tripping over our DNA.

When superoxide comes in contact with DNA, it can damage our genes, which, if not repaired, can cause mutations in our chromosomes that may lead to cancer.[386] Thankfully, the body calls in its defense squad, known as *antioxidants*, that proceeds to wrestle the supercharged electron away from the superoxide, leaving oxygen and its ripped jeans behind.

In scientific circles, the phenomenon by which oxygen molecules grab stray electrons and go wild is called *oxidant*, or *oxidative*, *stress*. According to the theory, the resulting cellular damage is what essentially causes aging. Those brown age spots that may be on the back of our hands? Oxidized fat and protein under the skin. Oxidant stress is thought to be why we get wrinkles[387] and become more forgetful,[388] and why our organ systems break down as we get older. In sum, the theory goes, we're rusting.[389] (Rust is the oxidation of metal.)

One of the diseases antioxidant-rich foods may help prevent is stroke. Swedish researchers followed more than thirty thousand older women over a period of a dozen years and found that those who ate the most antioxidant-rich foods had the lowest stroke risk.[390] Similar findings were reported in a younger cohort of men and women in Italy.[391] As with lung disease,[392] antioxidant *supplements* don't appear to help.[393] Mother Nature's powers cannot be stuffed into a pill.

Knowing this, scientists set out to find the most antioxidant-rich foods. Sixteen researchers spanning the globe published a database of the antioxidant power of more than a whopping three thousand foods, beverages, herbs, spices, and supplements. They tested everything from Cheerios cereal to the crushed dried leaves of the African baobab tree. They even tested dozens of brands of beer to see which has the most antioxidants. (Santa Claus beer from Eggenberg, Austria, tied for first place.)[394] Sadly, beer represents Americans' fourth-largest source of dietary antioxidants.[395] You can check out the list online to see where your favorite foods and beverages rank: see.nf/antioxidantlist.

No need to post the 138-page chart on your fridge, though. Here's the simple rule: On average, plant foods contain *sixty-four times* more antioxidants than animal foods. As the researchers put it, "[A]ntioxidant rich foods originate from the plant kingdom while meat, fish and other foods from the animal kingdom are low in antioxidants."[396] Even the least healthy plant food I can think of, good old American iceberg lettuce (which is 96 percent water[397]), contains 17 units (daµmol using a modified FRAP assay per 100-gram serving) of antioxidant power. Some berries have more than 1,000 units, to give you some perspective. But compare iceberg lettuce's 17 units to fresh salmon, which has only 3 units. Chicken? As few as 5 units of antioxidant power. Skimmed milk or a hard-boiled egg? Just 4 units, and Egg Beaters has a big old goose egg—0 units. "Diets comprised mainly of animal-based foods are thus low in antioxidant content," concluded the research team, "while diets based mainly on a variety of plant-based foods are antioxidant rich, due to the thousands of bioactive antioxidant phytochemicals found in plants which are conserved in many foods and beverages."[398] This may help explain why those eating more plant-based diets have a significantly lower stroke risk.[399]

There is no need to cherry-pick individual foods to boost our antioxidant intake (though cherries do have up to 714 units!); we can simply strive to include a variety of fruits, vegetables, herbs, and spices at every meal. This way, we can continuously flood our body with antioxidants to potentially help ward off stroke and other age-related diseases.

Antioxidants, in a Pinch

The food category that averages the most antioxidants is herbs and spices.

Let's say you prepare a nice healthy bowl of whole-wheat pasta with marinara sauce. Together, they may achieve a score of about 80 units of antioxidant power (approximately 20 units from the pasta and 60 from the sauce). Add in a handful of steamed broccoli florets, and you may end up with a delicious 150-unit meal. Not bad. Now sprinkle on a single teaspoonful of dried oregano or marjoram, oregano's sweeter and milder twin. That alone could double your meal's antioxidant power, up to more than 300 units.[400]

How about a morning bowl of oatmeal? By adding just half a teaspoon of cinnamon, you could bring up your breakfast's antioxidant power from 20 units to 120 units. And if you want even more flavor, adding a pinch of cloves could take your unassuming meal up to an antioxidant score of 160 units.

Plant-based dishes tend to be rich in antioxidants on their own, but taking a moment to spice up your life may make your meal even healthier.

Antioxidant-rich diets appear to protect against stroke by preventing the circulation of oxidized fats in the bloodstream that can damage the sensitive walls of small blood vessels in the brain.[401] They can also help decrease artery stiffness,[402] prevent blood clots from forming,[403] and lower blood pressure[404] and inflammation. Free radicals can disfigure proteins in our bodies to the extent they become unrecognizable by our immune systems.[405] The inflammatory response this triggers can be prevented by saturating our bodies with sufficient antioxidants. Whereas all whole plant foods may have anti-inflammatory effects,[406] some plants are better than others. High-antioxidant fruits and vegetables, such as berries and greens, have been found to douse systemic inflammation significantly better than the same number of servings of more common low-antioxidant fruits and veggies, such as bananas and lettuce.[407]

The foods we choose make a difference.

ALZHEIMER'S DISEASE

In my clinical practice, the one diagnosis I dreaded giving more than cancer was Alzheimer's. It wasn't just because of the psychological toll to come for the patient but because of the emotional toll that would be placed on loved ones. The Alzheimer's Foundation estimates that eleven million friends and family members supply more than eighteen billion unpaid hours annually caring for loved ones who may not even recognize them.[408]

Despite billions of dollars spent on research, a cure or even an effective treatment for the disease, which invariably progresses to death, has remained elusive. Alzheimer's is reaching a state of crisis—emotionally, economically, and even scientifically. Over the past decade, more than a hundred thousand research articles have been published on the disease—dozens of papers a day. Yet, over the years, very little clinical progress has been made in treating or even understanding it. And a total cure has been thought likely impossible, given that lost cognitive function in Alzheimer's patients may never be regained due to fatally damaged neuronal networks. Dead nerve cells cannot be brought back to life. Even if drug companies can figure out how to halt the disease's progression, for many patients, the damage has already been done, and the individual's personality may be forever lost.[409]

The good news, as a senior scientist at the Center for Alzheimer's Research entitled a review article, is that "Alzheimer's Disease Is Incurable but Preventable."[410] Diet and lifestyle changes could potentially prevent millions of cases a year.[411] How? There is an emerging consensus that "what is good for our hearts is also good for our heads,"[412] because clogging of the arteries inside of the brain with atherosclerotic plaque is thought to play a pivotal role in the development of Alzheimer's disease.[413]

Is Alzheimer's a Vascular Disorder?

In 1901, a woman named Auguste was taken to an insane asylum in Frankfurt, Germany, by her husband. She was described as a delusional, forgetful, disoriented woman who "could not carry out her homemaking duties."[414] She was seen by a Dr. Alzheimer and was to become the subject of the case that made Alzheimer a household name.

On autopsy, Dr. Alzheimer described the plaques and tangles in her brain that would go on to characterize the disease. But lost in the excitement of discovering a new disease, a clue may have been overlooked. He wrote, *"Die größeren Hirngefäße sind arteriosklerotisch verändert,"* which translates to "The larger cerebral vessels show arteriosclerotic change." He was describing the hardening of arteries inside his patient's brain.[415]

We generally think of atherosclerosis as a condition of the heart, but it's been described as "an omnipresent pathology that involves virtually the entire human organism."[416] We have blood vessels in every one of our organs, including our brain. The concept of "cardiogenic dementia," first proposed in the 1970s, suggested that because the aging brain is highly sensitive to a lack of oxygen, lack of adequate blood flow may lead to cognitive decline.[417] Today, we have a substantial body of evidence strongly associating atherosclerotic arteries with Alzheimer's disease.[418]

Autopsies have shown repeatedly that Alzheimer's patients tend to have significantly more atherosclerotic plaque buildup and narrowing of the arteries within the brain.[419,420,421] Normal resting cerebral blood flow—the amount of blood circulating to the brain—is typically about 950 ml per minute. Starting in adulthood, people appear to naturally lose about half a percent of blood flow per year. By age sixty-five, this circulating capacity could be down by as much as 20 percent.[422] While such a drop alone may not be sufficient to impair brain function, it can put us close to the edge. The clogging of the arteries inside, and leading to, the brain with cholesterol-filled plaque can drastically reduce the amount of blood—and therefore oxygen—our brain receives. Supporting this theory, autopsies have demonstrated that Alzheimer's patients had particularly significant arterial blockage in the arteries leading to the memory centers of their brains.[423] In light of such findings, some experts have even suggested that Alzheimer's be reclassified as a vascular disorder.[424]

There are limitations to how much we can glean from autopsy studies, however. For example, perhaps a person's dementia led to their poor diet rather than vice versa. To further assess the role of clogged brain arteries in the development of Alzheimer's, researchers followed about four hundred people who were just starting to lose their mental faculties, which is called *mild cognitive impairment*. Special brain-artery scans were employed to evaluate the amount of arterial blockage in each patient's brain. The researchers found that the cognition and daily functioning of those with the least narrowing of the arteries in their heads remained stable over the course of the four-year study. Meanwhile, participants with more arterial blockage lost significant brain function, and those with the worst cases of plaque buildup declined rapidly, doubling their likelihood of progressing to full-blown Alzheimer's. The researchers concluded: "An inefficient blood supply to the brain has very grave consequences on brain function."[425]

A study of three hundred Alzheimer's patients found that treating vascular risk factors, such as high cholesterol and blood pressure, may even slow the progression of the disease but not stop it.[426] That's why prevention is the key. Cholesterol doesn't just help generate atherosclerotic plaques within our brain arteries; it may help seed the amyloid plaques that riddle the brain tissue of Alzheimer's victims.[427] Cholesterol is a vital component of our cells, which is why our body makes all that we need.[428] Consuming excess cholesterol, and especially trans and saturated fats, can raise our blood cholesterol level.[429] Too much cholesterol in our blood is not only considered the primary risk factor for heart disease[430] but is also unanimously recognized as a risk factor for Alzheimer's disease.[431] Those with a total cholesterol of 5.82 mmol/L or more may have nearly twenty-five times the odds of ending up with amyloid plaques in their brain ten to fifteen years later.[432]

Autopsies have revealed that Alzheimer's brains have significantly more cholesterol buildup than unaffected brains.[433] We used to think that the pool of cholesterol in the brain was separate from the cholesterol circulating in the blood, but there is growing evidence to the contrary.[434] Excess cholesterol in the blood can lead to excess cholesterol in the brain, which may then help trigger the clumping of amyloid seen in Alzheimer's brains. Under an electron microscope, we can see the clustering of amyloid fibers on and around tiny crystals of cholesterol.[435] And indeed, advanced brain imaging techniques, such as PET scans, have shown a direct correlation between the amount of "bad" LDL cholesterol in the blood and amyloid buildup in the brain.[436] Drug companies have hoped to capitalize on this connection to sell cholesterol-lowering statin drugs to prevent Alzheimer's, but statins themselves can cause cognitive impairment, including short- and long-term memory loss.[437] For people unwilling to change their diets, the benefits of statins may outweigh the risks,[438] as we've discussed, but it's better to lower our cholesterol levels naturally by eating more healthfully to help preserve our heart, brain, and mind.

Genetics or Diet?

This dietary concept may be surprising, because most of the popular press today treats Alzheimer's as a genetic disease, saying our genes, rather than our lifestyle choices, determine whether we'll succumb. However, when we examine the distribution of Alzheimer's disease around the world, that argument begins to crumble.

The rates of Alzheimer's vary tenfold around the world, even taking into account the fact that some populations live longer than others.[439] For example, in rural Pennsylvania, of one hundred senior citizens, it is likely that an average of nineteen of them would develop Alzheimer's disease within the next decade. However, that number would probably be closer to only three out of one hundred in rural Ballabgarh in India.[440] How do we know some populations aren't just more genetically susceptible? Because of migration studies, in which disease rates within the same ethnic group are compared between their current locale and their homeland. The Alzheimer's rates among Japanese men living in the United States, for instance, are significantly higher than those of Japanese men living in Japan.[441] The Alzheimer's rates among Africans in Nigeria were found to be four times lower than those of African Americans in Indianapolis.[442]

Why does living in the United States increase dementia risk?

The balance of evidence suggests that the answer lies in the typical American diet. Of course, in our increasingly globalized world, one doesn't need to move to the West to adopt a Western diet. In Japan, the prevalence of Alzheimer's has shot up over the past few decades, thought to be due to the shift from a traditional rice-and-vegetable-based diet to one featuring triple the dairy and six times the meat. The closest correlation researchers found between diet and dementia was consumption of animal fat; animal fat intake shot up nearly 600 percent between 1961 and 2008.[443] A similar trend linking diet and dementia was found in China.[444] With diets Westernizing globally, Alzheimer's rates are expected to continue to increase, writes one researcher in the *Journal of Alzheimer's Disease*, "unless dietary patterns change to those with less reliance on animal products. . . ."[445]

The lowest validated rates of Alzheimer's disease in the world were found in rural India,[446] where people eat traditional, plant-based diets centered on grains and vegetables.[447] In the United States, those who don't eat meat (including poultry and fish) appear to cut their risk of developing dementia by as much as half. And the longer meat is avoided, the lower dementia risk may fall. Compared to those eating meat more than four times a week, those who have eaten vegetarian diets for thirty years or more had up to three times lower risk of developing dementia.[448]

Surely genetic factors play some part? They do. Back in the 1990s, scientists discovered a gene variant called *apolipoprotein E4*, or ApoE4, which makes us more susceptible to getting Alzheimer's. Everyone has some form of ApoE, but about one in seven people has a copy of the E4 gene that is linked to the disease. It's been shown that if we inherit one ApoE4 gene from our mother or father, our risk of getting Alzheimer's may triple. If we get the ApoE4 gene from both parents—which about one in fifty people do—we might end up with nine times the risk.[449]

What does the ApoE gene do? It makes the protein that's the principal cholesterol carrier in the brain.[450] The E4 variant may lead to an abnormal accumulation of cholesterol within brain cells, which could trigger Alzheimer's pathology.[451] This mechanism may explain the so-called *Nigerian paradox*. The highest frequency of the ApoE4 variant occurs in Nigerians,[452] who surprisingly also have some of the lowest rates of Alzheimer's.[453] How could the population with the highest rate of the "Alzheimer's gene" have one of the lowest rates of Alzheimer's disease? This contradiction may be explained by Nigerians' extremely low blood-cholesterol levels, thanks to a diet low in animal fat[454] and consisting mainly of grains and vegetables.[455] So, it seems, diet can trump genetics.

Consider that in one study of a thousand people over a period of two decades, the presence of the ApoE4 gene, unsurprisingly, was found to more than double the odds of Alzheimer's. But in those same individuals, high blood cholesterol was found to nearly *triple* the odds. The researchers suspect that controlling such risk factors as high blood pressure and cholesterol could substantially reduce the risk of Alzheimer's, dropping the odds from up around ninefold with the dreaded, double-barreled ApoE4 down to just twice the risk.[456]

Too often, doctors and patients have a fatalistic approach to chronic degenerative diseases, and Alzheimer's is no exception.[457] "It's all in your genes," they say, "and what will happen will happen." Research shows that although we might have been dealt some poor genetic cards, we may be able to reshuffle the deck with diet.

Preventing Alzheimer's with Plant Foods

Alzheimer's typically manifests as a disease of the elderly, but like heart disease and most cancers, it's a disease that may take decades to develop. At the risk of sounding like a broken record (or should I say an MP3 glitch?), it's never too early to start eating healthier and it's never too late. Dietary decisions we make now may directly influence our health much later in life, including the health of our brain.

Most Alzheimer's patients aren't diagnosed until they're in their seventies,[458] but we now know that their brains began deteriorating long before that. Based on thousands of autopsies, pathologists seemed to detect the first silent stages of Alzheimer's disease—what appear to be tangles in the brain—in half of people by age fifty and even 10 percent of those in their twenties.[459] The good news is that the clinical manifestation of Alzheimer's disease—just like heart disease, lung disease, and stroke—may be preventable.

Plant-based diets are recommended in Alzheimer's prevention guidelines because of the foods they tend to accentuate and the foods they tend to reduce.[460] The Mediterranean diet, for example, which is higher in vegetables, beans, fruits, and nuts, and lower in meats and dairy products, has been associated with slower cognitive decline and lower risk of Alzheimer's.[461] When researchers tried to tease out the protective components, the critical ingredients appeared to be the diet's high vegetable content and lower ratio of saturated to unsaturated fats.[462] This conclusion aligns with that of the Harvard Women's

Health Study, which found that higher saturated fat intake (sourced predominantly from dairy, meat, and processed foods) was associated with a significantly worse trajectory of cognition and memory. Women with the highest saturated fat intake had a 60 to 70 percent greater chance of cognitive deterioration over time, while women with the lowest saturated fat intake had the brain function, on average, of women six years younger.[463]

The benefits of a plant-based diet may also be due to the plants themselves. Whole plant foods contain thousands of compounds with antioxidant properties,[464] some of which can traverse the blood-brain barrier and may provide neuroprotective effects[465] by defending against free radicals—that is, protecting against the "rusting" of the brain. Our brain is only about 2 percent of our body weight but may consume up to 50 percent of the oxygen we breathe, potentially releasing a firestorm of free radicals.[466] Special brain-accessing antioxidant pigments in berries[467] and dark green leafy vegetables[468] may make them the brain foods of the fruit and vegetable kingdom.

The first human study to show that blueberries improve memory abilities in older adults exhibiting early cognitive deterioration was published in 2010.[469] Then, in 2012, researchers at Harvard University actually quantified these findings by using data from its Nurses' Health Study, in which the diets and health of sixteen thousand women were followed starting in 1980. They found that women who consumed at least one serving of blueberries and two servings of strawberries each week had slower rates of cognitive decline—by as much as two and a half years—compared with those who didn't eat berries. These results suggest that simply eating a handful of berries every day may slow our brain's aging by more than two years.[470]

Even just drinking fruit and vegetable juices may be beneficial. A study that followed nearly two thousand people for about eight years found that people who regularly drank fruit and vegetable juices appeared to have a 76 percent lower risk of developing Alzheimer's disease. "Fruit and vegetable juices may play an important role in delaying the onset of Alzheimer's disease," the researchers concluded, "particularly among those who are at high risk for the disease."[471]

The researchers suspect the active ingredient may be a class of powerful antioxidants called *polyphenols*. If that's the case, Concord (purple) grape juice may be the best choice,[472] although whole fruits are generally preferable to juices.[473] Concord grapes aren't always available, though, so look for cranberries, which are also packed with polyphenols[474] and can typically be found frozen year-round.

Beyond their antioxidant activity, polyphenols have been shown to protect nerve cells in vitro by inhibiting the formation of the plaques[475] and tangles[476] that characterize Alzheimer's brain pathology. In theory, they could also "pull out"[477] metals that accumulate in certain brain areas and may play a role in the development of Alzheimer's and other neurodegenerative diseases.[478] Polyphenols are one of the reasons I make specific recommendations for berries and green tea in Part 2.

Treating Alzheimer's with Saffron

Despite the billions poured into Alzheimer's research, no drugs have been found to reverse the progression of the disease. There are medications that can help manage the symptoms, though, and so can something found in our local supermarket.

Although some remarkable benefits have been reported in anecdotal case studies with the spice turmeric,[479] the best data we have on spice-based interventions for Alzheimer's are for saffron. A spice derived from the flower of *Crocus sativus*, saffron was found in a double-blind trial to help diminish the symptoms of Alzheimer's disease. In a sixteen-week study, Alzheimer's patients with mild to moderate dementia who took saffron capsules displayed significantly better cognitive function on average than a group of patients who took a placebo.[480]

How about pitting saffron head-to-head against one of the most popular Alzheimer's drugs on the market: donepezil (commonly marketed under the brand name Aricept)? A twenty-two-week double-blind study (meaning that neither the researchers nor the participants knew who was on the drug and who was on the spice until the study's conclusion) found that saffron appears just as effective at treating Alzheimer's symptoms as the leading drug.[481] Unfortunately, working just as well as medication isn't saying much,[482] but at least a person doesn't have to risk the drug's side effects, most typically nausea, vomiting, and diarrhea.[483] Pass the saffron-spiced paella!

Gerontotoxins

Each of us contains tens of billions of miles of DNA—enough for one hundred thousand round trips to the moon if each strand was uncoiled and placed end to end.[484] How do our bodies keep it from getting tangled? Enzymes known as *sirtuins* keep our DNA wrapped up nice and neat around spool-like proteins.

Although they were only discovered relatively recently, sirtuins represent one of the most promising areas of medicine, as they appear to be involved in promoting healthy aging and longevity.[485] Autopsy studies show the loss of sirtuin activity is closely associated with the hallmarks of Alzheimer's disease—namely, the accumulation of plaques and tangles in the brain.[486] Suppression of this key host defense is considered a central feature of Alzheimer's.[487] The pharmaceutical industry has been trying to develop drugs to increase sirtuin activity, but why not just prevent its suppression in the first place? We may be able to do this by reducing our dietary exposure to *advanced glycation end products*, or AGEs.[488]

AGE is an appropriate acronym, as they are considered "gerontotoxins,"[489] meaning aging toxins (from the Greek *geros*, meaning "old age," as in "geriatric"). AGEs are thought to accelerate the aging process by cross-linking proteins together, causing tissue stiffness, oxidative stress, and inflammation. This process may play a role in cataract formation and macular degeneration in the eye, as well as damage to the bones, heart, kidneys, and liver.[490] They may also impact the brain, appearing to accelerate the slow shrinkage of our brain as we age[491] and suppressing our sirtuin defenses.[492]

Older adults with high levels of AGEs in their blood[493] or urine[494] appear to suffer an accelerated loss of cognitive function over time. Elevated AGE levels are also found in the brains of Alzheimer's victims.[495] Where are these AGEs coming from? Some are produced and detoxified naturally in our body,[496] but other than cigarette smoke,[497] major sources are "meat and meat-derived products" exposed to dry-heat cooking methods.[498] AGEs are formed primarily when fat- and protein-rich foods are exposed to high temperatures.[499]

More than five hundred foods have been tested for AGE content, everything from Big Macs and M & M's to coffee and ketchup. In general, meat, cheese, and highly processed foods had the highest AGE content, and grains, beans, breads, vegetables, fruits, and milk had the least.[500]

The top-twenty most AGE-contaminated products per serving tested were various brands of:

1. BBQ chicken
2. Bacon
3. Grilled hot dog
4. Roasted chicken thigh
5. Roasted chicken leg
6. Pan-fried steak
7. Oven-fried chicken breast
8. Deep-fried chicken breast
9. Stir-fried steak strips
10. McDonald's Chicken Selects breast strips
11. Pan-fried turkey burger
12. BBQ chicken
13. Oven-fried fish
14. McDonald's Chicken McNuggets
15. Grilled chicken
16. Pan-fried turkey burger
17. Baked chicken
18. Pan-fried turkey burger
19. Boiled hot dog
20. Grilled steak[501]

You get the idea.

Yes, cooking methods matter. A baked apple has three times more AGEs than a raw apple, and a grilled hot dog has more than a boiled one. But the source is what matters most: A baked apple has 45 units of AGEs compared to a raw apple's 13 units, while a grilled hot dog has 10,143 units compared to a boiled hot dog's 6,736. The researchers recommend cooking meat using moist-heat cooking methods, such as steaming or stewing, but even boiled fish has more than ten times more AGEs than a sweet potato roasted for an hour. Meat averages about twenty times more AGEs than highly processed foods like breakfast cereals and about 150 times more than fresh fruits and vegetables. Poultry was the worst, containing about 20 percent more AGEs than beef. The researchers concluded that even a modest reduction in meat intake could realistically cut daily AGE intake in half.[502]

Because sirtuin suppression is both preventable and reversible by AGE reduction, avoiding high-AGE foods is seen as potentially offering a new strategy to combat the Alzheimer's epidemic.[503]

Halting Cognitive Decline with Exercise?

There is exciting news for people on the verge of losing their mental faculties. In a study published in the *Archives of Neurology,* researchers took a group of people with mild cognitive impairment—those who are starting to forget things, for example, or regularly repeating themselves—and had them engage in aerobic exercise for forty-five to sixty minutes a day, four days a week, for six months. The control group was instructed to simply stretch for the same time periods.[504]

Memory tests were performed before and after the study. Researchers found that in the control (stretching) group, cognitive function continued to decline. But the exercising group not only didn't get worse; they got *better.* The exercisers got more test answers correct after six months, indicating their memory had improved.[505]

Subsequent studies using MRI scans found that aerobic exercise can actually reverse age-related shrinkage in the memory centers of the brain.[506] No such effect was found in the stretching and toning control groups or a nonaerobic strength-training group.[507] Aerobic exercise can help improve cerebral blood flow, improve memory performance, and help preserve brain tissue. A 2024 systematic review concluded that the best regimen to preserve global cognitive function would involve at least three sessions a week of a minimum of thirty minutes of moderate-intensity exercise combining multiple modalities, such as aerobics with strength training.[508]

Can Alzheimer's Be Reversed with a Plant-Based Diet?

Dr. Dean Ornish was the first to show, in a randomized controlled trial,[509] that a plant-based diet and lifestyle program could reverse the progression of our number one killer, heart disease.[510] Then he showed that the same plant-based program could potentially reverse the course of early-stage prostate cancer[511] and elongate our telomeres, suggesting an anti-aging effect as well.[512] But when he told me he was going to see if he could reverse the progression of Alzheimer's disease, I was skeptical. Surely he was biting off a little more than he could chew.

The centerpiece of the "Dietary and Lifestyle Guidelines for the Prevention of Alzheimer's Disease," published in the journal *Neurobiology of Aging*, was "Vegetables, legumes (beans, peas, and lentils), fruits, and whole grains should replace meats and dairy products as primary staples of the diet."[513] In other words, the dietary pillar of lifestyle medicine: whole food, plant-based nutrition.[514] That may help explain why vegetarians may be up to three times less likely to develop dementia later in life.[515] But it's not all or nothing. Even just substituting 5 percent of animal protein with plant protein appears to significantly reduce the risk of dying from dementia.[516]

But prevention isn't sexy. When prevention works, nothing happens. But the same diet and lifestyle that help *prevent* heart disease were proven to help *reverse* it. Until then, it was believed that heart disease progression could only be slowed, not stopped or reversed, which is similar to the way we view Alzheimer's disease today. So, what if people with Alzheimer's follow the same plant-based program?

Dr. Ornish and his team conducted a randomized, controlled, phase 2 clinical trial to see if the progression of Alzheimer's disease may be slowed, stopped, or perhaps even reversed. They randomized about fifty men and women diagnosed with early-stage Alzheimer's to either make no lifestyle changes for twenty weeks or eat a whole food, plant-based diet (with supplements like vitamin B12), exercise moderately (like walking half an hour a day), practice stress management (like relaxing with breathing exercises), and get group support (over Zoom).[517]

The researchers measured standard tests of cognition and function before and after in each group, as well as objective experimental biomarkers of disease progression. On the Clinical Dementia Rating global scale, which is used to stage the severity of dementia, the control group continued to get worse, but those in the diet and lifestyle group started to get better. People diagnosed with Alzheimer's getting *better*? The same seemed to happen when measured with the Alzheimer's Disease Assessment Scale, though that did not reach statistical significance. Using what's called the Clinical Dementia Rating Sum of Boxes scoring, both groups continued to decline, but the decline was significantly less in the healthy-living group. Overall, using what's called the Clinical Global Impression of Change scoring, most of the people in the control group kept getting worse and none showed any improvement, whereas about 40 percent of those in the diet and lifestyle group appeared to get better within five months of eating and living more healthfully. In the control group, 100 percent of the individuals stayed the same or got worse, whereas in the diet and lifestyle group, 70 percent stayed the same or got better. I know which group I would have rather gotten randomized to!

Why did some people get better and others not? Well, the more the study participants complied with the recommendations, the greater the beneficial impact on their cognition and function. This helps to explain why studies of less-intensive lifestyle interventions were not sufficient to stop disease progression, let alone actually *improve* cognition and function. Healthy lifestyles only work if you actually live them.

No matter how significant the results, the dry statistics don't convey the human impact. Many patients who experienced improvement reported regaining cognition and function they had lost, but how does that translate into real life? Several patients in the intervention group, for instance, reported that they had been unable to read a book or watch a movie because they kept forgetting what they had just read or watched and had to keep starting over, but, after the plant-based diet and lifestyle intervention, they were able to read and watch films again and retain most everything. One individual reported that it used to take him weeks to finish reading a book, but after participating in the study, he was able to do so in a matter of days.[518]

Another participant, a former business executive, reported regaining the ability to manage his own finances and investments. He said, "It was so much a part of my life—who I am, and who I was—it was hard saying that part of me was just gone. But now I'm back to reconciling our finances monthly; I keep up to date on our investments. A lot of self-worth comes back."

Another said that for five years she had been unable to prepare their family business's financial reports but was once again able to—and to do so accurately. "A deep sense of identity is returning. It's given me a new lease on life, and yet it's a familiarity and something I've always prided myself on. I'm coming back like I was prior to the Alzheimer's disease being diagnosed. I feel like I'm me again—an older but better version of me."

But even words are insufficient to describe such transformations. One of Dr. Ornish's study participants gave us permission to share his story on camera. You can see the emotional video at see.nf/testimonial.

The biggest limitation of the study is that, unlike drug trials in which participants can be given a disguised placebo sugar pill, when a study involves major diet and lifestyle changes, the placebo effect can't be ruled out, especially for self-reported, subjective questions like "How's your memory been?" But the researchers also measured objective investigational biomarkers of disease progression and saw the same kind of trajectory—improvements in the interventional group and worsening in the control group, with the same apparent dose-response effect, meaning the more participants improved their diet and lifestyle, the more dramatic the effect.

Compare that to some of the latest Alzheimer's drugs, which may not even work at all.[519] For instance, all we may get for $56,000[520] is a one-in-three chance of swelling or bleeding in our brain.[521] When the U.S. Food and Drug Administration approved the drug aducanumab anyway, the head of the American Geriatrics Society replied, "My head just exploded."[522]

"In contrast," wrote the head of Harvard's brain center at Massachusetts General Hospital, "the intensive lifestyle changes implemented in this study have been shown here to improve cognition and function, at a fraction of the cost—and the only side effects are positive ones."[523]

Let's face it: A life without memories is not much of a life. Whether those memories are lost all at once from a massive stroke, chipped away by ministrokes that leave little holes in the brain, or destroyed by degenerative diseases like Alzheimer's, eating and living more healthfully can help eliminate some of the worst risk factors for the most serious brain diseases.

But the key is starting early. High cholesterol and high blood pressure may begin harming our brain as early as our twenties. By our sixties and seventies, when the damage can become apparent, it may already be too late.

Like so many other organs, the brain possesses a miraculous ability to heal itself, to forge new synaptic connections around old ones, to learn and relearn. That is, however, if we don't keep damaging it three times a day. A wholesome diet and exercise may offer our best hope for remaining sharp and healthy into our twilight years.

Thankfully, I can conclude this chapter on a happier note than how it began. Despite our family history, both my mom and my brother, Gene, now eat a healthy, plant-based diet, and my mom shows no signs of succumbing to the same fate of brain disease that claimed the lives of her parents. Although Gene and I know that one day we'll eventually lose her, given her healthy diet, our hope is that we won't lose our mom before she is gone.

4

How Not to Die from Infections

I was still in medical school when I got a call to help defend Oprah Winfrey, the legendary American talk show host and icon. She was being sued by a cattle rancher under a Texas food-disparagement law. (Thirteen states have so-called food-libel laws that make it illegal to make a comment that unfairly "implies that [a] perishable food product is not safe for consumption by the public."[524])

Oprah had been talking on her television show with Howard Lyman, a former fourth-generation cattle rancher who decried the cannibalistic feeding of cow parts to other cows, a risky practice blamed for the emergence and spread of mad cow disease. Repulsed by the thought, Oprah told the viewing audience, "It has just stopped me cold from eating another burger." The next day, cattle futures tumbled, and the Texas cattleman claimed to have lost millions.

My job was to help establish that Lyman's comments were "based on reasonable and reliable scientific inquiry, facts, or data."[525] Despite the ease with which we did just that, not to mention the blatant violation of First Amendment protections inherent in the law, the Texas cattleman was able to tie up Oprah in a long and harrowing appeals process. Finally, after five years, a federal judge dismissed the case with prejudice, ending Oprah's ordeal.

In a narrow legal sense, she won. But if the meat industry is able to drag one of the country's richest and most powerful people through the courts for years and cost her a small fortune in legal fees, what kind of chilling effect does that have on others who want to speak out? Now the meat industry has started to pass so-called ag-gag laws, which make it illegal to take pictures or videos inside their operations. Presumably, they fear people might be less inclined to buy their products if they knew how these products are made.[526]

Thankfully, humanity dodged a bullet with mad cow disease. Nearly an entire generation in Britain was exposed to infected beef, but only a few hundred people died. We weren't as lucky with swine flu, which the CDC estimates killed twelve thousand Americans,[527] or COVID, thought to have come originally from bats,[528] which has killed in excess of a million Americans.[529] Nearly three-quarters of all emerging and reemerging human diseases arise from the animal kingdom.[530]

Humanity's dominion over animals has unleashed a veritable Pandora's ark of infectious diseases. Most modern human infectious diseases were unknown before domestication led to a mass spillover of animal disease into human populations.[531] For example, tuberculosis appears to have been originally acquired through the domestication of goats[532] but now infects nearly one-third of humanity.[533] Meanwhile, measles[534] and smallpox[535] may have arisen from mutant cattle viruses. We domesticated pigs and got whooping cough, we domesticated chickens and got typhoid fever, and we domesticated ducks and got influenza.[536] Leprosy may have come from water buffalo and the cold virus from horses.[537] How often did wild horses have the opportunity to sneeze into humans' faces until they were broken and bridled? Before then, the common cold was presumably common only to them.

Once pathogens jump the species barrier, they can then transmit person-to-person. HIV, a virus thought to have originated from the butchering of primates in Africa for the bush-meat trade,[538] causes AIDS by weakening the immune system. The opportunistic fungal, viral, and bacterial infections AIDS patients contract—but to which healthy people are resistant—demonstrate the importance of baseline immune function. Our immune system is not just active when we're lying in bed sick spiking a fever—it's involved in a daily life-or-death struggle to save our life from the pathogens that surround and live inside us.

With every breath we take, we inhale thousands of bacteria,[539] and with every bite we eat, we can ingest millions more.[540] Most of these tiny germs are completely harmless, but some can cause serious infectious diseases, occasionally making headlines with sinister-sounding names like SARS or Ebola. Although many of these exotic pathogens receive a lot of press coverage, more lives are lost to some of our most common infections. For example, respiratory infections such as influenza, pneumonia, and COVID kill nearly one hundred thousand Americans each year.[541,542]

Bear in mind that we don't need to come in contact with a sick person to fall ill with an infection. There are latent infections that may exist within us, waiting to strike should our immune function falter. That is why it's not enough to just wash our hands; we have to keep our immune system healthy.

In Good Hands

To protect others when we're sick, we need to practice good respiratory etiquette by coughing or sneezing into the crook of our arm (into our bent elbow). (Adorably, my friends taught their toddler this by calling out, *Dracula!*, and he would pull an imaginary cape around himself and cough so politely.) This practice limits the dispersal of respiratory droplets and also avoids contaminating our hands. The Mayo Clinic has a slogan worth remembering: "The ten worst sources of contagion are our fingers." When we cough into our hand, we can transfer contagion to everything from elevator buttons and light switches to petrol pumps and toilet handles.[543] It's no surprise that during flu season, the influenza virus can be found on more than 50 percent of common household and day-care-center surfaces.[544]

Ideally, we should sanitize our hands after every bathroom visit and handshake, before all food preparation, and before touching our eyes, nose, or mouth after coming in contact with public surfaces. The latest recommendations from the World Health Organization favor the use of alcohol-based sanitizing rubs or gels over handwashing for routine disinfection of our hands throughout the day. (Products containing between 60 and 80 percent alcohol were found to be more effective than soap in every scientific study available for review.) The only time handwashing is preferable is when they are dirty or visibly contaminated with bodily fluids. For routine decontamination—that is, for all other times—alcohol-based products are the preferred method for hand sanitation,[545] though there are pathogens like the stomach bug norovirus that are relatively resistant to disinfectants like alcohol.[546]

Still, some germs will always get past our first line of defense of practicing good hand hygiene. This is why we need to keep our immune system functioning at peak performance with a healthy diet and lifestyle.

PREVENTING INFECTIOUS DISEASES WITH A HEALTHY IMMUNE SYSTEM

The term "immune system" is derived from the Latin word *immunis*, meaning "untaxed" or "untouched," which is fitting, given that the immune system protects the body from foreign invaders. Composed of various organs, white blood cells, and proteins called antibodies that form alliances against trespassing pathogens threatening the body, the immune system, apart from the nervous system, is the most complex organ system humans possess.[547]

Our first layers of protection against intruders are physical surface barriers like our skin. Beneath that are white blood cells, such as neutrophils that attack and engulf pathogens directly, and natural killer cells that put our cells out of their misery if they become cancerous or infected with a virus. How do natural killer cells recognize pathogens and infected cells? They are often marked for destruction by antibodies, which are special proteins made by another type of white blood cell, known as B cells, that zero in like smart bombs and stick to invaders.

Each B cell makes one type of antibody that's specific for one foreign molecular signature. We don't have one B cell that covers grass pollen and another that covers bacteria; instead, we have a B cell whose only job is to make antibodies against the pollen of purple Siberian onion grass and another whose only job is to make antibodies against the tail proteins of bacteria that live in the thermal vents at the bottom of the ocean. If each of our B cells produces only one type of antibody, then we need to have a billion different types of B cells, given the incredible variety of potential pathogens on our planet. And we do.

Let's suppose one day you're walking along and suddenly get attacked by a platypus. (They have poisonous spurs on their heels, in case you didn't know.) For your whole life up until that point, the B cell in your body that produces antibodies against duck-billed platypus venom was just waiting for that very moment. Just as the venom is detected, this specific B cell begins dividing madly, and soon you have a whole swarm of clones, each producing millions of antibodies against platypus poison. You fend off the toxin and go on to live platypus venom–free. That is how the immune system works. Aren't our bodies spectacular?

As we get older, though, our immune function declines. Is this just an inevitable consequence of aging? Or could it be because dietary quality also tends to go down in older populations? To test the theory that inadequate nutrition could help explain the loss in immune function as we age, researchers split eighty-three volunteers between the ages of sixty-five and eighty-five into two groups. The control group ate fewer than three daily servings of fruits and vegetables, while the experimental group consumed at least five servings a day. They were all then vaccinated against pneumonia, a practice recommended for all adults over the age of fifty.[548] The goal of vaccination is to prime our immune system to produce antibodies against a specific pneumonia pathogen should we ever become exposed. Compared with the control group, people eating five or more daily servings of fruits and vegetables had an 82 percent greater protective antibody response to the vaccine—and this was after only a few months of eating just a few extra servings of fruits and vegetables a day.[549] That is how much control the fork may exert over immune function.

Certain fruits and vegetables may give our immune system an extra boost.

Kale?

As a dark green leafy vegetable, kale is not only one of the most nutrient-dense foods on the planet, but it may also help fight off infection. Japanese researchers tried dripping a tiny quantity of kale onto human white blood cells in a petri dish, about one-millionth of a gram of kale protein. Even that minuscule quantity triggered a quintupling of antibody production in the cells.[550]

The researchers used raw kale, but the scant amounts of kale Americans consume are often cooked. Does cooking kale destroy its immune-boosting effects? It turned out that even boiling the greens nonstop for thirty minutes did not affect antibody production. In fact, the cooked kale appeared to work even better.[551]

However, this property was discovered in a test-tube study. Even kale aficionados don't mainline it like heroin, which is presumably the only way intact kale proteins would ever come in direct contact with our blood cells. Although there have been clinical studies (that is, studies on real people) showing that kale can reduce DNA damage, inflammation,[552] body weight,[553] and postoperative pain,[554] as well as improve constipation,[555] insulin resistance, and blood sugar control,[556,557] no such studies on immune function have been performed to date. (Maybe by the twentieth-anniversary edition! The original *How Not to Die* reported no clinical kale studies at all.) Big Kale, it seems, has yet to muster the research dollars. Currently, we have stronger evidence for the immune benefits of kale's less trendy cousin, broccoli.

Broccoli

As I've mentioned, one of the body's greatest exposures to the outside world is through the lining of our intestines, which may cover hundreds of square feet.[558] But the lining is extremely thin—just fifty-millionths of a meter. In other words, the barrier separating our bloodstream from the world is many times thinner than a single sheet of tissue paper. This is because our body needs to absorb nutrients from food: If our gut lining were any thicker, nutrients would have trouble passing through. It's a good idea for our skin to be waterproof so we don't start leaking, but the lining of the gut has to allow for the absorption of both fluids and nutrition. With such a fragile layer between our sterile core and the chaos outside, we need to have a good defense mechanism in place to keep out the bad.

This is where the immune system comes in, specifically a special type of white blood cell called *intraepithelial lymphocytes*. These cells serve two functions: They condition and repair the thin intestinal lining, and they also serve as its first line of gut defense against pathogens.[559] These lymphocytes are packed with "Ah receptors" that activate the cells.[560] For years, scientists couldn't find the key that fit into the Ah receptor lock. If we could figure out how to activate these cells, we might be able to boost our immunity.[561]

It turns out that key is contained in broccoli and other veggies in its cruciferous family, such as kale, cauliflower, cabbage, and brussels sprouts. This family of vegetables contains compounds necessary for the maintenance of the body's intestinal defenses. In short, broccoli and other crucifers are able to rally our immune-system foot soldiers.[562]

Why did our immune systems evolve to depend on certain vegetables? Well, when do we need to boost our intestinal defenses? When we eat. The body uses up a lot of energy to maintain its immune system, so why remain on high alert 24-7 when we only eat a few times a day? Why would our bodies specifically use vegetables as the bat signal to assemble the troops? We evolved over millions of years eating mostly weeds—wild plants, including dark green leafy vegetables (or, as they were known back then, *leaves*)—so our bodies may have evolved to equate vegetables with mealtime. The presence of veggies in our gut works as a signal to upkeep our immune systems.[563] So if we don't eat plants with each meal, we may be undermining our bodies' strategy to protect us.

Interestingly, the immune boost provided by cruciferous vegetables like broccoli not only protects us against the pathogens found in food but also against pollutants in the environment. These days, we're constantly exposed to a wide range of toxic substances—cigarette smoke, car exhaust, furnaces, cooked meat, fish, and dairy, and even mother's milk[564] (as a consequence of what the mother was exposed to). Because some of these pollutants, such as dioxins, exert their toxic effects through the Ah receptor system, cruciferous compounds may block them.[565]

Other plants may also defend against toxic invaders. Researchers in Japan found that phytonutrients in such plant foods as fruits, vegetables, tea leaves, and beans can block the effects of dioxins in vitro. For instance, researchers found that having phytonutrient levels in the bloodstream equivalent to eating three apples or a tablespoon of red onion daily appeared to cut dioxin toxicity in half. The only catch was that these phytonutrient effects lasted only a few hours, meaning we may have to keep eating healthy foods, meal after meal, if we want to maintain our defenses against pathogens as well as pollutants.[566]

The ability to block toxins isn't limited to plant foods, however. There is one animal product that has also been shown to potentially block the cancer-causing effects of dioxins—camel urine.[567] So next time your kids don't want to eat their fruits and veggies, you can just say, "It's either the broccoli or camel pee. Your choice."

Pretty in Pee-nk

Ever noticed that your urine turns a bit pink after you eat beetroot? Though the color looks a little unnatural, it's a completely harmless and temporary condition called *beeturia*.[568] It's a vivid reminder of an important fact: When we eat plant foods, many of the pigment phytonutrients that act as antioxidants in our body (such as lycopene and beta-carotene) are absorbed into the bloodstream and bathe our organs, tissues, and cells.

In other words, beetroot pigments find their way into our urine because they are absorbed through the gut and then travel into the bloodstream, where they circulate throughout the body until eventually being filtered out by the kidneys. During this trip through the body, even our blood becomes a bit pinker too.

The same principle causes garlic breath. It isn't just the residue in our mouth that's scaring everyone off; it's also the health-promoting compounds that were absorbed into our bloodstream after we swallowed the garlic, which are then exhaled pungently from our lungs in our breath. Even if garlic was taken as an enema, we'd *still* get garlic breath. For this reason, garlic can potentially be used as an adjunct treatment for critical cases of pneumonia, as it may help clear bacteria on its way out of the lungs.[569]

Boosting Natural Killer Cell Activity with Berries

For disease prevention, berries of all colors have "emerged as champions," according to the head of the Bioactive Botanical Research Laboratory.[570] The purported anticancer properties of berry compounds have been attributed to their apparent ability to counteract, reduce, and repair damage resulting from oxidative stress and inflammation.[571] But we now know that berries may also boost our levels of natural killer cells.

They may sound sinister, but natural killer cells are a type of white blood cell that's a vital member of the immune system's rapid-response team against virus-infected and cancerous cells. They're called natural killers because they don't require prior exposure to a disease to be activated, unlike some other parts of the immune system that can only respond effectively after a history of exposure, as in the case of, say, chicken pox.[572] After all, we don't want to wait until our *second* tumor appears before our immune system starts fighting back.

There are about two billion of these elite special-ops fighters patrolling the bloodstream at any one time, but research suggests that we can bolster their ranks by eating blueberries. In one study, researchers asked athletes to eat 250 grams of blueberries every day for six weeks to see if the berries could reduce the oxidative stress caused by long-distance running.[573] The blueberries succeeded, unsurprisingly, but a more important finding was their effect on natural killer cells. Normally, these cells decrease in number after a bout of prolonged endurance exercise, dropping by half to about one billion. But the athletes consuming blueberries actually *doubled* their killer cell counts, to more than four billion.

Blueberries can boost the number of natural killer cells, but are there any foods that can boost killer cell *activity*—that is, how effectively they fight cancer cells? Yes, it seems the aromatic spice cardamom may be one. Researchers put some lymphoma cells in a petri dish and added natural killer cells, which were able to wipe out about 5 percent of the cancer cells. But after researchers effectively sprinkled on some cardamom, the natural killer cells became supercharged and eradicated even more cancer cells—up to about ten times more than without cardamom.[574] No clinical trials have yet been done to try this out in cancer patients.

In theory, though, cardamom-infused blueberry muffins may increase the number of circulating natural killer cells in the body, as well as boost their cancer-killing instincts.

Forest Breathing

Exposure to nature can offer a variety of self-reported psychological benefits—a "natural high"—but there's been a dearth of data on changes in objective measurements.[575] That's why I was excited to see a paper on the effects of forest bathing—surrounding yourself with trees—on cortisol in the saliva, which is considered an indicator of our level of stress.[576] People's salivary cortisol levels were significantly lower while they walked in a forest or even after just hanging out in the woods compared to a city. But it turns out that those who had been told they were heading to the forest developed lower cortisol levels before they even left. Just the *thought* of spending the day in the forest relieved stress, so it wasn't really an effect of the forest per se. I was ready to dismiss it as just another nebulous psychological effect until I ran across literature on the effects of forest bathing on boosting the number and activity of natural killer cells. That got my attention.

Those randomized to visit a forest experienced a significant elevation in natural killer cell activity compared to the individuals randomized to visit a city instead.[577] Both trips were matched for physical activity, alcohol, and sleep—other factors that can affect immune function. Moreover, researchers found that the increased natural killer cell activity lasted for up to thirty days after the trip, suggesting a monthly trip to the woods may be able to maintain the enhanced immunity. The question is *why?*

The immune benefits of forest bathing could be from the reduction of stress,[578] but diminished stress hormone levels start to normalize within days, whereas the protective effect appeared to last for weeks.[579] Could it have something to do with our "old friends"? If we spend most of our time indoors, we may be missing the abundance of microorganisms floating around in the air outdoors. When outdoor air was sampled, microbes were picked up from the soil and water that are rare or absent in our indoor air, which is dominated by organisms that either live on us or try to attack us. So, to keep our immune system on ready alert, on a day-to-day basis, it might not be sufficient to encounter only the biased microbes of the modern, synthetic, indoor environment that likely bear little resemblance to the microbes we evolved to live with over millions of years.[580]

Or, maybe it's the trees themselves.

Trees produce aromatic volatile compounds called *phytoncides*,[581] like pinene, which we breathe into our lungs in the forest.[582] Do they actually get into our bloodstream? Spending just one hour in the woods gives us about a sixfold increase in pinene levels circulating throughout our system.[583] But, to fully connect all the dots, these tree essential oils would have to induce natural killer cell activity in humans. And indeed they do. When natural killer cells are in a petri dish with some unsuspecting leukemia cells, they can only wipe out some of the cancer cells; add a whiff of cypress, white cedar, eucalyptus, or pine, though, and the cancer cells don't stand a chance.[584]

A combination of wood aromas improved the recovery of mice from stress-induced immune suppression,[585] but is it really just the fragrance of the forest? Researchers investigated whether that same boost in natural killer cell activity could be achieved by just vaporizing some essential oil from one of the trees into a hotel room overnight—and it worked! There was a significant boost in natural killer cell activity, though just their activity was increased, rather than their numbers,[586] whereas being in an actual forest may do both. So, perhaps it's a combination of the tree fragrance and the lower cortisol levels working together.[587]

Ironically, these phytoncide compounds are part of the tree's *own* immune system, which we may be able to commandeer.[588] Researchers speculate these compounds may be playing some role in the fact that more heavily forested regions in Japan appeared to have lower death rates from breast cancer and prostate cancer.[589] Being out in nature has been found

> to be an important coping strategy among cancer patients.[590] It turns out this could potentially help more than just with the coping, thanks to the fragrance of trees.

Preventing the Common Cold with Probiotics?

Babies delivered via cesarean section appear to be at increased risk for various allergic diseases, including allergic runny nose, asthma, eczema, and even food allergies.[591] (Allergy symptoms are caused when our immune system overreacts to normally harmless stimuli, such as tree pollen.) Typical vaginal delivery leads to the colonization of the baby's gut with the mother's vaginal bacteria. Babies delivered via C-section, on the other hand, are deprived of this natural exposure. The resulting difference in gut flora may affect the way the baby's immune system develops, accounting for the difference in allergy rates. This explanation is supported by research showing that a disturbance in a mother's vaginal flora during pregnancy due to sexually transmitted infections or douching, for example, may result in higher asthma risk for the infant.[592]

These findings raise a broader question about the effects the good bacteria in our gut may have on our immune system. Some studies have shown that supplementing with good bacteria (probiotics) might have immunity-enhancing effects. The first such study demonstrated that white blood cells extracted from individuals on a probiotic regimen for a few weeks showed a significantly enhanced ability to engulf and destroy potential invaders. This effect lasted for at least three weeks after the probiotics were discontinued. Natural killer cell activity against cancer cells in vitro was improved as well.[593]

Improving cell function in a petri dish is nice, but do these results translate into fewer infections? It took another ten years before a randomized, double-blind, placebo-controlled study was performed. (Considered the gold standard of research, a randomized, double-blind, placebo-controlled study is a trial in which neither the participants nor the researchers know who is receiving an experimental treatment and who is receiving a placebo until the end of the study.) The study showed that people who take probiotic supplements may indeed have significantly fewer colds, fewer sick days, and fewer overall symptoms.[594] The evidence to date suggests probiotics may reduce the risk of upper-respiratory-tract infections but is insufficient for recommending that people start popping probiotic pills.[595]

It may be best to focus on feeding the good bacteria already living in our gut.[596] What do our friendly flora eat? Fiber and a certain type of starch concentrated in beans. These substances are called *prebiotics*. Probiotics are the good bacteria themselves, whereas *prebiotics* are what our good bacteria eat. So, the best way to keep our good bacteria happy and well fed is to eat lots of whole plant foods.

When we eat fresh produce, we can get *both* pre- and probiotics into our gut. Fruits and veggies are covered with millions of lactic acid bacteria, some of which are the same types used in probiotic supplements. When we make sauerkraut, for example, we don't need to add a starter culture because the bacteria are already naturally present on cabbage leaves. Including raw fruits and vegetables in our daily diet may therefore offer the best of both worlds.[597]

Plant-Based Pandemic Protection

The COVID-19 pandemic offered a good opportunity to see if eating more healthfully could help stave off infection. A study of frontline health care workers across six countries found that those eating plant-based diets had 73 percent lower odds of suffering a moderate or severe course of COVID-19. Pescatarians, those who eat fish but no other meat, enjoyed an intermediate level of protection. The biggest spread was between those eating plant-based and those eating low-carb. Compared to health care workers eating vegetarian or whole food, plant-based diets, those on low-carb, high-protein diets had nearly four times greater odds of suffering a serious infection.[598]

This may not seem surprising, given that many of the underlying risk factors for COVID-19 severity and death—obesity, heart disease, hypertension, and type 2 diabetes[599]—can be controlled or even reversed with a healthy enough plant-based diet and lifestyle.[600] But the apparent plant-based protection went above and beyond. The greatly reduced risk was independent of all those conditions. The researchers also controlled for smoking status, physical activity, weight, and lung disease. They concluded: "Our results suggest that a healthy diet rich in nutrient-dense foods may be considered for protection against severe COVID-19."[601] The one food group most associated with lower symptom severity in a study of outpatients in Mexico was legumes, followed by grains, the top sources of dietary fiber. The investigators suggest that the anti-inflammatory effects of the short-chain fatty acids released by our good fiber-feeding gut bugs may be playing a role.[602]

The health care worker study only enrolled a couple thousand people, though. Harvard researchers collected data from nearly 600,000 participants using a plant-based-diet scoring system. They found that those who ate the most healthful plant foods and the least meat, eggs, dairy, and junk not only had a significantly lower risk of suffering a severe course of COVID-19, but they also had a significantly lower risk of getting infected in the first place. Again, this was after taking comorbidities into account, alongside other nondietary lifestyle risk factors, such as exercise, smoking, and socioeconomic status.[603] In terms of dealing with the aftermath, "large-scale promotion of plant-based eating" has been suggested as a way to manage the physical and mental impacts of "long COVID" syndrome, but this has yet to be tested.[604]

Boosting the Immune System with Exercise

What if there were a drug or supplement that could halve the number of sick days we take due to such upper-respiratory infections as the common cold? It would make some pharmaceutical company billions of dollars. But there is already something that can boost our immune system for free and by so much that we can achieve a 25 to 50 percent reduction in sick days. And it has only good side effects. What is it?

Exercise.[605]

What's more, it doesn't take much of a workout to get results. Studies find that if kids run around for just six minutes, the levels of immune cells circulating in their blood increases by nearly 50 percent.[606] At the other end of the life cycle, regular exercise can also help prevent age-related immune decline. One study found that while older sedentary women have a 50 percent chance of getting an upper-respiratory illness during the autumn season, those randomized to begin a half-hour-a-day walking program dropped their risk down to 20 percent. Among conditioned runners, though, the risk was just 8 percent.[607] Exercising appeared to make their immune systems more than five times better at fighting infection.

What's going on here? How does the simple act of moving our body decrease the chance of contracting an infection? Approximately 95 percent of all infections start in the mucosal (moist) surfaces, including the eyes, nostrils, and mouth.[608] These surfaces are protected by antibodies called *IgA* (short for *immunoglobulin, type A*), which provide an immunological barrier by neutralizing and preventing viruses from penetrating into the body. The IgA in saliva, for instance, is considered the first line of defense against such respiratory-tract infections as pneumonia and influenza.[609] Moderate exercise may be all it takes to boost IgA levels and significantly reduce the chance of coming down with flu-like symptoms. Compared to a sedentary control group, those who performed aerobic exercises for thirty minutes three times a week for twelve weeks had a 50 percent increase in the levels of IgA in their saliva and reported significantly fewer respiratory infection symptoms.[610]

While regular physical activity improves immune function and lowers respiratory infection risk, sustained and intense exertion may have the opposite effect. As we go from inactive to active, infection risk declines, but at a certain point, overtraining and excessive stress can *increase* the risk of infection by impairing immune function.[617] In the weeks following marathons or ultramarathons, runners report a two- to sixfold increase in upper-respiratory-tract infections.[618] Within a day of starting an international competition, elite soccer players were found to suffer a significant drop in their IgA production.[619] This drop has been tied to upper-respiratory-tract infections during training. Other studies have found that IgA levels can drop after even just single bouts of overstrenuous exercise.[620]

What can we do, then, if we're hardcore athletes? How can we reduce our chance of infection? Traditional sports medicine recommendations don't appear to have much to offer: They'll tell us to get a flu shot, avoid touching our eyes or picking our nose, and stay away from sick people.[621] Gee, thanks. The reason these steps may be insufficient is that respiratory infections are often triggered by reactivations of latent viruses already inside the body, such as Epstein-Barr virus, the cause of mononucleosis. So even if we never came in contact with anyone else, as soon as our immune function dips, these dormant viruses can reawaken and make us sick.

Thankfully, a number of foods may help maintain our immunity to keep the germs at bay.

One option for athletes who want to sustain their immune function is nutritional yeast. A 2013 study reported that we may more effectively maintain our levels of white blood cells after exercise by consuming a special type of fiber, called *beta-glucan*, found in baker's, brewer's, and nutritional yeasts.[622] Brewer's yeast is bitter, but nutritional yeast has a pleasant cheese-like flavor. (It tastes particularly good on popcorn.)

The study found that after two hours of intense cycling, the number of monocytes (another type of immune system white blood cell) in participants' bloodstreams took a dip. But those who were given the equivalent of about three-quarters of a teaspoon of nutritional yeast before they exercised ended up with even higher levels of monocytes than when they started working out.[623]

That's all well and good on a lab report, but does consuming yeast fiber actually translate to fewer illnesses? Researchers put that question to the test at the Carlsbad Marathon in California.

Runners who were given the daily equivalent of about a spoonful of nutritional yeast in the four weeks after the race appeared to have just half the rates of upper-respiratory infection compared to runners consuming a placebo. Remarkably, the runners on yeast reported feeling better too. When asked how they felt on a scale of one to ten, with ten being the best, the people taking the placebo reported about a four or five. On the other hand, the participants on the nutritional yeast consistently reported feeling better, around a six or seven. Elite athletes normally experience mood deterioration before and after a marathon, but this study revealed that a little nutritional yeast may improve a wide range of emotional states, reducing feelings of tenseness, fatigue, confusion, and anger, while at the same time increasing perceived "vigor."[624] Pass the popcorn!

Boosting Immunity with Mushrooms

Do you suffer from seasonal allergies? Runny nose, itchy eyes, sneezing? While our allergies may make us feel lousy because our immune system is busy attacking things left and right, that same heightened state of alertness may have benefits for our overall health.

Individuals suffering from allergies appear to have a decreased risk for certain cancers.[625] Yes, our immune system might be in overdrive striking out at harmless things like pollen or dust, but that same overvigilance may also take down budding tumors in the body. It would be nice if there were a way to boost the part of the immune system that fights infections while down-regulating the part that results in chronic inflammation (and all those annoying symptoms).

Mushrooms may just do the trick.

Thousands of edible mushrooms grow naturally, with worldwide annual commercial production in the millions of tons.[626] But check the nutrition label on a carton of mushrooms and not much is listed beyond some B vitamins and minerals. Is that all mushrooms have? No. What we don't see listed is the array of unique myconutrients that may boost our immune function.[627]

Researchers in Australia split people into two groups. One group ate its regular diet, while the other ate its regular diet plus 100 grams of cooked white button mushrooms every day. After just a week, the mushroom eaters showed a 50 percent boost in the IgA levels in their saliva. These antibody levels remained elevated for about a week before dropping.[628] So, for sustained benefits, we should try to make mushrooms a steady part of our diet.

But wait. If mushrooms trigger such a dramatic rise in antibody production, shouldn't we be concerned they may worsen the symptoms of allergic or autoimmune diseases? On the contrary, it seems mushrooms may have an *anti*-inflammatory effect. In vitro studies have shown that a variety of mushrooms, including plain white button mushrooms, appear to blunt the inflammatory response, potentially offering a boost in immune and anticancer function without aggravating diseases of inflammation.[629] The first randomized, double-blind, placebo-controlled clinical study of its kind, published in 2014, confirmed an apparent anti-allergy effect in children with a history of recurrent upper-respiratory-tract infections.[630]

Note that it is best not to eat white, cremini, and portobello mushrooms raw.[631] (They are all the same mushroom, just at different stages of maturity.[632]) Oyster mushrooms can be eaten raw, but shiitake[633] and morel[634] mushrooms should also be fully cooked.

Food Poisoning

Pathogens (from the Greek *pathos*, for "suffering," and *genes*, meaning "producer of") can also be found in what we eat. Foodborne illness, or food poisoning, is an infection caused by eating contaminated food. According to the CDC, about one in seven Americans develops food poisoning every year. Roughly forty-eight million people are sickened annually—more than the combined populations of California and Massachusetts. More than one hundred thousand of them are hospitalized, and thousands die, just because of something they ate.[635]

In terms of healthy years of life lost, the top five most devastating pathogen-food combinations are *Campylobacter* and *Salmonella* bacteria in poultry, *Toxoplasma* parasites in pork, and *Listeria* bacteria in deli meats and dairy products.[636] One of the reasons animal foods are the leading culprits is that most foodborne pathogens are fecal pathogens. Because plants don't poop, the *E. coli* we may get from spinach didn't actually originate in the spinach; *E. coli* is an intestinal pathogen, and spinach doesn't have intestines. The application of manure to crops has been found to increase the odds of *E. coli* contamination by more than fiftyfold.[637]

Eggs and *Salmonella*

The single greatest public health burden in the United States in terms of food poisoning is *Salmonella*. It's the leading cause of food poisoning–related hospitalizations, as well as the number one cause of food poisoning–related deaths.[638] Within twelve to seventy-two hours after infection, the most common symptoms appear—fever, diarrhea, and severe abdominal cramps.[639] The illness typically lasts between four and seven days, but among children and the elderly, the disease can be severe enough to require hospitalization—or funeral arrangements.

Many people associate *Salmonella* with eggs—and for good reason. However, the egg industry mantra is "completely cooked eggs are completely safe eggs."[640] But what exactly does "completely cooked" mean?

The egg industry itself funded research on *Salmonella* and the various ways to cook eggs. What did it find? *Salmonella* in eggs can survive scrambled, over-easy, and sunny-side-up cooking methods. Sunny-side up was found to be the riskiest. The industry-funded researchers bluntly concluded: "The sunny-side-up method should be considered unsafe."[641] In other words, even the egg industry itself knows that its product, prepared in a manner that millions of Americans eat on any given day across the country, is *unsafe*. Actually, we've known this for some time. Thirty years ago, Purdue University researchers determined that *Salmonella* can survive in cooked omelets and French toast.[642] *Salmonella* may even survive in eggs boiled up to eight minutes.[643]

Given all of this, it should come as no surprise that, according to the U.S. Food and Drug Administration, an estimated 133,000 Americans are sickened each year by *Salmonella*-tainted eggs.[644] That's an egg-borne epidemic each year in the United States. But eggs are "only" number ten on the worst pathogen-food combination list.

Poultry and *Salmonella*

Eating chickens, not their eggs, is the most common source of *Salmonella* poisoning.[645] When a car manufacturer's brakes malfunction, it announces a recall due to safety concerns. Why isn't *Salmonella*-tainted chicken recalled? The U.S. Department of Agriculture once tried to shut down a company found to be repeatedly violating *Salmonella* standards. The company sued and won. "Because normal cooking practices for meat and poultry destroy the *Salmonella* organism," the judges in the case concluded, "the presence of *Salmonella* in meat products does not render them 'injurious to health.'"[646]

If proper cooking kills the bug, then why do hundreds of thousands of Americans continue to be sickened by *Salmonella*-contaminated poultry every year? It's not like *E. coli* and medium-rare hamburgers. Who undercooks chicken? The problem here is cross-contamination. Between the time the fresh or frozen bird is picked up from the store and when it's slid into the oven, the germs on the chicken can contaminate hands, utensils, and kitchen surfaces. Studies have shown that up to 80 percent of the time, placing fresh chicken on a cutting board for a few minutes can transfer disease-causing bacteria.[647] Then, if cooked chicken is put back on the same cutting board, there's about a 30 percent chance that the meat will become recontaminated.[648]

"It is not unusual for raw poultry from any producer to have *Salmonella* bacteria," one of the nation's largest poultry producers wrote in a press release after its chicken sickened an estimated ten thousand people. "Consumers must use proper preparation, handling and cooking practices."[649] In other words, it should be considered normal for chicken to be contaminated with *Salmonella*. Eat at your own risk.

Why are American consumers placed at such peril? Some European countries have gotten *Salmonella* contamination in poultry down as low as 2 percent. How? Because there, it's illegal to sell chicken tainted with *Salmonella*. What a concept! They don't allow the sale of fowl fouled with a pathogen that sickens more than a million Americans a year.[650] In a meat industry trade publication, an Alabama poultry science professor explained why we don't have such a "heavy-handed" policy: "The American consumer is not going to pay that much. It's as simple as that." If the industry had to pay to make it safer, the price would go up. "The fact," he said, "is that it's too expensive not to sell salmonella-positive chicken."[651]

Fecal Bacteria on Meat

Consumer Reports published a study on the true cost of cheap chicken. It discovered that 97 percent of chicken breasts found in retail stores were contaminated with bacteria that could make people sick.[652] Thirty-eight percent of the *Salmonella* found was resistant to multiple antibiotics. The CDC has been raising the alarm as antibiotic-resistant strains continue to spread, and it considers *Salmonella* to be one of the foodborne pathogens that is a "serious threat" to public health.[653]

As the Mayo Clinic rather indelicately put it, "Most people are infected with *Salmonella* by eating foods that have been contaminated by feces."[654] How does it get there? In slaughter plants, birds are typically gutted by a metal hook, which too often punctures their intestines and can expel feces onto the flesh itself. According to the latest national FDA retail-meat survey, about 90 percent of retail chicken showed evidence of contamination with fecal matter.[655]

Using the presence of bugs like *E. faecalis* and *E. faecium* as markers of fecal contamination, 85 percent of ground beef and turkey, about half of chicken, and one-third of pork are tainted on the retail level nationally.[656]

While outbreaks of *Salmonella* infection have increased, *E. coli* infection from fecal matter in beef has decreased.[657] Why is beef getting safer but chicken getting riskier?[658] One likely factor is that the government was able to enact a ban on the sale of beef contaminated with a particularly dangerous strain of *E. coli*. But why is it illegal to sell beef known to be contaminated with a potentially deadly pathogen but perfectly legal to sell contaminated chicken? After all, *Salmonella* in chicken kills far more people than *E. coli* in beef.[659]

The problem dates back to a famous case in 1974 when the American Public Health Association sued the U.S. Department of Agriculture for putting its stamp of approval on meat contaminated with *Salmonella*. Defending the meat industry, the USDA pointed out that because "there are numerous sources of contamination which might contribute to the overall problem," it would be "unjustified to single out the meat industry and ask that the [USDA] require it to identify its raw products as being hazardous to health."[660] In other words, because *Salmonella* has also been linked to dairy and eggs, it wouldn't be fair to force only the meat industry to make its products safer. That's like the tuna industry arguing there's no need to label cans of tuna with mercury warnings because we could also get exposed by eating a thermometer.

The Washington, D.C., Circuit Court of Appeals upheld the meat industry's position, asserting that the USDA can allow potentially deadly *Salmonella* in meat because "American housewives and cooks normally are not ignorant or stupid and their methods of preparing and cooking of food do not ordinarily result in salmonellosis."[661] That's like saying minivans don't need airbags or seat belts, and kids don't need car seats, because soccer moms don't *ordinarily* crash into things.

Avoiding Chicken to Avoid Urinary Tract Infections

Where do bladder infections come from? Back in the 1970s, studies of women over time found that movement of bacteria from the rectum into the vaginal area preceded the appearance of bladder infections.[662] It took another twenty-five years, though, before DNA fingerprinting techniques proved that *E. coli* strains residing in the gut serve as the reservoir for urinary tract infections (UTIs).[663]

Another fifteen years passed before scientists tracked down the ultimate culprit, the original source of some of the UTI-associated bacteria in the rectum: chicken. McGill University researchers were able to capture UTIcausing *E. coli* at slaughter plants, tracing them to the meat supply and, eventually, to urinary specimens obtained from infected women.[664] As a result, we now have direct proof that bladder infections can be a zoonosis—an animal-to-human disease.[665] This is a critical discovery, since UTIs affect more than ten million women each year in the United States at the cost of more than $1 billion.[666] Even worse, it turns out that many of the strains of *E. coli* in chicken that cause UTIs are now resistant to some of our most powerful antibiotics.[667]

Can't we solve this crisis by simply distributing meat thermometers and making sure people cook chicken thoroughly? No—because of the cross-contamination issue. Studies have shown that handling raw chicken can lead to intestinal colonization even if we don't eat any of it.[668] In that case, it doesn't matter how well we cook chicken. We could incinerate it to ash and still walk away infected. After infection, the drug-resistant chicken bacteria were then found to multiply to the point of becoming a major part of the research subject's gut flora.[669]

The reason most people have more fecal bacteria in their kitchen sinks than their toilet seats[670] is likely because they prepare their chickens in the kitchen, not the bathroom. But what if we're really careful? A landmark study, published as "The Effectiveness of Hygiene Procedures for Prevention of Cross-Contamination from Chicken Carcasses in the Domestic Kitchen," put this question to the test. Researchers visited five dozen homes, gave each family a raw chicken, and asked them to cook it. After the bird was cooked, researchers returned to find bacteria from chicken feces—*Salmonella* and *Campylobacter*, both serious human pathogens—all over the families' kitchens: on the cutting board, utensils, cupboard, the refrigerator handle, the oven handle, the doorknob, and so on.[671]

Did those families just not know what they were doing? The researchers repeated the experiment but the second time gave the families specific instructions. After cooking the chicken, the participants were told to wash surfaces with hot water and detergent, specifically the cutting board, utensils, cupboard, handles, and knobs. Yet the researchers *still* found pathogenic fecal bacteria all over.[672]

Reading the study, it's clear the researchers were getting a bit exasperated. Finally, they insisted the participants use bleach. The dishcloth to be used for cleaning was first to be immersed in bleach disinfectant; then the subjects were to spray a bleach solution on all surfaces and let it sit for five minutes. However, the researchers returned to still find *Salmonella* and *Campylobacter* on some utensils, the dishcloth, the counter around the sink, and the cupboards.[673] The extent of the kitchen contamination was much less, but it appears that unless we treat our kitchen like a biohazard laboratory, the only way to guarantee we're not going to leave fecal pathogens around the kitchen is to not bring them into our house in the first place.

There is some good news: It's not as if we eat chicken once and our gut is colonized for life. In the study in which volunteers became infected after just handling the meat, the chicken bacteria that tried to take over their gut only seemed to survive about ten days.[674] The good bacteria in their guts seemed able to muscle the bad guys out of the way. The problem, unfortunately, is that people tend to eat chicken more than once every ten days, so they may be constantly reintroducing these chicken bugs into their systems.

Yersinia in Pork

Nearly one hundred thousand Americans are sickened each year by *Yersinia* bacteria.[675] In every outbreak for which a source has been found, the culprit was contaminated pork.[676]

In most cases, *Yersinia* food poisoning leads to little more than acute gastroenteritis, but the symptoms can become severe and mirror appendicitis, resulting in unnecessary emergency surgeries.[677] Long-term consequences of *Yersinia* infection include chronic inflammation of the eyes, kidneys, heart, and joints.[678] Studies have found that within a year of contracting *Yersinia* food poisoning, victims appear forty-seven times more likely to come down with autoimmune arthritis,[679] and the bacteria may also play a role in triggering an autoimmune thyroid condition known as Graves' disease.[680]

How contaminated are U.S. pork products? *Consumer Reports* magazine tested nearly two hundred samples from cities across the country and found that more than two-thirds of the pork was contaminated with *Yersinia*.[681] This may be because of the intensification and overcrowding that characterizes most of today's industrial pig operations.[682] As noted in an article in *National Hog Farmer* entitled "Crowding Pigs Pays," pork producers can maximize their profits by confining each pig to a six-square-foot space. This basically means cramming a two-hundred-pound animal into an area equivalent to about two feet by three feet. The authors acknowledged that overcrowding presents problems, including inadequate ventilation and increased health risks, but they concluded that "crowding pigs a little tighter will make you more money."[683]

Unfortunately, this situation is not expected to change anytime soon. Why? *Yersinia* bacteria do not cause clinical disease in pigs.[684] In other words, it's a public health problem, not an animal production problem. It doesn't affect the industry's bottom line. So instead of giving these animals a little more breathing room, the pork industry just largely passes along to society the estimated $250 million cost of sickening tens of thousands of Americans every year.[685]

C. *Difficile* Superbugs in Meat

A newer superbug is *Clostridium difficile*. *C. diff*, as it's commonly known, is one of our most urgent bacterial threats, infecting an estimated half-million Americans annually, killing tens of thousands, and costing billions of dollars a year.[686] It causes a condition called *pseudomembranous colitis*, which manifests as painful, crampy diarrhea. *C. diff* has traditionally been considered a hospital-acquired infection—something we pick up in health care settings—but only about one-third of *C. diff* cases can be linked to contact with an infected patient.[687] What's going on?

Well, another source of infection may be meat. The CDC found that 42 percent of the sampled packaged meat products sold at three national chain supermarkets contained toxin-producing *C. diff* bacteria.[688] The United States, it turns out, has the highest reported levels of *C. diff* meat contamination in the world.[689]

C. diff has also been found in chicken, turkey, and beef, but pork contamination has received the greatest attention from health officials, as it most closely matches the same strain found in non-hospital-related human infections.[690] Since 2000, *C. diff* has increasingly been reported as one of the leading causes of intestinal infections among baby piglets.[691] Carcass contamination with this diarrheal pathogen at the time of slaughter is considered the most likely source of the contamination of retail pork.[692]

Normally, *C. diff* won't do anything to us. Even if it gets into our gut, our good bacteria can usually muscle it into submission. It can lie in wait, though, until the good guys are out of the way. The next time we have to take an antibiotic that disrupts our normal gut flora, *C. diff* can rear its ugly head and cause a range of inflammatory bowel conditions, including a life-threatening condition that's as bad as it sounds: toxic megacolon.[693] (It carries a mortality rate as high as a flip of a coin.[694])

Doesn't cooking wipe out most bugs? *C. diff* isn't like most bugs. For most meat, 71°C (160°F) is the recommended internal cooking temperature. But *C. diff* can survive two hours of cooking at that temperature.[695] In other words, we could grill chicken at the recommended cooking thermometer temperature for two hours straight and still not kill the bug.

You've probably seen advertisements for those alcohol-based hand sanitizers that advertise they kill 99.99 percent of all germs. Well, *C. diff* falls into that 0.01 percent. It isn't called a *superbug* for nothing. Residual spores of the pathogen have been shown to be readily transmitted with a handshake even after using hand sanitizer.[696] As one of the lead researchers who discovered MRSA, another superbug in the U.S. meat supply,[697] has advised,[698] people who handle raw meat may want to wear gloves.

Facing a Post-Antibiotic Age

Dr. Margaret Chan, former director-general of the World Health Organization, warned that we may be facing a future in which many of our miracle drugs no longer work. She stated, "A post-antibiotic era means, in effect, an end to modern medicine as we know it. Things as common as strep throat or a child's scratched knee could once again kill."[699] We may soon be past the age of miracles.

The former director-general's prescription to avoid this catastrophe included a global call to "restrict the use of antibiotics in food production to therapeutic purposes." In other words, only use antibiotics in agriculture to treat sick animals. But that isn't happening. In the United States, meat producers feed millions of kilos of antibiotics each year to farm animals just to promote growth or prevent disease in the often cramped, stressful, and unhygienic conditions of industrial animal agriculture. Yes, physicians overprescribe antibiotics as well, but 66 percent of antibiotics important to human medicine sold in the United States every year now go to the meat industry.[700]

> Antibiotic residues can then end up in the meat we eat. Studies have revealed that traces of such antibiotics as Bactrim, Cipro, and enrofloxacin have been found in the urine of people eating meat—even though none of them was taking those drugs. The researchers concluded: "Consumption amounts of beef, pork, chicken, and dairy products could explain the daily excretion amount of several antibiotics in urine."[701] These antibiotic levels can be lowered, however, after merely five days of removing meat from the diet.[702]
>
> Nearly every major medical and public health institution has come out against the dangerous practice of feeding antibiotics to farm animals by the ton just to fatten them faster.[703] Yet the combined political might of agribusiness and the pharmaceutical industries that profit from the sales of these drugs has thwarted any effective legislative or regulatory action, all to save the industry less than a penny per half kilo of meat.[704]

Healthy living may help protect us against both airborne and foodborne illnesses. Eating more fruits and vegetables and exercising more frequently can boost our immune system to help us fight off respiratory infections like the common cold. And sticking to mostly plant foods can help prevent us from becoming another food-poisoning statistic by reducing our exposure to some of the deadliest fecal pathogens. For more on maintaining your body's defenses as you get older, see the "Preserving Your Immune System" chapter of my book *How Not to Age*.

Six years after I helped defend Oprah against her meat-defamation lawsuit, I received my own legal threat. The Atkins corporation accused me of "defamatory" statements in my book *Carbophobia: The Scary Truth About America's Low-Carb Craze*. Its lawyer claimed my words "continue to harm Atkins' reputation and cause injury to Atkins." My book certainly couldn't have caused more injury to Dr. Atkins than his own diet. You see, he had died the year before, overweight and—according to his autopsy report—suffering from a history of heart attack, congestive heart failure, and hypertension.[705]

However, the lawyers were talking about damage to Atkins Nutritionals,

Inc. Rather than let them silence me, I posted their legal threat online with a point-by-point rebuttal.[706] Thankfully, under the law, the truth is considered an absolute defense against defamation.

Atkins's attorneys never made good on their threat. Within four months of my book's publication, the Atkins corporation filed for bankruptcy.

How Not to Die from High Blood Pressure

The Global Burden of Disease Study is the most comprehensive and systematic analysis of the causes of death ever undertaken.[707] Funded by the Gates Foundation, it involves more than 8,000 researchers and analysts examining more than 150,000 data sources.[708] The results allow us to answer such questions as "How many lives could we save if people around the world cut back on fizzy drinks?" The best answer? 75,700.[709] So soft drinks and their empty calories don't just fail to promote health—they actually seem to promote death. But apparently fizzy drinks aren't nearly as deadly as bacon, ham, and hot dogs. Processed meat is blamed for the deaths of nearly 300,000 people every year.[710]

The study also noted which foods, if added to the diet, might *save* lives. Eating more legumes like beans could potentially save 390,000 lives a year.[711] More nuts and seeds? 660,000 lives.[712] How about vegetables? 860,000 lives.[713] More whole grains could potentially save an incredible 1.6 million lives a year.[714] And the food the world needs most? Fruits. Worldwide, if humanity ate more fruits, we might save an estimated 1.7 million lives. That's more than a million lives hanging in the balance, and our salvation isn't medication or a new vaccine—it may be just more fruit.[715]

The number one risk factor for death in the world that the study identified is high blood pressure. Also known as hypertension, high blood pressure lays waste to more than ten million people worldwide every year.[716] It kills so many because it contributes to deaths from a variety of causes, including aneurysms, heart attacks, heart failure, kidney failure, and stroke.

You've probably had your blood pressure taken at the doctor's office. The nurse reads off two numbers, say, for example, "115 over 75." The first number ("systolic") represents the pressure in our arteries as our blood pumps from the heart; the second number ("diastolic") is the pressure in our arteries while the heart is resting between beats. The American Heart Association defines "normal" blood pressure as a systolic pressure under 120 and a diastolic pressure under 80—or 120/80.[717] Anything above 130/80 is considered hypertensive.[718]

Increased blood pressure puts a strain on the heart and can damage the sensitive blood vessels in our eyes and kidneys, cause bleeding in the brain, and even lead certain arteries to balloon and rupture. The fact that hypertension can damage so many organ systems and increase the risk of heart disease and stroke, two of our leading killers, explains why it is the number one killer risk factor worldwide.

In the United States, nearly half of all adults have high blood pressure, and only 41 percent are even aware of their hypertension when diagnosed. As we age, our blood pressure tends to get higher and higher. In fact, after age sixty, more than 70 percent of Americans can expect to be diagnosed with the condition.[719] This has led many people, including doctors, to assume that high blood pressure, like wrinkles or gray hair, is just an inevitable consequence of getting older. However, we've known for nearly a century that this isn't true.

In the 1920s, researchers measured the blood pressure of a thousand native Kenyans who ate a low-sodium diet centered around whole plant foods—whole grains, beans, fruits, and leafy greens and other vegetables.[720] Up until age forty, the blood pressure of the rural Africans was similar to that of Europeans and Americans, about 125/80. However, as the Westerners aged, their blood pressure began to surge past the Kenyans'. By age sixty, the average Westerner was hypertensive, with blood pressure exceeding 140/90. And the Kenyans? By age sixty, their average blood pressure had *improved* to an average of about 110/70.[721]

The 130/80 threshold for hypertension is considered an arbitrary cutoff.[722] Just like having too much cholesterol or body fat, there are benefits to having a blood pressure that is even lower than the "normal" range. So even people who start out with a so-called normal blood pressure of 120/80 appear to benefit from going down to 110/70.[723] But is it possible to do that? Look at the Kenyans—not only is it possible, but it appears *typical* for people who live healthy enough lifestyles.

Over a two-year period, 1,800 patients were admitted into a rural

Kenyan hospital. How many cases of high blood pressure did they find? Zero. There also wasn't a single case found of America's number one killer, atherosclerosis.[724]

High blood pressure, then, appears to be a choice. We can continue eating the artery-bursting Western diet, or we can choose to take off the pressure. The truth is that eliminating humanity's primary risk factor for death may be simple. No drugs, no scalpels. Just forks.

Beans, Beans, They're Good for Your Heart

In chemistry and physics, there are constants—physical quantities thought to be both universal and unchanging. Biology, though, was considered too complex and too messy to be governed by simple, natural laws. In 1997, however, a theoretical high-energy physicist from Los Alamos joined two biologists to describe universal scaling laws that appear to apply across the board.[725] For example, the number of heartbeats per lifetime is remarkably similar whether you're a hamster or a whale. Mice, which typically live less than two years, have a heart rate of about five hundred to six hundred beats per minute—up to ten beats per second. In contrast, the heart of a Galapagos tortoise beats a hundred times more slowly, but they live about a hundred times longer.[726]

There's such a remarkable consistency in the number of heartbeats mammals get in their lifetimes that a group of researchers started to ask a provocative question: "Can human life be extended by cardiac slowing?" In other words, "[i]f humans are predetermined to have ~3 billion heart beats/lifetime, would a reduction in average heart rate extend life?"[727] This isn't just an academic question. If it turns out to be true, then we may be able to estimate that a reduction in resting heart rate—how fast our heart beats when we're just sitting at rest—from an average of more than seventy beats per minute down to sixty beats per minute, which is what many athletes have, could theoretically increase lifespan by more than a decade.

This reasoning may seem a bit off the wall, but that's how the scientific method works: We start out with an observation, such as these striking heartbeat data, and then make an educated guess, or hypothesis, which we go on to put to the test. How might one demonstrate a life-prolonging effect of cardiac slowing? Unfortunately, most drugs that lower heart rate have other effects. For example, drugs like beta-blockers lower both heart rate and blood pressure, so they wouldn't be ideal for testing the question at hand.[728] We could at least start by seeing whether people with slower heart rates live longer lives.

A high resting heart rate is indeed associated with an increase in mortality in the general population, suggesting a faster heart rate may lead to a faster death rate.[729] At first, I thought the explanation was painfully obvious. Of course lower resting heart rates are associated with a longer lifespan. After all, who has a really slow pulse? Athletes. The more physically fit we are, the lower our resting pulse. But no. Researchers found that those with higher resting heart rates fared worse irrespective of their level of physical fitness.[730] And now that we have medications that affect only heart rate, we have direct evidence from drug trials that lowering our heart rate may at least reduce the risk of heart attack in those who start out with a resting heart rate of seventy or higher.[731]

The thought is that if our heart rate is elevated twenty-four hours a day, even when we're sleeping, the stress of all the pulsations may break some of the elastic fibers within the arterial walls, causing our arteries to become stiff.[732] What's the target heart rate we should aim for? Based on a dozen studies, we know that risk rises as resting heart rate exceeds sixty-five beats per minute, so we don't want our heart to beat more than about one beat per second while at rest. (You can measure your pulse right now.) But don't worry if your heart is beating too fast. Heart rate is a modifiable risk factor,[733] thanks to exercise and beans.

Ironically, we make our heart go faster for short periods of time so that it beats more slowly the rest of the time. A twelve-week aerobic conditioning program of cycling, stair-climbing, and running on a treadmill can make our resting heart rate drop about three beats per minute. Of course, you have to keep it up. Stop exercising, and resting heart rate goes right back up.[734]

Exercise is only one way to lower our heart rate, though. Another way to our heart may be through our stomach. What if, instead of exercising for three months, we ate legumes for three months, like 200 grams a day of beans, chickpeas, or lentils? The first randomized controlled trial of beans for the treatment of diabetes showed that legumes do in fact successfully improve long-term blood-sugar control, with a side benefit of producing a drop of 3.4 beats per minute in heart rate[735]—just as much as about fifty hours on a treadmill.[736] That may help explain why a single daily serving of beans, chickpeas, or lentils may be associated with a 10 percent decrease in all-cause mortality risk.[737]

Sodium

The two most prominent dietary risks for death and disability in the world may be not eating enough fruits and getting too much salt. As I mentioned, not eating enough fruits appears to kill 1.7 million people a year,[738] whereas consuming too much salt kills an estimated 1.9 million.[739]

Salt is a compound made up of about 40 percent sodium and 60 percent chloride. Sodium is an essential nutrient, but vegetables and other natural foods provide the small amounts of sodium we need in our diet. If we consume too much, it can cause water retention, and our body may respond by raising our blood pressure to push the excess fluid and salt out of our system.[740]

For the first 90 percent of human evolution, we likely ate diets containing less than the equivalent of a quarter teaspoon of salt's worth of sodium a day.[741] Why? Because anthropological evidence shows we ate mostly unprocessed plants.[742] We went millions of years without saltshakers, so our bodies evolved into sodium-conserving machines. That served us well until we discovered that salt could be used to preserve foods.[743] Without refrigeration, this was a boon to human civilization. It didn't matter that the addition of salt to our food resulted in a general rise in blood pressure—the alternative was starving to death because all our food rotted away.

But where does that leave us now? After all, we no longer have to live off pickles and jerky. Humans are genetically programmed to eat ten times less sodium than we do now.[744] Many so-called low-salt diets can actually be considered high-salt diets. That's why it's critical to understand what the concept of "normal" is when it comes to sodium. Having a "normal" salt intake can lead to a "normal" blood pressure, which can contribute to us dying from all the "normal" causes, like heart attacks and strokes.[745]

The American Heart Association recommends everyone consume less than 1,500 mg of sodium daily[746]—that's about three-quarters of a teaspoon of salt. The average American adult consumes more than double that amount, about 3,500 mg daily.[747]

If we could cut our salt intake by about half a teaspoon a day, which is achievable by avoiding salty foods and not adding salt to our food, we might prevent 22 percent of stroke deaths and 16 percent of fatal heart attacks. That's potentially more lives saved than if we were able to successfully treat people with blood pressure pills.[748] Simply put, reducing salt is an easy at-home intervention that may be more powerful than filling a prescription from the pharmacy. In the United States alone, up to ninety-two thousand lives could be saved each year simply by eating less salt.[749]

The evidence that sodium raises blood pressure is clear, including double-blind, randomized trials dating back decades.[750] If we take study participants with high blood pressure and put them on a sodium-restricted diet, their blood pressure drops. If we keep them on the low-salt diet and add a placebo, nothing happens. However, if we instead give them salt in the form of a time-release sodium pill, their blood pressure goes back up again.[751] The more sodium we give them secretly, the higher their blood pressure climbs.[752]

Even just a single meal can do it. If we give people with normal blood pressure a bowl of soup containing the amount of salt that may be found in an average American meal,[753] their blood pressure climbs over the next three hours compared to eating the same soup without any added salt.[754] Dozens of similar studies demonstrate that if we reduce our salt intake, we reduce our blood pressure. And the greater the reduction, the greater the benefit. But if we don't cut down, chronic high salt intake can lead to a gradual increase in blood pressure throughout life.[755]

Doctors used to be taught that a "normal" systolic blood pressure is approximately 100 plus age. Indeed, that's about what we're born with. Babies start out with a blood pressure around 95/60. But, as we age, that 95 can go up to 120 by our twenties. By the time we're in our forties, it can be up to 140—past the official cutoff for high blood pressure—and then continue to climb as we get older.[756]

What would happen if, instead of consuming ten times more sodium than what our bodies were designed to handle, we just ate the natural amount found in whole foods? Is it possible our blood pressure would stay low our whole life? To test that theory, we'd have to find a population in modern times who doesn't use salt, eat processed food, or go out to eat. To find a no-salt culture, scientists had to go deep into the Amazon rainforest.[757]

Strangers to saltshakers, Cheetos, and KFC, the Yanomamo Indians were found to have the lowest sodium intake ever recorded—which is to say the sodium intake we evolved eating.[758] Lo and behold, researchers found that the blood pressures among older Yanomamo were the same as those of adolescents.[759] In other words, they start out with an average blood pressure of about 100/60 and stay that way for life. The researchers couldn't find a single case of high blood pressure.[760]

Why do we suspect it was the sodium? After all, the Yanomamos studied didn't drink alcohol; ate a high-fiber, plant-based diet; exercised; and were not obese.[761] An interventional trial could prove that sodium was the culprit. Imagine if we took people literally dying from out-of-control high blood pressure (known as *malignant hypertension*), a condition from which you go blind from bleeding into your eyes, your kidneys shut down, and your heart eventually fails. What if these patients were put on a Yanomamo-level salt intake—in other words, a normal-for-the-human-species salt intake?

Enter Dr. Walter Kempner and his rice-and-fruit diet. Without drugs, he brought patients with eye-popping blood pressures like 240/150 down to 105/80 with dietary changes alone. How could he ethically withhold medication from such seriously ill patients? Modern high-blood-pressure pills hadn't been invented yet—Dr. Kempner conducted his work back in the 1940s.[762] Back then, malignant hypertension was a death sentence, with a life expectancy of about six months,[763] but he was able to reverse the course of the disease with diet in more than 70 percent of cases.[764] Though the diet wasn't merely extremely low sodium—it was also strictly plant-based and low in fat and protein—Dr. Kempner is now recognized as the person who established, beyond any shadow of doubt, that high blood pressure can often be lowered by a low-sodium diet.[765]

In addition to high blood pressure, salty meals can significantly impair artery function,[766] even among people whose blood pressure tends to be unresponsive to salt intake.[767] In other words, salt itself can injure our arteries independent of its impact on blood pressure. And that harm begins within thirty minutes.[768]

Using a technique called laser Doppler flowmetry, researchers can measure blood flow in the tiny vessels in our skin. After a high-sodium meal, there is significantly less blood flow—unless vitamin C is injected into the skin, which appears to reverse much of the sodium-induced suppression of blood vessel function.[769] So, if an antioxidant helps block the sodium effect, then the mechanism by which salt impairs arterial function may be oxidative stress, the formation of free radicals in our bloodstream.[770] It turns out that sodium intake appears to suppress the activity of a key antioxidant enzyme in the body called *superoxide dismutase*,[771] which has the ability to detoxify one million free radicals per second.[772] With the action of this workhorse of an enzyme stifled by sodium, artery-crippling levels of oxidative stress can build up.

After one salty meal, not only does blood pressure increase but the arteries begin to stiffen.[773] This may be how we figured out thousands of years ago that too much salt was bad for us. Quoting from a translation of *The Yellow Emperor's Classic of Internal Medicine*, an ancient Chinese medical text, "If too much salt is used in food, the pulse hardens . . ."[774] It turns out that we may not need a double-blind trial; we may just have to give someone a bag of crisps and take their pulse.

Unsurprisingly, the salt industry isn't thrilled about the idea of us cutting back on salt. Back in 2009, the American Heart Association quoted the chair of the U.S. Dietary Guidelines Advisory Committee as saying that Americans should reduce their sodium intake. The Salt Institute, a salt industry trade organization, accused her of having an "unhealthy prejudice" against salt, arguing that she had "pre-judged the salt issue."[775] This is like the tobacco industry complaining that people at the American Lung Association are biased against smoking. Of course, the Salt Institute wasn't the only aggrieved party. Cheese, it turns out, ranks as a leading contributor of sodium in the American diet,[776] and the National Dairy Council stood shoulder-to-shoulder with Big Salt in its condemnation of the Dietary Guidelines Advisory Committee recommendations.[777]

The salt industry has its own PR and lobbying firms to play tobacco-industry-style tactics to downplay the dangers of its product.[778] But the real villains aren't necessarily the salt-mine barons—it's the processed food industry. The trillion-dollar processed food industry uses dirt-cheap added salt and sugar to sell us their junk.[779] That's why it's not easy avoiding sodium on the typical American diet, since three-quarters of our sodium intake comes from processed foods rather than a saltshaker.[780] By getting hooked on hypersweet and hypersalty foods, our taste buds get so dampened that natural foods can taste like cardboard. Indeed, the ripest fruit may taste sour after a bowl of Frosties.

But there are two other major reasons the food industry adds salt to foods. If salt is added to meat, it draws in water. This way, a company can increase the weight of its product by nearly 20 percent. Since meat is sold by the pound, that's 20 percent more profits for very little added cost. Second, as everyone knows, eating salt makes us thirsty. There's a reason bars often put out free baskets of salted nuts and pretzels, and it's the same reason soft-drink conglomerates own snack-food companies. A cold drink and a salty snack go hand in hand. It may be no coincidence that Pepsi and Frito-Lay are part of the same corporation.[781]

Which has been reported to contain the most sodium: a serving of beef, a serving of baked all-natural chicken, a large order of McDonald's french fries, or a serving of salted pretzels? Chicken. The poultry industry commonly injects chicken carcasses with salt water to artificially inflate their weight, yet they can still be labelled "100 percent natural." *Consumer Reports* found that some chickens in supermarkets were pumped so full of salt that they had an incredible 840 mg of sodium per serving—that could mean more than a full day's worth of sodium in just one chicken breast.[782]

The number one source of sodium for American kids and teens is pizza.[783] A single slice of Pizza Hut pepperoni pizza can contain half our recommended sodium intake limit for the entire day.[784] For adults over fifty, it's bread, but between the ages of twenty and fifty, the greatest contributor of sodium to the diet is chicken—not the canned soups, pretzels, or crisps one might expect.[785]

How can we overcome our built-in craving for salt, sugar, and fat? Just give it a few weeks, and our taste buds will start to change. When researchers put people on a low-salt diet, over time, the participants increasingly enjoyed the taste of salt-free soup and became turned off by the salt-heavy soup they had previously craved. As the study progressed, when participants were allowed to salt their own soup to taste, they preferred less and less salt as their taste buds became acclimated to healthier levels.[786]

The same may be true for sugar and fat. It's likely that humans actually taste fat, just like we taste sweet, sour, and salty flavors.[787] People placed on low-fat diets start preferring low-fat foods over fatty options.[788] Our tongue may actually become more sensitive to fat, and the more sensitive our tongue becomes, the less butter, meat, dairy, and eggs we eat. On the flip side, if we eat too much of these foods, we may blunt our taste for fat, which can cause us to eat more calories and more fat, dairy, meat, and eggs—and ultimately gain weight.[789] This can all happen in just a matter of weeks.[790]

There are four things we can do to shake the salt habit.[791] First, don't add salt at the table. (One out of three people may add salt to their food before even tasting it.)[792] Instead, try using potassium salt—a salt substitute readily available in supermarkets that's made of potassium chloride instead of sodium chloride. A massive randomized controlled trial of more than twenty thousand people found that replacing salt with even just a 25-percent potassium chloride blend (with which one wouldn't even taste a difference) led to 13 percent fewer cardiovascular events.[793] In the United States, that would mean potentially preventing hundreds of thousands of heart attacks and strokes every year.[794] However, those with advanced kidney disease or on medications that block the kidney from excreting potassium may not be able to take advantage of this potentially lifesaving tweak.[795]

Second, stop adding salt when cooking. The food may taste bland at first, but within two to four weeks, the salt-taste receptors in our mouth become more sensitive, and food tastes better. Believe it or not, after two weeks, you may actually *prefer* the taste of food with less salt.[796] Try any combination of such fantastic flavorings as pepper, onions, garlic, tomatoes, sweet peppers, basil, parsley, thyme, celery, lime, chili powder, rosemary, smoked paprika, curry, coriander, and lemon instead.[797] Also, it's probably a good idea to avoid eating out as much as possible. Even non-fast-food restaurants tend to oversalt.[798] Finally, do what you can to avoid processed foods.

In most countries studied, processed foods provide only about half of people's sodium intake, but in the United States, we consume so much sodium from processed foods that even if we completely stopped adding salt in the kitchen and at the dining table, we'd still only reduce our salt intake by a small fraction.[799] Try to buy foods with fewer milligrams of sodium on the label than there are grams in the serving size. For example, if it's a 100 g serving size, the product should have less than 100 mg of sodium.[800] Alternatively, aim for fewer milligrams of sodium per serving than there are calories. That's a trick I learned from one of my favorite dietitians, Jeff Novick. Most people get around 2,200 calories a day, so if everything you ate had more calories than sodium, you would probably make it at least under the Dietary Guidelines for Americans' upper limit of 2,300 mg of sodium a day.[801]

Ideally, though, we'd buy mostly food without any labels at all. It is considered almost impossible to come up with a diet consisting of unprocessed natural plant foods that exceeds the strict 1,500 mg a day American Heart Association guideline for sodium reduction.[802]

> ## Savory Spice Blend 2.0
> from *The How Not to Age Cookbook*
>
> **Makes about ½ cup (100 g)**
>
> Similar to the spice blend recipes in *The How Not to Die Cookbook* and *The How Not to Diet Cookbook*, this updated variety is a great seasoning to boost flavors or use in place of salt. I always have this on hand.
>
> 3 tablespoons nutritional yeast
> 1 tablespoon onion powder or granules
> 2 teaspoons garlic powder or granules
> 2 teaspoons ground paprika
> 1 teaspoon ground black cumin (nigella seeds)
> ½ teaspoon ground ginger
> ½ teaspoon ground thyme
> ½ teaspoon mustard powder
> ½ teaspoon ground turmeric
> ½ teaspoon celery seeds
> ½ teaspoon ground pippali or black pepper
>
> In a spice grinder or small food processor, combine all the ingredients, then mix well and grind into a powder. Transfer the mixture to a jar or bottle with a tight-fitting lid. Store in a cool, dry place.

Whole Grains

On average, high blood pressure medications reduce the risk of heart attack by 15 percent and the risk of stroke by 25 percent.[803] But in a randomized, controlled trial, three portions of whole grains a day were able to help people achieve the same blood-pressure-lowering benefit.[804] The study revealed that a diet rich in whole grains can yield the same benefits without the adverse side effects commonly associated with antihypertensive drugs, such as electrolyte disturbances in those taking diuretics (also known as water pills);[805] increased breast cancer risk for those taking calcium-channel blockers (like amlodipine or diltiazem);[806] lethargy and impotence for those on beta-blockers (like metoprolol and nadolol);[807] sudden, potentially life-threatening swelling for those taking ACE inhibitors (like enalapril and ramipril);[808] and an increased risk of serious fall injuries for apparently any class of these blood pressure drugs.[809]

Whole grains do have side effects, though. Good ones! Whole-grain intake is associated with lower risks of type 2 diabetes, coronary heart disease, weight gain,[810] and colon cancer.[811] Take note of the *whole*, however. While whole grains, such as oats, whole wheat, and brown rice, have been shown to reduce our risk of developing chronic disease,[812] *refined* grains may *increase* our risk. Harvard University researchers, for example, found that while regular consumption of brown rice was associated with a lower risk of type 2 diabetes, consuming white rice was associated with a higher risk. Daily servings of white rice were associated with a 17 percent greater risk of diabetes, whereas replacing one-third of a serving a day of white rice with brown rice might lead to a 16 percent *drop* in risk. And it looks like replacing white rice with oats and barley may be an even more powerful step, associated with a 36 percent drop in diabetes risk.[813]

Given the improvements in cardiac risk factors seen in interventional trials of whole grains,[814] it's not surprising to see a reduction in the progression of arterial disease among those who regularly eat them. In studies of two of the most important arteries in the body, the coronary arteries that feed the heart and the carotid arteries that feed the brain, people who ate the most whole grains had significantly slower narrowing of their arteries.[815,816] Since atherosclerotic plaque in the arteries is our leading killer, ideally, we should not just slow down the process but actually stop or even reverse it altogether. As we saw in chapter 1, this appears to require more than just whole grains; whole vegetables, whole fruits, whole beans, and other whole plant foods are needed, along with a significant reduction in our intake of trans fats, saturated fats, and cholesterol, the food components that contribute to clogging our arteries shut.

What About the DASH Diet?

What if you are among the 120 million Americans[817] who already have high blood pressure? How can you bring it down?

The American Heart Association (AHA), the American College of Cardiology (ACC), and the Centers for Disease Control and Prevention (CDC) all recommend that patients first try lifestyle modifications, such as reducing body weight, limiting sodium and alcohol intake, getting more exercise, and eating a healthier diet.[818]

However, if those recommended lifestyle changes don't work, then it's off to the pharmacy. First up is a diuretic (water pill), and before we can spell "pharmaceutical cocktail," the medications begin piling up until our blood pressure comes down. High blood pressure patients commonly end up on three different antihypertensive drugs at a time,[819] yet only about half tend to stick to even the first-line drugs.[820] (This is due in part to all their side effects, which can include erectile dysfunction, fatigue, and leg cramps.[821]) At the end of all this, the drugs still haven't gotten to the root cause of the problem. The cause of high blood pressure isn't medication deficiency. The underlying cause is what we eat and how we live.

As we discussed earlier, the ideal blood pressure, defined as the level at which lowering it further yields no additional benefit, is probably around 110/70.[822] Can we really get it that low without medication? Remember, this was the *average* blood pressure of men more than sixty years old in rural Africa on no treatment other than their traditional, healthier diets and lifestyles.[823] In rural China, we find similar results: 110/70 throughout life without any increase with age.[824] The reason we suspect that the plant-based nature of their diets is responsible is because, in the Western world, the only group able to routinely achieve these blood pressure readings is vegetarians.[825]

So, do the AHA/ACC/CDC guidelines recommend that people with high blood pressure eat a meat-free diet? No. They recommend the DASH diet, which stands for Dietary Approaches to Stop Hypertension, an eating plan specifically designed to lower blood pressure.[826] Although it's been described as a lactovegetarian diet[827] (dairy but no meat or eggs), that isn't accurate. The DASH diet emphasizes fruits, vegetables, and low-fat dairy, but meat is still present—we're just supposed to eat less of it.[828]

Why not recommend an even more plant-based diet? We've known for decades that "food of animal origin was highly significantly associated with systolic and diastolic B[lood] P[ressure] after the age and weight effects were removed."[829] That's a quote from a series of studies performed by renowned physician Frank Sacks and colleagues in the 1970s, but there are studies going all the way back to the 1920s demonstrating that adding meat to a plant-based diet can significantly elevate blood pressure in a matter of days.[830]

Why isn't the DASH diet meatless? Based on Dr. Sacks's work at Harvard University, the American Heart Association acknowledged that "[s]ome of the lowest B[lood]P[ressure]s observed in industrialized countries have been documented in strict vegetarians. . . ."[831] Were the designers of the DASH diet just not aware of Dr. Sacks's research? No, the chair of the committee that designed the diet *was* Dr. Sacks.[832]

The reason that the DASH diet was modeled explicitly after vegetarian diets but was not meat-free itself might surprise you. The primary design goal of the DASH diet was to explicitly create eating patterns "that would have the blood pressure lowering benefits of a vegetarian diet yet contain enough animal products to make them palatable to nonvegetarians . . ."[833] Dr. Sacks had even shown that the more dairy vegetarians consumed, the higher their blood pressure appeared to rise,[834] but he figured there was no point in calling for a diet he believed few would follow. This is a recurring theme in official dietary recommendations. Instead of simply telling us what the science shows and then letting us make up our own mind, experts patronize the population by advocating for what they think is practical rather than ideal. By making the decision for us, they undermine those willing to make even greater changes for optimal health. As Dr. Joel Fuhrman wrote, "Information should not be muddled and watered down to meet the objections of those people who seek mediocrity."[835]

The DASH diet does help to bring down blood pressure, but the primary effect seems to arise not from the switch to low-fat dairy and white meat or the reduction in sugary snacks and added fats but from the added fruits and vegetables.[836] If the benefits are due to the added plant foods, why not strive to center people's diets more around these healthiest of foods in the first place?

A recent systematic review concluded: "The overwhelming majority of intervention studies demonstrate that plant-based diets result in lower blood pressure readings when compared to diets that are based on animal products."[837] And the more plants, perhaps, the better. Meat-free diets in general "confer protection against cardiovascular diseases . . . some cancers and total mortality," but completely plant-based diets "seem to offer additional protection for obesity, hypertension, type-2 diabetes, and cardiovascular mortality."[838] Even just switching from cow's milk to soya milk can significantly lower blood pressure.[839]

There appears to be a stepwise drop in hypertension rates the more plant-based foods we eat. Based on the same study of eighty-nine thousand Californians that will be featured in chapter 7, compared with people who eat meat more than once a week, flexitarians (those who eat less meat, perhaps just a few times a month) had 23 percent lower rates of high blood pressure. Those who cut out all meat except for fish had a 38 percent lower risk of high blood pressure, and those who cut out all meat completely had a 55 percent lower rate. People who cut out all meat, eggs, and dairy did the best, with a 75 percent reduced risk of high blood pressure. Those eating completely plant-based diets appeared to have thrown three-quarters of their risk for developing this major killer out the window.[840]

When scientists looked at diabetes and body weight, they found the same apparent progressive improvements as consumption of animal products decreased and plant foods increased. Those eating plant-based diets had only a fraction of the diabetes risk even after factoring out the weight benefits,[841] but what about hypertension? On average, those who eat completely plant-based foods are about thirty pounds lighter than those eating conventional diets.[842] Might they have such great blood pressure just because they're so much thinner? In other words, do omnivores who are as slim as vegans enjoy the same blood pressure?

To answer this question, researchers would have to find a group of individuals who eat the standard American diet but are also as thin as people eating plant-based diets. To find an omnivorous group that fit and trim, researchers recruited long-distance endurance athletes who had run, on average, forty-eight miles per week for twenty-one years. Running almost two marathons a week for twenty years, pretty much anyone can become as slim as a plant eater no matter what they eat! The researchers then compared these hardcore athletes to two groups: sedentary meat eaters who exercised less than an hour per week and sedentary vegans who ate mostly unprocessed, uncooked plant foods.

How did the numbers come out? Not surprisingly, the endurance runners on a standard American diet had a better blood pressure average than their sedentary, meat-eating counterparts: 122/72 compared with 132/79, which fits the definition of high blood pressure. But the sedentary vegans? They averaged an extraordinary 104/62.[843] Apparently, eating standard American fare even when running two thousand miles a year may not bring down blood pressure as much as being a vegan couch potato.

Foods for Additional Hypertension Protection

A low-sodium diet centered around whole plant foods appears to be the best way to bring down high blood pressure, but what if you're already eating this way and that 110/70 still eludes you? There are a few foods in particular you can try that may offer additional protection.

I've already touched on whole grains and will go into detail below about hibiscus tea, nitrate-rich vegetables, and ground flaxseeds, which, on their own, "induced one of the most potent blood-pressure-lowering effects ever achieved by a dietary intervention."[844] In one study, eating just a few tablespoons of ground flaxseeds a day appeared to be two to three times more powerful than adopting an aerobic endurance exercise program[845] (not that we shouldn't do both—incorporate flaxseeds into our diet *and* exercise).

Consumption of both raw and cooked vegetables is associated with lower blood pressure, but raw veggies may be slightly more protective.[846] Studies have also found that loading up on beans, split peas, chickpeas, and lentils may help a little,[847] so add those to your shopping list. Red wine may help, but only nonalcoholic brands. Only wine that has had the alcohol removed appears to lower blood pressure.[848]

Watermelon appears to offer protection, which is great (and delicious) news, but you may have to eat about two pounds of it per day to achieve an effect.[849] Kiwifruits flopped, though. In a study funded by a kiwifruit company, kiwi failed to offer any protection.[850] Perhaps the kiwi industry should take a cue from the California Raisin Marketing Board, which funded a study designed to show that raisins can reduce blood pressure. To inflate the benefits of raisins, they used junk food as the control group. So the study found raisins may lower blood pressure, but only, apparently, compared to fudge cookies, Cheez-Its, and Chips Ahoy![851]

Flaxseeds

In chapters 12 and 14, we will see how effective flaxseeds may be against breast and prostate cancers, but we should be a little skeptical when scientists throw around words like "miraculous" to describe them. (One medical journal published a review titled "Flaxseed: A Miraculous Defense Against Some Critical Maladies.")[852] However, a remarkable intervention trial published in the journal *Hypertension* suggests that in this case, the term "miraculous" may not be too far off.

Rarely does one see a dietary study of this caliber: It was a prospective, double-blind, placebo-controlled, randomized trial. That's hard to pull off with food. With a drug trial, a blinded study is easy: Researchers administer a sugar pill that looks identical to the drug, so neither the study participant nor the researcher giving the pill knows which is which. (Hence, double-blind.) But how do you do that with food? People tend to notice if you try to sneak 25 grams of ground flaxseeds into their lunch.

The researchers tried a clever tactic to overcome this problem. They created a number of recipes for common foods including muffins and pasta in which they could disguise placebo ingredients like bran and molasses to match the texture and color of the flax-laden foods. This way, they could randomize people into two groups and secretly introduce tablespoons of daily ground flaxseeds into the diets of half the participants to see if it made any difference.

After six months, those who ate the placebo foods started out hypertensive and stayed hypertensive, despite many of them being on a variety of blood pressure pills. On average, they started the study at 155/81 and ended it at 158/81. What about the hypertensives who were unknowingly eating flaxseeds every day? Their blood pressure dropped from 158/82 down to 143/75. A seven-point drop in diastolic blood pressure may not sound like a lot, but that would be expected to result in 46 percent fewer strokes and 29 percent less heart disease over time.[853]

How does that result compare with taking drugs? The flaxseeds managed to drop systolic and diastolic blood pressures by up to fifteen and seven points, respectively. Compare that to the effect of powerful antihypertensive drugs, such as calcium-channel blockers (for example, amlodipine, diltiazem, nifedipine), which have been found to reduce blood pressure by only eight and three points, or to ACE inhibitors (such as enalapril, benazepril, lisinopril, ramipril), which drop patients' blood pressure by only five and two points.[854] Ground flaxseeds may work two to three times better than these medicines, and they have only good side effects. In addition to their anticancer properties, flaxseeds have been demonstrated in clinical studies to help control cholesterol, triglyceride, and blood sugar levels; reduce inflammation; and successfully treat constipation.[855]

Hibiscus Tea for Hypertension

Hibiscus tea, derived from the flower of the same name, is also known as roselle, sorrel, jamaica, or sour tea. With a distinct tart, cranberry-like flavor and bright red color, this herbal tea is served and enjoyed both hot and cold around the world. In a comparison of the antioxidant content of 280 common beverages, hibiscus ranked number one, beating out other heavyweights, including the oft-lauded green tea.[856] Within an hour of consumption, the antioxidant power of our bloodstream shoots up, demonstrating that the antioxidant phytonutrients in the tea are absorbed into our system.[857] What effects might this infusion have on our health?

Unfortunately, efficacy against obesity has been disappointing. After giving hibiscus tea for months to individuals who are overweight, researchers have only been able to show about an extra half pound of weight loss per month over a placebo.[858] Early studies on cholesterol-lowering effects looked promising, suggesting that drinking two cups of hibiscus tea a day for a month may provide as much as an 8 percent drop in cholesterol,[859] but when all such studies were put together, the results were pretty much a wash.[860] This may be because, for some reason, hibiscus tea only seemed to have an effect on about half the study participants. If you're in the lucky half, you may be able to get as much as a 12 percent drop in cholesterol.[861]

High blood pressure is where hibiscus really shines.[862] A double-blind, placebo-controlled study out of Tufts University that compared hibiscus tea with an artificially colored and flavored look-alike showed that three cups of hibiscus tea a day significantly lowered blood pressure in prehypertensive adults better than the placebo beverage.[863] But by how much? How does drinking hibiscus tea compare with other interventions?

The PREMIER Clinical Trial randomized hundreds of men and women with elevated blood pressure into an "advice only" control group or an active lifestyle intervention group. The control group was given a brochure and told to lose weight, reduce their salt intake, get more exercise, and eat more healthfully (i.e., go on the DASH diet). Those in the behavioral intervention group received the same instruction but also participated in in-person sessions, attended group meetings, kept food diaries, and monitored their physical activity, calories, and sodium intake. Within six months, the intervention group achieved a four-point drop in systolic blood pressure compared with the advice-only group. That may not seem like a lot, but on a population scale, a five-point drop may lead to 14 percent fewer stroke deaths, 9 percent fewer fatal heart attacks, and 7 percent fewer deaths overall each year.[864] Meanwhile, in the Tufts study, a cup of hibiscus tea with each meal managed to lower subjects' systolic blood pressure by six points over the control group.[865]

To lower blood pressure, we should still lose any excess weight, reduce our salt intake, get more exercise, and eat more healthfully, but the evidence shows that adding hibiscus tea to our daily routine may offer an additional benefit, comparable even to that provided by antihypertensive drugs. Tested head-to-head against a leading blood pressure drug, two cups of strong hibiscus tea every morning (using a total of five tea bags) was as effective in lowering participants' blood pressure as a starting dose of the drug Captopril taken twice a day.[866]

However, there are differences: Captopril can have side effects, most commonly rash, cough, and taste impairment, and it can even cause fatal swelling of the throat, though extremely rarely.[867] No side effects were reported for hibiscus tea, though there's a reason it's called sour tea. If you drink it, be sure to rinse your mouth with water afterward to keep the natural acids in the tea from softening the enamel on your teeth.[868] And given the extraordinary manganese content in hibiscus tea,[869] to be on the safe side, I wouldn't recommend drinking more than a liter of it a day.

The Power of NO

Nitric oxide (NO) is a key biological messenger within the body, and its message is: "Open sesame!" When released by our endothelium (the cells lining our arteries), it signals the muscle fibers within our arterial walls to relax, allowing them to open up and for more blood to flow. That's how nitroglycerin pills work: The nitroglycerin people take when they're experiencing chest pain is converted into NO, which dilates the coronary arteries, allowing more blood to flow to the heart muscle. Erectile dysfunction (ED) pills like Viagra work the same way; they boost nitric oxide signaling, which relaxes penile arteries and improves blood flow to the penis.

The ED we really need to be concerned about, though, is endothelial dysfunction, the failure of the linings of our arteries to produce enough NO to properly dilate them. Nitric oxide is produced by an enzyme called *NO synthase*. Its enemy is free radicals, which not only gobble up nitric oxide but can hijack NO synthase and force it to start pumping out *additional* free radicals.[870] Without enough NO, our arteries can stiffen, become dysfunctional, and raise our blood pressure and our risk for heart attack.

So we need to flood our body with antioxidant-rich plant foods throughout the day to extinguish the free radicals and let NO synthase get back to its job of keeping our arteries fully functional. There's an ultrasound device researchers use to measure the NO-induced dilation of the arteries. One study using this device found that when people following a standard Western diet ate even fewer antioxidants, their artery dilation got only a little bit worse. It seems they were already near the bottom of the barrel arterial-function-wise, so there wasn't much room for further decline. But when people were put on a high-antioxidant diet by, among many other things, switching their bananas for berries and their white chocolate for dark, within just two weeks, they experienced a significant boost in their arteries' ability to relax and dilate normally.[871]

In addition to eating antioxidant-rich foods that can boost our body's ability to produce NO, we can also eat certain vegetables, such as beetroot and greens, that are rich in natural nitrates that our body can then convert into nitric oxide. (For the difference between nitrates and nitrites, see chapter 10.) This process explains why researchers have been able to show a ten-point systolic blood pressure drop in volunteers within hours of their consuming beetroot juice—an effect that lasted throughout the day.[872]

That study was performed on a group of healthy subjects, though. Obviously, we need to test the power of beetroot where it counts most—in people with high blood pressure. If nitrate-rich vegetables can so powerfully modulate humanity's leading risk factor for dying, why did it take until 2015 before such a study was published? Well, who was going to fund it? Big Beetroot? Drug companies rake in more than $10 billion a year from blood pressure medications.[873] You can't make billions on beetroot. That's why we are fortunate to have charities like the British Heart Foundation, which funded a beetroot juice study involving people with high blood pressure.

Half the participants were provided 250 ml of beetroot juice daily for four weeks, while the other half were given an indistinguishable, nitrate-free placebo drink. The researchers found that not only was systolic blood pressure reduced by about eight points in the beetroot-juice drinkers, but the benefits grew week by week, suggesting their blood pressure might have continued to improve even further. The scientists concluded that "nitrate-rich vegetables may prove to be both cost-effective, affordable, and favorable for a public health approach to hypertension."[874]

The optimal dose appears to be 125 ml,[875] but beetroot juice is perishable, processed, and hard to find. A typical 250-gram packet of beetroot would provide the same dose of nitrate, but the most concentrated sources of the compound are dark green leafy vegetables. The following is a top-ten list of nitrate-rich foods. As you'll see in the chart below, eight out of the top ten are greens.

Top-Ten Food Sources of Nitrates

1. Rocket
2. Rhubarb
3. Coriander
4. Butterhead lettuce
5. Mixed salad leaves
6. Basil
7. Beetroot greens
8. Oak leaf lettuce
9. Swiss chard
10. Beetroot

Rocket comes out on top with a whopping 480 mg of nitrate per hundred-gram serving, which is more than four times the content of beetroot.[876]

The healthiest way we can get our nitrate fix is to eat a big salad every day. We could take nitrate- and nitric-oxide-boosting supplements, but they have questionable safety[877] and efficacy[878] records and should be avoided. What about V8 juice, which boasts both beetroot and spinach juice? It must not have much, because we'd have to drink eighteen liters of it each day to reach our daily nitrate intake target.[879]

The benefits of nitrates may explain why eating our greens is associated with reduced rates of heart disease[880] and a longer lifespan,[881] not to mention the "veggie Viagra" effect. You read that right. There's a link between vegetable consumption and improved sexual function,[882] as well as improved blood flow to the most important organ of the body, the brain.[883] And the only side effect of *beeting* your brains out may be a little extra color in your life—namely, stools and urine with a rosy hue.

Doping with Beetroot Juice

A Lamborghini goes faster than a lemon not because the chemistry of petrol combustion is somehow different in a sports car than a banger. It's because the Lambo has a more powerful engine. Similarly, athletes may have bigger muscles and be able to get more oxygen to those muscles faster. But fundamentally, the amount of energy a body can extract from oxygen remains the same . . . or so we thought.

About fifteen years ago, one of the gospels of sports physiology got turned on its head—all because of beetroot juice.

Nitrates, concentrated in dark green leafy vegetables and beetroot, not only help deliver oxygenated blood to our muscles by helping to dilate our arteries but also enable our body to extract more energy from that oxygen—something never before thought possible. For example, one little shot of beetroot juice has been found to allow free divers to hold their breath for half a minute longer than usual.[884] After sipping beetroot juice, cyclists were able to perform at the same level of intensity while consuming 19 percent less oxygen than the placebo group. Then, when they ramped up their bike resistance for an intense bout of what they called "severe cycling," the time to exhaustion was extended from 9:43 minutes to 11:15 minutes. The beetroot-juice-drinking group exhibited greater endurance while using less oxygen. In short, the beetroot juice made the cyclists' bodies' energy production significantly more efficient. No drug, steroid, supplement, or intervention had ever before been shown to do what beetroot juice could do.[885]

This effect works with whole beetroot too. In another study, men and women eating 200 grams of baked beetroot seventy-five minutes before running a 5K race improved their running performance while maintaining the same heart rate and even reported less exertion.[886] Faster time with less effort? Can't beet that!

To maximize athletic performance, the ideal dose and timing appears to be 140 ml of beetroot juice (or three 8-cm beetroots, or 180 grams of cooked spinach[887]) two to three hours before a competition.[888]

It seems sports news programs are always talking about steroids and other illegal performance-enhancing drugs. Why don't we hear more about these mighty and perfectly legit performance-enhancing vegetables? Beets me.

A blood pressure checkup is easy to ignore or postpone. Unlike the case with many of our other leading killers, the insidious consequences of hypertension may not be apparent until we're lifted into an ambulance or lowered into a grave. So go to your local pharmacy, fire station, or doctor's office, and get your blood pressure checked. If it's too high, the bad news is that you'll join the one billion people living with this condition.[889] The good news is that you *don't* have to join the millions who die from it every year. Try eating and living healthfully for even just a few weeks, and you may be amazed by the results.

6

How Not to Die from Digestive Cancers

Every year, Americans lose more than five million years of life from cancers that may have been prevented.[890] Only a small percentage of all human cancers are attributable to purely genetic factors. The rest involve external factors, particularly our diet.[891]

Our skin covers about twenty square feet, but our intestines, counting all the little folds, would flatten out to blanket hundreds of square feet, making it a much greater interface with any carcinogens lurking in the outside world.[892]

Three of the most common cancers of the digestive tract kill more than 110,000 Americans each year. Colorectal (colon and rectal) cancer, which claims more than 50,000 lives annually,[893] ranks among the most commonly diagnosed of all cancers. Thankfully, it is also among the most treatable if caught early enough. Pancreatic cancer, on the other hand, is virtually a death sentence for the approximately 56,000 people who develop it every year.[894] Only about 10 percent survive beyond a year after diagnosis, which means prevention is paramount. Esophageal cancer, which affects the tube between our mouth and stomach, is also frequently fatal for its 16,000 annual victims.[895] The foods we eat can indirectly affect cancer risk, for example, by exacerbating acid reflux, a risk factor for esophageal cancer, or through direct contact with the lining of the digestive tract.

COLORECTAL CANCER

The average American has about a one-in-twenty-five chance of developing colorectal cancer over the course of their lifetime.[896] Fortunately, it is among the most treatable cancers, as regular screening has enabled doctors to detect and remove the cancer before it spreads. There are about three-quarters of a million colorectal cancer survivors in the United States alone,[897] and, among those diagnosed before the cancer has spread beyond the colon, the five-year survival rate is about 90 percent.[898]

But, in its early stages, colorectal cancer rarely causes symptoms. If the cancer is not caught until later stages, treatment is more difficult and less effective. Starting at age forty-five until age seventy-five, most of us should either get stool testing every year for hidden blood, stool DNA testing at least every three years, a "virtual" colonoscopy (CT colonography) or sigmoidoscopy every five years, or a colonoscopy every ten years.[899] (If you have a family history of colorectal cancer or are otherwise at particularly high risk, talk with your doctor about a personalized screening schedule.) For more on the risks and benefits of these options, see chapter 15. While regular screenings are certainly sensible to detect colorectal cancer, preventing it in the first place is even better.

Turmeric

Based on data collected between 1993 and 2001, women in the United States appeared to have ten times more colorectal cancer than women in India, seventeen times more lung cancer, nine times more endometrial cancer and melanoma, twelve times more kidney cancer, eight times more bladder cancer, and five times more breast cancer. Men in the United States appeared to have eight times more colorectal cancer than men in India, twenty-five times more prostate cancer, ten times more kidney cancer, and six times more lung cancer and bladder cancer.[900] Why such a discrepancy? Though underreporting of cancer cases in India may be the major factor,[901] the regular use of the spice turmeric in Indian cooking has been proposed as a partial explanation.[902]

In chapter 2, we saw how curcumin, the yellow pigment in the spice turmeric, may be effective against cancer cells in vitro. Very little of the curcumin we eat gets absorbed into our bloodstream, however, so it may never come in sufficient contact with tumors outside the digestive tract.[903] But what doesn't get absorbed into our blood ends up in our colon, where it could impact the cells lining our large intestine where cancerous polyps develop.

The emergence of colorectal cancer can be broken up into three stages. The first sign may be what are called *aberrant crypt foci*, or abnormal clusters of cells along the lining of the colon. Next come polyps that grow from that inner surface. The final stage is thought to occur when a benign polyp transforms into a cancerous one. The cancer can then eat through the wall of the colon and spread throughout the body. To what degree can curcumin block each stage of colorectal cancer?

Studying smokers, who tend to have a lot of aberrant crypt foci, investigators found that curcumin consumption could reduce the number of those cancer-associated structures in their rectums up to nearly 40 percent, from eighteen down to eleven, within just thirty days. The only reported side effect was a yellow tint to their stools.[904]

What if polyps have already developed? Six months of curcumin, along with another phytonutrient called *quercetin*, which is found naturally in such fruits and vegetables as red onions and grapes, were found to decrease the number and size of polyps by more than half in patients with a hereditary form of colorectal cancer. Again, virtually no side effects were reported.[905]

What if the polyps have already transformed into cancer? In a last-ditch attempt to save the lives of fifteen patients with advanced colorectal cancer who didn't respond to any of the standard chemotherapy agents or radiation, oncologists started them on a turmeric extract. In the two to four months of treatment, it appeared to help stall the disease in one-third of the patients, five out of fifteen.[906]

If we were talking about some new kind of chemotherapy drug that only helped one in three people, we'd have to weigh that against all the serious side effects. But when it's just some plant extract shown to be remarkably safe, even if it helped only one person in a hundred, it would be worth considering. With no serious downsides, wouldn't it seem that a one-in-three potential benefit for end-stage cancer would spark further research? But who's going to pay for a study of something that can't be patented?[907]

The lower cancer rates in India may be due in part to the spices commonly used in their cuisine, but it may also stem from the types of foods they are putting those spices on. India is one of the world's largest producers of fruits and vegetables, and only about 7 percent of the adult population eats meat on a daily basis. What most of the population does eat every day are dark green leafy vegetables and legumes,[908] such as beans, split peas, chickpeas, and lentils, which are packed with another class of cancer-fighting compounds called *phytates*.

Stool Size Matters

The bigger and more frequent our bowel movements are, the healthier we may be. Based on a study of twenty-three populations across a dozen countries, the incidence of colon cancer appears to skyrocket as the average daily stool weight drops below about half a pound. Populations dropping quarter pounders appear to have three times the rate of colon cancer.[909] You can measure the weight of your stools with a simple bathroom scale. No, not that way—by weighing yourself before and after you "go."

The link between stool size and colon cancer may be related to "intestinal transit time," the number of hours it takes for food to travel from mouth to toilet. The larger the stool, the quicker the transit time, as it's easier for our intestines to move things along.[910] Many don't realize that we can have daily bowel movements and still effectively be constipated; what we're flushing today may have been eaten the week before.

How long it takes food to get from one end to the other can depend on gender and dietary habits. Food goes through men eating plant-based diets in just a day or two, but this transit time takes as long as five or more days among those eating more conventional diets. Women eating plant-based diets also average a day or two, but the typical intestinal transit time in most women eating conventional diets may be four days.[911] So we can be regular but four days "late." You can measure your own oral-anal transit time by eating some beetroot and noting when your stools turn pink. If that takes less than twenty-four to thirty-six hours, you're probably meeting the healthy half-pound target.[912]

Constipation is the most common gastrointestinal complaint in the United States, leading to millions of doctor visits each year.[913] But beyond just the discomfort, the straining associated with trying to pass small, firm stools may play a role in a host of health problems, including hiatal hernia, varicose veins, hemorrhoids,[914] and painful conditions like anal fissure.[915]

Constipation can be considered a nutrient-deficiency disease, and that nutrient is fiber.[916] Just as we can get scurvy if we don't get enough vitamin C, we can get constipation if we don't get enough fiber. Since fiber is found only in plant foods, it's no surprise that the more plants we eat, the less likely we are to be constipated. For example, a study comparing thousands of omnivores, vegetarians, and vegans found that those eating strictly plant-based diets are three times more likely to have daily bowel movements.[917] Looks like vegans are just regular people.

Phytates

Colorectal cancer is the second-leading cause of cancer-related death in the United States,[918] yet in some parts of the world, it's practically unheard of. The highest rates were recorded in Connecticut, and the lowest in Kampala, Uganda.[919] Why is colorectal cancer so much more prevalent in Western cultures? Seeking answers to this question, renowned surgeon Denis Burkitt spent twenty-four years in Uganda. Many of the Ugandan hospitals Dr. Burkitt visited had never even seen a case of colon cancer.[920] He eventually came to the conclusion that fiber intake was the key,[921] as most Ugandans consumed diets centered around whole plant foods.[922]

Subsequent research has suggested that dietary prevention of cancer may involve something other than just fiber. For instance, colorectal cancer rates were higher in Denmark than Finland,[923] yet Danes consumed slightly more dietary fiber than Finns.[924] What other protective compounds might explain the low cancer rates among plant-based populations? Well, fiber isn't the only thing found in whole plant foods that's missing from processed and animal-based foods.

The answer might lie in natural compounds called *phytates*, which are found in the seeds of plants—in other words, in all whole grains, beans, nuts, and seeds. Phytates have been shown to detoxify excess iron in the body, which otherwise can generate a particularly harmful kind of free radical called *hydroxyl radicals*.[925] The standard American diet may therefore be a double whammy when it comes to colorectal cancer: Meat contains the type of iron (heme) particularly associated with colorectal cancer[926] but lacks, as do refined plant foods, the phytates to extinguish these iron-forged free radicals.

For many years, phytates were maligned as inhibitors of mineral absorption, which is why you might have heard advice to roast, sprout, or soak nuts before eating them to get rid of the phytates. In theory, this would allow you to absorb more minerals, such as calcium. This belief stemmed from a series of laboratory experiments on puppies from 1949 that suggested that phytates had a bone-softening, anticalcifying effect,[927] as well as from subsequent studies with similar findings on rats.[928] But more recently, in light of actual human data, phytates' image has undergone a complete makeover.[929] Those who eat more high-phytate foods actually tend to have a greater bone mineral density,[930] less bone loss, and fewer hip fractures.[931] Phytates appear to protect bone in a manner similar to that of antiosteoporosis drugs like Fosamax,[932] but without the risk of osteonecrosis (bone rot) of the jaw, a rare, potentially disfiguring side effect associated with that class of drugs.[933]

Phytates may also help protect against colorectal cancer. A six-year study of about thirty thousand Californians found that higher meat consumption was associated with higher risk of colon cancer. Unexpectedly, white meat appeared to be worse. Indeed, those who ate red meat at least once each week had about double the risk of developing colon cancer; that risk appeared to triple, however, for those who ate chicken or fish once or more a week. Eating beans, an excellent source of phytates, was found to help mediate some of that risk, so our colon cancer risk may be determined by our meat-to-vegetable ratio.[934]

There may be as much as an eightfold difference in colorectal cancer risk between the two extremes—high-vegetable, low-meat diets and low-vegetable, high-meat diets.[935] So it may not be enough to just cut down on how much meat is in our diet; we also need to eat more plants. The National Cancer Institute's Polyp Prevention Trial found that those who increased their bean consumption by less than just 40 grams a day appeared to cut their odds of precancerous colorectal polyp recurrence by up to 65 percent.[936]

Of all the wonderful nutrients in beans, why do we credit the phytates with reduced risk? Petri-dish studies have shown that phytates inhibit the growth of virtually all human cancer cells tested so far—including cancers of the colon, breast, cervix, prostate, liver, pancreas, and skin[937]—while leaving normal cells alone.[938] This is the mark of a good anticancer agent, the ability to discriminate between tumor cells and normal tissue. When we eat whole grains, beans, nuts, and seeds, phytates are rapidly absorbed into our bloodstream and readily taken up by tumor cells. Tumors concentrate these compounds so efficiently that phytate scans can be used to trace the spread of cancer within the body.[939]

Phytates target cancer cells through a combination of antioxidant, anti-inflammatory, and immune-enhancing activities. Besides affecting the cancer cells directly, phytates have been found to boost the activity of *natural killer cells*, which are the white blood cells that form our first line of defense by hunting down and disposing of cancer cells.[940] Phytates can also play a role in our last line of defense, which involves starving tumors of their blood supply. There are many phytonutrients in plant foods that can help block the formation of new blood vessels that feed tumors, but phytates also appear able to disrupt existing tumor supply lines.[941] Similarly, many plant compounds appear able to help slow down and even stop cancer cell growth,[942] but phytates can sometimes also cause cancer cells to apparently revert back to their normal state—in other words, to stop behaving like cancer. This cancer cell "rehabilitation" has been demonstrated in vitro in colon cancer cells,[943] as well as in cancer cells of the breast,[944] liver,[945] and prostate.[946]

Phytates do have side effects, but they all appear to be good. High phytate intake has been associated with less heart disease, less diabetes, and fewer kidney stones. In fact, some researchers have suggested that phytates be considered an essential nutrient. Like vitamins, phytates participate in important biochemical reactions in the body. Our levels fluctuate with dietary intake, and insufficient consumption is associated with diseases that can be moderated by eating adequate amounts. Maybe phytates should be considered "Vitamin P."[947]

Reversing Rectal Polyps with Berries?

There are many ways the healthfulness of different fruits and vegetables can be compared, such as by nutrient content or antioxidant activity. Ideally, we would use a measure involving actual biological activity. One way to do this is by measuring the suppression of cancer cell growth. Eleven common fruits were tested by dripping their extracts on cancer cells growing in a petri dish. The result? Berries came out on top.[948] Organically grown berries in particular may suppress cancer cell growth better than those grown conventionally.[949] But a laboratory is different from real life. These findings are only applicable if the active components of the food are absorbed into our system and manage to find their way to budding tumors. Colorectal cancer, however, grows out of the inner lining of our intestines, so what we eat may have a direct effect regardless. Researchers decided to give berries a try.

Familial adenomatous polyposis is an inherited form of colorectal cancer caused by a mutation in our tumor-suppression genes. People who are affected develop hundreds of polyps in their colons, some of which inevitably turn cancerous. Treatment can involve prophylactic colectomy, where the colon is removed early in life as a preventive step. There was a drug that appeared able to cause polyps to regress, but it was pulled from the market after it killed tens of thousands of people.[950] Could berries also cause polyps to retreat without the fatal side effects? Yes. After nine months of daily treatment with black raspberries, the polyp burden of fourteen patients with familial adenomatous polyposis was cut in half.[951]

Normally, polyps would have to be surgically removed, but the berries seemed to have made them disappear naturally. The method by which the berries were administered, though, was anything but natural. The researchers used a shortcut, giving the berries as suppositories. Don't try this at home! After they inserted the equivalent of eight pounds of raspberries into patients' rectums over those nine months, some of the patients suffered from torn anuses.[952] The hope is that research will one day show similar cancer-fighting effects of berries taken the old-fashioned way—through the mouth.

Too Much Iron?

In 2012, the results from two major Harvard University studies were published. The first, known as the Nurses' Health Study, began following the diets of about 120,000 women aged thirty to fifty-five starting back in 1976; the second, the Health Professionals Follow-Up Study, followed about 50,000 men aged forty to seventy-five. Every four years, researchers checked in with the study participants to keep track of their diets. By 2008, a total of about 24,000 subjects had died, including approximately 6,000 from heart disease and 9,000 from cancer.[953]

After the results were analyzed, the researchers found that the consumption of both processed and unprocessed red meat was associated with an increased risk of dying from cancer and heart disease and shortened lifespans overall. They reached this conclusion even after controlling for (factoring in) age, weight, alcohol consumption, exercise, smoking, family history, caloric intake, and even the intake of whole plant foods, such as whole grains, fruits, and vegetables. In other words, the study participants apparently weren't dying early because they ate less of some beneficial compound like phytates in plants. The findings suggest there may be something harmful in the meat itself.

Imagine the logistics of following more than 100,000 people for decades. Now imagine a study five times that size. The largest forward-looking study of diet and health in history is the NIH-AARP study, cosponsored by the National Institutes of Health and the American Association of Retired Persons. Over the course of a decade, researchers followed about 545,000 men and women aged fifty to seventy-one. The largest study of meat and mortality ever conducted came to the same conclusion as the Harvard studies: Meat consumption was associated with increased risk of dying from cancer, dying from heart disease, and dying prematurely in general. Again, this was after controlling for other diet and lifestyle factors, effectively excluding the possibility that people who ate meat also smoked more, exercised less, or failed to eat their fruits and veggies.[954] The accompanying editorial in the American Medical Association's *Archives of Internal Medicine* (titled "Reducing Meat Consumption Has Multiple Benefits for the World's Health") called for a "major reduction in total meat intake."[955]

What does meat contain that may raise the risk of premature death? One of the possibilities is heme iron, the form of iron found predominantly in blood and muscle. Because iron can generate cancer-causing free radicals by acting as a pro-oxidant,[956] iron can be considered a double-edged sword—too little of it and we risk anemia; too much and we may increase risk of cancer and heart disease.

The human body has no specific mechanism to rid itself of excess iron.[957] Instead, we have evolved to tightly regulate the amount of iron absorbed. If we don't have enough iron circulating in our body, our intestines begin boosting iron absorption; if we have too much iron in circulation, our intestines decrease absorption. But this thermostat-like system only works effectively with the primary source of iron in the human diet: the nonheme iron variety found predominantly in plant foods. Once we have a sufficient amount of iron in our blood, our body is about five times more effective at blocking the absorption of excess iron from plant foods than from animal foods.[958] This may be why heme iron is associated with cancer[959] and heart disease risk.[960] Similarly, heme iron is associated with higher risk of diabetes, but nonheme iron is not.[961]

If we remove iron from people's bodies, can we decrease cancer rates? Studies have found that people randomized to give regular blood donations to reduce their iron stores appear to cut their risk of getting and dying from new gut cancers by about half over a five-year period.[962] The findings were so remarkable that an editorial in the *Journal of the National Cancer Institute* responded that "these results almost seem too good to be true."[963]

Donating blood is great, but we should also try to prevent the excess buildup of iron in the first place. The meat industry has been working on coming up with additives that "suppress the toxic effects of heme iron,"[964] but a better strategy may be to emphasize plant sources in our diet, which our body can better manage.

Getting Enough Iron on a Plant-Based Diet

Compared with people who eat meat, vegetarians tend to consume more iron (as well as more of most nutrients),[965] but the iron in plant foods is not absorbed as efficiently as the heme iron in meat. While this can be an advantage in preventing iron overload, about one in thirty menstruating women in the United States lose more iron than they take in, which can lead to anemia.[966]

Regardless of diet, heavy menstrual bleeding is the most common cause of iron-deficiency anemia in high-income countries.[967] There are numerous medical treatments, both hormonal and nonhormonal, to treat the cause of the anemia by lightening menstrual flow.[968] In terms of treating the anemia itself, oral iron supplements are considered the first-line remedy, but in serious cases, rapid repletion of blood levels using IV iron can be used.[969]

Intravenous iron may also be used for inflammatory bowel disease, since oral iron can be toxic to the lining of the intestine, potentially worsening the disease process.[970] Iron supplements cause adverse gastrointestinal effects such as abdominal pain, constipation, or nausea in nearly 75 percent of users, ultimately resulting in one in four of them to cease treatment.[971]

> Even if you don't experience symptoms, iron supplements may exacerbate inflammation or hurt your microbiome, reducing the abundance of beneficial microbes while increasing the abundance of deleterious ones.[972] Dietary interventions are a better long-term strategy.[973]
>
> Iron-deficiency anemia can be successfully treated with diet alone, usually with an increase in iron-rich foods like iron-fortified grains, along with vitamin C-rich foods or beverages that help with iron absorption.[974] The healthiest iron sources are legumes (beans, split peas, chickpeas, and lentils), whole grains, dark green leafy vegetables, certain fruits like dried apricots, and nuts and seeds.[975] Although dietary factors such as not drinking tea with meals or adding vitamin C-rich foods don't have as much effect on iron absorption as we used to think,[976] when we eat, it can't hurt to drink tea separately and include vitamin C-rich foods, such as citrus, tropical fruits, bell peppers/capsicum, and broccoli, to improve iron absorption.

PANCREATIC CANCER

My grandfather died of pancreatic cancer. By the time the first symptom arose—a dull ache in his gut—it was too late. That's why we need to prevent it in the first place.

Pancreatic cancer is among the most lethal forms of cancer, with just 13 percent of Americans surviving five years after diagnosis.[977] Thankfully, it's relatively rare, killing about forty-eight thousand people in the United States each year.[978] As many as 20 percent of pancreatic cancer cases may be a result of tobacco smoking.[979] Other modifiable risk factors include obesity and heavy alcohol consumption.[980] As we'll see, specific dietary factors may also play a significant role in the development of this deadly disease.

How the fat in one's diet may contribute to pancreatic cancer risk has long been a subject of debate. The inconsistency of research findings on the impact of total fat intake may be partly because different fats affect risk differently. The previously mentioned NIH-AARP study was large enough to be able to tease out what kind of fat was most associated with pancreatic cancer. It was the first to separate out the role of fats from plant sources, such as those found in nuts, seeds, avocados, and olive and vegetable oils, versus all animal sources, including meats, dairy products, and eggs. The consumption of fat from all animal sources was significantly associated with pancreatic cancer risk, but no correlation was found with the consumption of plant fats.[981]

Chicken and Pancreatic Cancer Risk

Starting in the early 1970s, a series of laws has restricted the use of asbestos, yet thousands of Americans continue to die every year from exposure to it. The Centers for Disease Control and Prevention, the American Academy of Pediatrics, and the U.S. Environmental Protection Agency have estimated that over a period of thirty years, approximately one thousand cases of cancer will occur among people exposed to asbestos in school buildings as children.[982]

It all started generations ago with the asbestos workers. The first asbestos-related cancers occurred in the 1920s among miners who dug it up. Then came a second wave among shipbuilders and construction workers who used asbestos. We are now in the third wave of asbestos-related disease, as buildings constructed with asbestos are beginning to deteriorate.[983]

As the history of asbestos shows, to see if something causes cancer, scientists first study those who have the greatest exposure to it. That's how we're learning about the potential cancer-causing effects of poultry viruses. There has been long-standing concern about the possibility that wart-causing chicken cancer viruses are being transmitted to the general population through the handling of fresh or frozen chicken.[984] These viruses are known to cause cancer in the birds, but their role in human cancers is unknown. This concern arises out of studies that show that people who work in poultry slaughtering and processing plants have increased risk of dying from certain cancers.

A study of thirty thousand poultry workers was designed specifically to test whether "exposure to poultry cancer-causing viruses that widely occurs occupationally in poultry workers—not to mention the general population—may be associated with increased risks of deaths from liver and pancreatic cancers." The study found that those who slaughter chickens have about *nine times* the odds of both pancreatic cancer and liver cancer.[985] To put this result in context, the most carefully studied risk factor for pancreatic cancer is cigarette smoking. Even if we smoked for fifty years, we'd have "only" doubled our odds of getting pancreatic cancer.[986]

What about people who eat chicken? The largest study to address that question is the European Prospective Investigation into Cancer and Nutrition

(EPIC) study, which followed 477,000 people for about a decade. The researchers found a 72 percent increased risk of pancreatic cancer for every fifty grams of chicken consumed daily.[987] And that's not much meat, under two ounces a day—just about a quarter of a chicken breast.

The researchers expressed surprise that it was the consumption of poultry—not red meat—that was more closely tied to cancer. When a similar result was found for lymphomas and leukemias, the same EPIC research team acknowledged that while the growth-promoting drugs fed to chickens and turkeys could be playing a role, it might also be cancer viruses found in poultry.[988] A systematic review of all such studies (a total of ten others) found greater poultry consumption was indeed significantly associated with greater pancreatic cancer risk.[989]

The reason the connection between asbestos and cancer was comparatively easy to nail down is that asbestos caused a particularly unusual cancer (mesothelioma), which was virtually unknown before widespread asbestos use.[990] But because the pancreatic cancer one might get from eating chicken is the same pancreatic cancer one might get from smoking cigarettes, it's more difficult to tease out a cause-and-effect relationship. There are diseases unique to the meat industry, such as "salami brusher's disease" that only affects people whose full-time job is to wire-brush off the white mold that naturally grows on salami.[991] But most diseases suffered by meat industry workers are more universal. So, despite the compelling evidence linking poultry exposure to pancreatic cancer, don't expect an asbestos-type ban on KFC anytime soon.

Treating Pancreatic Cancer with Curry

Pancreatic cancer is among the most aggressive forms of cancer. Untreated, most patients die two to four months after diagnosis. Unfortunately, as few as 10 percent of patients appear to respond to chemotherapy, with the majority suffering severe side effects.[992]

Curcumin, the colorful component of the spice turmeric, appears able to reverse precancerous changes in colon cancer and has been shown in laboratory studies to be effective against lung cancer cells. Similar results were obtained using pancreatic cancer cells.[993] So why not try using curcumin to treat patients with pancreatic cancer? In a study funded by the

National Cancer Institute and performed at the MD Anderson Cancer Center, patients with advanced pancreatic cancer were given large doses of curcumin. Of the twenty-one patients the researchers were able to evaluate, two responded positively to the treatment. One had a 73 percent reduction in their tumor size, though eventually a curcumin-resistant tumor developed in its place.[994]

The other patient, however, showed steady improvement over the course of eighteen months. The only time cancer markers bumped up was during a brief three-week period when the curcumin therapy was halted.[995] Yes, the tumors of only two out of twenty-one participants responded, but that's about the same as the chemo regimen, and zero adverse effects were reported with the curcumin treatment. As a result, I'd certainly suggest curcumin to pancreatic cancer patients regardless of what other treatments they choose. Given the tragic prognosis, though, prevention is critical. Until we know more, our best bet is to avoid tobacco, excess alcohol intake, and obesity and to eat a diet that is low in animal products, refined grains, and added sugars[996] and rich in beans, lentils, split peas, dried fruits,[997] and cruciferous vegetables.[998]

ESOPHAGEAL CANCER

Esophageal cancer occurs when cancer cells develop in the esophagus, the muscular tube carrying food from our mouth to our stomach. Typically, the cancer arises in the lining of the esophagus and then invades the outer layers before metastasizing (spreading) to other organs. Early on, there may be few symptoms—if any at all. But as the cancer grows, swallowing difficulties can develop.

Every year, there are nearly nineteen thousand new cases of esophageal cancer and sixteen thousand deaths.[999] The primary risk factors include smoking, heavy alcohol consumption, and gastroesophageal reflux disease (GERD, also called acid reflux), in which acid from the stomach gurgles up into the esophagus, burning the inner layer and causing inflammation that can eventually lead to cancer. Besides avoiding tobacco and alcohol (even light drinking appears to increase risk),[1000] the most important thing we can do to prevent esophageal cancer is to eliminate acid reflux disease—and that can often be accomplished through diet.[1001]

Acid Reflux and Esophageal Cancer

Acid reflux is one of the most common disorders of the digestive tract. The usual symptoms include heartburn as well as the regurgitation of stomach contents back up toward the throat, which can leave a sour taste in the mouth. GERD causes millions of doctor visits and hospitalizations each year and represents the highest annual cost of all digestive diseases in the United States.[1002] Chronic inflammation caused by acid reflux can lead to Barrett's esophagus, a precancerous condition that involves changes in the esophageal lining.[1003] To prevent adenocarcinoma, the most common type of esophageal cancer in the United States, this sequence of events must be stopped—and that means halting acid reflux in the first place.

That's a tall order in the United States. Over the past five decades, the incidence of the most common type of esophageal cancer in Americans has increased sevenfold[1004]—an increase greater than that of breast or prostate cancer, and it may be chiefly because acid reflux is on the rise.[1005] In the United States, about one in four people (28 percent) suffer at least weekly heartburn and/or acid regurgitation, compared to just 5 percent of the population in Asia.[1006] This suggests that dietary factors may play a key role.

Dozens of studies have examined the link between diet, Barrett's esophagus, and esophageal cancer. The most consistent association with these cancers may be the consumption of meat and high-fat meals.[1007] Interestingly, different meats were associated with cancers in different locations. Red meat is strongly associated with cancer in the esophagus itself, whereas poultry was more strongly associated with cancer down around the stomach-esophagus border.[1008]

How does this happen? Within five minutes of eating fat, our sphincter muscle at the top of our stomach—which acts like a valve to keep down food inside the stomach—relaxes, allowing acids to creep back up into the esophagus.[1009] In one study, for example, volunteers consuming a high-fat meal (McDonald's sausage, egg, and cheese sandwich) experienced more acid squirting up into their esophagus than those eating a lower-fat meal (McDonald's hotcakes).[1010] Part of this effect may be due to the release of a hormone called *cholecystokinin*, which is triggered by both meat[1011] and eggs[1012] and may also relax the sphincter.[1013] This helps explain why those who eat meat have been found to have twice the odds of reflux-induced esophageal inflammation compared with vegetarians.[1014]

Even without the cancer risk, GERD itself can cause pain, bleeding, and scar-tissue narrowing of the esophagus that can interfere with swallowing. Billions of dollars are spent on medications to alleviate heartburn and acid reflux by reducing the amount of stomach acid produced, but these drugs can contribute to nutrient deficiencies and increase the risk of pneumonia, intestinal infections, and bone fractures.[1015] Perhaps the better strategy would be to just keep the acid in its place by minimizing the intake of foods that allow acid to escape.

The protection afforded by plant-based eating may not be based just on the foods that are reduced, though. Centering our diet around antioxidant-rich plant foods may cut in half our odds of esophageal cancer.[1016] The most protective foods for cancer at the esophagus-stomach border appear to be vegetables that are dark green and leafy, red, or orange; berries; apples; and citrus fruits.[1017] But *all* unprocessed plant foods have the advantage of containing fiber.

Acid Blockers May Be Bad to the Bone

Stomach acid-blocking "proton pump inhibitor" (PPI) drugs with brand names like omeprazole, lansoprazole, esomeprazole, pantoprazole, and rabeprazole are among the most popular medications in the world, raking in billions of dollars a year.[1018] Many people take them to reduce acid reflux, but that comes at a cost. In 2006, two observational studies out of Europe suggested an association between intake of this class of drugs and increased risk of hip fracture.[1019] By 2010, the growing evidence forced the U.S. Food and Drug Administration to issue a safety alert implicating PPI use with fractures of the hip, wrist, and spine.[1020] By now, there have been dozens of such studies totaling more than two million people that, overall, show higher hip fracture rates among both long- and short-term users at all dose levels.[1021]

The irony is that most people taking these drugs shouldn't even be on them in the first place. The FDA approves the use of PPIs for ten days for the treatment of *Helicobacter pylori* (a kind of stomach infection), up to two weeks for heartburn, up to eight weeks for acid reflux disease, and two to six months for ulcers. Yet, most participants in a community survey said they remained on the drugs for more than a year, and more than 60 percent of patients in another survey were taking them for inappropriate reasons; they're often wrongly prescribed for indigestion, for example.[1022] The risks of these drugs almost always exceed the benefits over the long run. Calls from regulatory authorities to stop this overuse have fallen on deaf doctor ears.[1023] Now that they're available over the counter, the problem of overuse is likely even worse.[1024]

What's more, once you start taking them, it can be hard to stop. Between 44 and 59 percent of patients experience withdrawal symptoms that can last for weeks.[1025] When healthy, symptom-free volunteers were placed on these drugs for two months and then covertly switched to a placebo without their knowledge, 44 percent of them suddenly developed acid-related symptoms, such as heartburn or acid regurgitation.[1026]

In addition to bone fractures, this class of drugs has been linked to increased risk of other possible long-term adverse effects, such as pneumonia,[1027,1028] intestinal infections, kidney failure,[1029,1030] stomach cancer,[1031] and cardiovascular disease.[1032] (Their effect on blood vessels explains the recent case report "Abrupt-Onset, Profound Erectile Dysfunction in a Healthy Young Man After Initiating Over-the-Counter Omeprazole."[1033]) They also increase the risk of premature death.[1034]

There are individuals with rare conditions like Zollinger-Ellison syndrome, where tumors cause excess stomach acid secretion, for whom the risk-benefit of long-term use may be acceptable,[1035] but that's a far cry from the 100 million PPIs prescribed annually in the United States alone.[1036]

Fiber and Hiatal Hernia

While fat intake is associated with increased risk of reflux, fiber intake appears to decrease that risk.[1037] High fiber intake may reduce the incidence of esophageal cancer by as much as one-third[1038] by helping to prevent the root cause of many cases of acid reflux: the herniation of part of the stomach up into the chest cavity.

Hiatal hernia, as this condition is known, occurs when part of the stomach is pushed up through the diaphragm into the chest. More than one in five

Americans suffer from hiatal hernias. In contrast, hiatal hernias are almost unheard of among populations whose diets are plant-based, with rates closer to one in a thousand.[1039] This is thought to be because they smoothly pass large, soft stools.[1040]

People who don't eat an abundance of whole plant foods have smaller, firmer stools that can be difficult to pass. (See box on page 128.) If we regularly strain to push out stool, over time the increased pressure can push part of the stomach up and out of our abdomen, allowing acid to flow up toward the throat.[1041]

This same pressure from straining on the toilet week after week can cause other problems. Similar to the way squeezing a stress ball causes a balloon bubble to pop out, the pressure from straining at the toilet may herniate outpouchings from the wall of the colon, a condition known as *diverticulosis*. The increased abdominal pressure may also back up blood flow in the veins around the anus, causing hemorrhoids, and even push blood flow back into the legs, resulting in varicose veins.[1042] But a fiber-rich diet can relieve the pressure in both directions. Those who eat diets that revolve around whole plant foods tend to pass such effortless bowel movements that their stomachs stay where they're supposed to,[1043] which can reduce the acid spillover implicated in one of our deadliest cancers.

Can Strawberries Reverse the Development of Esophageal Cancer?

Esophageal cancer joins pancreatic cancer as one of the gravest diagnoses imaginable. The five-year overall survival rate is 22 percent,[1044] with about half of those diagnosed dying within the first year.[1045] This underscores the need to prevent, stop, or reverse the progression of this disease as early as possible.

Researchers decided to put berries to the test. In a randomized clinical trial of powdered strawberries in patients with precancerous lesions in their esophagus, study participants ate 30–60 grams of freeze-dried strawberries every day for six months—that's the equivalent of about half a kilo of fresh strawberries a day.[1046]

All the participants started out with either mild or moderate precancerous disease, but, amazingly, the progression of the disease was *reversed* in

> about 80 percent of the patients in the high-dose strawberry group. Most of these precancerous lesions either regressed from moderate to mild or disappeared entirely. Half of those on the high-dose strawberry treatment walked away disease-free.[1047]

Fiber consumption doesn't just take off the pressure. Humans evolved eating huge amounts of fiber, likely in excess of one hundred grams a day.[1048] That's up to about ten times what the average person eats today.[1049] Because plants don't tend to run as fast as animals, the bulk of our diet used to be made up of a lot of bulk. In addition to keeping us regular, fiber binds to toxins, such as lead and mercury, and flushes them away.[1050] (Pun intended!) Our bodies were designed to expect an ever-flowing fiber stream, so it dumps such unwanted waste products as excess cholesterol and estrogen into the intestines, assuming they will be swept away. But if we aren't constantly filling our bowels with plant foods, the only natural source of fiber, unwanted waste products can get reabsorbed and undermine our body's attempts at detoxifying itself. Only 6 percent of Americans may even reach the recommended minimum daily intake of fiber, making it the single most widespread nutritional deficiency in the United States.[1051]

How Not to Die from Diabetes

Millan, a member of the NutritionFacts.org community, was kind enough to share her story with me. When she was thirty years old, she was diagnosed with type 2 diabetes. Millan had struggled with obesity all her life and suffered through the highs and lows of years of yo-yo dieting. She had tried nearly every fad diet she could find but, not surprisingly, would quickly gain back whatever weight she'd lost. Diabetes wasn't a stranger to her. Millan's parents, brothers, and aunt were all diabetic, so she figured that her own diagnosis was inevitable. It's age related. It's genetic. There was nothing she could do. Or so she thought.

Millan's initial diagnosis was back in 1970, and she lived with diabetes for two decades. Then, in the 1990s, she switched to an entirely plant-based diet and completely turned her life around. Today, her energy levels are better than ever, she looks and feels younger, and she's finally been able to maintain a healthy weight. More than five decades after being diagnosed with diabetes, Millan, now in her eighties, is fit as a fiddle. She still even teaches Zumba classes! She didn't find some wonder drug or trademarked diet. She simply decided to eat healthier food.

The disease called diabetes mellitus comes from two words: *diabetes* (Greek for "to pass through or siphon") and *mellitus* (Latin for "honey sweet"). Diabetes mellitus is characterized by chronically elevated levels of sugar in the blood. This is because either the pancreas gland isn't making enough insulin (the hormone that keeps our blood sugar in check) or because our body becomes resistant to insulin's effects. The insulin-deficiency disease is called *type 1 diabetes*, and the insulin-resistance disease is called *type 2 diabetes*. If too much sugar builds up in our blood, it can overwhelm the kidneys and spill into our urine.

How did people test urine before there were modern laboratory techniques? They tasted it. Diabetic urine can evidently taste as sweet as honey. Hence the name.

Type 2 diabetes has been called the "Black Death of the twenty-first century" in terms of its exponential spread around the world and its devastating health impacts. Instead of the bubonic plague, though, the pathological agents in obesity and type 2 diabetes are identified as "high-fat and high-calorie diets," and instead of fleas and rodents, the causes are "advertisements and inducements to poor lifestyle."[1052] Thirty-eight million Americans are currently diagnosed with diabetes, and the CDC estimates that one in five people don't even know they are diabetic.[1053] At this rate, the CDC predicts that one in three Americans will be diabetic by midcentury.[1054] Currently in the United States, about one in every ten people with diabetes suffer severe vision difficulty or blindness, compounded with the annual toll of about 62,000 cases of kidney failure, 160,000 lower extremity amputations, and 400,000 deaths.[1055]

Our digestive system breaks down the carbohydrates we eat into a simple sugar called glucose, which is the primary fuel powering all the cells in our body. To get from the bloodstream into our cells, glucose requires insulin. Think of insulin as the key that unlocks the doors to our cells to allow glucose to enter. Every time we eat a meal, insulin is released by our pancreas to help shuttle the glucose into our cells. Without insulin, our cells can't accept glucose, and, as a result, the glucose builds up in our blood. Over time, this extra sugar can damage the blood vessels throughout the body. That's why diabetes can lead to blindness, kidney failure, heart attacks, and stroke. High blood sugar can also damage our nerves, creating a condition known as neuropathy that can cause numbness, tingling, and pain. Because of the damage to their blood vessels and nerves, people with diabetes may also suffer from poor circulation and lack of feeling in the legs and feet, which can lead to poorly healing injuries that can, in turn, end as amputations.

Type 1 diabetes, previously known as juvenile-onset diabetes, represents approximately 5 percent of all diagnosed diabetes cases.[1056] In most people with type 1 diabetes, the immune system mistakenly destroys the insulin-producing beta cells in the pancreas. Without insulin, blood sugar rises to unsafe levels. Type 1 diabetes is therefore treated with injections of insulin, a type of hormone-replacement therapy, to make up for the lack of production. The exact cause of type 1 diabetes is unknown, though a genetic predisposition combined with exposure to such environmental triggers as viral infection and/or cow's milk may play a role.[1057]

Type 2 diabetes, previously known as adult-onset diabetes, accounts for nearly 95 percent of diabetes cases.[1058] In type 2 diabetes, the pancreas can make insulin, but it doesn't work as well. The accumulation of fat inside the cells of muscles and the liver interferes with the action of insulin.[1059] If insulin is the key that unlocks the doors to our cells, saturated fat is what appears to gum up the locks. With glucose denied entry into our muscles, the primary consumer of such fuel, blood sugar can rise to damaging levels. The fat inside these muscle cells can come from the fat we eat or the fat we wear (i.e., our body fat). The prevention, treatment, and reversal of type 2 diabetes therefore depends on diet and lifestyle.

The good news: Type 2 diabetes is almost always preventable, often treatable, and sometimes even reversible through diet and lifestyle changes. Like other leading killers—especially heart disease and high blood pressure—type 2 diabetes is an unfortunate consequence of our dietary choices. But even if you already have diabetes and its complications, there is hope. Through lifestyle changes, you may be able to achieve a complete remission of type 2 diabetes, even if you've been suffering with the disease for decades. In fact, by switching to a healthy diet, you can start improving your health within a matter of hours.

What Causes Insulin Resistance?

The hallmark of type 2 diabetes is insulin resistance in our muscles. As we've learned, insulin normally enables blood sugar to enter the cells, but when the cells are resistant and don't respond to insulin as they should, it can lead to dangerous levels of sugar remaining in the bloodstream.

What causes insulin resistance in the first place?

Studies dating back nearly a century note a striking finding. In 1927, researchers divided healthy young medical students into multiple groups to test out the effects of different diets. Some were given a fat-rich diet composed of olive oil, butter, egg yolks, and cream, and others were given a carbohydrate-rich diet of sugar, candy, pastry, white bread, baked potatoes, syrup, bananas, rice, and oatmeal. Surprisingly, insulin resistance skyrocketed in the fat-rich diet group; within a matter of days, their blood sugar levels doubled in response to a sugar challenge, far more than those on the sugar and starch diet.[1060] It took scientists another seven decades to unravel the mystery of why this happened, but the answer would provide the key to what causes type 2 diabetes.

To understand the role of diet, we must first understand how the body stores fuel. When athletes talk about "carb loading" before a competition, they're referring to the need to build a fuel supply in their muscles. Carb loading is a more extreme version of what we do every day: Our digestive system breaks down the starch we eat into glucose, which enters our circulatory system as blood sugar and is then stored in our muscles to be used for energy as needed.

Blood sugar, though, is a little like a vampire: It needs an invitation to come into our cells. And that invitation is insulin, the key that unlocks the front door of our muscle cells so glucose can enter. When insulin attaches to insulin receptors on a cell, it activates a series of enzymes that escort in the glucose. Without insulin, blood glucose is stuck out in the bloodstream, banging on our cells' front doors, unable to enter. Blood sugar levels then rise, damaging vital organs in the process. In type 1 diabetes, the body destroys the insulin-producing beta cells of the pancreas, so very little insulin is present to let blood sugar enter our cells. But with type 2 diabetes, insulin production isn't the problem. The key is there, but something has gummed up the lock. This is called insulin resistance. Our muscle cells become resistant to the effect of insulin.

So what's jamming the locks on our muscle cells, preventing insulin from letting glucose enter? Fat—more specifically, *intramyocellular lipid*, the fat inside our muscle cells.

Fat in our bloodstream, either from our own fat stores or from our diet, can build up inside our muscle cells, where it can create toxic breakdown products and free radicals that block the insulin-signaling process.[1061] No matter how much insulin we produce, our fat-compromised muscle cells can't use it effectively.

This mechanism by which fat interferes with insulin function has been demonstrated by either infusing fat into people's bloodstreams and watching insulin resistance shoot up[1062] or by removing fat from people's blood and seeing insulin resistance drop.[1063] We can now even visualize the amount of fat in the muscles using MRI technology.[1064] Researchers are able to track the fat going from our blood into our muscles and watch insulin resistance rise.[1065] One hit of fat, and within 160 minutes, the absorption of glucose into our cells becomes compromised.[1066]

Researchers don't have to give their study participants fat through an IV, though. All they have to do is feed them.

Even among healthy individuals, a high-fat diet can impair the body's ability to handle sugar. But we can lower our insulin resistance by lowering our fat intake. Research has clearly shown that as the amount of fat in our diet becomes increasingly lower, insulin works increasingly better.[1067] Unfortunately, given the current diets of American children, we're seeing both obesity and type 2 diabetes occur earlier and earlier in life.

Prediabetes in Children

Prediabetes is defined by elevated blood sugar levels that are not yet high enough to reach the official diabetes threshold. Commonly found among those who are overweight and obese, in the past, prediabetes was regarded as a high-risk state that presaged diabetes, but it was not thought to be a disease in itself. However, we now know that prediabetic individuals may already be experiencing organ damage.

People with prediabetes may already have sugar damage to their kidneys, eyes, blood vessels, and nerves even before diabetes is diagnosed.[1068] Evidence from numerous studies suggests that chronic complications of type 2 diabetes begin occurring during the prediabetic state.[1069] To prevent diabetic damage, therefore, we need to prevent prediabetes—and the earlier, the better.

Forty years ago, virtually all diabetes in children was assumed to be type 1. But since the mid-1990s, we've seen an increase in type 2 diabetes among kids.[1070] What was once called "adult-onset diabetes" is now known as type 2 diabetes because children as young as four are developing the disease.[1071] This trend can have devastating consequences: A fifteen-year follow-up study of children who were diagnosed with type 2 diabetes found an alarming prevalence of blindness, amputation, kidney failure, and death by the time these kids had reached young adulthood.[1072]

Why the dramatic rise in childhood diabetes? It's likely due to the dramatic rise in childhood obesity.[1073] Over recent decades, the number of children considered to be overweight has increased such that now one in five American kids have obesity.[1074] Children who are obese at age six are more likely than not to stay that way, and 75 to 80 percent of obese adolescents will remain obese as adults.[1075]

Childhood obesity is a powerful predictor of adult disease and death. For example, being overweight as a teenager was found to predict disease risk fifty-five years later. Such individuals may end up with twice the risk of dying from heart disease and a higher incidence of other diseases, including colorectal cancer, gout, and arthritis. Researchers have found that being overweight as a teen could be an even more powerful predictor of disease risk than being overweight as an adult.[1076]

To prevent childhood diabetes, we need to prevent childhood obesity. How do we do that?

The former chair of the nutrition department at Loma Linda University has suggested that giving up meat entirely is an effective way to combat childhood obesity, pointing to population studies demonstrating that people eating plant-based diets are consistently thinner than those who eat meat.[1077]

To study body weight, we usually rely on body mass index (BMI), which is a measure of weight that also takes height into account. For adults, a BMI over 30 is considered obese. Between 25 and 29.9 is considered overweight, and a BMI between 18.5 and 24.9 is considered "ideal weight." In the medical profession, we used to call a BMI of under 25 "normal weight." Sadly, that's no longer normal.

What's your BMI? Visit one of the many online BMI calculators or grab a calculator and divide your weight in kilos twice by your height in meters. For example, if you weigh 90.5 kilos and are 1.8 meters tall (five foot eleven), that would be $90.5 \div 1.8 \div 1.8 = 27.9$, a BMI indicating that you would be, unfortunately, significantly overweight.

The largest study ever to compare the obesity rates of those eating plant-based diets was published in North America. Meat eaters topped the charts with an average BMI of 28.8—close to being obese. Flexitarians (people who ate meat more on a weekly basis rather than daily) did better at a BMI of 27.3 but were still overweight. With a BMI of 26.3, pesco-vegetarians (people who avoid all meat except fish) did better still. Even U.S. vegetarians tend to be marginally overweight, coming in at 25.7. The only dietary group found to be of ideal weight were the vegans, whose BMI averaged 23.6.[1078]

So why aren't more parents feeding their kids plant-based diets? There's a common misconception in the United States that their growth will be stunted. However, sometimes the opposite may be true. Loma Linda University researchers found that children who eat vegetarian diets not only grow up leaner than kids who eat meat but taller too, by about an inch.[1079] In contrast, meat intake is associated more with horizontal growth: The same researchers found a strong link between consumption of animal foods and increased risk of being overweight.[1080]

Developing diabetes in childhood appears to cut life expectancy by about twenty years.[1081] Who among us wouldn't go to the ends of the earth to enable our kids to live two decades longer?

Hating Their Guts

The size-acceptance movement is definitely right about one thing: the extraordinary scourge of weight stigma. Described as the last "acceptable" form of bias,[1082] weight stigma is the rampant discrimination and stereotyping of individuals who are overweight. Fifty overweight women were asked to keep a diary of all the times they felt they were stigmatized for their weight. Over just one week, more than a thousand instances were recorded.[1083] A woman who is overweight may expect to be harassed (such as called names or insulted), encounter physical barriers (like being unable to fit into public seats), or be discriminated against (such as receiving perceived poorer service at restaurants or stores) on average about three times a day. Men who are obese report three times less discrimination than women of the same size,[1084] so it may be only a daily occurrence for them.

This weight stigma starts surprisingly early. Children as young as three years old label overweight peers as "mean," "stupid," "lazy," and "ugly."[1085] One of the most poignant illustrations comes from a famous study published in 1961. Children in summer camps and schools across a swath of different social, cultural, and ethnic backgrounds in California, Montana, and New York were asked to rank the following images as to whom they liked best:

1. a child in crutches with one leg in a brace
2. a child in a wheelchair
3. a child with one hand missing
4. a facially disfigured child
5. an obese child

In every population of kids they tested, there was "remarkable uniformity."[1086] The obese child always came in dead last.

But that was ages ago. What happened when the original study was repeated? Researchers published the forty-year follow-up in 2003, and guess what they found? The title of the study gives it away: "Getting Worse: The Stigmatization of Obese Children." The obese child was liked even less.[1087] This parallels trends throughout society with a 70 percent jump in perceived weight discrimination recorded in national surveys since the mid-1990s.[1088]

Attitudes among educators may not be helping. More than a quarter of teachers and other school staff surveyed felt that becoming obese is "one of the worst things that could happen to a person."[1089] Even parents can be biased, providing less support for college for their overweight daughters compared to thinner siblings.[1090] As two prominent obesity researchers commented, "It is strong prejudice indeed when parents discriminate against their own children."[1091]

What about doctors? One representative national survey found that more than half of physicians viewed patients with obesity as "awkward, unattractive, ugly, and noncompliant."[1092] About a quarter of nurses agreed or strongly agreed with the statement "Caring for an obese patient usually repulses me."[1093] This antagonism can have serious health consequences for those who may need care the most. For example, women who are obese are at higher risk for developing cervical,[1094] endometrial, and ovarian cancers,[1095] yet they are less likely to be screened. Morbidly obese patients only have about half the odds of getting their recommended pelvic exams.[1096] Though some of this may be avoidance on the part of the patient, some doctors just turn away patients with obesity. The *Sun Sentinel* polled OB-GYN practices in Florida and found that as many as one in seven refused to see heavier women, for example, setting weight cutoffs for new patients starting at two hundred pounds.[1097]

Even doctors who welcome obese patients have been found to give them short shrift. Physicians randomized to receive a medical chart of a migraine patient who either presented as average weight or obese said they would give the obese patient about 28 percent less of their time[1098]—and it's less quality time too. Recorded doctor visits found physicians tend to build less emotional rapport with overweight patients.[1099]

> At least the doctors appear able to hide their disdain. In a study entitled "Obese Patients Overestimate Physicians' Attitudes of Respect," despite the negative attitudes doctors harbored toward their obese patients, the same patients expressed their satisfaction with their providers. The researchers concluded, "While physicians may be successfully playing the part, the lack of true respect suggests . . . the authenticity of the patient–physician relationship should be questioned."[1100]

THE FAT WE EAT AND THE FAT WE WEAR

Carrying excess body fat is the number one risk factor for type 2 diabetes; up to 90 percent of those who develop the disease are overweight.[1101] What's the connection? In part, a phenomenon known as the spillover effect.

Interestingly, the number of individual fat cells in our body doesn't change much in adulthood, no matter how much weight we gain or lose. They just swell up with fat as the body gains weight, so when our belly gets bigger, we aren't necessarily creating new fat cells; rather, we're just cramming more fat into existing ones.[1102] In people who are overweight and obese, these cells can get so bloated that they actually spill fat back into the bloodstream, potentially causing the same clogging of insulin signaling one would experience from eating a fatty meal.

Doctors can actually measure the level of freely floating fat in the bloodstream. Normally, it's between about one hundred and five hundred micromoles per liter. But people who are obese have blood levels between roughly six hundred and eight hundred. People eating low-carb, high-fat diets can reach the same elevated levels. Even a trim person eating a high-fat diet can average eight hundred, so that sky-high number isn't exclusive to obese patients. Because those eating high-fat diets are absorbing so much fat into their bloodstreams from their digestive tract, the level of free fat in their blood is as high as someone who's grossly obese.[1103]

Similarly, being obese can be like gorging on bacon and butter all day even if you are actually eating healthfully. That's because an obese person's body may be constantly spilling fat into the bloodstream, regardless of what goes into the mouth. No matter the *source* of fat in our blood, as fat levels rise, our ability to clear sugar from the blood drops due to insulin resistance—the cause of type 2 diabetes.

People who eat a plant-based diet, on the other hand, have just a small fraction of the rate of diabetes seen in those who regularly eat meat. As you can see in figure 1 below, as diets become increasingly plant-based, there appears to be a stepwise drop in diabetes rates.[1104] Based on a study of eighty-nine thousand Californians, flexitarians appear to cut their rate of diabetes by 28 percent, good news for those who eat meat maybe once a week rather than every day. Those who cut out all meat except fish appear to cut their rates in half. What about those eliminating all meat, including fish? They appear to eliminate 61 percent of their risk. And those who go a step further and drop eggs and dairy foods too? They may drop their diabetes rates by 78 percent compared with people who eat meat on a daily basis.

Why would this be?

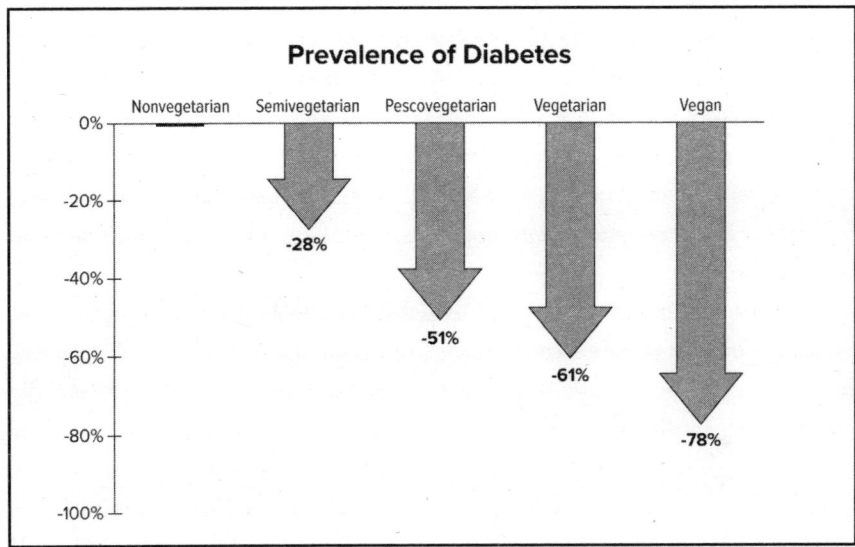

Figure 1

Is it just because people eating plant-based diets are better able to control their weight? Not entirely. Even at the same weight as omnivores, vegans appear to have less than half the risk of diabetes.[1105] The explanation may lie in the difference between plant fats and animal fats.

Saturated Fat and Diabetes

Not all fats affect our muscle cells in the same way. For example, palmitate, the kind of saturated fat found mostly in meat, dairy, and eggs, causes insulin resistance. On the other hand, oleate, the monounsaturated fat found mostly in nuts, olives, and avocados, may actually protect against the detrimental effects of the saturated fat.[1106] Saturated fats can wreak all sorts of havoc in muscle cells and may result in the accumulation of more toxic breakdown products (such as ceramide and diacylglycerol)[1107] and free radicals, as well as cause inflammation and even mitochondrial dysfunction—that is, interference with the little power plants (mitochondria) within our cells.[1108] This phenomenon is known as lipotoxicity (*lipo* meaning "fat," as in liposuction).[1109] If we take muscle biopsies from people, saturated fat buildup in the membranes of their muscle cells correlates with insulin resistance.[1110] Monounsaturated fats, however, are more likely to be detoxified by the body or safely stored away.[1111]

This discrepancy may explain why individuals eating plant-based diets are better protected from diabetes. Researchers have compared the insulin resistance and muscle-fat content of vegans versus omnivores. Because people eating plant-based diets have the advantage of being so much slimmer on average, the researchers recruited omnivores who weighed the same as the vegans they were studying so that they could see whether plant-based diets had a direct effect beyond the indirect benefit of pulling fat out of the muscles by helping people to lose weight.

The result? There was significantly less fat trapped in the deep calf muscles of vegans than in those of comparably slim omnivores.[1112] Those eating plant-based diets have been found to have better insulin sensitivity, better blood sugar levels, better insulin levels,[1113] and even significantly improved function of their beta cells—the cells in the pancreas that produce insulin in the first place.[1114]

In other words, people eating plant-based diets appear to be better at both producing and using insulin.

Preventing Diabetes by Eating More

Many population studies have shown that people who eat significant amounts of legumes (beans, split peas, chickpeas, and lentils) tend to weigh less. They also have slimmer waists, less obesity, and lower blood pressure compared to people who don't eat many legumes.[1115] But couldn't these benefits be due not to the legumes themselves but to the fact that people who eat more legumes may eat a healthier diet in general? To tease out the connection, researchers used the most powerful tool in nutrition research: the interventional trial. Instead of just observing what people eat, change their diets to see what happens. In this case, researchers put legumes to the test by comparing extra legume consumption head-to-head against caloric restriction.

Reducing belly fat may be the best way to prevent prediabetes from turning into full-blown diabetes. Though calorie cutting has been the cornerstone of most weight-loss strategies, evidence suggests that the majority of individuals who lose weight by portion control eventually regain it. Starving ourselves almost never works long term, so wouldn't it be great if instead we could find a way to eat more food to get the same weight-loss benefit?

The researchers divided overweight subjects into two groups. The first group was asked to eat one kilo per week of lentils, chickpeas, split peas, or haricot beans—but not to change their diets in any other way. The second group was asked to simply cut out five hundred calories a day from their diets. Guess who got healthier? The group directed to eat *more* food. Eating legumes was shown to be just as effective at slimming waistlines and improving blood sugar control as calorie cutting. The legume group also gained additional benefits in the form of improved cholesterol and insulin regulation.[1116] This is encouraging news for overweight individuals at risk for type 2 diabetes. Instead of just eating smaller portions and reducing the quantity of the food they eat, they can also improve the *quality* of their food by eating legume-rich meals.

Saturated fats may also be toxic to the cells in the pancreas that produce insulin. At around age twenty, the body stops making new insulin-producing beta cells. After that, if they are lost, they may be lost for good.[1117] Autopsy studies have shown that by the time type 2 diabetes is diagnosed later in life, we may have already killed off half our beta cells.[1118]

The toxicity of saturated fats can be demonstrated directly. If we expose beta cells to saturated fat[1119] or to "bad" LDL cholesterol in a petri dish, the beta cells begin to die.[1120] The same effect is not observed with the monounsaturated fats concentrated in fatty plant foods, such as nuts.[1121] When we eat saturated fat, both insulin action and insulin secretion are impaired within hours.[1122] The more saturated fat we have in our blood, the higher our risk may be for developing type 2 diabetes.[1123]

Of course, just as everyone who smokes doesn't develop lung cancer, everyone who eats excessive saturated fat doesn't develop diabetes. There is a genetic component. But for those who already have a genetic predisposition, a diet with too many calories and rich in saturated fat is considered a cause of type 2 diabetes.[1124]

Losing Weight with a Plant-Based Diet

As noted earlier, even if we don't eat extra fat, the extra fat we *wear* may cause the spillover effect—the tendency for overstretched fat cells to spill fat into the bloodstream. The advantage of a whole food, plant-based approach to weight loss is that there may be no need for portion control, skipping meals, or counting calories, because most plant foods are naturally nutrient dense and low in calories. (See my book *How Not to Diet* for a comprehensive investigation into *why* and *how* we are in the midst of an epidemic of obesity and *what*, *when*, and *how* we can eat to maximize weight loss with minimal effort.)

Fruits and vegetables, on average, contain about 80 to 90 percent water. Just as fiber can bulk up the volume of foods without adding calories, so can water. Experiments have shown that people tend to eat the same amount of food at a meal, regardless of calorie count—probably because stretch receptors in the stomach send signals to the brain after a certain volume of food has been ingested. When much of that volume is a zero-calorie component like fiber or water, that means we can eat more food but gain less weight.[1125]

Figure 2 (page 157) shows the amounts of broccoli, tomatoes, and strawberries that contain one hundred calories, compared with the quantities of one hundred calories of chicken, cheese, and fish. You'll notice that even though the calorie content is the same, the volume of these foods is different. So it makes sense that one hundred calories of the plants would be more likely to fill us up, while the same one hundred calories from animal or processed foods may leave us half-empty.

That's why whole food, plant-based diets are great for people who like to eat, since we can basically eat as much as we want without worrying about counting calories. Compared to any other way of eating that didn't involve portion control, a whole food, plant-based diet has been shown in a randomized

Figure 2

controlled trial to lead to greater average weight loss than any other diet in the medical literature.[1126] (For in-depth coverage of the pros and cons of taking the new class of injectable anti-obesity drugs, check out my book *OZEMPIC: Risks, Benefits, and Natural Alternatives to GLP-1 Weight-Loss Drugs*.)

In addition to weight loss, individuals consuming plant-based meals experienced improved blood sugar control as well as reduced risk of cardiovascular disease compared with people who followed diets that included more animal products.[1127] Such are the benefits of a plant-based diet.

People with diabetes are more likely to suffer from strokes and heart failure.[1128] In fact, diabetic patients without a history of coronary heart disease may have the same risk of heart attack as nondiabetic individuals with confirmed heart disease.[1129] In addition to improving insulin sensitivity better than conventional diabetic diets, the plant-based approach can also lead to a significant drop in LDL cholesterol, thereby reducing risk of heart disease, the number one killer of people with diabetes.[1130] But how do people feel about making such a major shift in their diets? As Dr. Dean Ornish has quipped, are we all going to live longer, or is it just going to *seem* longer?[1131]

Apparently, most people who switch to a plant-based diet are happy they did. One of the reasons there's been such great compliance with plant-based dietary interventions is that people not only tend to get measurably better, but they also tend to *feel* much better. In a randomized, clinical weight-loss trial, people with diabetes were split into two groups. Half were put on the conventional diabetic diet as recommended by diabetes organizations; the other half were prescribed a plant-based diet consisting mostly of vegetables, grains, legumes, fruits, and nuts. At the end of six months, the plant-based group reported both a significantly better quality of life and significantly higher mood scores than those assigned to the conventional diet. Patients consuming the plant-based diet also felt less constrained than those consuming the conventional diet. Moreover, disinhibition decreased, meaning patients eating vegetarian food were less likely to binge, and the plant-based folks tended to feel less hungry as well—both of which could help these individuals sustain this way of eating in the long run.[1132] So not only do plant-based diets appear to work better, but they may be easier to adopt long term. And with the improvements in mood they seem to bring, there may be benefits for both physical and mental health. (See chapter 11 for more on this topic.)

When it comes to maximally lowering diabetes risk, does it matter if we eat just a little meat? Researchers in Taiwan sought to answer that question. Traditionally, Asian populations have enjoyed very low rates of diabetes. In the twenty-first century, however, diabetes has emerged on a near-epidemic scale, coinciding with the Westernization of Asian diets. Rather than compare vegetarians to modern-day omnivores, these researchers compared vegetarians to those eating a traditional Asian diet, which customarily included very little fish and other meat. The women ate the equivalent of just a single serving of meat each week, while the men had a serving every few days.[1133]

Both the vegetarian and traditional Asian diet groups were following healthy eating patterns, avoiding fizzy drinks, for example. Despite the similarities in diet among the four thousand study participants, and after accounting for weight, family history, exercise, and smoking, the researchers found that the vegetarian men had only half the odds of diabetes as the occasional meat eaters. The vegetarian women had 75 percent lower odds of diabetes. Those who avoided meat altogether appeared to have significantly lower risk of both prediabetes and diabetes than those who ate plant-based diets with an occasional serving of meat, including fish. The researchers were unable to compare the diabetes rates of the more than one thousand vegetarians in the study to the sixty-nine vegans in the group, however, because the prevalence of diabetes among those eating strictly plant-based was zero.[1134]

Diabetes-Promoting Pollutants

The dramatic rise in obesity has been blamed squarely on overeating and inactivity. But could there be something else about the food we're eating that's plumping us up? Scientists have begun identifying "obesogenic" chemical pollutants released into the environment that may disrupt our metabolism and predispose us to obesity. Contaminated food is the main source of exposure to these chemicals, and 95 percent of that exposure may come through the consumption of animal fat.[1135] What's the big deal? A nationwide study found that people with the highest levels of pollutants in their bloodstreams had an astounding thirty-eight times the odds of diabetes.[1136] Harvard University researchers identified one chemical in particular, hexachlorobenzene, as a potent risk factor for the disease.[1137]

Where is this toxin found? Apparently, at the supermarket. In a supermarket survey of a variety of foods, canned sardines were found to be the most heavily tainted with hexachlorobenzene, though salmon was found to be the most contaminated food overall. Two dozen pesticides were detected in the salmon fillets.[1138] Farmed salmon may be the worst, containing ten times more of a class of toxic chemicals called PCBs than wild-caught salmon.[1139]

Industrial toxins like hexachlorobenzene and PCBs were largely banned decades ago. So how could they account for any of our increasing rates of diabetes? The answer to this paradox may be our obesity epidemic. The association between these toxic chemicals and diabetes was much stronger among obese subjects than in lean subjects studied, raising the possibility that our own fat stores are acting as reservoirs for these pollutants.[1140] Overweight individuals may be effectively carrying around a personal toxic waste dump on their hips. Without significant weight loss, people whose bodies contain salmon pollutants may take between fifty to seventy-five years to clear the chemicals from their bodies.[1141]

Do those who avoid meat completely get enough nutrients? To find out, researchers looked at a day in the life of thirteen thousand people across the United States. They compared the nutrient intake of those who ate meat to those who didn't. The study found that, calorie for calorie, those eating vegetarian diets were getting higher intakes of nearly every nutrient: more fiber, more vitamin A, more vitamin C, more vitamin E, more of the B vitamins thiamin, riboflavin, and folate, as well as more calcium, magnesium, iron, and potassium. Furthermore, many of the nutrients that are so rich in plant-based diets are among the very ones that most Americans normally don't get enough of—namely, vitamins A, C, E, not to mention fiber, calcium, magnesium, and potassium. At the same time, people who avoided meat also ingested fewer harmful substances, such as sodium, saturated fat, and cholesterol.[1142]

In terms of weight management, those eating meat-free diets consumed an average of 364 fewer calories daily.[1143] That's about what most people on traditional weight-loss programs strive to cut out, meaning a meatless diet could be considered an all-you-care-to-eat version of a calorie-restricted weight-loss diet, without having to count calories or restrict portion intake.

Those who eat plant-based diets may even have an 11 percent higher resting metabolic rate.[1144] That means vegetarians could be burning more calories even in their sleep. Why? One of the reasons could be that vegetarians have a higher gene expression of a fat-burning enzyme called *carnitine palmitoyltransferase*, which effectively shovels fat into the mitochondrial furnaces in our cells.[1145]

So a calorie may not be a calorie when it comes to meat. A massive study with an equally massive name, the European Prospective Investigation into Cancer–Physical Activity, Nutrition, Alcohol, Cessation of Smoking, Eating Out of Home, and Obesity—commonly known as EPIC-PANACEA—was comprised of hundreds of thousands of men and women who were followed for years. It's the largest study ever to investigate eating meat and body weight, and it found that meat consumption was associated with significant weight gain even after adjusting for calories. This means that if two people ate the *same* number of calories, it appears the person eating more meat would, on average, gain significantly more weight.[1146]

REVERSING DIABETES

Individuals with type 2 diabetes are at elevated risk for such serious health problems as heart disease, premature death, blindness, kidney failure, and amputations, as well as fractures, depression, and dementia, as noted earlier.

And the higher people's blood sugar levels, the more heart attacks and strokes they tend to have, the shorter their lifespans, and the higher their risk of complications. Diabetes must be addressed, but how?

What About Drugs and Surgery?

To see if these serious health outcomes could be averted, a study was performed in which ten thousand individuals with diabetes were randomized into one of two groups: the standard therapy group (in which the goal was just to lower blood sugar levels) and an intensive blood-sugar-lowering group (in which the researchers put individuals with diabetes on up to five different classes of oral drugs at the same time) with or without insulin injections. The goal was not just to drive down blood sugars, as is the case with standard therapy, but to drive them down consistently into the normal range.[1147]

Considering that type 2 diabetes is a disease of insulin resistance, high blood sugar is just a symptom of that disease, not the disease itself. So even by artificially forcing down blood sugars by any means necessary, we aren't treating the *cause*—just like blood-pressure-lowering drugs aren't treating the cause. By lowering one of the disease's effects, however, scientists hoped they could prevent some of its devastating complications.

The results of this study, published in *The New England Journal of Medicine*, sent shock waves through the medical community. The intensive blood-sugar-lowering therapy actually *increased* subjects' mortality, requiring the researchers to halt the study prematurely for safety reasons.[1148] The drug combinations may have been more dangerous than the high blood sugars they were trying to treat.[1149]

Insulin treatments themselves may accelerate aging, worsen diabetic vision loss, and promote cancer, obesity, and atherosclerosis.[1150] Insulin can promote inflammation in the arteries, which may help explain the increased death rate in the intensively treated group.[1151] So rather than trying to overcome insulin resistance by brute force—just pumping in more and more insulin—isn't it better to treat the disease itself by eliminating the unhealthy diet that caused it? That reminds me of people who undergo bypass surgery for clogged arteries. If they keep eating unhealthfully, their bypasses will eventually get clogged too. It's better to treat the cause than the symptoms.

How about surgery for diabetes? Gastric bypass surgery—which effectively reduces the size of the stomach by 90 percent or more—is one of the most successful treatment methods for type 2 diabetes, with reported long-term remission rates of up to 83 percent. These results had led to the suggestion that gastric bypass surgery improves diabetes by somehow altering digestive hormones, but this interpretation ignores the fact that patients are placed on a severely limited diet for up to two weeks following the procedure to recover from the surgery. Extreme caloric restriction alone can reverse diabetes. So, is the success of surgery the result of the operation itself or due to the restrictive diet?

Once again, researchers designed a study to uncover the answer.[1152] They compared people with diabetes placed on the same postoperative diet before and after they had the actual surgery. Amazingly, they found that the diet alone worked *better* than the surgery even in the same group of patients: The study participants' blood sugar control was better in the absence of the operation. This means the benefits of major surgery may be obtained without ever having to go under the knife and getting our internal organs rearranged.[1153]

The bottom line: Blood sugar levels can normalize within a week of eating six hundred calories daily, because fat is pulled out of the muscles, liver, and pancreas, allowing them to function normally again.[1154]

This reversal of diabetes can be accomplished either by voluntary caloric restriction[1155] or involuntarily, by having most of our stomach removed, a form of compulsory food restriction. Undergoing surgery may be easier than starving ourselves, but major surgery carries major risks, both during the operation and afterward. These risks include bleeding, leakage, infections, erosions, herniation, and severe nutritional deficiencies.[1156]

Surgery or starvation? There's got to be a better way, and, in fact, there is. Instead of changing the quantity of food we eat, it's possible to reverse diabetes by changing the *quality* of that food.

Does Eating Obesity Cause Obesity?

The EPIC-PANACEA study, which found that meat consumption is associated with weight gain even independent of calories, identified poultry as potentially the most fattening meat,[1157] a finding that has since been confirmed in another study. Men and women eating just 28 grams of chicken a day (think two chicken nuggets) had a significantly greater gain in body mass index over the fourteen-year follow-up period than those who consumed no chicken at all.[1158] Perhaps this news shouldn't be surprising, considering how fat chickens themselves are now genetically manipulated to become.

According to the U.S. Department of Agriculture, about one hundred years ago, a single serving of chicken may have contained only sixteen fat calories. Nowadays, one serving of chicken may have more than two hundred calories of fat. The fat content in poultry has ballooned from less than two grams per serving a century ago to up to twenty-three grams today. That's ten times more fat. Chicken now contains two to three times more calories from fat than from protein, leading nutrition researchers to ask, "Does eating obesity cause obesity in the consumer?"[1159] As the beef industry is proud of pointing out, even skinless chicken can have more fat, and more artery-clogging saturated fat, than a dozen different cuts of steak.[1160]

Reversing Diabetes with Food

We've known since the siege of Paris in 1870 that type 2 diabetes can be reversed by an extreme reduction in food intake. Parisian doctors documented how glucose disappeared from their patients' urine after people went weeks without food.[1161] Diabetes specialists have long known that iron-willed patients who are able to lose up to one fifth of their body weight can reverse their diabetes and bring their metabolic function back to normal.[1162]

Instead of starving by eating less food, though, what if people with diabetes just ate better food, as in a 90 percent or more plant-based diet of all-you-can-eat greens, lots of other vegetables and beans, whole grains, fruits, nuts, and seeds? In a pilot study, thirteen men and women with diabetes were told to eat at least one big salad every day, as well as veggie-bean soup, a handful of nuts and seeds, fruit at every meal, 450 grams of cooked greens, and some whole grains; to restrict their animal product consumption; and to eliminate refined grains, junk food, and oil. Then the researchers measured their hemoglobin

A1c levels, considered the best measure of how poorly blood sugars have been controlled over time.

At the onset of the study, the participants had A1c levels averaging 8.2. An A1c level under 5.7 is considered normal, between 5.7 and 6.4 is considered prediabetic, and above 6.5 is considered diabetic. However, the American Diabetes Association's target is just to get most diabetics down below 7.0.[1163] (Recall that intensive blood-sugar-lowering trials using drugs, which tried to push A1c levels under 6.0, unfortunately ended up pushing many diabetics six feet under.)

After about seven months of eating a diet centered on whole plant foods, the study participants' A1c levels dropped to a nondiabetic 5.8—and this was after they were able to stop taking most of their medications.[1164] We've known diabetes can be reversed with an extremely low-calorie diet.[1165] Now we know that it can also be reversed with an extremely healthy diet, but is that because it was also low in calories? The participants lost about as much weight on the vegetable-packed, plant-based diet as people who went on semi-starvation diets based on liquid meal replacements.[1166] But even if this type of diabetes reversal was just about caloric restriction, which would be healthier? Subsisting on mostly diet shakes made of sugar, powdered milk, corn syrup, and oil, or eating a plant-based diet where real food—and lots of it—can be enjoyed?

Surprisingly, even participants who temporarily didn't lose weight on the plant-based diet, or who actually gained weight, still appeared to improve their diabetes. In other words, the beneficial effects of plant-based diets may extend beyond weight loss.[1167] However, the study described just a handful of people, had no control group, and included only those who stuck to the eating plan. To prove plant-based diets could actually improve diabetes independent of weight loss, researchers would need to design a study in which they switched people to a healthy diet but one that had them eat so much that they didn't lose any weight.

Just such a study was published more than forty-five years ago. People with type 2 diabetes were placed on a plant-based diet and weighed every day. If they started losing any weight, they had to eat more food—so much more food that some of the participants actually had trouble eating it all! The result: Even with no weight loss, subjects on the plant-based diet saw their insulin requirements cut by about 60 percent, meaning the amount of insulin they had to inject dropped by more than half. Furthermore, half of the individuals with diabetes were able to get off insulin altogether, despite no change in body weight—just by eating a healthier diet.[1168]

This wasn't over the course of months or years, either. This was after eating a plant-based diet for an average of only sixteen days. Some of the participants had been diabetic for two decades and had been injecting twenty units of insulin a day. Yet within two weeks of eating a plant-based diet, they were off insulin altogether. One patient was on thirty-two units of insulin per day at the onset of the study. After eighteen days, his blood sugar levels plummeted so low that insulin injections were no longer necessary. Even at approximately the same body weight, he had lower blood sugars on a plant-based diet using no insulin than when he had been on a regular diet using thirty-two units of insulin daily.[1169] That's the power of plants.

An expert consensus statement put out by the American College of Lifestyle Medicine in 2022, endorsed by the American Association of Clinical Endocrinology, supported by the Academy of Nutrition and Dietetics, and co-sponsored by the Endocrine Society, states that "diet as a primary intervention for T2D [type 2 diabetes] can achieve remission in many adults with T2D" and that diet "is most effective in achieving remission when emphasizing whole, plant-based foods with minimal consumption of meat and other animal products."[1170]

Curing Diabetic Neuropathy

Up to 50 percent of people with diabetes eventually develop neuropathy, or damage to their nerves.[1171] Neuropathy can be very painful, and that pain is frequently resistant to conventional treatments. No medical treatment is considered effective for the condition,[1172] so doctors are left with only steroids, opiates, and antidepressants to try to ease our patients' suffering. But then a remarkable study was published, entitled "Regression of Diabetic Neuropathy with Total Vegetarian (Vegan) Diet." Twenty-one people with diabetes who had been suffering from painful neuropathy for up to ten years were placed on a whole food, plant-based diet. After years of suffering, seventeen out of the twenty-one patients reported that they felt complete relief from their pain—*within days*. Their numbness noticeably improved too. And the side effects were all good: They lost an average of 4.5 kilos, their blood sugar levels dropped, their insulin needs dropped in half, and, in five of the patients, not only was their painful neuropathy cured, so was, apparently, their diabetes. After having been diabetic for up to twenty years, they were off all blood sugar drugs in less than a month.[1173]

On top of that, their triglyceride and cholesterol levels improved on average as well. High blood pressures dropped by so much that half the study participants also appeared cured of their hypertension. Within three weeks, their need for high blood pressure medications dropped by 80 percent.[1174] (This is why it is critically important to work with your doctor when radically improving your diet, because if they don't reduce or eliminate your medications accordingly, your blood sugar levels or blood pressure may drop too low.)

We've long known that plant-based diets can reverse diabetes[1175] and hypertension,[1176] but reversing nerve damage pain with diet was new.

This study involved a live-in program in which patients were provided meals. What happened after they were sent home, back into the real world? These seventeen people were followed for years, and in all cases but one, the relief from their painful neuropathy continued—or improved even further. How were the researchers able to achieve such a high degree of dietary compliance even in an uncontrolled setting? "Pain and ill health," the researchers wrote, "are strong motivating factors."[1177] In other words: Because plant-based diets work.

Think about it. Patients walk in with one of the most painful, frustrating, and hard-to-treat conditions in all of medicine, and three-quarters of them were cured in a handful of days using a natural, nontoxic treatment—namely, a diet composed of whole plant foods. This should have been front-page news.

How could nerve damage pain be reversed so suddenly? It didn't appear to involve the improvement in blood sugar control. It took approximately ten days for the diet to control the diabetes itself, but the pain was gone in as few as four days.[1178]

The most interesting speculation was that trans fats naturally found in meat and dairy could be causing an inflammatory response in the patients' bodies. The researchers found that a significant percentage of the fat under the skin of those who ate meat, or even just dairy and eggs, was composed of trans fats, whereas those who had been on a strictly whole food, plant-based diet had no detectable trans fat in their tissues.[1179]

The researchers stuck needles into the buttocks of individuals who had been eating different diets and discovered that people who had been on a whole food, plant-based diet for nine months or more appeared to have removed all the trans fat from their bodies (or at least from their butts).[1180] But their neuropathy pain didn't take nine months to get better. It improved in closer to nine *days*. It's more likely that this amazing reversal was due to an improvement in blood flow.[1181]

Nerves contain tiny blood vessels that may become clogged, depriving the nerves of oxygen. Indeed, biopsies of leg nerves in diabetics with severe progressive neuropathy have shown arterial disease within the sural nerve in the leg.[1182] However, within days of eating healthier meals, blood flow may improve to the extent that neuropathy disappears.[1183] Within an average of two years of eating a plant-based diet composed mostly of rice and fruits, even diabetic vision loss can be reversed in as many as 30 percent of patients.[1184]

So why didn't I learn about any of this in medical school? There's little money to be made from prescribing plants instead of pills. The neuropathy pain reversal study was published more than thirty years ago, and the blindness reversal studies more than sixty years ago. As one commentator wrote, "The neglect of this important work by the broader medical community is little short of unconscionable."[1185]

BMI vs. WHtR

The body mass index (BMI) is a better predictor of disease than body weight alone, as BMI takes height into account. But BMI has long been criticized for not considering the location or the nature of our weight. Bodybuilders, for instance, have extremely low body fat but can have off-the-chart BMIs, because muscle is heavier than fat.

Today, it's generally accepted that health risks can be determined as much by the relative distribution of body fat as by its total amount.[1186] What's the worst kind? Abdominal fat—the kind that builds up around our internal organs. Having a potbelly may be a strong predictor of premature death.[1187]

Figure 3

Both of the men in figure 3 have the same BMI, but the distribution of weight is different. People with the so-called apple shape, with body fat concentrated in the abdominal region, may have the lowest life expectancy.[1188]

Fortunately, there may be an even better tool than BMI that we can use to gauge the health risks of body fat. It's called Waist-to-Height Ratio, or WHtR.[1189] Instead of stepping on a scale, grab a simple measuring tape. Stand up straight and take a deep breath, exhale, and let it all hang out. The circumference of our belly (halfway between the top of our hip bones and the bottom of our rib cage) should be half our height—ideally, less. If that measurement is more than half our height, it's time to start eating healthier and exercising more regardless of our weight.[1190]

Type 2 diabetes in the United States is reaching epidemic proportions. The CDC estimates that 38 percent of U.S. adults—and 49 percent of adults over sixty-five—have prediabetes. That's ninety-eight million people,[1191] most of whom will develop full-blown diabetes.[1192] But type 2 diabetes can be prevented, arrested, and even reversed with a healthy-enough diet. Unfortunately, doctors don't tend to educate their patients about diabetes prevention. Only about one in three prediabetic patients reports ever being told by their doctors to exercise or improve their diets.[1193] Possible reasons for not counseling patients include a lack of insurance reimbursement for the extra time spent, a lack of resources, a lack of time, and a lack of knowledge.[1194] We're just not training doctors how to empower the people they serve.

The current medical education system has yet to adapt to the great transformation of disease from acute to chronic. Medicine is no longer just about setting broken bones or curing strep throat. Such chronic diseases as diabetes are now the principal cause of death and disability in America, consuming three-quarters of the nation's health care budget. Medical education has yet to recognize and respond to the changing nature of disease patterns, which now requires a focus on prevention and lifestyle change.[1195] How far behind the times is the medical profession? A report by the Institute of Medicine on medical training concluded that the fundamental approach to medical education has not changed since 1910.[1196]

I still remember an email I received that helps sum up where we are. Tonah, then a sixty-five-year-old Native American, had been on insulin for type 2 diabetes for twenty-seven years. He was told by his doctor that Native Americans were "genetically predisposed" to the disease. He just had to live with it, including the excruciating nerve pain, three heart stents, and erectile dysfunction. After watching my "Uprooting the Leading Causes of Death" video on NutritionFacts.org, his granddaughter convinced him to try a plant-based diet.

It wasn't easy, since, at the time, the nearest store with fresh food was fifty miles away. Nevertheless, in less than two weeks, he turned his life around. His nerve pain diminished dramatically, to the point where it no longer kept him up at night. He lost thirty pounds in a matter of months and no longer needed insulin. His own doctor couldn't believe this was possible and ordered a CT scan to check for tumors. There weren't any. He felt better than he had in years.

"I'm grateful that my granddaughter has stopped seeing me as a sick old man," Tonah concluded his note. "I feel young again, Doc."

How Not to Die from Liver Diseases

There are some patients you never forget. It was the first day of my GI rotation. GI stands for *gastrointestinal*, which means I was about to come face-to-face with any issues in the digestive tract from mouth to tush. I reported in and was told to go observe my team of senior doctors in one of the endoscopy rooms, where physicians use a scope to look into the GI tract for all manner of routine procedures. I expected to walk into a colonoscopy looking at a rectal polyp or maybe an upper endoscopy looking at a stomach ulcer. But I'll never forget what I saw. It fuels me to this day in my mission to help people understand the connection between lifestyle and health.

A sedated patient was lying on a trolley, surrounded by a team of doctors using a scope with a camera. I looked at the monitor, trying to find anatomical landmarks to understand where the scope was. It was definitely down her throat, but the esophagus was snaked with what looked like throbbing varicose veins. They were everywhere. They looked like worms trying to emerge from under the smooth surface of the esophagus. Several had eroded through the lining and were spurting blood. I watched as more blood surged out with every one of the patient's heartbeats. She was basically bleeding to death into her stomach. The doctors tried desperately to cauterize and tie off these fountains of fresh red blood, but it was like a game of Whac-A-Mole. Every time one was cut off, another sprang up.

These were known as *esophageal varices*—veins swollen with backed-up blood due to a cirrhotic liver. Watching this nightmare unfold, I wondered how the patient first came down with cirrhosis. Was she an alcoholic? Did she contract hepatitis? I remember thinking how devastated she must have felt when she found out she had end-stage liver disease. How was her family coping? I was jerked back from my thoughts by screeching monitor alarms. She was bleeding out.

The doctors couldn't transfuse blood faster than the patient was losing it internally. Her blood pressure fell, and her heart stopped. The staff jumped into action with chest compressions, paddles delivering shocks, and injections of adrenaline, but within minutes, she was gone.

It was my job to talk with the patient's family. I learned that her cirrhosis was not due to drinking too much or from being an IV drug user. Her liver had scarred over because she was obese and had developed a fatty liver. Everything I had just witnessed was preventable, a direct result of lifestyle choices. As we've discussed, when people are overweight, they can suffer from social stigma, knee problems, and increased risk for metabolic disorders like diabetes, but this was the first person I saw bleed to death before my eyes.

The family cried. I cried. I swore to myself I'd do whatever was necessary to help prevent this from ever happening to anyone under my care.

We can make do with only one kidney. We can survive without a spleen or a gallbladder. We can even get by without a stomach. But we can't live without a liver, the body's largest internal organ.

What exactly does the liver do? Up to five hundred different functions have been attributed to this vital organ.[1197] First and foremost, it plays the role of bouncer, keeping unwanted guests out of our bloodstream. Whatever we absorb through our digestive tract isn't immediately circulated throughout our body. The blood from our intestines first goes straight to the liver, where nutrients are metabolized and toxins are neutralized. It's no surprise, then, that what we eat can and does play a critical role in liver health and disease.

About eighty thousand Americans die of liver disease every year.[1198,1199] That's a distressing increase of twenty thousand more lives lost annually since the first edition of this book, and the death rate continues to rise.[1200] Liver dysfunction can run in families, like the iron-overload disease hemochromatosis. It can be caused by infections that can lead to liver cancer, or it can stem from drugs—most often inadvertent or intentional overdoses of paracetamol.[1201] The most common causes, however, are drink and food: alcoholic liver disease and fatty liver disease.

ALCOHOLIC LIVER DISEASE

Alcohol use appears to be the eleventh leading risk factor for dying globally,[1202] potentially leading to millions of deaths annually[1203] and resulting in more than twice as many healthy years of life lost than all illicit drug use combined.[1204] About half of all alcohol-related deaths may be due to sudden causes, such as vehicular accidents; the other half are slower, with alcoholic liver disease the leading cause.[1205] Over the last twenty years or so in the United States, there has been about a 50 percent increase in alcoholism rates, annual alcohol-related emergency room visits,[1206] and alcohol-related death rates.[1207] Alcohol appears to kill about 100,000 Americans every year.[1208]

Excessive alcohol consumption can lead to an accumulation of fat in the liver (what's known as fatty liver), which can cause inflammation and result in liver scarring and, eventually, liver failure. The CDC defines *excessive drinking* as the regular consumption of more than one drink a day for women and more than two a day for men. A drink is defined as 355 ml of beer, 237 ml of high-strength beer, 148 ml of wine, or 44 ml (a "shot") of spirits.[1209] Progression of the disease can usually be halted by stopping drinking, but sometimes it's too late.[1210]

Heavy alcohol consumption can cause a fatty liver in less than three weeks,[1211] but it usually resolves within four to six weeks after stopping drinking.[1212] But in 5 to 15 percent of cases, the disease continues to progress, and the liver starts to scar despite alcohol cessation.[1213]

Similarly, once alcohol-induced hepatitis (liver inflammation) is diagnosed, three-year survival rates can be as high as 90 percent among people who stop drinking after diagnosis.[1214] But as many as 18 percent of them go on to develop cirrhosis, an irreparable scarring of the liver.[1215]

The best strategy to avoid alcoholic liver disease is to not drink so much in the first place. But if you do drink excessively, help is available. Though most people who drink may not have an alcohol abuse problem,[1216] there is convincing evidence that twelve-step programs such as Alcoholics Anonymous can be effective for those who do suffer from alcohol dependence.[1217]

Isn't Moderate Drinking Beneficial?

Everyone agrees that heavy drinking, drinking during pregnancy, and binge drinking are bad ideas, but what about "moderate" drinking? In large populations followed over time, in general, the more people drink, the higher their risk of dying prematurely. However, those with the lowest risk, those who tend to live the longest, are not the abstainers who drink zero alcohol but those who imbibe a few drinks a week.[1218] The mortality-versus-drinking curve, therefore, resembles the letter J rather than being a straight diagonal line that goes up like a slash.

I describe our evolution in understanding in my video see.nf/jcurve, but, long story short, this appears to be an artifact of the "sick quitter effect" arising from the systematic misclassification of former drinkers as lifelong abstainers.[1219] It's the same reason studies can find higher mortality rates among those who quit smoking compared to those who continue to smoke. It's not that abstention led to poor health but rather that poor health led to abstention.[1220]

When researchers went back and controlled for the error of misclassifying former drinkers as if they were lifelong abstainers, the J-shaped curve disappeared. In other words, the death-versus-alcohol relationship became more consistent with a linear dose response, meaning more alcohol, more death, with no protection at low levels of consumption.[1221]

Given the known harms and vanishing evidence of benefit, the most comprehensive analysis on the overall effect of alcohol use[1222] echoed the clear and unambiguous conclusion of the World Health Organization[1223] and the World Heart Federation[1224] and many national drinking guidelines[1225] that the "safest level of drinking is none."[1226]

NONALCOHOLIC LIVER DISEASE

The most common cause of a fatty liver is not alcohol but *nonalcoholic fatty liver disease*, recently renamed *metabolic dysfunction-associated steatotic liver disease* (MASLD), since the words "alcoholic" and "fatty" might be considered stigmatizing.[1227] (*Steatotic* is just doctor-speak for fatty.) You may remember the blockbuster documentary *Super Size Me*, in which the film's director, Morgan Spurlock, ate exclusively at McDonald's for a month. Predictably, Spurlock's weight, blood pressure, and cholesterol all went up—but so did his liver enzymes. That was a sign that his liver cells were dying and spilling their contents into his bloodstream. How was his diet causing liver damage? Let's put it this way: He was beginning to turn his liver into human foie gras (fatty liver pâté).

Some critics wrote off the film as overly sensational, but researchers in Sweden took it seriously enough to formally replicate Spurlock's one-man experiment. In their study, a group of men and women agreed to eat two fast-food meals a day. At the start, their liver enzyme levels were normal, but after just one week of this diet, more than 75 percent of the volunteers' liver function test results became pathological.[1228] If an unhealthy diet can cause liver damage within just seven days, it should be no surprise that MASLD has quietly become the most common cause of chronic liver disease in the United States, afflicting an estimated one hundred million people.[1229] That's about one in three adults. Nearly 100 percent of those with severe obesity may be affected.[1230]

Like alcoholic fatty liver, MASLD starts with a buildup of fat deposits in the liver that cause no symptoms. In rare cases, this can progress to inflammation and, over years, end up scarring the liver into a state of cirrhosis, resulting in liver cancer, liver failure, and even death—as I saw in that endoscopy suite.[1231]

Fast food is so effective at instigating the disease because MASLD is associated with the intake of soft drinks and meat. Drinking just one can of fizzy drink a day appears to raise the odds of getting fatty liver disease by 45 percent.[1232] Meanwhile, those who eat the meat equivalent of fourteen chicken nuggets or more daily have nearly triple the rate of fatty liver disease compared to people who eat seven nuggets' worth or less.[1233]

MASLD has been characterized as a "tale of fat and sugar,"[1234] but not all fat affects the liver similarly. People suffering from fatty liver inflammation were found to be consuming more animal fat (and cholesterol) but less plant fat (and less fiber and antioxidants).[1235] This may explain why adherence to a Mediterranean-style diet with plenty of fruits, vegetables, whole grains, and beans has been associated with less severe fatty liver disease even though it is not typically a low-fat diet.[1236]

MASLD may also be caused by cholesterol overload.[1237] The dietary cholesterol found in eggs, meat, and dairy can become oxidized and then set off a chain reaction that results in excess fat in the liver.[1238] When the concentration of cholesterol in our liver cells gets too high, it can crystallize like rock candy and result in inflammation. This process is similar to the way uric acid crystals cause gout (as we'll see in chapter 10).[1239] Our white blood cells try to engulf the cholesterol crystals but then die in the process, spilling out inflammatory compounds. This may explain how benign fatty liver cases can turn into serious hepatitis.[1240]

To explore the relationship between diet and serious liver disease, about nine thousand American adults were studied for thirteen years. The researchers noted that their most important finding may be that cholesterol consumption was a strong predictor of cirrhosis and liver cancer. Those consuming the amount of cholesterol found in two Egg McMuffins[1241] or more each day appeared to double their risk of hospitalization or death.[1242]

Our best bet for avoiding MASLD, the most common cause of liver disease, may be to avoid excess calories, sugar, saturated fat, and cholesterol.

VIRAL HEPATITIS

Another common cause of liver disease is viral hepatitis, which is triggered by one or more of five different viruses: hepatitis A, B, C, D, or E. The mode of transmission and prognosis differs for each of these viruses. Hepatitis A is spread primarily through food or water that is tainted with contaminated feces. It can be prevented through vaccination, avoiding raw and undercooked shellfish, and trying to ensure that everyone who handles our food washes their hands after changing diapers or using the toilet.

While hepatitis A virus is foodborne, hepatitis B virus is bloodborne and is transmitted sexually. As with hepatitis A, an effective vaccine is available against hepatitis B. Hepatitis D virus infection can only occur in someone who is already infected with hepatitis B, so it can be prevented by preventing hepatitis B. So get vaccinated for hepatitis B if you haven't already and refrain from intravenous drug use and unsafe sex. Unfortunately, there is currently no vaccine for the hepatitis C virus, but there are now successful treatments that prevent the infection from progressing to liver scarring, cancer, and death.[1243]

Hepatitis C is transmitted via blood, usually through sharing needles rather than via blood transfusions, now that the blood supply is screened for the virus. However, sharing personal-care items that can be contaminated with trace amounts of blood, such as toothbrushes and razors, may also present a risk.[1244]

Although a case was once reported involving a woman who contracted hepatitis C from sharing a supermarket meat slicer with an infected coworker,[1245] the virus would not naturally be present in the meat itself, as humans and chimpanzees are the only animals who appear susceptible to it.

The same cannot be said for hepatitis E virus.

Preventing Hepatitis E Through Diet

As one of the CDC's Division of Viral Hepatitis laboratory chiefs explained in a paper entitled "Much Meat, Much Malady: Changing Perceptions of the Epidemiology of Hepatitis E," hepatitis E virus is now considered a zoonotic disease, able to spread from animals to humans, and pigs may be the primary viral reservoir.[1246]

The shift in thinking began in 2003 when researchers in Japan linked the hepatitis E virus (HEV) with the consumption of grilled pork liver. After testing pig livers from Japanese supermarkets, the researchers determined that nearly 2 percent of the meat tested positive for HEV.[1247] In the United States, it was even worse: Eleven percent of commercial pig livers purchased from supermarkets were contaminated with HEV.[1248]

That's alarming, but how many people really eat pig livers? What about plain pork?

Unfortunately, pork may harbor HEV as well. Experts suspect that much of the U.S. population has been exposed to this virus, as there is known to be a relatively high prevalence of HEV antibodies among U.S. blood donors. This exposure may be a result of individuals consuming HEV-contaminated pork.[1249]

So do more people die of liver disease in countries where pork is more popular? It appears so. The relationship between national per capita pork consumption and deaths from liver disease correlates as tightly as per capita alcohol consumption and liver fatalities. Each pork chop consumed per capita may be associated with about two beers' worth of increased liver mortality risk on a countrywide scale.[1250]

Aren't viruses deactivated by cooking? Usually, but there's always the problem of cross-contaminating our hands or kitchen surfaces while handling raw meat. Once meat is in the oven, most foodborne pathogens can be destroyed by cooking the meat to proper internal cooking temperatures, with an emphasis on *proper*. Researchers at the National Institutes of Health subjected the hepatitis E virus to various levels of heat and found that HEV can survive the internal temperature of meat cooked rare.[1251] So if you cook pork, invest in a meat thermometer and make sure to follow proper handling techniques, including washing kitchen surfaces with a bleach solution.[1252]

Though most people who develop hepatitis E recover completely, it can be deadly for pregnant women. The risk of death during the third trimester can reach as high as 30 percent.[1253] If you are pregnant, please be especially careful about pork preparation. And if there are people in the household who like their pork pink in the middle, they should be sure to wash their hands thoroughly after using the bathroom.

Weight-Loss Supplements and Liver Disease

We've all seen those marketing schemes involving products espousing all sorts of health claims. And given the pyramid-like multilevel structure of those types of distribution programs—you earn money by selling products and also for recruiting others to sell—word can spread pretty fast, which is particularly troubling when PR outruns the truth.

Indeed, while the vast majority of drug-induced liver injuries are caused by conventional medications, liver damage caused by certain classes of dietary supplements can be even more serious and may lead to higher rates of liver transplants and death.[1254] Multilevel marketers of products later linked to toxic reactions (such as noni juice[1255] and Herbalife[1256]) have pointed to scientific studies to support their health claims. However, a public health review found that such studies often seemed "deliberately created for marketing purposes" and were presented in such a way as to appear "designed to mislead potential consumers." Often, multilevel marketing study researchers didn't disclose their funding sources, but a little detective work can expose a web of financial conflicts of interest.[1257]

These suspect studies were the same ones cited to provide proof of safety for their products. For example, a multilevel marketing company that sells mangosteen juice cited a study it paid for to support its assertion that its product is "safe for everyone." The study involved exposing just thirty people to its product, with another ten people given a placebo. With so few people tested, the stuff could literally kill 1 or 2 percent of users and we wouldn't know.[1258]

A study that the multilevel marketing company behind a supplement called Metabolife cited for safety placed thirty-five people on its pills.[1259] Metabolife has since been withdrawn from the market after being linked to heart attacks, strokes, seizures, and deaths.[1260] Hydroxycitric acid, a component of such products as Hydroxycut, was studied on forty people.[1261] No serious adverse effects were found, but the story ended the same way: Hydroxycut was withdrawn after dozens of verified cases of organ damage were brought to light—including massive liver failure requiring transplantation and even death.[1262] Until the multibillion-dollar herbal supplement industry is better regulated, we're better off saving our money—and our health—by sticking to real food.

PROTECTING THE LIVER AT BREAKFAST

Specific plant foods have been found to be protective of the liver. For instance, starting out the day with a bowl of oatmeal and (surprisingly) coffee may help safeguard our liver function.

Oatmeal

In numerous population studies, consumption of whole grains has been associated with reduced risk of a range of chronic diseases,[1263] but it's hard to tease out whether eating whole grains may just be a marker for a healthier lifestyle in general. For example, people who eat whole grains, such as oatmeal, whole wheat, and brown rice, also tend to be more physically active, smoke less, and eat more fruits, vegetables, and dietary fiber[1264] than those who might prefer a breakfast of, say, Coco Pops. No wonder the former group may have lower disease risk. Fortunately, researchers can control for these factors, effectively comparing nonsmokers only to nonsmokers with similar diet and exercise habits. When that's done, whole grains still appear to be protective.[1265]

In other words, the evidence seems clear that oatmeal eaters may have lower rates of disease, but that's not the same as showing that our risk will drop if we start eating more oatmeal. To prove cause and effect, we need to put it to the test by performing an interventional trial: Change people's diets and see what happens. Ideally, researchers would randomly split people into two groups and give half of them oatmeal and the other half a placebo—a fake, similar-tasting and -looking oatmeal. Neither the study participants nor the researchers themselves can know who's in which group until the end. This robust, double-blind method is easy to use when studying drugs, as you just give people a sugar pill that looks like the drug in question. As we've discussed, it's not as easy to make placebo food.

But in 2013, a group of researchers published the first double-blind, randomized, placebo-controlled trial of oatmeal in overweight men and women.[1266] They found a significant reduction in liver inflammation in the real oatmeal group, but that may have been because they lost so much more weight than those in the control group eating the placebo oatmeal. Nearly 90 percent of the real-oatmeal eaters had lost weight, compared with no weight loss, on average, among the control group. So it may be that the benefits of whole grains on liver function are indirect.[1267] A follow-up study in 2014 helped confirm the findings of a protective role for whole grains in MASLD patients in reducing the risk of liver inflammation. In this study, refined grain consumption was associated with increased risk of the disease.[1268] So lay off the sliced, white loaf and stick to truly wonderful whole-grain foods, including oatmeal.

Make Your Own Whole-Cranberry Cocktail

A specific class of plant compounds called *anthocyanins*—the purple, red, and blue pigments in such plants as berries, grapes, plums, red cabbage, and red onions—have been found to prevent fat accumulation in human liver cells in in vitro studies.[1269] A single confirmatory clinical (human) trial has been published in which a purple sweet potato concoction successfully dampened liver inflammation better than a placebo.[1270]

When it came to suppressing the growth of human liver cancer cells in a petri dish,[1271] cranberries beat out the other most common fruits in the United States: apples, bananas, grapefruits, grapes, lemons, oranges, peaches, pears, pineapples, and strawberries. Other studies have found that cranberries are also effective in vitro against additional cancers, including those of the brain,[1272] breast,[1273] colon,[1274] lung,[1275] mouth,[1276] ovary,[1277] prostate,[1278] and stomach.[1279] Unfortunately, there have yet to be clinical studies of the effects of cranberries on cancer outcomes that confirm these findings.

Moreover, to the drug industry's chagrin, scientists have been unable to pin down the active ingredients involved in cranberries' special effects. Extracts concentrating individual components fail to match the anticancer effects of the cranberry as a whole,[1280] which of course can't be patented. More proof that it's nearly always best to give preference to whole foods.

How do you do that with cranberries, though, since they're so tart?

It's not easy at the supermarket. Ninety-five percent of cranberries are sold in the form of processed products, such as juices and sauces.[1281] In fact, to get the same amount of anthocyanins found in 140 grams of fresh or frozen cranberries, we'd have to drink 4 liters of cranberry juice cocktail, eat 1.1 kilos of dried cranberries, or make our way through 9.2 liters of cranberry sauce.[1282] The ruby-red phytonutrient found in cranberries is a powerful antioxidant, but the high-fructose corn syrup typically added to cranberry cocktail acts as a pro-oxidant, canceling out some of the benefit.[1283]

I just put defrosted cranberries in my oatmeal, but here's a simple recipe for a whole food version of a tasty cranberry beverage, what I call my Pink Juice:

1 handful fresh or frozen cranberries
500 ml water
2 tablespoons date powder (a whole food composed of straight powdered dates)

Place all the ingredients in a blender and blend at high speed. Pour over ice and serve.

This recipe has three times fewer calories and at least eight times more phytonutrients than typical cranberry juice drinks.[1284]

For an extra boost, blend in some fresh mint leaves. It'll give your drink an exotic green foam on top, and not only will it taste good, but you'll be happy to know that you're sipping berries and leafy greens, two of the healthiest foods on the planet. Bottoms up!

Coffee

Back in 1986, a group of Norwegian researchers came across an unexpected finding: Alcohol consumption was associated with liver inflammation (no surprise there), but coffee consumption was associated with *less* liver inflammation.[1285] These results were replicated in subsequent studies performed around the world. In the United States, a study was done with people at high risk for liver disease—for example, those who were overweight or drank too much alcohol. Subjects who drank more than two cups of coffee a day appeared to have less than half the risk of developing chronic liver problems as those who drank less than one cup.[1286]

What about liver cancer, one of the most feared complications of chronic liver inflammation? It is now the fifth-leading cause of cancer-related death,[1287] and expected to worsen, driven largely by increases in alcoholic liver disease and MASLD.[1288]

Recent review studies involving more than two million participants found that people who drank more coffee had only about half the risk of liver cancer compared to those who drank less.[1289] One study found the consumption of four or more cups of coffee a day was associated with 92 percent lower risk among smokers dying from chronic liver disease.[1290] Of course, quitting smoking would have helped as well; smoking may multiply by as much as tenfold the odds of those with untreated hepatitis C dying from liver cancer.[1291] Similarly, heavy alcohol drinkers who consume more than four cups of coffee per day appear to reduce their risk of liver inflammation—but not by nearly as much as people who cut down on alcohol.[1292]

Liver cancers are among the most avoidable cancers, through hepatitis B vaccination, treatment of hepatitis C infection, and reduction of alcohol consumption. These three measures could, in principle, eliminate 90 percent of liver cancers worldwide. It remains unclear whether drinking coffee has an additional role to play, but such a role would be limited compared with preventing liver damage in the first place.[1293]

But what if you're already among the more than one in three adults[1294] with MASLD, a liver diseased with excess fat? To see if coffee could dampen liver inflammation, researchers placed forty patients with chronic hepatitis C into two groups: The first group consumed four cups of coffee daily for a month, while the second group drank no coffee at all. After thirty days, the groups switched. Of course, two months is not long enough to detect changes in cancer outcomes, but during that time, the researchers were able to demonstrate that coffee consumption may reduce DNA damage, increase the clearance of virus-infected cells, and slow the scarring process.[1295] These results help explain the role coffee appears to play in reducing the risk of liver disease progression.

A commentary in the journal *Gastroenterology* entitled "Is It Time to Write a Prescription for Coffee?" explored the pros and cons.[1296] Some insist that we must first identify the active ingredient in coffee beans that's protective. After all, more than one thousand different compounds have already been found in coffee.[1297] More studies are needed, but meanwhile, moderate daily ingestion of unsweetened coffee should be considered a reasonable adjunct to medical therapy for people at high risk for liver damage, such as those with fatty liver disease.[1298] See the section about coffee in the Beverages chapter for the potential downsides of coffee consumption.

With liver disease, as always, prevention is the key. All the most serious liver conditions—liver cancer, liver failure, and cirrhosis—can start with an inflamed liver. That inflammation can be caused by an infection or the buildup of fatty deposits. Liver viruses can be prevented by common-sense measures: Don't inject drugs, do get vaccinated, and do practice safe sex. Liver fat can also be prevented by common sense measures: Avoid excess consumption of alcohol, calories, cholesterol, saturated fat, and sugar.

How Not to Die from Blood Cancers

Eleven-year-old Missy had leukemia. It was in remission, thanks in part to the yellow bags of chemo that hung from the IV pole she rolled down the hospital halls. Missy was one of my first patients in my pediatrics rotation during medical school at the Eastern Maine Medical Center in Bangor—home to Stephen King, moose-crossing signs, and billboards advertising lobster ice cream.

During this time, I was in full Patch Adams regalia, from the fuzzy pink rabbit ears on my head down to the plastic rainbow Slinkys trailing at my feet. On every button of my white doctor's coat hung a Beanie Baby, and a plushie animal's foot was crammed into every buttonhole. Robin Williams may have portrayed the famed physician on the big screen, but I channeled him in real life. Missy drew a smiley face on my beanie hippo and named the rooster attached to my stethoscope "Elvis."

She loved to paint pictures for me and signed each one of them, in all caps: FROM MISSY. In these pictures, she still had her curly brown locks. In reality, her head was completely bald. She refused to wear a wig, which only made her smile seem brighter.

I painted her nails a pale pink, and she painted mine a lovely purplish brown.

I remember the morning after she gave me the manicure. My senior resident took me aside after rounds. "Your fingernails are getting in people's way," he said.

"Huh?" I asked.

"The attending physicians are complaining," he replied. "This is a conservative profession."

I tried to explain that I didn't paint them myself, upset that I even felt the need to explain at all. The senior resident knew that Missy had done it, but he didn't seem to care. "Medicine," he said, "is also an anti-emotion profession."

Later, the chair of the department had a talk with me. A number of the attending physicians were concerned I was "too enthusiastic," "too dramatic," and "too sensitive."

My wife remarked they probably just had Slinky envy.

The next day, head down, I walked into Missy's room.

"I'm sorry," I told her. "The doctors made me take off the nail polish."

I held up my hands to show her. She inspected them and said, with great indignation, "If you can't wear it, then I'm not going to either!" So I helped her take off her polish, bemused and empowered by such solidarity from an eleven-year-old. (Then I let her paint my toenails.)

I remember the last note I wrote in Missy's medical chart. Hospital progress notes are written in SOAP format, a mnemonic for Subjective findings, Objective findings, Assessment, and Plan. I wrote: "Assessment: 11yo girl finishing last round of maintenance chemotherapy. Plan: Disney World."

Childhood leukemia is one of the few success stories in our war on cancer, with ten-year survival rates as high as 90 percent.[1299] Yet it still affects more children than any other cancer and is ten times more likely to be diagnosed in adults, among whom current treatments are much less effective.[1300]

What can we do to help prevent blood cancers in the first place?

Blood cancers are sometimes referred to as liquid tumors, since the cancer cells often circulate throughout the body rather than concentrate in a solid mass. These cancers typically begin undetected in the bone marrow, that spongy tissue in the interior of our bones where red blood cells, white blood cells, and platelets are born. When healthy, our red blood cells deliver oxygen throughout our body, our white blood cells fight off infections, and our platelets help our blood to clot. Most blood cancers involve mutations of the white cells.

Blood cancers can be categorized into three types: leukemia, lymphoma, and myeloma. Leukemia (from the Greek roots *leukos*, or "white," and *haima*, or "blood") is a disease in which the bone marrow feverishly produces abnormal white blood cells. Unlike normal ones, these imposters aren't able to fight infection. They also impair the ability of our bone marrow to produce normal red and white cells by crowding out healthy ones, creating a diminished healthy blood cell count that can lead to anemia, infection, and, eventually, death. According to the CDC and the National Cancer Institute, every year, nearly 53,000 Americans are diagnosed with leukemia, and 23,000 die from it.[1301]

Lymphoma is a blood cancer of lymphocytes, which are specialized types of white blood cells. Lymphoma cells multiply quickly and can collect in our lymph nodes, small immune organs that are spread throughout the body, including the armpits, neck, and groin. Lymph nodes help to filter our blood. Like leukemia, lymphoma can crowd out healthy cells and impair our ability to fight infections. You may have heard of non-Hodgkin's lymphoma. Hodgkin's lymphoma can strike young adults, but it's a rare and usually treatable form of lymphoma. As its name suggests, non-Hodgkin's lymphoma (NHL) includes all the other dozens of types of lymphoma. They're more common and can be harder to treat, and their risk increases with age. There are 72,000 new diagnoses of non-Hodgkin's lymphoma and about 19,000 deaths each year just in the United States.[1302]

Finally, myeloma is a cancer of plasma cells, which are white blood cells that produce antibodies, the proteins that stick to invaders and infected cells to neutralize or tag them for destruction. Cancerous plasma cells can displace healthy cells from our bone marrow and make abnormal antibodies that can clog the kidneys. About 90 percent of myeloma sufferers are discovered with masses of cancer cells growing in multiple bones of their bodies, hence the common term for this condition, *multiple myeloma*. Each year, more than 24,000 Americans are diagnosed with multiple myeloma, and 12,000 lose their lives to it.[1303]

Though treatable, multiple myeloma is considered incurable. That's why prevention is key. Fortunately, dietary changes may reduce our risk of all these blood cancers.

FOODS ASSOCIATED WITH DECREASED RISK OF BLOOD CANCERS

After following more than 60,000 people for more than a dozen years, University of Oxford researchers found that those who consume a plant-based diet are less likely to develop all forms of cancer combined. The greatest protection appeared to be against blood cancers. The incidence of leukemia, lymphoma, and multiple myeloma among those eating vegetarian diets is nearly half that of those eating meat.[1304] Why is this greatly reduced risk of blood cancers associated with a more plant-based diet? As the British Journal of Cancer concluded at the time, "More research is needed to understand the mechanisms behind this."[1305] While they are figuring out the reasons, why not get a head start and try adding more healthy plant foods to your plate today?

Greens and Cancer

The key to cancer prevention and treatment is to keep tumor cells from multiplying out of control while allowing healthy cells to grow normally. Chemotherapy and radiation can do a great job of wiping out cancer cells, but healthy cells can get caught in the crossfire. Some compounds in plants, though, may be more discriminating.

For instance, sulforaphane, considered one of the more active components in cruciferous vegetables, kills human leukemia cells in a petri dish while having little impact on the growth of normal cells.[1306] As we've discussed, cruciferous vegetables include broccoli, cauliflower, and kale, but there are many others in this family, such as collard greens, watercress, pak choi, kohlrabi, swede, turnips, rocket, radishes (including horseradish), wasabi, and all types of cabbage.

It's intriguing that dripping cabbage compounds on cancer cells affects them in a laboratory, but what really matters is whether people with blood cancers who eat lots of vegetables actually live longer than those who don't. For about eight years, Yale University researchers followed more than 500 women with non-Hodgkin's lymphoma. Those who started out eating three or more servings of vegetables daily had a 42 percent improved survival rate over those who ate less. Leafy green vegetables, including salad and cooked greens, and citrus fruits appeared most protective.[1307] It's not clear, though, whether the survival benefit arose from helping to keep the cancer at bay or from improving patients' tolerance to the chemotherapy and radiation treatments they were receiving. The accompanying editorial in the journal *Leukemia & Lymphoma* suggested that a "lymphoma diagnosis may be an important 'teachable' moment to improve diet . . ."[1308] I would suggest we not wait until a cancer diagnosis to clean up our diet.

The Iowa Women's Health Study, which followed more than thirty-five thousand women for decades, found that higher broccoli and other cruciferous vegetable intake was associated with lower risk of getting non-Hodgkin's lymphoma in the first place.[1309] Likewise, a study at the Mayo Clinic found that those who ate about five or more servings of leafy green vegetables a week had roughly half the odds of getting lymphoma compared with those who ate less than one serving a week.[1310]

Some of the plant-based protection might have been due to the antioxidant properties of fruits and vegetables. Higher dietary intake of antioxidants is associated with significantly lower lymphoma risk. Note I said *dietary* intake, not supplementary intake. Antioxidant supplements don't appear to work.[1311] For example, getting lots of vitamin C in our diet is associated with lower lymphoma risk, but taking in even more vitamin C in pill form did not seem to help. The same was found for carotenoid antioxidants like beta-carotene.[1312] Apparently, pills do not have the same cancer-fighting effects as produce.

When it comes to certain other cancers, like those of the digestive tract, antioxidant supplements may even make things worse. Combinations of antioxidants like vitamin A, vitamin E, and beta-carotene in pill form were associated with increased risk of death in those who took them.[1313] Supplements contain only a select few antioxidants, whereas our body relies on hundreds of them, all working synergistically to create a network to help the body dispose of free radicals. High doses of a single antioxidant may upset this delicate balance and may actually diminish our body's ability to fight cancer.[1314]

When you buy antioxidant supplements, you may be doling out money to live a shorter life. Save your cash and your health by eating the real thing: food.

Açai Berries and Leukemia

Açai berries gained celebrity status in 2008 when television personality Dr. Mehmet Oz talked about them on *The Oprah Winfrey Show*. This spawned a frenzy of knockoff supplements, powders, shakes, and other dubious products bearing the açai berry label but not necessarily containing any of the actual berry.[1315] Even major corporations jumped on the açai bandwagon, including Anheuser-Busch with its 180 Blue "with Açai Energy" drink and Coca-Cola with its Bossa Nova beverage. This is an all-too-common practice in the "superfruit" supplement and beverage market, where less than a quarter of products sold may even contain the ingredients their labels claim.[1316,1317] The benefits of these products are suspect at best, but there is some preliminary research on real açai berries, which can be purchased as unsweetened frozen pulp.

The first study published in the medical literature on the effects of açai on human tissue was performed on leukemia cells. Researchers dripped an açai berry extract on leukemia cells taken from a thirty-six-year-old woman. It appeared to trigger self-destruct reactions in up to 86 percent of the cells.[1318] Also, sprinkling some freeze-dried açai berries on immune cells called *macrophages* (from the Greek words *makros* and *phagein*, meaning "big eater") in a petri dish appeared to enable the cells to engulf and devour up to 40 percent more microbes than usual.[1319]

Though the leukemia study was done using açai extract at the concentration one might expect to find in the bloodstream after eating the berries, no studies have yet been performed on cancer patients themselves (just cancer cells in a test tube), so more testing is needed.

In terms of antioxidant bang for our buck, açai berries get honorable mention, beating out other superstars, such as walnuts, apples, and cranberries. The bronze for best bargain, though, goes to cloves, the silver to cinnamon, and the gold for most antioxidants per dollar—according to a USDA database of common foods—goes to red cabbage.[1320] Açai berries, however, would probably make a tastier smoothie.

Curcumin and Multiple Myeloma

Multiple myeloma is one of the most dreaded cancers. It is practically incurable even with aggressive medical treatment. As myeloma cells take over the bone marrow, healthy white blood cells continue to decline in number, which increases our susceptibility to infection. Reduced levels of red blood cells can lead to anemia, and reduced platelet counts can lead to serious bleeding.

Multiple myeloma does not occur out of the blue. It appears to be nearly always preceded by a precancerous condition known as *monoclonal gammopa-*

thy of undetermined significance, or MGUS.[1321] When scientists first discovered MGUS, it was aptly named because, at that time, the significance of finding elevated levels of abnormal antibodies in someone's body was unclear. We now know it's a precursor to multiple myeloma, and about 3 percent of Caucasians over age fifty have it,[1322] while the rate among African Americans may be triple that.[1323]

MGUS causes no symptoms. You won't even know you have it unless your doctor finds it incidentally during routine blood work. The chance of MGUS progressing into myeloma is about 1 percent per year, which means many MGUS-stricken people may die of other causes before they develop myeloma.[1324] However, since multiple myeloma is so deadly serious, scientists have been desperate to find ways to stop MGUS in its tracks.

Given the safety and efficacy of the turmeric spice component curcumin against other types of cancer cells, researchers from the University of Texas collected multiple myeloma cells and put them in a petri dish. Without any intervention, the cancer cells quadrupled within a few days—that's how fast this cancer can grow. But when a little curcumin was added to the solution they were bathing in, the myeloma cells' growth was either stunted or stopped altogether.[1325]

As we've covered, stopping cancer in a laboratory is one thing. What about in people? In 2009, a pilot study found that half (five out of ten) of the participants with MGUS who had particularly high abnormal antibody levels responded positively to curcumin supplements. None (zero out of nine) of those given a placebo experienced a similar drop in antibody levels.[1326] Buoyed by this success, scientists conducted a randomized, double-blind, placebo-controlled trial and achieved similarly encouraging results in both patients with MGUS and those with "smoldering" multiple myeloma, an early stage of the disease.[1327] This result suggests that a simple spice found in the supermarket might have the ability to slow or stop this horrific cancer in a certain percentage of patients, though we won't know more until longer studies are performed to see if these hopeful changes in blood work biomarkers translate into changes in patient outcomes. There was another randomized clinical trial published in 2022 with patients with full-blown multiple myeloma in which curcumin supplementation appeared to double remission rates during chemotherapy compared to placebo. Long-term outcomes have yet to be reported.[1328] In the meantime, it couldn't hurt to spice up our diet.

ARE ANIMAL VIRUSES INVOLVED IN HUMAN BLOOD CANCERS?

The reason people eating plant-based diets appear to have much lower rates of blood cancers[1329] may be due to the foods they're choosing to eat and/or choosing to avoid. To tease out the role different animal products might play in the myriad blood cancers, we would need to conduct a very large study. Enter the aptly named EPIC study, the European Prospective Investigation into Cancer and Nutrition, which did just that. As we saw in chapter 6, researchers recruited more than four hundred thousand men and women across ten countries and followed them for about nine years. If you recall, regular chicken consumption was associated with an increased risk for pancreatic cancer. Similar findings were seen for blood cancers. Of all the animal products studied (including unusual categories, such as offal, or entrails and organs), poultry tended to be associated with the greatest increased risk of non-Hodgkin's lymphoma, all grades of follicular lymphoma, and B-cell lymphomas, such as B-cell chronic lymphatic leukemia (including small lymphocytic leukemia and prolymphocytic lymphocytic leukemia).[1330] The EPIC study found that risk increased between 56 percent and 280 percent for every 50 grams of poultry consumed daily. For comparison, a cooked, boneless chicken breast may weigh as much as 384 grams.[1331]

Why is there so much lymphoma and leukemia risk associated with eating such relatively small amounts of poultry? The researchers suggested this result could be a fluke, or it could be due to the drugs, such as antibiotics, that are often fed to chickens and turkeys to promote their growth. Or it might be the dioxins found in some poultry meat, which have been linked to lymphoma.[1332] But dairy can also contain dioxins, and milk consumption was not linked to NHL. The researchers surmised it may be the cancer-causing viruses in poultry, given that lower risk of NHL has been associated with eating meat cooked well done (and thereby inactivating any viruses) instead of rare.[1333] This suggestion is consistent with the results of the NIH-AARP study (see page 133), which found an association between eating just-done chicken and one type of lymphoma and *lower* risk of another blood cancer tied to greater exposure to the cooked meat carcinogen MeIQx.[1334]

How could less cancer be linked to *more* carcinogen exposure? MeIQx is one of the heterocyclic amines created by cooking meat at high temperatures, such as baking, grilling, and frying.[1335] If, in the case of blood cancers, one cause is a poultry virus, then the more the meat was cooked, the more likely it is that the virus was destroyed. Cancer-causing poultry viruses—including the avian herpesvirus that causes Marek's disease, several retroviruses like reticuloendotheliosis virus, the avian leukosis virus found in chickens, and the lymphoproliferative disease virus found in turkeys—may explain the higher rates of blood cancers among farmers,[1336] slaughter plant workers,[1337] and butchers.[1338] Viruses can cause cancer by directly inserting a cancer-causing gene into a host's DNA.[1339]

Animal viruses can infect people who prepare meat with unpleasant skin diseases, such as contagious pustular dermatitis.[1340] There's even a well-defined medical condition commonly known as "butchers' warts" that affects the hands of those who handle fresh meat, including poultry and fish.[1341] Even the wives of butchers appear to be at higher risk for cervical cancer, a cancer definitively associated with wart-virus exposure.[1342]

Workers in poultry slaughter plants have been found to have higher rates of cancers of the mouth, nasal cavities, throat, esophagus, rectum, liver, and blood. On a public health level, the concern here is that the cancer-causing viruses present in poultry and poultry products may then be transmitted to those in the general population who handle or eat inadequately cooked chicken.[1343] These results were replicated in the largest investigations to date, studying tens of thousands of workers in poultry slaughtering and processing plants. They confirmed the findings of three other studies: Workers in these facilities do have increased risk of dying from certain cancers, including cancers of the blood.[1344,1345]

Researchers are finally starting to connect the dots. The high levels of antibodies to avian leukosis/sarcoma viruses[1346] and to reticuloendotheliosis viruses[1347] found in poultry workers provide evidence of human exposure to these cancer-causing poultry viruses. Even line workers in slaughter plants who simply cut up the finished product and are never exposed to live birds had elevated levels of antibodies in their blood.[1348] Beyond just occupational safety, the potential threat to the public, the researchers concluded, "is not trivial."[1349]

Elevated blood cancer rates can even be traced back to the farm. An analysis of more than one hundred thousand death certificates found that those who grew up on a farm raising animals appeared significantly more likely to develop a blood cancer later in life, whereas growing up on a farm growing only crops was not. Worst was growing up on a poultry farm, which was associated with nearly three times the odds of developing blood cancer.[1350]

Exposure to cattle and pigs has also been associated with non-Hodgkin's lymphoma.[1351] A 2003 study by University of California researchers revealed that nearly three-quarters of human subjects tested positive for exposure to the bovine leukemia virus, likely through the consumption of meat and dairy products.[1352] Approximately 85 percent of U.S. dairy herds have tested positive for the virus (and 100 percent on industrial-scale operations).[1353]

However, just because people are exposed to a virus that causes cancer in cows does not mean that humans themselves can become actively infected with it. In 2014, researchers supported in part by the U.S. Army Breast Cancer Research Program published a remarkable report in a journal of the Centers for Disease Control and Prevention. They reported that the bovine leukemia virus DNA was found to be incorporated into human breast tissue, effectively proving that people can also become infected with this cancer-causing animal virus.[1354] Subsequent research comparing infection rates in normal versus cancerous breast tissue offer "strong support" that bovine leukemia virus found in milk and meat[1355] may be a risk factor for breast cancer.[1356] To date, however, the role poultry and other farm animal viruses play in the development of human cancers remains unknown.

What about the *feline* leukemia virus? Thankfully, pet companionship is associated with *lower* rates of lymphoma, which is a personal relief given how many animals I've shared my life with. And the longer people have had cats or dogs in their lives, the lower their risk. In one study, the lowest risk of lymphoma was found in people who had had pets for twenty years or longer. The researchers suspect the reason is connected to the fact that having pets may have beneficial effects on the immune system.[1357]

Who Is Rescuing Whom?

More than two-thirds of U.S. households, including mine, include a pet.[1358] In an "awwww"-inspiring paper published in the prestigious journal *Science* entitled "Oxytocin-Gaze Positive Loop and the Coevolution of Human-Dog Bonds," researchers found that petting or looking into the eyes of a canine companion leads to oxytocin release in the brains of both the humans and the dogs—the same "love hormone" that bonds breastfeeding mothers to their infants.[1359]

I was reading about the potential mechanisms by which our animal companions might improve our survival after a heart attack when I ran across a passage about a "profound" cardiovascular response when petting dogs or horses. "This response usually takes the form of a significant reduction in the heart rate and blood pressure." I could totally see that. But then the next sentence made me do a double take: "Unfortunately, we have no information about the physiological responses of the person doing the petting."[1360] The researchers were talking about the heart rate and blood pressure of the animals!

To my surprise, studies of the effects of companion animals on human health have, as one review put it, produced a "mishmash of conflicting results."[1361] A meta-analysis of studies involving more than three million people followed for an average of a decade did find that having a canine companion, for example, was associated with a 24 percent reduction in risk of premature death. The authors suggested that enhanced survival may be a result of the increased physical activity we get when we take our dogs for walks.[1362] That could also help explain why sharing our lives and homes with animals (or grandchildren) has been associated with a lower risk of frailty.[1363] Of course, this too could be reverse causation, where people who are already active are more likely to get a dog in the first place, but the greater issue may be confounding factors.[1364]

People with pets tend to be younger, wealthier, more educated, and more often married.[1365] Sadly, when these types of elements are taken into account, the significant mortality risk reduction disappears.[1366] The same seems to be true for pet ownership in general. The higher survival rate becomes statistically insignificant once confounding factors, like socioeconomic characteristics, are considered.

When it comes specifically to cats, though, confounding can work in the opposite direction. Given evidence that social support may help with survival after a heart attack, a number of studies have been undertaken to see if animal companionship can help.[1367] One study found that people living with cats had a significantly *greater* risk of death.[1368] This may be because they appear to be not only more likely to be sedentary than people with dogs, who may be taking more walks, but cat owners may also be more sedentary than people without any pets at all.[1369]

> Given the pitfalls of trying to impute cause and effect from observational studies, I was so excited to see a randomized controlled trial that actually put animal companionship to the test. Don't get your hopes up too much, though. The title of the study was "Effect of Pet Insects on the Psychological Health of Community-Dwelling Elderly People: A Single-Blinded, Randomized, Controlled Trial." Pet insects? Yes. Crickets. Nevertheless, older individuals (average age of seventy-two) randomized to take care of crickets experienced a significantly greater improvement in depression, cognitive status, and mental health quality of life, compared to the control group.[1370] So, maybe there's hope for Fido yet.
>
> Most investigations on pets and human health are snapshot-in-time studies where it's impossible to know which came first, but longitudinal studies, which take place over time, have shown that people who walk their dogs are indeed more likely to achieve recommended activity levels.[1371] Sadly, only a minority of older dog owners (36 percent) took their dogs for walks even three times a week.[1372] To maximize the benefits for pooch and person alike, we should heed this wise advice from a medical journal article published in 1925: "The best prescription to be written for a walk is to take a dog, a cane and a friend."[1373]

A pair of Harvard University studies suggested that diet fizzy drink consumption may increase the risk of non-Hodgkin's lymphoma and multiple myeloma,[1374] but this association was only seen among men and was not confirmed in two other large studies on aspartame-sweetened fizzy drinks.[1375,1376] Artificially sweetened beverage consumption is associated with leukemia,[1377] though, so we should eliminate fizzy drinks from our diets for this reason—and many others.

Plant-based diets are associated with nearly half the risk of blood cancers, protection likely derived both from the avoidance of foods tied to liquid tumors, such as poultry, as well as the additional consumption of fruits and vegetables. Greens may be particularly useful for non-Hodgkin's lymphoma and turmeric for multiple myeloma. The role tumor-promoting farm animal viruses play in human cancers is not known, but this should be a research priority given the potential extent of public exposure.

How Not to Die from Kidney Disease

Letters and emails from patients never fail to inspire me. One note that came to mind as I was writing this chapter was from Dan, a retired NFL player. I first met him when he was forty-two. Even at that relatively young age, the former professional athlete was already taking three separate blood pressure medications. Still, his blood pressure was elevated. He was a little overweight, maybe by twenty-five pounds. He and his significant other waited around after one of my talks to see me.

Dan's physician had just told him that his kidneys were starting to show signs of damage due to his blood pressure. The first thing I asked was if he was taking his meds as prescribed, since many people skip their blood pressure medications because of their unpleasant side effects. Yes, he assured me, he was. He showed me a checklist he carried around to keep track of his meds. He asked me what supplements he could add to the list to help his kidneys.

I told him that no matter what he might have seen on the internet, there's no such magic pill, but if he filled up his plate with lots of whole, healthy foods each day, the damage might be stopped or even reversed. Well, Dan took this advice to heart (and to kidney!), and he allowed me to share his email:

Well, I went home that night and we cleaned house. Got rid of everything that didn't grow out of the ground, everything processed. And guess what, over the next year, I lost my beer belly and the high blood pressure. Life is so much better without those medications—they made me feel so tired all the time. And my kidney function is back to normal. It makes me mad that no one told me this sooner and that I had to feel so bad before I felt better.

It's easy to take our kidneys for granted, but they work around the clock, like a high-tech, nonstop water filter for our blood. They process up to 142 liters of blood every twenty-four hours just to make the 1 to 2 liters of urine we pee out each day.

If our kidneys do not function properly, metabolic waste products can accumulate in the blood and eventually lead to such symptoms as weakness, shortness of breath, confusion, and abnormal heart rhythms. Most people with deteriorating kidney function, however, don't experience any symptoms at all. If our kidneys fail completely, we will either need a new one (i.e., need a kidney transplant) or have to go on dialysis, a process by which a machine artificially filters the blood. But kidney donors can be difficult to come by, and the average life expectancy of a person on dialysis is around four years.[1378] It's better to keep our kidneys healthy in the first place.

Although our kidneys can fail suddenly in response to certain toxins, infections, or urinary blockage, most kidney disease is characterized by a gradual loss of function over time. According to the Centers for Disease Control and Prevention, about forty million Americans have chronic kidney disease (CKD), but, astoundingly, as many as nine out of ten of them don't even know it. The risk of impaired kidney function increases with age, such that one in three people over the age of sixty-four may suffer with CKD.[1379] More than half of American adults currently aged thirty to sixty-four are expected to develop chronic kidney disease during their lifetimes.[1380]

Why, then, aren't millions of people on dialysis? Because kidney malfunction can be so damaging to the rest of the body that most people don't live long enough to reach that stage. In a study in which more than a thousand Americans over age sixty-four with CKD were followed for a decade, only one in twenty developed end-stage kidney failure. Most of the others had already died, with cardiovascular disease killing more than all other causes combined.[1381] That's because our kidneys are so critical to proper heart function that patients under age forty-five with kidney failure can be a hundred times more likely to die of heart disease than those with working kidneys.[1382]

The good news? The diets that are healthiest for our hearts—those centered around unprocessed plant foods—may be the best way to prevent and treat kidney disease as well.

Damaging Our Kidneys with Diet

Kidneys are highly vascular organs, meaning they're packed with blood vessels, which is why they look so red. We've already seen that the standard American diet can be toxic to blood vessels in the heart and the brain—so what might it be doing to our kidneys?

Putting that question to the test, researchers at Harvard University followed thousands of healthy women, their diets, and their kidney function for more than a decade[1383] to look for the presence of protein in the women's urine. Healthy kidneys work hard to retain protein and other vital nutrients, preferably filtering toxic or useless wastes out of the bloodstream via our urine. If the kidneys are leaking protein into urine, it's a sign that they may be starting to fail.

The researchers found three specific dietary components associated with this sign of declining kidney function: animal protein, animal fat, and cholesterol. Each of these is found in only one place: animal products. The researchers found no association between kidney function decline and the intake of protein or fat from plant sources.[1384]

One hundred and sixty years ago, Rudolf Virchow, the father of modern pathology, first described fatty degeneration of the kidney.[1385] This concept of lipid nephrotoxicity, or the idea that fat and cholesterol in the bloodstream could be toxic to the kidneys, has since been formalized,[1386] based in part on studies that found plugs of fat clogging up the works in autopsied kidneys.[1387]

The link between cholesterol and kidney disease has gained such momentum in the medical community that cholesterol-lowering statin drugs have been recommended to slow its progression.[1388] But wouldn't it be better (not to mention safer and cheaper) to treat the underlying cause of the disease by eating healthier?

Which Type of Protein Is Better for Our Kidneys?

In the two decades between 1990 and 2010, the leading causes of death and disability remained relatively constant. As noted in chapter 1, heart disease is still the leading cause of loss of health and life. Some diseases, such as HIV/AIDS, have slid down the list, but among the diseases whose incidence has increased the most over the past generation is chronic kidney disease. The number of deaths has doubled.[1389]

. This has been blamed on our "meat-sweet" diet.[1390] Excess table sugar and high-fructose corn syrup consumption is associated with increased blood pressure and uric acid levels, both of which can damage the kidney. The saturated fat, trans fat, and cholesterol found in animal products and junk food are also associated with impaired kidney function, and meat protein increases the acid load to the kidneys, boosting ammonia production and potentially damaging our sensitive kidney cells.[1391] This is why a restriction of protein intake is often recommended to chronic kidney disease patients to help prevent further functional decline.[1392]

But all protein isn't created equal. It's important to understand that not all protein has the same effect on our kidneys.

High animal protein intake can have a profound influence on normal human kidney function by inducing a state called *hyperfiltration*, a dramatic increase in the workload of the kidney. Hyperfiltration isn't harmful if it occurs only occasionally. We all have built-in reserve kidney function—so much so that people can live with only one kidney. The human body is thought to have evolved the capacity to handle intermittent large doses of protein from our remote hunting and scavenging days. But now many of us are ingesting large doses of animal protein day after day, forcing our kidneys to call on their reserves continuously. Over time, this unrelenting stress may explain why kidney function tends to decline as people age, predisposing even otherwise healthy people to progressive deterioration of kidney function.[1393]

The reason those who eat a plant-based diet appear to have better kidney function was originally thought to be due to their lower overall protein intake.[1394] However, we now know that it's more likely due to the fact that our kidneys appear to handle plant protein very differently from animal protein.[1395]

Within hours of consuming meat, our kidneys rev up into hyperfiltration mode. This is true of a variety of animal proteins—beef, chicken, and fish appear to have similar effects.[1396] But an equivalent amount of plant protein causes virtually no noticeable stress on the kidneys.[1397] Eat some tuna, and within three hours, kidney filtration rate can shoot up 36 percent. But eating the same amount of protein in the form of tofu doesn't appear to place any additional strain on the kidneys.[1398]

Could substituting plant protein for animal protein help slow the deterioration of kidney function? Yes, half a dozen clinical trials have shown that plant protein replacement can reduce hyperfiltration and/or protein leakage,[1399,1400,1401,1402,1403,1404] but all these studies were short-term, lasting fewer than eight weeks. It wasn't until 2014 that a six-month, double-blind, randomized, placebo-controlled clinical trial was performed examining how the kidneys process soya protein versus dairy protein. Consistent with the other studies, plant protein was found to help preserve function in ailing kidneys.[1405]

Why does animal protein cause the overload reaction while plant protein doesn't? Apparently because of the inflammation animal products can cause. Researchers discovered that after giving study participants a powerful anti-inflammatory drug along with animal protein, the hyperfiltration response and protein spillage disappeared.[1406]

Reducing Dietary Acid Load

Another reason animal protein may be so detrimental to kidney function is that it is generally more acid-forming. This is because animal protein tends to have higher levels of sulfur-containing amino acids, such as methionine, which produce sulfuric acid when metabolized in the body. Fruits and vegetables, on the other hand, are generally base-forming, which helps neutralize acids in our kidneys.[1407]

Dietary acid load is determined by the balance of acid-inducing foods (such as meats, eggs, and cheeses) and base-inducing foods (such as fruits and vegetables). Most studies of diets and kidney function found that a higher dietary acid load was associated with significantly higher risk of both developing[1408] and exacerbating[1409] chronic kidney disease.

Ancient human diets largely consisted of plants, so they likely produced more base than acid in the kidneys of our ancestors. Humans and prehumans evolved eating these alkaline (base-forming) diets over millions of years. Most contemporary diets, on the other hand, produce acid in excess. This switch from base- to acid-forming diets may help explain our modern epidemic of kidney disease.[1410] Acid-inducing diets are believed to impact the kidney through "tubular toxicity," damage to the tiny, delicate, urine-making tubes in the kidneys. To buffer the excess acid formed by our diet, kidneys produce ammonia, which is a base and can neutralize some of that acid. Counteracting the acid is beneficial in the short term, but over the long run, all the extra ammonia in the kidneys may have a toxic effect.[1411] The decline in kidney function over time may be a consequence of a lifetime of ammonia overproduction.[1412] Kidneys may start to deteriorate in our twenties,[1413] and by the time we reach our eighties, we may be down to half capacity.[1414]

The chronic, low-grade, metabolic acidosis attributed to a meat-rich diet[1415] helps explain why people eating plant-based diets appear to have superior kidney function[1416] and why various plant-based diets have been so successful in treating chronic kidney failure.[1417,1418] Under normal circumstances, a vegetarian diet alkalinizes the kidneys, whereas a nonvegetarian diet carries an acid load. This proved to be true even among vegetarians who consumed ultra-processed meat alternatives, such as veggie burgers.[1419]

Ultra-Processed Meat Alternatives Are Better than the Alternative

Ultra-processed foods are products that can't be made in home kitchens because they are chemically or physically transformed using industrial processes.[1420] They typically contain little or no whole foods, are ready-to-consume or just need to be heated up, and are fatty, salty, or sugary and depleted in dietary fiber and other nutrients. Think sweet, fatty, or salty snacks, like crisps, ice cream, fizzy drinks, candy, french fries, chicken nuggets, fish sticks, hot dogs, and deli meat.[1421]

The link between ultra-processed food consumption and premature death appears to be limited to only two categories of ultra-processed foods: sweetened beverages and ultra-processed animal products.[1422] However, the association between more ultra-processed foods and higher mortality appears to be present even among vegetarians.[1423]

Plant-based diets are associated with a reduced risk of a variety of chronic diseases, but that doesn't mean we can live off vegan donuts. Whole plant foods, like fruits and vegetables, are associated with lower risk of disease, but ultra-processed "plant-based" foods like Oreos and Mountain Dew are associated with higher risks.[1424] What about plant-based meats, like veggie burgers?

The EPIC study, true to its name, was large enough to answer that question. More than a quarter million people were followed for more than a decade. Higher consumption of ultra-processed foods in general was associated with an increased risk of chronic diseases, such as cancer, cardiovascular disease, and diabetes, but when the researchers drilled down, they found that only fizzy drinks and the animal-based ultra-processed products, like processed meat, were to blame. They looked specifically at ultra-processed plant-based foods and found no increased risk. Beverages aside, the only ultra-processed food that appears to be killing people is meat.[1425] In that case, instead of being a contributor, plant-based meats may be the *solution* to the ultra-processed foods problem.

In my forthcoming 2026 book *Ultra-Processed Foods: Concerns, Controversies, and Exceptions*, I take a deep dive into all the interventional trials that study the health effects of randomizing people to try replacing some of their meat with plant-based meat. The Stanford SWAP-MEAT study, for example, found that switching out a few servings a day of meat for plant-based meat for two months significantly decreased circulating levels of the microbiome toxin TMAO, as well as lowered LDL cholesterol and body weight.[1426] The longest study was a four-year, randomized clinical trial in which people with diabetes and ailing kidneys either replaced half their animal protein intake with an ultra-processed plant-based meat replacement called TVP (textured vegetable protein) or continued eating their regular diet. The researchers saw significant improvements in blood sugar control, cholesterol, triglycerides, inflammation, and kidney function in those who swapped out some of their meat for TVP.[1427]

Diets high in processed and red meats are also the two leading causes of diet-related disability in the United States, responsible for more than a million years lived in disability annually. That's three times more than diets high in sugar-sweetened beverages and translates into more than two million years of lost life.[1428] How is "high" defined? A diet "high" in processed meat is defined as having *any* intake of processed meat.[1429] And a diet "high" in red meat? Any intake above *zero* grams a day.[1430] Millions of years of life are lost annually in the United States alone because people are eating more than zero red and processed meats.

Higher intake of meat in general—whether red meat, white meat, processed, or unprocessed—is also associated with an increased risk of death from all causes put together.[1431] If the whole world cut out meat, we'd save an estimated seven million lives a year. If humanity cut out all animal-sourced foods, we might save eight million lives annually.[1432]

If people are unwilling to reduce their meat consumption, they should be encouraged to eat more fruits and vegetables to balance out that acid load.[1433] "However," one kidney doctor editorialized, "many patients find it difficult to follow a diet high in fruits and vegetables and might therefore be more adherent to a supplement."[1434]

So what did researchers try? Giving people sodium bicarbonate pills. Instead of treating the primary cause of the excess acid formation (too many animal products and too few fruits and vegetables), they preferred to treat the consequences. Too much acid? Here's some base to neutralize it. Sodium bicarbonate can effectively buffer the acid load,[1435] but, rather obviously, sodium bicarbonate contains sodium, which over the long term may itself contribute to kidney damage.[1436]

Unfortunately, this type of sticking-plaster approach is all too typical of today's medical model. Cholesterol too high from eating a diet unnaturally high in saturated fat and cholesterol? Take a statin drug to cripple our cholesterol-making enzyme. Diet unnaturally high in acid-forming foods? Swallow some sodium bicarbonate pills to balance that right out.

These same researchers also tried giving people fruits and vegetables instead of sodium bicarbonate and found that they offered similar protections, with the additional advantage of lowering the study participants' blood pressure. The title of the accompanying commentary in the medical journal was telling: "The Key to Halting Progression of CKD Might Be in the Produce Market, Not in the Pharmacy."[1437]

Kidney Stones

Eating a plant-based diet to alkalinize our urine may also help prevent and treat kidney stones—those hard mineral deposits that can form in our kidneys when the concentration of certain stone-forming substances in our urine becomes so high they start to crystallize. Eventually, these crystals can grow into pebble-sized rocks that block the flow of urine, causing severe pain that tends to radiate from one side of the lower back toward the groin. Kidney stones can pass naturally (and often painfully), but some become so large that they must be removed surgically.

The incidence of kidney stones has increased dramatically since World War II[1438] and even just in the last twenty-five years. Approximately one in nine Americans will experience a kidney stone,[1439] compared with only one in twenty just three decades ago.[1440] What accounts for this rising incidence? The first clue to an answer came in 1979 when scientists reported a striking relationship between the prevalence of kidney stones since the 1950s and increasing consumption of animal protein.[1441] As in all observational studies, though, the researchers couldn't prove cause-and-effect, so they decided to perform an interventional trial: They asked the study participants to add extra animal protein to their daily diets, the equivalent of about an extra can's worth of tuna fish. Within two days of eating the extra tuna, the levels of stone-forming compounds—calcium, oxalate, and uric acid—shot up such that their risk of kidney stones increased by 250 percent.[1442]

Note the experimental "high" animal protein diet was designed to recreate the animal protein intake of the average American,[1443] suggesting that Americans could considerably lower their risk of kidney stones by lowering their meat consumption.

By the 1970s, enough evidence had accumulated that researchers began to ask whether people suffering from recurrent kidney stones should stop eating meat altogether.[1444] A study on the kidney stone risk of vegetarians wasn't published until 2014, though. Oxford University researchers found that people who didn't eat meat at all had a significantly lower risk of being hospitalized for kidney stones, and for those who did eat meat, the more they ate, the higher their associated risk.[1445]

Is some meat worse than others? People who form kidney stones are commonly advised to restrict their intake of red meat, but what about chicken or fish? We didn't know until another 2014 study compared salmon and cod to chicken breasts and burgers. It found that gram for gram, fish might be slightly worse than other meat in terms of the risk of certain kidney stones, but they concluded that, overall, "[s]tone formers should be counseled to limit the intake of all animal proteins."[1446]

Most kidney stones are composed of calcium oxalate, which forms like rock candy when urine becomes supersaturated with calcium and oxalates. For many years, doctors assumed that because the stones are made of calcium, they should counsel their patients to simply reduce their calcium intake.[1447] As with so much in medicine, clinical practice often flies blind without solid experimental support. This changed with a landmark study, published in *The New England Journal of Medicine*, which pitted the traditional, low-calcium diet against a diet low in animal protein and sodium. After five years, the study found that eating less meat and salt was about twice as effective as the conventionally prescribed low-calcium diet; it cut the risk of kidney stones in half.[1448]

What about cutting down on oxalates, which are concentrated in certain vegetables? Reassuringly, a recent study found there was no increased risk of stone formation with higher vegetable intake. In fact, greater consumption of fruits and vegetables was associated with a reduced risk independent of other known risk factors, meaning there may be additional benefits to bulking up on plant foods above and beyond restricting animal foods.[1449] You can overdo it, though. We should avoid consuming multiple portions a day of spinach, beetroot greens, Swiss chard, or rhubarb,[1450] more than a few star fruits,[1451] or even spoonsful of chaga mushroom powder.[1452] Reference see.nf/oxalaterisk to see who is at particular risk and see.nf/oxalatefood for other risky doses, including sixteen glasses of iced tea a day[1453,1454] and regularly eating in excess of a handful of cashews[1455] or almonds.[1456]

Another reason a reduction in animal protein is helpful is that it lowers uric acid buildup, which can form crystals that seed calcium stones or form stones on its own. Indeed, uric acid stones are the second most common type of kidney stones. So, it makes sense that to reduce our risk, we should try to reduce excess uric acid production. This can be accomplished one of two ways: by adding drugs or by subtracting meat.[1457] Uric acid-blocking medications like allopurinol may be effective, but they can have serious side effects.[1458] On the other hand, removing all meat from a standard Western diet appears to reduce the risk of uric acid crystallization by more than 90 percent within as few as five days.[1459]

Bottom line: When urine is more alkaline, stones are less likely to form. This helps explain why less meat and more fruits and vegetables appear so protective. The standard American diet yields acidic urine. When people are placed on a plant-based diet, however, their urine can be alkalinized up to a near neutral pH in less than a week.[1460]

Not all plant foods are alkalinizing, though, and not all animal foods are equally acidifying. The LAKE (Load of Acid to Kidney Evaluation) score takes into account both the acid load of foods and their typical serving sizes in order to help people modify their diets for the prevention of kidney stones and other acid-related diseases, such as gout. As you can see in figure 4, the single most acid-producing food is fish, including tuna, followed by pork, poultry, cheese, and beef. Eggs are more acid-producing than beef, but people tend to eat less eggs than beef at one sitting. Some grains can be a little acid-forming, such as bread and rice, but not pasta, interestingly. Beans are significantly acid-*reducing*, but not as much as fruits are, with vegetables crowned the most alkaline-forming of foods.[1461]

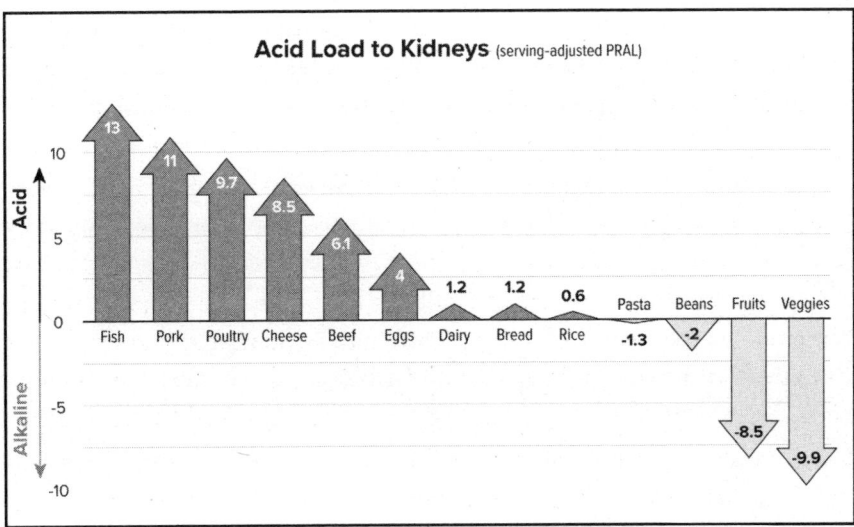

Figure 4

Dietary changes can be so powerful they can not only help prevent kidney stones but also, in some cases, cure them without drugs or surgery. Uric acid stones can apparently be dissolved away completely with a combination of eating more fruits and vegetables, restricting animal protein and salt intake, and drinking at least ten glasses of fluid a day.[1462]

Testing Your "Pee-H" with Red Cabbage

We know that the average Western diet is acid-producing, while the average plant-based diet is acid-reducing.[1463] Eating an acid-forming diet can not only affect kidney stone risk but may also produce the systemic, chronic, low-grade metabolic acidosis[1464]—excess acid in the bloodstream—that is thought to contribute to muscle breakdown as we age.[1465] So what's the best way to determine how acid-forming our diet really is? Perhaps the easiest (and most boring) method is to order some pH paper strips to pee on. Alternatively, why not use what you (should) have right now in your refrigerator's crisper: red cabbage. Red, or purple, cabbage provides one of the single best nutritional bangs for our buck, and it can even be used to perform kitchen chemistry experiments, or in this case, bathroom chemistry.

Boil some red cabbage until the water turns deep purple, or blend raw cabbage with some water and then strain out the solids. Pee into your toilet then take your red-cabbage cocktail and pour it into the toilet bowl. (Low-flow toilets work best, because there's less water in the bowl.) If the liquid in the toilet bowl remains purple or, even worse, turns pink, your urine is too acidic. Blue is the target. If your pee-and-cabbage water turns blue, your urine is not acidic but neutral or even basic.

Preventing Excess Phosphorus Intake

Having too much phosphorus in the blood may increase the risk of kidney failure, heart failure, heart attacks, and premature death. Excess phosphorus also appears to damage our blood vessels and accelerate aging and bone loss.[1466] As such, elevated levels appear to be an independent risk factor for early death among the general population.[1467]

Phosphorus is found in a variety of plant and animal foods. Most Americans consume about twice as much phosphorus as they need,[1468] but it's not just about how much we eat but how much we absorb. By switching to a plant-based diet, we can achieve a significant drop in our blood phosphorus levels even as our intake levels of the mineral remains constant.[1469] This occurs because the phosphorus in animal foods appears in the form of a compound called *phosphate*, which is absorbed into the bloodstream more readily than *phytate*, the predominant form of phosphorus in plant foods.[1470] As you may remember from chapter 6, this situation is similar to the case of iron, another essential mineral of which we can get too much. Our body can better protect itself from absorbing too much plant-based iron, but it can't as effectively stop surplus muscle or blood-based (heme) iron from slipping through the intestinal wall.

The worst type of phosphorus, though, is that which is found in phosphate food additives. These phosphorus compounds are added to cola drinks and meat to enhance their color.[1471] (Without added phosphate, Coca-Cola would be pitch black.[1472]) Less than half of most plant phosphorus[1473] and about three-quarters of phosphorus naturally found in animal products gets into our bloodstream,[1474] but added phosphate can be absorbed at a rate of nearly 100 percent.[1475]

Phosphate additives play an especially important role in the meat industry. Chicken meat is often injected with phosphates to improve its color, to add water weight (and thus to increase profitability since chicken can be sold by the kilo), and to reduce "purge," the term used to describe the liquid that seeps from meat as it ages.[1476] The problem with this additive is that it can nearly double the phosphorous levels in meat.[1477] Phosphate additives have been described as "a real and insidious danger" for kidney patients, since they have diminished capacity to excrete it,[1478] but given what we now know about excess phosphorus, it's a concern for us all.

In the United States, eleven different types of phosphate salts are allowed to be injected into raw meat and poultry,[1479] a practice that's long been banned in Europe.[1480] This is because phosphates found in meat and processed foods are considered "vascular toxins,"[1481] capable of impairing our arterial function within hours of consuming a high-phosphate meal.[1482] In meat, there's an additional food safety concern, as adding phosphate may increase the growth of a leading food poisoning bacteria *Campylobacter* in poultry purge up to a millionfold.[1483]

It's easy to avoid added phosphorus in processed foods—just don't buy anything containing ingredients with the word "phosphate" in their names, including pyrophosphate and sodium triphosphate.[1484] With meat, it's more difficult to determine the phosphate content, as producers aren't required to disclose injected additives. Added phosphate may be labeled as "flavorings" or "broth" or not labeled at all.[1485] Meat already contains highly absorbable phosphates; adding more may just add insult to kidney injury. Chicken appears to be the worst offender: A supermarket survey found more than 90 percent of chicken products contained phosphate additives.[1486]

Who Determines Whether Food Additives Are Safe?

In 2021, the U.S. Food and Drug Administration finally announced its plans to all but eliminate trans fats from processed foods,[1487] citing a CDC estimate that as many as twenty thousand heart attacks each year could be prevented by eliminating partially hydrogenated oils.[1488] Until June 16,

2015, trans fats enjoyed so-called GRAS status: "generally recognized as safe."

Why were these killer fats deemed safe in the first place?

Guess who makes the "generally recognized as safe" determination? It's not the government or a scientific body. It's the manufacturer. You read that right. The food maker gets to determine whether its own product is safe for the public, a process the FDA refers to as "GRAS self-determination." What's more, manufacturers can legally add things to our food supply without informing the FDA—or us as consumers.[1489] An estimated one thousand food-additive safety decisions have never even been reported to the FDA or the public.[1490]

But sometimes food manufacturers do notify the FDA when they introduce a new additive. Sounds responsible of them, doesn't it? Presumably they found some independent third-party panel to evaluate the safety of their product so as to avoid a financial conflict of interest, right?

Well, not exactly.

Of all the GRAS safety determinations that were voluntarily submitted to the FDA over a fifteen-year period, 22.4 percent were made by someone directly employed by the manufacturer itself, 13.3 percent were made by someone directly employed by a firm handpicked by the manufacturer, and 64.3 percent were made by a panel either appointed by the manufacturer or chosen by a firm hired by the manufacturer.[1491] Are you doing the maths? Yes, *zero* food safety decisions were made independently.

How could regulators let companies decide for themselves whether the food additives they use in their own products are safe? Follow the money. Three of Washington's largest lobbying firms reportedly work for the food industry.[1492] For example, PepsiCo alone spent more than $9 million in a single year to lobby Congress.[1493] The deeper we dig, the less surprising it is that such food additives as trans fats have been allowed to kill thousands year after year.

But, according to the manufacturer, they're safe . . .

Can Diet Protect Against Kidney Cancer?

Each year, sixty-eight thousand Americans are diagnosed with kidney cancer, and about fifteen thousand die from it.[1494] Approximately 4 percent of these cases are hereditary,[1495] but what about the other 96 percent?

Historically, the only accepted risk factor for kidney cancer has been tobacco use.[1496] A class of carcinogens in cigarette smoke called *nitrosamines* are considered to be so harmful that even so-called thirdhand smoke is a concern. The risks of tobacco smoke do not end when a cigarette is extinguished, as residual smoke can stick to walls and other surfaces.[1497] Around 80 percent of nitrosamines from cigarette smoke can remain in a room, even with normal ventilation,[1498] so always try to choose smoke-free hotel rooms. Nitrosamines are one of the reasons you can't smoke indoors without endangering others, even if you smoke without anyone present. As one of the leading scholars in the tobacco control movement recently wrote, "Carcinogens of this strength in any other consumer product designed for human consumption would be banned immediately."[1499]

Except for one: meat.

One hot dog has as many nitrosamines (and nitrosamides, which are similar tobacco carcinogens[1500]) as four cigarettes, and these carcinogens are also found in fresh meat, including beef, chicken, and pork.[1501] This may help explain the rising rates of kidney cancer over the last few decades despite the falling rates of smoking.

Clearing the Confusion: Nitrates, Nitrites, and Nitrosamines

Although fresh meat contains nitrosamines, processed or cured meats like bacon, ham, hot dogs, sausage, and lunch meat may be particularly harmful. In Europe, the world's second-largest prospective study on diet and cancer calculated that a reduction in processed meat consumption to less than twenty grams a day—less than a small matchbook-sized portion—would prevent more than 3 percent of all deaths.[1502] In the largest such investigation, the NIH-AARP study of more than five hundred thousand Americans (see page 133) found the preventable fraction of deaths may be even higher. The researchers suggested, for example, that 20 percent of heart disease deaths among American women could be averted if the highest consumers of processed meat would cut down to the equivalent of less than a half strip of bacon a day.[1503]

Since *How Not to Die* was originally published, processed meat has been officially classified as a known human carcinogen.[1504] Each fifty grams a day of processed meat intake is associated with an 18 percent higher risk of colorectal cancer, the leading cancer killer of nonsmokers. The risk of developing colorectal cancer from eating a single daily serving of processed meat is similar to the increased risk of lung cancer from breathing in secondhand cigarette smoke living with a smoker.[1505] We try not to smoke around our children but may send them to school with a ham sandwich.

In response, global nutrition and health organizations have flat out recommended avoiding processed meats. This includes the World Health Organization, the American Institute for Cancer Research, Harvard University's Medical School and School of Public Health, the World Cancer Research Fund, and the leading cancer centers Memorial Sloan Kettering and MD Anderson.[1506]

Nitrites are added to cured meat as a "color fixative" and to help prevent the growth of the bacteria that causes botulism (a rare but serious paralytic illness).[1507] What about "uncured" bacon? It says right on the package: "No nitrites or nitrates added." But study the fine print and you may see a footnote that reads something like "except those naturally occurring in celery juice." Vegetables do contain nit*r*ates that can be fermented into nit*r*ites, so adding fermented celery juice to bacon is just a sneaky way of adding nitrites. Even commentators in the journal *Meat Science* have realized this may be perceived by consumers as "incorrect at best or deceptive at worst."[1508]

But the same fermentation that converts nitrates to nitrites can happen when we eat vegetables, thanks to bacteria on our tongue. So why are vegetable nitrates and nitrites okay but the same compounds from meat are linked to cancer?[1509] Because nitrites themselves are not carcinogenic; they *turn into* carcinogens. Nitrites only become harmful when they turn into nitros*amines* and nitros*amides*. For them to do that, amines and amides must be present, and amines and amides are found in abundance in animal products. This transformation can happen in the meat itself or in our stomach after we eat it. In the case of plant foods, the vitamin C and other antioxidants that are found naturally in them block the formation of these carcinogens in our body.[1510] This process would explain why intake of both nitrate and nitrite from processed meats has been linked to kidney cancer, but no increased risk was found for nitrate or nitrite intake from plant sources.[1511]

While nitrite from animal sources—not just processed meats—was associated with an increased risk of kidney cancer, some of the highest nitrate-containing vegetables, such as rocket, kale, and collards, are associated with significantly reduced risk for kidney cancer.[1512]

Kidneys are tasked with the monumental responsibility of filtering our blood all day, every day. That's a lot of work for two fist-sized organs. Kidneys are extremely resilient, but they aren't indestructible. When they begin to fail, the body can start failing too. Toxic substances that healthy kidneys would ordinarily filter out can pass through and build up in the bloodstream.

To keep our kidneys strong and our blood clean, we must carefully consider what we eat. The typical meat-sweet Western diet can slowly damage our kidneys one meal at a time, forcing the kidneys into a state of hyperfiltration. Imagine how long your car engine would last if you always revved it near the red line? Thankfully, medical science has shown that we can reduce our kidneys' workload (and acid load) by moving toward a more plant-based diet.

11

How Not to Die from Suicidal Depression

How can you prevent death by suicide? For those unfamiliar with the ravages of mental illness, the flippant answer is: Just don't do it. In fact, death from other leading killers, such as heart disease, type 2 diabetes, and hypertension, may be just as much a choice as death from suicide, since psychiatric disorders can cloud our judgment. Nearly fifty thousand Americans take their own lives each year,[1513] and depression appears to be a leading cause.[1514] Thankfully, lifestyle interventions can help heal our mind as well as our body.

In 1946, the World Health Organization defined health as "a state of complete physical, mental and social well-being and not merely the absence of disease or infirmity."[1515] In other words, we can be in excellent physical shape—enjoying low cholesterol, a healthy body weight, and good overall physical fitness—but that doesn't necessarily mean we're healthy. Mental health can be just as important as physical health.

Major depression is one of the most commonly diagnosed mental illnesses. An estimated 7 percent of American adults suffer from serious depression—that's about sixteen million people who have at least one depressive episode each year.[1516] Now, everyone feels sad occasionally. A full range of emotions is part of what makes us human. Depression, however, is not just sadness. It is usually characterized by weeks of such symptoms as low or sad mood, diminished interest in activities that used to be pleasurable, weight gain or loss, fatigue, inappropriate guilt, difficulty concentrating, and recurrent thoughts of death.

Indeed, major depression can be a life-threatening ailment.

Good mental health isn't "merely the absence of disease," though. Just because we aren't depressed doesn't necessarily mean we're happy. There are twenty times more studies published on health and depression than there are on health and happiness.[1517] In recent years, however, the field of "positive psychology" has emerged, focusing on the relationship between optimal mental and physical health.

Growing evidence indicates that positive psychological well-being is associated with reduced risk of physical illness, but which came first? Are people healthier because they're happy, or are people happier because they're healthy?

Prospective studies that follow individuals over time have found that people starting out happier do indeed end up healthier. An analysis of seventy such studies on mortality concluded that "positive psychological well-being has a favorable effect on survival in both healthy and diseased populations."[1518] Those who are happier appear to live longer.

Not so fast, though. While positive mental states may be associated with less stress and more resilience to infection, positive well-being might also be accompanied by a healthy lifestyle. In general, people who feel satisfied appear to smoke less, exercise more, and eat more healthfully.[1519] So is being happier just a marker of good health and not a cause of it? To find out, researchers set out to make people sick.

Scientists at Carnegie Mellon University took hundreds of individuals—some happy, some unhappy—and paid them $800 each to be allowed to drip the common cold virus into their noses. Even if someone with a cold sneezes right into our face and the virus gets into our nose, we won't get sick automatically, because our immune system may be able to fight it off. So the study question was: Whose immune system would be better at fighting off a common virus—those in the group initially rated as happy, peppy, and relaxed, or those in the group who were anxious, hostile, and depressed?

About one in three of the negative-emotion individuals failed to successfully fight off the virus and came down with a cold. But only one in five of the happy individuals became sick, even after the researchers took into account such factors as their sleep patterns, exercise habits, and stress levels.[1520] In a subsequent study, the researchers even exposed participants (who had also been paid) to the influenza virus, a more serious infection. Once again, increased positive emotions were associated with decreased verified illness rates.[1521] Happier people, it seems, are less likely to get sick.

So mental health does appear to play a part in physical health. That's why it's crucial that the food we eat supports both our mind and our body. As you'll see, common foods, from leafy green vegetables to your basic garden-variety tomato, may positively affect our brain chemistry and help ward off depression. In fact, even simply *smelling* a common spice may improve our emotional state.

But avoiding the blues is not just about eating our greens. There are also components in certain foods that may increase the risk of depression, such as arachidonic acid, an inflammation-promoting compound found mostly in chicken and eggs in the diet that is blamed for potentially impairing mood by inflaming the brain.

Arachidonic Acid

Studies on the emotional health and mood states of those eating plant-based diets suggest that eating less meat isn't just good for us physically; it's good for us emotionally too. Researchers employed two psychological tests, the Profile of Mood States (POMS) and the Depression and Anxiety Stress Scale (DASS). POMS measures levels of depression, anger, hostility, fatigue, and confusion. The DASS gauges other negative mood states as well, including hopelessness, lack of interest, anhedonia (lack of pleasure), agitation, irritability, and impatience with other people. Study participants eating plant-based diets appeared to experience significantly fewer negative emotions than omnivores. Those eating more healthfully also reported feeling more "vigor."[1522]

The researchers offered two explanations for their findings. First, people eating better diets may be happier because they're healthier.[1523] Those eating plant-based diets don't just have lower rates of many of the leading killer diseases but also appear to have lower rates of such aggravating ills as hemorrhoids, varicose veins, and ulcers; fewer surgeries; fewer hospitalizations; and only about half the odds of being on drugs, including tranquilizers, aspirin, insulin, blood pressure pills, pain medications, antacids, laxatives, or sleeping pills.[1524] (Being able to avoid doctor visits and health insurance hassles would make anyone less irritable, stressed, and depressed!)

The researchers also suggested a more direct explanation for their results: Maybe the pro-inflammatory compound arachidonic acid found in animal products can "adversely impact mental health via a cascade of neuroinflammation."[1525] The body metabolizes arachidonic acid into an array of inflammatory chemicals. In fact, that's how anti-inflammatory drugs like aspirin and ibuprofen work to relieve pain and swelling—by blocking the conversion of arachidonic acid into these inflammatory end products. Maybe the mental health of omnivores was being comparatively compromised by inflammation in their brains.

Inflammation isn't always bad, of course. When the area around a splinter gets red, hot, and swollen, it's a sign that the body is using arachidonic acid to mount an inflammatory response to help fight off infection. But our body already makes all the arachidonic acid we need, so we don't need to take in any more via our diet.[1526] In this way, arachidonic acid resembles cholesterol, another essential component that the body makes all on its own: When we add excess amounts through diet, it may upset our system's internal balance.[1527] In this particular case, the researchers suspected arachidonic acid intake might impair the body's emotional state. There are data suggesting that people with higher levels of arachidonic acid in their blood may end up at significantly higher risk of suicide and episodes of major depression.[1528]

The top-five sources of arachidonic acid in the American diet are chicken, eggs, beef, pork, and fish, although chicken and eggs alone contribute more than the other top sources combined.[1529] Just a single egg's worth of arachidonic acid a day may significantly raise arachidonic acid levels in the blood.[1530] Overall, omnivores appear to consume about nine times more arachidonic acid than those eating plant-based diets.[1531]

The study showing improved moods and emotional states in those eating plant-based diets was a cross-sectional study, meaning it was a snapshot in time. What if people who start out mentally healthier go on to eat healthier too, and not the other way around? Who needs comfort food if you're already comforted? To show cause and effect, researchers would have to perform an interventional study: Gather subjects, change their diets, and see what happens. The same research team did just that. They took men and women who ate meat at least once a day and took away their eggs and chicken, along with other meats, to see what would happen to their moods. Within just two weeks, the study subjects experienced a significant improvement in measures of their mood states.[1532] The researchers concluded: "Perhaps eating less meat can help protect mood in omnivores, particularly important in those susceptible to affective [mood] disorders."[1533]

Given these results, another research team decided to put a healthy diet to the test in a workplace setting, where healthy bodies and minds could potentially translate into improved productivity—and elevate the mood of shareholders as well. At a major insurance company, a group of employees who were overweight and had diabetes was encouraged to follow a whole food, plant-based diet, cutting out all meat, eggs, dairy, oil, and junk foods. There was no portion-size restriction, no calorie counting, and no carb tracking, and participants were explicitly told not to change their exercise habits. Meals were not provided, but the company cafeteria did start offering such daily options as bean burritos and lentil and minestrone soups. A control group of employees received no dietary advice.[1534]

Despite the dietary restrictions, over the course of about five months, the plant-based group reported greater diet satisfaction than the control group and experienced improved digestion, increased energy, and better sleep, as well as significant improvement in their physical functioning, general health, vitality, and mental health. No surprise, then, that they showed measurable improvements in work productivity too.[1535]

Based on this success, a much larger study of plant-based nutrition was conducted at ten corporate locations across the country from San Diego, California, to Macon, Georgia. The same resounding success was reported, showing improvements not only in the participants' body weight, blood sugar levels, and ability to control cholesterol[1536] but also in their emotional states, including depression, anxiety, fatigue, sense of well-being, and daily functioning.[1537]

Treating Major Depression with Diet

The limitation with all these studies is that they involved people who started out mentally healthy. Proponents of the field of *nutritional psychiatry* claim that diet may be as important to psychiatry as it is to cardiology.[1538] To support such a bold claim, we'd have to show diet can help people with major mental illness. To date, only two trials have put dietary interventions to the test for diagnosed major depression: the SMILES trial and the HELFIMED trial.[1539]

The SMILES trial was the first randomized controlled trial to explicitly seek to answer the question: *If I improve my diet, will my mental health improve?* Over twelve weeks, study participants starting out with poor diets either received nutritional consulting sessions delivered by a clinical dietician or followed a control group "social support protocol" called *befriending*. So, instead of seeing a dietician, those in the control group socialized with someone to talk sport, news, or music or to play cards or board games, with the intention of keeping the participants engaged and positive. Befriending aims to control for factors such as time, expectancy, and therapeutic alliance. It's like placebo therapy and is indeed often used as a control condition for clinical trials of psychotherapy.[1540]

What did the dieticians tell people to eat? It was a Mediterranean*ish* diet with lots of whole grains—five to eight servings a day—and lots of vegetables and fruits, nuts and olive oil every day, with restrictions on meat, eggs, sugary snacks, refined cereals, fried foods, fast foods, and sugary and alcohol-containing drinks. All the participants began the study diagnosed with major depression, and while those in the social support control group improved, they still ended up, on average, with moderate depression. The diet group, however, ended up only mildly depressed on average. They were four times as likely to score under 10 on the 0 to 60 MADRS depression rating scale (32.3 percent in the diet group, compared to only 8 percent in the control group), indicating at most the lower end of mild depression.[1541]

The HELFIMED study was a similar Mediterranean-style dietary intervention versus social support trial with a three-month duration. The diet group successfully consumed more vegetables, fruits, nuts, legumes, and whole grains, as well as a greater diversity of vegetables, while eating fewer unhealthy snacks and less red meat and chicken. Compared to the social support control group, the diet change group appeared to reap significant mental health benefits in terms of reduced depression and improved quality of life, which were notably sustained at least at six months.[1542] They also supplemented with fish oil, but omega-3s have not been convincingly shown to have a meaningful antidepressant effect.[1543] Indeed, HELFIMED study researchers found no correlation between increased omega-3 levels and improved symptoms. However, improvements in a range of mental health outcomes *were* significantly correlated with the greater diversity of vegetables and fruits, intake of legumes and nuts, and reduced consumption of unhealthy snacks, takeout, and meat.[1544]

Fighting the Blues with Greens

Here's a statistic you probably haven't heard: Higher consumption of vegetables may cut the odds of developing depression by as much as 62 percent.[1545] A review in the journal *Nutritional Neuroscience* concluded that, in general, eating lots of fruits and veggies may present "a non-invasive, natural, and inexpensive therapeutic means to support a healthy brain."[1546]

But how, exactly?

The traditional explanation of how depression works, known as the *monoamine theory*, proposes that the condition arises out of a chemical imbalance in the brain. The billions of nerves in our brain communicate with each other using chemicals called neurotransmitters. Our nerve cells don't physically touch one another. Instead, they manufacture and deploy neurotransmitters to bridge the gap between them. The levels of an important class of neurotransmitters called monoamines, which includes serotonin and dopamine, are controlled by an enzyme called monoamine oxidase (known as MAO) that breaks down any excess monoamines. Some people who are depressed appear to have elevated levels of this enzyme in their brains.[1547] Thus, the theory goes, depression is caused by abnormally low levels of monoamine neurotransmitters due to elevated levels of the neurotransmitter-breakdown enzyme.

Antidepressant medications were developed to try to boost the levels of neurotransmitters to offset their accelerated breakdown. But if the excess MAO is responsible for depression, why not just develop a drug that blocks this enzyme? Such drugs do exist, but they have serious risks—not the least of which is the dreaded "cheese effect," in which eating certain foods (such as certain cheeses, cured meats, and fermented foods) while on the drug can potentially cause fatal brain hemorrhaging.[1548]

If only there were a way to safely tamp down the monoamine oxidase enzyme. Well, it turns out that many plant foods, including apples, berries, grapes, onions, and green tea, contain phytonutrients that appear to naturally inhibit MAO, as do such spices as cloves, oregano, cinnamon, and nutmeg.[1549] This may help explain why those eating plant-rich diets have lower rates of depression.[1550]

Even on a day-to-day basis, studies have shown that the more fruits and vegetables we eat, the happier, calmer, and more energetic we may feel that day—and this positivity can spill over into the next day. For our diet to have a meaningful psychological impact, though, we may need to consume approximately seven servings of fruits or eight servings of vegetables each day.[1551]

Seeds and Serotonin

Although some plant foods contain significant amounts of serotonin,[1552] the so-called happiness hormone, serotonin can't cross the blood-brain barrier. This means that dietary sources of serotonin can't make it into the brain, but the building block of serotonin, an amino acid called tryptophan, can get from our mouth to our blood to our brain. Tryptophan depletion experiments in the 1970s showed that people given specially concocted tryptophan-deficient diets suffered from irritability, anger, and depression.[1553] So if you give people extra tryptophan, will they feel better?

That's the theory. However, in the 1980s, certain tryptophan supplements created a debacle, causing a rash of deaths.[1554] But if tryptophan is an amino acid and if proteins are made out of amino acids, why can't we just give people high-protein meals to boost their serotonin levels by delivering extra tryptophan to the brain? It's been tried, and it's failed,[1555] likely because other amino acids in protein-rich foods crowd out the tryptophan for access to the brain. However, carbohydrate ingestion does the opposite: It helps shunt many non-tryptophan amino acids out from the bloodstream and into the muscles, allowing tryptophan greater access into the brain. For example, having a carb-rich breakfast like waffles and orange juice resulted in higher tryptophan levels in those studied than did a protein-rich breakfast of turkey, eggs, and cheese.[1556]

This principle may explain why women suffering from premenstrual syndrome (PMS) sometimes crave carbohydrate-rich food. Consumption of even a single carb-rich, protein-poor meal has been shown to improve depression, tension, anger, confusion, sadness, fatigue, alertness, and calmness scores among women with PMS.[1557] In a yearlong study, about one hundred men and women were randomly assigned to eat either a low-carb or high-carb diet. By the end of the year, the subjects eating the high-carb diets experienced significantly less depression, hostility, and mood disturbance than those in the low-carb group. This result is consistent with studies finding better moods and less anxiety among populations eating diets higher in carbohydrates and lower in fats and protein.[1558]

Carbohydrates may facilitate tryptophan transport into the brain, but we would still need a dietary source. Ideally, it would have a high tryptophan-to-protein ratio to facilitate brain access.[1559] Such seeds as sesame, sunflower, or pumpkin may fit the bill. Indeed, a double-blind, placebo-controlled trial of butternut squash seeds for social anxiety disorder reported a significant improvement in an objective measurement in anxiety within an hour of consumption.[1560] All of these factors may contribute to the comprehensive improvement in mood one may achieve after just a few weeks on a plant-based diet.[1561]

Saffron

The earliest recorded medical use of a spice appears to be more than 3,600 years ago, when saffron was evidently first used for healing.[1562] A few thousand years later, scientists finally put saffron to the test in a head-to-head trial against the antidepressant drug Prozac for the treatment of clinical depression. Both the spice and the drug worked equally well in reducing depression symptoms.[1563] As you can see in the box on pages 225–26, this may not be saying much, but at the very least, the saffron was safer in terms of side effects. For example, 20 percent of people in the Prozac group suffered sexual dysfunction, a common occurrence with many antidepressant medications, whereas no one in the saffron group did.

However, saffron may be one of those rare cases in which the natural remedy is more expensive than the drug. Saffron is the world's most expensive spice. It is harvested from crocus flowers, specifically the dried stigmas (the threadlike tips inside the flower), which are ground up to make the spice. More than fifty thousand crocuses—enough to cover an American football field—are needed to produce just 500 grams of saffron.[1564]

A Prozac-equivalent dose of saffron may cost more than twice as much as the drug, but a subsequent study found that even just smelling saffron appeared to have psychological benefits. Though researchers diluted the spice so much that the study participants couldn't detect its odor, they still noted a significant drop in stress hormones measured in women who sniffed the saffron for twenty minutes compared with those who spent twenty minutes smelling a placebo, along with significant improvement in the women's symptoms of anxiety.[1565]

So if you're feeling anxious, perhaps wake up and smell the saffron.

More Flower Power

Men and women diagnosed with major depression were randomized to receive either about two-thirds of a teaspoon of lavender flower powder or lemon balm leaf powder—both disguised in capsules—or an identical-looking capsule filled with a typical dose of Prozac twice a day. Both of the herbs appeared to work as well as the drug.[1566] Unfortunately, the study didn't include a placebo group with participants essentially taking nothing, but there are placebo-controlled trials of lemon balm showing it can significantly improve anxiety and depression symptoms.[1567]

There was also a trial with seniors that used lavender flower tea for anxiety and depression. Twice the amount was used—two grams, but this time in a tea bag—given twice a day. The control group didn't receive anything, though, so the reduction in depression and anxiety symptoms found with the lavender tea may have been a placebo effect. But, since it's cheap, safe, simple, and side-effect free, it might be worth giving lavender tea a try.[1568]

Coffee and Aspartame

Speaking of waking up to pleasant aromas, a cup of coffee may be doing more for the brain than making it feel less groggy in the morning. Researchers from Harvard University looked at data from three large-scale cohort studies of more than two hundred thousand American men and women. They found that people who drank two or more cups of coffee daily appeared to have about only half the suicide risk compared to non-coffee drinkers.[1569] What about drinking more than four cups a day? A Kaiser Permanente study of more than one hundred thousand people found that suicide risk seemed to continue to drop with increases in coffee dose. People who drank more than six cups a day were 80 percent less likely to commit suicide,[1570] though drinking *eight* or more cups a day has been associated with increased suicide risk.[1571]

What we put in our coffee may also make a difference. The NIH-AARP study, which followed hundreds of thousands of Americans for a decade, found that frequent consumption of sweetened beverages may increase the risk of depression among older adults. Indeed, adding sugar to coffee may negate many of its positive effects on mood, and adding the artificial sweetener aspartame (found in Canderel, Equal and NutraSweet) or saccharine (in Sweet'N Low and Sweetex) was associated with an increased risk of depression.[1572]

The controversy surrounding the neurological effects of aspartame began in the 1980s.[1573] At first, concern was limited to those with preexisting mental illness. An early study at Case Western Reserve University was halted prematurely for safety reasons because participants with a history of depression appeared to be experiencing such severe reactions to the sweetener. The researchers concluded that "individuals with mood disorders are particularly sensitive to this artificial sweetener and its use in this population should be discouraged."[1574]

Only more recently were the neurobehavioral effects of aspartame investigated in a population free from mental illness. Healthy individuals were split into two groups—half were given a higher dose of aspartame (the equivalent of about three liters of Diet Coke's worth) and the other half received a lower dose (a single liter of Diet Coke's worth). Then the groups switched.[1575] Bear in mind that the higher-aspartame diet contained just half the acceptable daily intake of aspartame, as determined by the U.S. Food and Drug Administration.[1576] After only eight days on the higher-aspartame dose, participants exhibited more depression and irritability and performed worse on certain brain function tests.[1577] So not only may aspartame cause adverse mental effects in sensitive populations, but it may also harm the general public at sufficient doses.

In 2023, aspartame was officially classified as *possibly carcinogenic*, offering another reason to stay away from it.[1578] Avoiding diet fizzy drinks and those pastel paper packets seems easy enough, but artificial sweeteners are also present in more than six thousand products,[1579] including breath mints, cereals, chewing gums, jams and preserves, juice drinks, desserts, and yogurts.[1580] This prevalence has led researchers to assert that aspartame "is impossible to completely eradicate from daily encounters."[1581] But, of course, that's only true for people who eat processed foods. Discriminating shoppers make it a priority to read ingredients lists, but the healthiest foods in the supermarket—found in the produce aisle—don't even have them.

Exercise vs. Antidepressants

We've known for decades that even a single workout can elevate mood[1582] and that physical activity is associated with decreased symptoms of depression. For example, one study of nearly five thousand people across the United States found that people who exercised regularly had 25 percent lower odds of a major depression diagnosis.[1583]

Of course, studies like these may not mean that exercise reduces depression. Maybe it means that depression reduces exercise. In other words, if we're depressed, we might feel like we can't get out of bed and go for a walk. What was needed to test this idea was an interventional study, one in which depressed subjects were split at random (randomized) into two groups, one who exercised and one who didn't.

That's what a team of researchers from Duke University attempted. They randomly assigned depressed men and women aged fifty or older to either begin an aerobic exercise program or take the antidepressant drug sertraline (Zoloft). Within four months, the mood of those in the drug group improved so much that they were, on average, no longer depressed. But the same powerful effect was found in the exercise group—that is, the group of people who weren't taking any drugs. Exercise, it seemed, works about as well as medication.[1584]

Let's play devil's advocate for a moment: The drug-free group in the Duke study met three times each week for an exercise class. Could the social stimulation rather than the exercise have improved their mood? With this question in mind, the same researchers subsequently conducted the largest-ever exercise trial of patients with depression. This time, they added a group: one group took antidepressants, one group took an exercise class, and a new third group exercised by themselves at home. The results? No matter the setting—whether subjects were alone or in a group—exercise appeared to work about as well as drugs at bringing depression into remission.[1585]

So before your doctor writes you a prescription for an antidepressant, ask about prescribing a daily workout instead.

Antioxidants and Folate

Accumulating evidence suggests that free radicals—those highly unstable molecules that cause tissue damage and contribute to aging—may play an important role in the development of various psychiatric disorders, including depression.[1586] Modern imaging techniques confirm autopsy studies showing a shrinkage of certain emotion centers in the brains of depressed patients that may be due to death of nerve cells in these areas caused by free radicals.[1587]

This phenomenon may help explain why those who eat more fruits and vegetables, which are rich in the antioxidants that extinguish free radicals, appear protected against depression. A study of nearly three hundred thousand Canadians found that greater fruit and vegetable consumption was associated with lower risk of depression, psychological distress, mood and anxiety disorders, and poor perceived mental health. The researchers concluded that eating antioxidant-rich plant foods "may dampen the detrimental effects of oxidative stress on mental health."[1588]

The Canadian study relied on questionnaires asking people to self-report fruit and vegetable intake, a method that's not always accurate. A nationwide American study took it one step further and measured the level of carotenoid phytonutrients in people's bloodstreams. These phytonutrients include some of the yellow, orange, and red antioxidant pigments found naturally in some of our healthiest foods, including sweet potatoes and dark green leafy vegetables. Not only did people with higher levels of these nutrients in their bloodstreams have a lower risk of depression symptoms, but there was also an apparent "dose-response relationship," meaning that the higher the level of phytonutrients, the better people seemed to feel.[1589]

Among the carotenoids, lycopene (the red pigment in tomatoes) has the highest antioxidant activity. Indeed, a study of nearly one thousand older men and women found that people who ate tomatoes or tomato products daily had just half the odds of depression compared with those who ate them once a week or less.[1590]

In an interventional trial, adolescents were randomized to about five teaspoons a day of wild blueberry powder or a placebo powder matched for sugars and vitamin C. Those getting the real blueberries had a significantly greater drop in depression scores compared to the placebo group.[1591]

If antioxidants are so helpful, why can't we just pop a few antioxidant pills?

Well, only food sources of antioxidants appear to be protectively associated with depression. The same can't be said for dietary supplements.[1592] This finding may indicate that the form and delivery of the antioxidants we consume are crucial to ensure their best effects. Alternatively, antioxidants may just be a marker for other components of plant-rich diets, such as folate.

Folate is a B vitamin concentrated in beans and greens. (Its name comes from the Latin word *folium*, meaning "leaf," because it was first isolated in spinach.) Early studies linking depression to low folate levels in the blood were cross-sectional in nature, meaning they were only snapshots in time. For this reason, we didn't know whether low folate intake led to depression or if depression itself led to low folate intake.[1593] However, more recent studies following people over time suggest that low dietary folate intake may indeed increase the risk of severe depression by as much as threefold.[1594] However, once again, folate *supplements* (folic acid) do not appear to help.[1595]

Vegetables—including antioxidant-rich tomatoes and folate-packed greens—may be good for the body and the mind.

How Well Do Antidepressant Drugs Work?

We've seen that saffron and exercise compare favorably to drugs in treating depression, but how much is that really saying? Thousands of published studies seem to have demonstrated that antidepressant drugs are effective.[1596] The key word here, though, may be *published*. What if drug companies decided to publish only those studies that showed a positive effect but quietly shelved and concealed any studies showing the drugs didn't work? To find out if this was the case, researchers applied to the Food and Drug Administration under the U.S. Freedom of Information Act (FOIA) to get access to the published *and* unpublished studies submitted by pharmaceutical companies. What they found was shocking.

According to the published literature, the results of nearly all antidepressant trials were positive. In contrast, FDA analysis of trial data—including the unpublished studies—demonstrated that roughly half of the trials showed the drugs didn't appear to work after all. When all the data—published and unpublished—were combined, antidepressants failed to show a clinically significant advantage over placebo sugar pills.[1597] This finding suggests that the placebo effect explains the apparent clinical effectiveness of antidepressants.

In other words, improvements in mood may be a result of the patient's *belief* in the power of the drug—not the drug itself.[1598]

Even worse, the FOIA documents revealed that the FDA knew that these drugs—such as Paxil and Prozac—didn't work much better than placebo yet made an explicit decision to shield drug companies by keeping this information from the public and prescribing physicians.[1599] How could drug companies get away with this? The pharmaceutical industry is considered one of the most profitable and politically powerful industries in the United States, and mental illness is considered a golden goose: chronic, common, and often treated with multiple drugs.[1600] Indeed, antidepressants are currently prescribed to more than 13 percent of the U.S. population.[1601]

Just because antidepressant drugs may not work better than fake pills doesn't mean they don't work at all. Antidepressants offer substantial benefits to millions of people suffering from depression. And although the placebo effect is real and powerful, antidepressants do seem to beat out sugar pills in reducing symptoms in the most severely depressed—perhaps about 10 percent of patients (although admittedly, this statistic also means that about 90 percent of depressed patients may be prescribed medication with negligible benefit).[1602]

If doctors are willing to give patients placebo-equivalent treatments, some argue that it would be better for them to just lie to patients and give them actual sugar pills.[1603] Unlike the drugs, sugar pills do not cause side effects. Antidepressants cause sexual dysfunction in up to three-quarters of users, for example. Other problems may include long-term weight gain and insomnia. And about one in five people have withdrawal symptoms when they try to quit.[1604]

Perhaps most tragically, antidepressants may make people more likely to become depressed in the future. Studies show that patients are more likely to become depressed again after treatment with antidepressants than after treatment by other means, including placebos.[1605] So even if the mood-boosting benefit of exercise is also a placebo effect, at least it's one with benefits rather than risks.

Our mental health can be as important as our physical health, and our overall well-being is interconnected, so it's vital that we choose foods to nourish our body as well as our mind.

How Not to Die from Breast Cancer

"You have breast cancer."

These are among the most feared words a woman can hear, and for a good reason. Breast cancer is the leading cause of cancer death among nonsmoking American women,[1606] taking the lives of more than forty thousand every year. The incidence of breast cancer continues to rise by about 1 percent each year, and now one in eight women in the United States can expect to be diagnosed with the disease.[1607]

Breast cancer does not occur overnight. That lump felt in the shower one morning may have started forming decades ago. By the time doctors detect a tumor, it may have been present for forty years or even longer.[1608] The cancer has been growing, maturing, and acquiring hundreds of new survival-of-the-fittest mutations that allow it to grow even more quickly as it tries to outmaneuver our immune system.

The scary reality is that what doctors call "early detection" is actually late detection. Modern imaging simply isn't good enough to detect cancer at its earliest stages, so it can spread long before it's ever spotted. A woman is considered "healthy" until she shows signs or symptoms of breast cancer. But if a person has been harboring a malignancy for two decades, can they truly be considered healthy?

People who are doing the right thing by improving their diets in hopes of preventing cancer may in fact be successfully treating cancer as well. Autopsy studies have shown that as many as 20 percent of women aged twenty to fifty-four who died from unrelated causes, such as car accidents, had so-called "occult" (or hidden) breast cancers growing inside them.[1609] Sometimes there's nothing we can do to prevent the initiation stage of cancer, when that first normal breast cell mutates into a cancerous one. Some breast cancers may even start in the womb and be related to our mother's diet.[1610] For this reason, we all need to choose a diet and lifestyle that not only prevents the initiation stage of cancer but also hampers the promotion stage, during which the cancer grows to a size large enough to pose a threat.

The good news is that no matter what our mom ate or how we lived as a child, by eating and living healthfully, we may be able to slow the growth rate of any hidden cancers. In short, we can die *with* our tumors rather than *from* them. This is how dietary cancer prevention and treatment can end up being the same thing.

One or two cancer cells never hurt anyone. But how about a billion cancer cells? That's how many may be in a tumor[1611] by the time it's picked up by a mammogram.[1612] Like most tumors, breast cancer starts with just one cell, which divides to become two, four, and then eight. Every time breast cancer cells divide, the tumor can effectively double in size.[1613]

How many times does a tiny tumor have to double to become a billion cells? Take out a calculator. Multiply one times two. Then multiply that number by two. Keep doing that until you reach one billion. Don't worry. It won't take long. It's only thirty doublings. In just thirty doublings, a single cancer cell can turn into a billion.

The key to how quickly we'd be diagnosed with cancer, then, is the doubling time. How long does it take tumors to double once? Breast cancers can double in size in anywhere from as few as twenty-five days[1614] to a thousand days or more.[1615] In other words, it could be two years or more than a hundred years before a tumor starts to cause problems.

Where we fall on that timescale—two years or a century—may depend in part on what we eat.

When I was a teen, I ate a lousy diet. One of my favorite meals was—no joke—chicken-fried steak. During my youth, I may have caused one of the cells in my colon or prostate to mutate. But I've been eating much more healthfully for the last thirty-five years. My hope is that even if I did initiate a cancerous growth, if I don't promote it, I may be able to slow down its growth. I don't care if I get diagnosed with cancer a hundred years from now. I don't expect to be around at that point to worry about it.

Controversy over the cost and effectiveness of mammograms[1616] misses an important point: Breast cancer screening, by definition, does not prevent breast cancer. It can just pick up existing breast cancer. Based on autopsy studies, as many as 39 percent of women in their forties already have cancers growing in their breasts that may simply be too small to be detected by mammograms.[1617] That's why we can't just wait until diagnosis to start eating and living more healthfully. We should start tonight.

The Risks and Benefits of Mammograms

Contradictory recommendations have been published about mammograms—for example, getting them from age forty versus fifty, screening annually versus every other year,[1618] or not getting them routinely at all.[1619] Nine out of ten women surveyed vastly overestimated the benefits of mammograms or had no idea how beneficial they are. One survey found that "if women knew how small the real effectiveness of breast cancer screening in preventing breast cancer deaths is, 70% said they would not submit to it."[1620] You may be in that 30 percent, though, and you have every right to decide for yourself.

Decisions with completely one-sided consequences—all risk or all benefit—are easy. For example, should doctors teach women to do breast self-exams? The answer is no. It was put to the test. Hundreds of thousands of women were randomized to perform self-exams or not. Researchers not only didn't find any benefit to doing them; they found harms, including double the number of women who had to get biopsies taken. Self-exams were not shown to decrease the risk of getting breast cancer, dying from it, or catching tumors in earlier stages. That's why the U.S. Preventive Services Task Force (USPSTF) came out explicitly recommending against teaching women to do breast self-exams in 2015.[1621]

To be clear, the USPSTF didn't come out against breast self-examination—only against teaching women to do them. That's because reminding women to perform self-exams only appeared to cause harm with no benefit. If you do discover an abnormality, then definitely tell your doctor, but being told to get in the practice of looking seems to do more harm than good. Yet, most doctors continue to teach women to perform self-exams. If self-exams haven't been shown to help and, in fact, have been shown to harm, why do physicians keep calling for them? Because that's just what they've been telling women forever. Medical inertia may trump women's health, even without a multibillion-dollar industry tipping the scales to push for the practice to continue, which brings us to mammograms.

Over the last half century, more than half a million women have participated in ten randomized trials of mammography, each with about a decade of follow-up.[1622] What does the science have to say? Let's imagine that one thousand asymptomatic women at average risk were randomized to either skip mammograms or get screened following the recommendation to get mammograms every other year starting at age fifty. Over the next twenty years, we would expect two hundred false alarms (though resulting in only thirty biopsies) and three cancers would be missed, but fifteen gratuitous cases would be found, meaning women would be diagnosed with—and treated for—breast cancer unnecessarily. (A third potential harm, getting radiation-induced breast cancer from the mammogram x-rays, is not included in the model because only rough indirect estimates exist—on the order of one to five cancer cases per ten thousand women).[1623] On the other side of the scale, thanks to mammograms, two breast cancer deaths would be averted, though no lives would apparently be saved overall.

When surveyed, women think mammograms cut the risk of dying from breast cancer in half, saving the lives of about one in twelve. In reality, about five women in a thousand die per decade from breast cancer without regular mammogram screening compared to four in a thousand dying with screening. Doesn't saving the life of even a single woman in a thousand make it all worth it? But even that may not be true. None of the ten randomized trials have ever shown an overall mortality benefit, meaning it appears that no lives are actually saved.[1624] How does that make sense? If a decade of mammograms prevents one in a thousand women from dying from breast cancer, then the only way for no lives to be saved is if mammograms somehow led to the deaths of one in a thousand *healthy* women. This is where the overdiagnosis may come in.

The fact is that some of the tiny tumors picked up on mammograms may have never progressed,[1625] and some might have even disappeared on their own.[1626] Autopsy studies of accident victims show that 7 to 39 percent of women aged forty to seventy have tiny breast cancers, 96 percent of which will never go on to spread or kill them. So, had those tumors not been picked up during screening, the women may have been none the wiser, may have never been affected by them or even known they had them. But once cancer is detected on a mammogram, the inclination is to treat it, because you don't know what it's going to do.[1627] And this treatment comes with all the attendant harms of unnecessary surgery, chemotherapy, and radiation.[1628]

Unnecessary radiation treatments to the chest increase the risk of dying from heart disease and lung cancer,[1629] which could explain why mammograms may kill as many as are saved.[1630] Those who survive become mammography's biggest cheerleaders, thinking mammograms saved their lives.[1631] In actuality, the more likely scenario—in fact, the two to ten times more likely scenario—is that the treatment didn't do anything because the cancer wouldn't have been harmful anyway.[1632] So, women may have gone through all that pain and suffering for nothing. That's the irony about mammograms: The people who are harmed the most are the ones who claim the greatest benefit.

I am not opposed to mammograms. I *am* opposed to the patronizing attitude that women should be pressured into getting them without being fully informed about the benefits and risks. Some women will still choose to get them, but others will not. It's for you to decide.

RISK FACTORS FOR BREAST CANCER

The American Institute for Cancer Research (AICR) is considered one of the world's leading authorities on diet and cancer. Based on the best available research, it came up with ten recommendations for cancer prevention.[1633] Beyond never chewing tobacco, its bottom-line dietary message is: "Diets that revolve around whole plant foods—vegetables, whole grains, fruits and beans—cut the risk of many cancers, and other diseases as well."[1634]

To demonstrate how dramatically lifestyle choices can impact breast cancer risk, over the course of about seven years, researchers followed a group of around thirty thousand postmenopausal women with no history of breast cancer. Achieving just three of the ten AICR recommendations—limiting alcohol, eating mostly plant foods, and maintaining a normal body weight—was associated with a 62 percent lower risk of breast cancer.[1635] Only three simple health behaviors appeared to cut risk by more than half.

Remarkably, eating a plant-based diet along with walking every day can improve our cancer defenses within just two weeks. Researchers dripped blood taken from women before and after fourteen days of healthy living onto breast cancer cells growing in petri dishes. The blood taken after they started eating healthier suppressed cancer growth significantly better and killed 20 to 30 percent more cancer cells than the blood taken from the same women just two weeks prior, before they switched to a more healthful diet.[1636] The researchers attributed this effect to a decrease in levels of a cancer-promoting growth hormone called IGF-1,[1637] likely due to the reduced intake of animal protein.[1638]

What kind of blood do you want in your body? What kind of immune system? The kind of blood that just rolls over when new cancer cells pop up, or blood that circulates to every nook and cranny in our body with the power to slow down and even stop cancer cells in their tracks?

Alcohol

In 2025, the U.S. Surgeon General released an advisory highlighting alcohol as a leading preventable cause of cancer, a fact that most Americans are not aware of, and calling for cancer warning labels on all alcoholic beverages.[1639] Alcohol is metabolized in the body into a toxic metabolite called *acetaldehyde,* which is a known human carcinogen.[1640] The advisory points to this metabolite as one of the reasons alcohol is believed to increase the risk of several different cancers,[1641] including breast cancer and colorectal cancer—even among light drinkers who only have up to one alcoholic beverage a day.[1642] A 2023 comprehensive systematic review and meta-analysis of cancer risk based on alcohol consumption levels found that even less than *half* a drink per day significantly increases the risk of breast cancer,[1643] the number one cancer killer of women aged twenty-five to fifty-four.[1644] Every year around the world, nearly five thousand breast cancer deaths may be attributable to light drinking.[1645]

Scientists have been unable, based on hundreds of studies, to identify a "threshold level of alcohol consumption below which no increased risk for cancer is evident."[1646] When it comes to alcohol and cancer, less is better,[1647] and total abstention is considered the "scientifically best solution."[1648] According to the American Cancer Society, it is "best not to drink alcohol."[1649]

The carcinogenic product acetaldehyde can form in our mouth almost immediately after we take a sip. Experiments show that even holding a single teaspoon of spirits in our mouth for five seconds before spitting it out results in the production of potentially carcinogenic levels of acetaldehyde that lingers for more than ten minutes.[1650]

If just a single sip of alcohol might produce cancer-causing levels of acetaldehyde in the mouth, what about using mouthwash that contains alcohol? Researchers who tested the effects of a variety of retail mouthwashes and oral rinses concluded that, although the risk is slight, it is probably best to refrain from using such products if they contain alcohol.[1651]

Red Wine vs. White Wine

The Harvard Nurses' Health Study found that less than one alcoholic drink a day may be associated with a small increase in breast cancer risk.[1652] Interestingly, drinking only red wine was *not* associated with breast cancer risk. Why? A compound in red wine appears to suppress the activity of an enzyme called *estrogen synthase*, which breast tumors can use to create estrogen to fuel their own growth.[1653] This compound is found in the skin of the dark-purple grapes used to make red wine, which explains why white wine appears to provide no such benefit,[1654] since it's produced without the skin.

The researchers concluded that red wine may "ameliorate the elevated breast cancer risk associated with alcohol intake."[1655] In other words, the grapes in red wine may help cancel out some of the cancer-causing effects of the alcohol. But we can reap the benefits without the risks associated with imbibing alcoholic beverages by simply drinking grape juice or, even better, eating the purple grapes themselves—preferably ones with seeds, as they appear to be most effective at suppressing estrogen synthase.[1656]

It's good (and delicious) to know that strawberries,[1657] pomegranates,[1658] and plain white mushrooms[1659] may also suppress this potentially cancer-promoting enzyme.

Melatonin and Breast Cancer Risk

For billions of years, life on planet Earth evolved under conditions of about twelve hours of light and twelve hours of darkness. Humans controlled fire for cooking about a million years ago, but we've only been using candles for about five thousand years and electric lights for a mere century. In other words, our ancient ancestors lived half their lives in the dark.

These days, though, because of the electric-light pollution at night, the only Milky Way we may see is inside a candy wrapper. Electric lighting has enabled us to remain productive well into the wee hours, but might this unnatural nighttime light exposure have any adverse health effects?

In philosophy, there's a flawed argument called the *appeal-to-nature fallacy*, in which someone proposes that something is good merely because it's natural. In biology, however, this may hold some truth. The conditions under which our bodies were finely tuned over millions of years can sometimes give us insight into our optimal functioning. For example, we evolved running around naked in equatorial Africa. Therefore, it's not surprising that many of us modern humans become deficient in vitamin D (the "sunshine vitamin") if we live in northern climes or in countries where the culture dictates full-body coverings for women.[1660]

Could something as ubiquitous as the lightbulb be a mixed blessing? Right in the middle of our brain sits the pineal gland, our so-called "third eye." It's connected to our actual eyes and has just one function: to produce a hormone called *melatonin*. During the day, the pineal gland is inactive. But once the sky darkens, it activates and begins pumping melatonin into our bloodstream. We begin to tire, feel less alert, and start thinking about sleep. Melatonin secretion may peak between 2:00 A.M. and 5:00 A.M. and then shuts off at daybreak, which is our cue to wake up. The level of melatonin in our bloodstream is one of the ways our internal organs know what time it is. It functions as one hand on our circadian clock.[1661]

Slave to the Rhythm

The 2017 Nobel Prize in Medicine was awarded for elucidating the molecular mechanisms of our internal circadian clocks.[1662] For billions of years, life on Earth evolved to the twenty-four-hour cycle of light and dark, so it's no surprise our bodies are finely attuned to that pattern. When people are in total darkness without any external time cues, their bodies still continue to cycle in about a twenty-four-hour circadian rhythm.[1663] In fact, we can even take tissue biopsies from people and show that the cells continue to cycle outside the body in a petri dish.[1664] Nearly every tissue and organ in our body has its own internal clock.[1665]

An intricate system of intrinsic clocks drives not only some of our behavioral patterns, such as eating, fasting, sleeping, and wakefulness,[1666] but also our internal physiology, including our digestion, body temperature, blood pressure, hormone production, and immune activity.[1667] Most of our genes exhibit daily fluctuations in expression, making the circadian rhythm the largest known regulatory system in our body.[1668] This cycling is thought to allow for a level of predictability and functional division of labor so that each of our body processes can run at the best time.[1669] At night while we're sleeping, a whole array of internal housekeeping activities can be switched on, such as clearing accumulated waste products from the brain, for example, and as dawn approaches, our body can shift back into activity mode.

Anyone who's ever had jet lag knows what throwing off our cycle by even just a few hours can do, but now we know our circadian rhythm can literally be the difference between life and death. A study of more than fourteen thousand suicide attempts using poison (such as drinking pesticides) found that those who tried killing themselves in the late morning were more than twice as likely to die than those who ingested a similar dose in the evening.[1670] In the same vein, properly timed chemotherapy can not only end up being five times less toxic but twice as effective against cancer.[1671] The same drugs, at the same doses, but with different effects depending on the time they're taken. Our body absorbs, distributes, metabolizes, and detoxifies what we ingest differently depending on when the processes are occurring during the twenty-four-hour cycle.

We're just beginning to figure out the optimal timing for different medications. Randomize people suffering from hypertension into taking their blood pressure pills at bedtime instead of the morning, and not only does the bedtime group achieve better blood pressure control and suffer fewer heart attacks and strokes, but they also cut their risk of death in half.[1672] (Sadly, most physicians and pharmacists still tell patients to take their blood pressure meds in the morning.[1673])

If chronotherapy—the optimal timing of drugs—can have such an impact, it may come as no surprise that *chronoprevention*—the scheduling of lifestyle interventions like mealtimes—can also make a difference.[1674] For example, check out my video on the benefits of early time-restricted eating at see.nf/earlytre.

Besides helping to regulate our sleep, melatonin is thought to play another role—suppressing cancer growth. Think of melatonin as helping to put cancer cells to sleep at night.[1675] To see if this function applies to preventing breast cancer, researchers from Brigham and Women's Hospital in Boston and elsewhere came up with the clever idea of studying blind women. The thought was that because blind women can't see sunlight, their pineal glands never stop secreting melatonin into their bloodstreams. Sure enough, the researchers found that blind women may have just half the odds of breast cancer as sighted women.[1676]

Conversely, women who interrupt their melatonin production by working night shifts appear to be at increased risk for breast cancer.[1677] Even living on a particularly brightly lit street may affect the risk. Studies comparing nighttime satellite photos against breast cancer rates have found that people living in brighter neighborhoods tend to have a higher breast cancer risk.[1678,1679,1680] Therefore, it's probably best to sleep without any lights on and with the blinds down, though the evidence to support these strategies is limited.[1681]

Melatonin production can be gauged by measuring the amount of melatonin excreted in our first pee in the morning. And, indeed, women with higher melatonin secretion have been found to have lower rates of breast cancer.[1682] Other than minimizing nighttime light exposure, is there anything else we can do to keep up our production of melatonin? Apparently so. In 2005, Japanese researchers reported an association between higher vegetable intake and higher melatonin levels in the urine.[1683] Is there anything in our diet that may lower melatonin production, thereby potentially increasing breast cancer risk? We didn't know until a comprehensive study of diet and melatonin was published in 2009. Researchers at Harvard University asked nearly a thousand women about their consumption of thirty-eight different foods or food groups and measured their morning melatonin levels. Meat consumption was the only food significantly associated with lower melatonin production, for reasons that are yet unknown.[1684]

Minimizing melatonin disruption may therefore mean putting curtains on our windows, eating more vegetables, and lowering the curtain on eating too much meat.

Exercise and Breast Cancer

Physical activity is considered a promising preventive measure against breast cancer[1685] not only because it helps with weight control but because exercise tends to lower circulating estrogen levels.[1686] Five hours a week of vigorous aerobic exercise can lower estrogen and progesterone exposure by about 20 percent.[1687] But do we need to work out that long for it to be protective?

Although even light exercise is associated with lowered risk of some other types of cancer, for breast cancer, leisurely strolls don't appear to cut it.[1688] Even an hour a day of activities such as slow dancing or light housework may not help.[1689] According to the largest study ever published on the subject, only women who worked up a sweat at least five or more times a week appeared to get significant protection.[1690] Moderately intense activity may offer as much benefit as vigorous exercise, though.[1691] Walking at a moderate pace for an hour a day is considered a moderately intense level of exercise, but it wasn't put to the test until a 2013 study reported that, indeed, walking an hour or more a day is associated with significantly lower breast cancer risk.[1692]

Darwin was right: It's survival of the fittest—so get fit!

Heterocyclic Amines

In 1939, a curious finding was published in a paper titled "Presence of Cancer-Producing Substances in Roasted Food." A researcher described how he could induce breast cancers in mice by painting their heads with extracts of roasted horse muscle.[1693] These "cancer-producing substances" have since been identified as heterocyclic amines (HCAs), described by the National Cancer Institute as "chemicals formed when muscle meat, including beef, pork, fish, and poultry, is cooked using high-temperature methods."[1694] These cooking methods include roasting, pan frying, grilling, and baking. Eating boiled meat is probably the safest. People who eat meat that never goes above 212°F (100°C) produce urine and feces that are significantly less DNA-damaging compared to those eating meat dry-cooked at higher temperatures.[1695] This means they have fewer mutagenic substances flowing through their bloodstreams and coming into contact with their colons. On the other hand, baking chicken for as few as fifteen minutes at about 350°F (177°C) leads to HCA production.[1696]

These carcinogens are formed in a high-temperature chemical reaction between some of the components of muscle tissue. (This explains why even fried veggie burgers may not contain measurable HCAs.)[1697] The longer meat is cooked, the more HCAs form, which may be why eating well-done meat is associated with increased risk of cancers of the breast, colon, esophagus, lung, pancreas, prostate, and stomach.[1698] The situation creates what the *Harvard Health Letter* called a meat preparation "paradox":[1699] Cooking meat thoroughly reduces the risk of contracting foodborne infections (see chapter 4), but cooking meat *too* thoroughly may increase the risk of foodborne carcinogens.

Just because heterocyclic amines cause cancer in rodents doesn't mean they cause cancer in humans. In this case, though—it turns out people may be even *more* susceptible. The livers of rodents have shown an uncanny ability to detoxify 99 percent of the HCAs scientists have forced down the animals' throats (a technique known as *gavage*).[1700] But then, in 2008, researchers discovered that the livers of humans fed cooked chicken were only able to detoxify about half these carcinogens, suggesting that the cancer risk is far higher than was previously thought based on experiments in rats.[1701]

The carcinogens found in cooked meat are thought to explain why, as the Long Island Breast Cancer Study Project reported in 2007, women who eat more grilled, barbecued, or smoked meats over their lifetimes may have as much as 47 percent higher odds of breast cancer.[1702] And the Iowa Women's Health Study found that women who ate their bacon, steak, and burgers "very well done" had nearly five times the odds of getting breast cancer compared with women who preferred these meats served rare or medium.[1703]

To see what was happening inside the breast, researchers asked women undergoing breast-reduction surgery about their meat-cooking methods. The scientists were able to link the consumption of fried meat with the amount of DNA damage found within the women's breast tissue,[1704] the type of damage that can potentially cause a normal cell to mutate into a cancer cell.[1705]

HCAs appear to be able to initiate cancer growth and promote it. PhIP, one of the most abundant HCAs in cooked meat, was found to have potent estrogen-like effects, fueling human breast-cancer cell growth almost as powerfully as pure estrogen,[1706] on which most human breast tumors thrive.

But that result was based on research in a petri dish. How do we know that cooked-meat carcinogens find their way into human breast ducts, where most breast cancers arise? We didn't, until researchers measured the levels of PhIP in the breast milk of nonsmoking women. (HCAs are also found in cigarette smoke.[1707]) In this study, PhIP was found in the breast milk of women who ate meat at the same concentration known to significantly boost breast cancer cell growth.[1708] No trace of PhIP was found in the breast milk of the one vegetarian participant.[1709]

A similar finding was reported in a study comparing the levels of PhIP in people's hair. The chemical was detected in hair samples of all six of the meat eaters tested, but in only one of the six vegetarians.[1710] (HCAs can also be found in fried eggs.[1711])

Our body can rapidly rid itself of these toxins once exposure ceases. In fact, urine levels of PhIP can drop to zero within twenty-four hours of refraining from eating meat.[1712] So if you practice Meatless Mondays, the level of PhIP passing through your body may become undetectable by Tuesday morning. But diet is not the only source of PhIP. HCA levels in vegetarians who smoke may approach those of nonsmoking meat eaters.[1713]

The heterocyclic amine PhIP is not just a so-called *complete carcinogen*, able to both initiate cancers and promote their growth. PhIP may also facilitate cancer spread. Cancer develops in three major stages: 1) initiation, the irreversible DNA damage that starts the process; 2) promotion, the growth and division of the initiated cell into a tumor; and 3) progression, which can involve the invasion of the tumor into surrounding tissue and metastasis (spread) to other areas of the body.

Scientists can test how invasive, or aggressive, a certain cancer is by putting its cells into an instrument called an *invasion chamber*. They place cancer cells on one side of a porous membrane and then gauge their ability to penetrate and spread through the membrane. When researchers placed metastatic breast cancer cells from a fifty-four-year-old woman in an invasion chamber all by themselves, relatively few were able to breach the barrier. But within seventy-two hours of adding PhIP to the chamber, the cancer cells became more invasive, crawling through the membrane at an accelerated rate.[1714]

PhIP in meat may therefore represent a three-strikes-you're-out type of carcinogen, potentially involved in every stage of breast cancer development. Staying away from PhIP isn't easy, though, when eating the standard American diet. As the researchers note: "Exposure to PhIP is difficult to avoid because of its presence in many commonly consumed cooked meats, particularly chicken, beef and fish."[1715]

PREVENTING (AND TREATING) BREAST CANCER BY EATING PLANTS

Given all the studies I read, it's easy for me to forget that the statistics refer to people's lives, but when real people make real changes, they can see real results.

Sadly, even after a breast cancer diagnosis, most women may not make the dietary changes that could help them most, such as consuming less meat and more fruits and vegetables.[1716] Maybe they don't realize (or their doctors never told them) that a healthier lifestyle may improve their survival chances. For example, a study of nearly 1,500 women found that remarkably simple behavior changes—such as eating just five or more servings of fruits and veggies per day along with walking for thirty minutes six days a week—were associated with a significant survival advantage. Those who followed these recommendations appeared to have nearly half the risk of dying from their cancer in the two years following diagnosis.[1717]

Over time, what to eat and feed our families are life-or-death decisions. How else can we decide but based on the best available balance of evidence?

Relieving Ourselves of Excess Estrogen

In the Harvard Nurses' Health studies that followed more than 150,000 women and their diets for decades, researchers found that those who ate more plant foods and fewer animal foods were significantly less likely to cultivate breast cancer—and that was even after controlling for factors such as body weight, family history, alcohol use, and exercise habits. Furthermore, plant-based eating appeared particularly protective against the deadliest[1718] types of tumors.[1719] The California Teachers Study, with more than 90,000 women, found similar results, including significantly reduced breast cancer risk associated with a plant-based dietary pattern, particularly for the hardest-to-treat tumors.[1720]

Circulating estrogen levels in both pre-[1721] and postmenopausal[1722] women are strongly associated with breast cancer risk, potentially explaining virtually the entire relationship between excess body fat and breast cancer.[1723] (Estrogen produced by fatty tissue spills into the bloodstream.[1724]) Does that explain why plant-based eaters, who tend to be thinner on average, have lower breast cancer risk? There are studies finding lower average estrogen levels in pre-[1725] and postmenopausal vegetarians that don't appear to be explained solely by their slimmer frames. That may be due to greater fiber intake.[1726]

Our body gets rid of excess estrogen the same way we evolved to get rid of excess cholesterol—by dumping it into the digestive tract, where it expects that there will be a lot of fiber to grab it, hold on to it, and flush it out of the body.[1727] Without fiber, excess hormones (and cholesterol) can wind up getting reabsorbed into the bloodstream,[1728] but our body just assumes our intestines are going to be packed with fiber all day long because that's the context in which we evolved. Our ancient ancestors got an estimated seven times more fiber than we're getting now.[1729]

Researchers at my medical alma mater published a study in *The New England Journal of Medicine* in which vegetarian and nonvegetarian women were "provided with plastic bags and insulated boxes filled with dry ice for three 24-hour fecal collections." (You've heard of popsicles; these were more like poopsicles.) Vegetarians excrete two to three times more estrogens every day because they produce two[1730] to three[1731] times greater "fecal output." So, passing on hormone pills is just one way to reduce breast cancer risk. The other is to rid ourselves of estrogen excess the way nature intended.

Researchers at Yale University and elsewhere found that premenopausal women who ate more than about six grams of soluble fiber a day (the equivalent of about 200 grams of black beans) had 62 percent lower odds of breast cancer compared with women who consumed less than around four grams a day. Fiber's benefits appeared even more pronounced for estrogen-receptor-negative breast tumors, which are harder to treat: Premenopausal women on a higher-fiber diet had *85 percent* lower odds of that type of breast cancer.[1732]

How did the researchers arrive at these figures? The Yale study was what's called a case-control study. Scientists compared the past diets of women who had breast cancer (the cases) to the past diets of similar women who did not have breast cancer (the controls) to try to tease out if there is something distinctive about the eating habits of women who developed the disease. The researchers found that certain women with breast cancer reported eating significantly less soluble fiber on average than the cancer-free women. Hence, soluble fiber may be protective.

The women in the study weren't getting their fiber from supplements, though; they were getting it from food. But this could mean that eating more fiber is merely evidence that the cancer-free women are eating more plant foods, the only place fiber is found naturally. Therefore, fiber itself might not be the active ingredient. Maybe there's something else protective in plant foods. "On the other hand," noted the researchers, "an increased consumption of fiber from foods of plant origin . . . may reflect a reduced consumption of foods of animal origin . . ."[1733] In other words, maybe it's not what they were eating *more* of but what they were eating *less* of. The reason high fiber intake is associated with less breast cancer may be because of more beans—or less bacon.

Either way, an analysis of a dozen other breast cancer case-control studies reported similar findings, with lower breast cancer risk associated with indicators of fruit and vegetable intake, such as vitamin C intake, and higher breast cancer risk associated with higher saturated-fat intake (an indicator of meat, dairy, and processed food intake). And according to these studies, the more whole plant foods we eat, the better it is for our health: Every twenty grams of fiber intake per day was associated with a 15 percent lower risk of breast cancer.[1734]

One problem with case-control studies, though, is that they rely on people's memory of what they've been eating, potentially introducing what's known as "recall bias." For example, if people with cancer are more likely to selectively remember more of the unhealthy things they ate, this skewed recall could artificially inflate the correlation between eating certain foods and cancer. Prospective cohort studies avoid this problem by following a group (cohort) of healthy women and their diets forward (prospectively) in time to see who gets cancer and who doesn't. A compilation of ten such prospective cohort studies on breast cancer and fiber intake came up with similar results to the dozen case-control studies mentioned above, a 14 percent lower risk of breast cancer for every twenty grams of fiber intake per day.[1735] The relationship between more fiber and less breast cancer may not be a straight line, though. Breast cancer risk may not significantly fall until at least twenty-five grams of fiber a day is reached.[1736]

Unfortunately, the average American woman appears to eat less than fifteen grams of fiber per day—only about half the *minimum* daily recommendation.[1737] Even the average vegetarian in the United States may only get about twenty grams daily.[1738] Healthier vegetarians, though, may average thirty-seven grams a day, and vegans forty-six grams daily.[1739] Meanwhile, the *whole* food, plant-based diets used therapeutically to reverse chronic disease contain upward of sixty grams of fiber.[1740]

Peeling Back Breast Cancer

"Does an Apple a Day Keep the Oncologist Away?" This was the title of a study published in the *Annals of Oncology* that set out to determine if eating an apple (or more) a day was associated with lower cancer risk. The results: Compared with people who average less than one apple a day, daily apple eaters had 24 percent lower odds of breast cancer, as well as significantly lower risks of ovarian cancer, laryngeal cancer, and colorectal cancer. The protective associations persisted even after considering these participants' intake of vegetables and other fruits, suggesting daily apple consumption was more than just an indicator of eating a healthier diet.[1741]

The cancer protection apples appear to offer is assumed to arise from their antioxidant properties. Apple antioxidants are concentrated in the peel, which makes sense: The skin is the fruit's first line of defense against the outside world. The antioxidant power of the peel may be between two times (Golden Delicious) to six times (Idared) greater than the pulp.[1742]

Beyond protecting against the initial free-radical hit to our DNA, apple extract has been shown to suppress the growth of both estrogen-receptor-positive and -negative breast cancer cells in a petri dish.[1743] When researchers at my undergrad alma mater, Cornell University, separately dripped extracts of peel and flesh from the same apples on cancer cells, the peel stopped cancer growth ten times more effectively.[1744]

Researchers found something in the peels of organic apples (presumably present in conventional ones as well) that appears to reactivate a tumor-suppressor gene called *maspin* (an acronym for *mammary serine protease inhibitor*). Maspin is one of the tools our body appears to use to keep breast cancer at bay. Breast cancer cells find a way to turn off this gene, but apple peels appear to be able to turn it back on. The researchers concluded that "apple peels should not be discarded from the diet."[1745]

Preventing Breast Cancer by Any Greens Necessary

Earlier, I discussed the 2007 study of Long Island women that linked breast cancer risk to the heterocyclic amines formed in meat. Older women consuming the most grilled, barbecued, or smoked meat over their lifetimes were found to have 47 percent increased odds of breast cancer. Those with high meat intake who *also* had low fruit and vegetable intake had 74 percent higher odds.[1746]

Low fruit and vegetable intake may just be a sign of unhealthy habits overall, but increasing evidence suggests that there may be something in produce that is actively protective against breast cancer. For example, cruciferous vegetables like broccoli boost the activity of detoxifying enzymes in our liver. Research has shown that when we eat broccoli and brussels sprouts, caffeine clears more quickly—meaning that if we eat a lot of cruciferous vegetables, we'd have to drink more coffee to get the same buzz because our liver (the body's purifier) has become so revved up.[1747] Might this process work for those cooked meat carcinogens as well?

To find out, researchers gave a group of nonsmokers pan-fried meat. They then measured the levels of heterocyclic amines circulating in their bodies by sampling their urine. For two weeks, the study participants added about 500 grams of broccoli and brussels sprouts to their daily diets and then ate the same meat meal. Though they consumed the same quantity of carcinogens, significantly less showed up in their urine, consistent with their broccoli-boosted liver detox ability.[1748]

What happened next was unexpected. The participants stopped eating their veggies and, two weeks later, ate the meat meal again. Presumably, by then, their ability to detox carcinogens would have reverted down to baseline. But instead, their liver function remained enhanced even weeks later.[1749] This finding suggests that not only might a heaping side of broccoli with that steak decrease carcinogen exposure, but eating our veggies days or even weeks before the big barbecue may help shore up our defenses. Choosing the veggie burger may be the safest choice, though, as it may have no heterocyclic amines to detoxify.[1750]

So are women who eat a lot of green vegetables less likely to get breast cancer? A study of fifty thousand African American women (a sadly neglected demographic in medical research, but a population group who tends to regularly eat more greens) found that those who ate two or more servings of vegetables a day had a significantly decreased risk of a kind of breast cancer that's hard to treat, estrogen- and progesterone-receptor-negative.[1751] Broccoli appeared especially protective among premenopausal women, but collard green consumption was associated with less breast cancer risk at all ages.[1752]

Breast Cancer Stem Cells

What if you're already fighting breast cancer or are in remission? Green vegetables may still be protective. Over the past decade, scientists have been developing a new theory of cancer biology based on the role of stem cells. Essentially the body's raw materials, stem cells are the "parents" from which all other cells with specialized functions are generated. As a result, stem cells are a critical component of the body's repair system, including regrowing skin, bone, and muscle. Breast tissue naturally has many stem cells in reserve, which are used during pregnancy to create new milk glands.[1753] However, as miraculous as stem cells are, their immortality can also work against us. Instead of rebuilding organs, if they turn cancerous, they can build tumors.[1754]

Cancerous stem cells may be why breast cancer can return, even up to twenty-five years after having been fought off successfully the first time.[1755] When people are told they are cancer-free, it may mean their tumors are gone, but if they harbor cancerous stem cells, the tumors still might reappear many years later. Sadly, someone who has been cancer-free for ten years might consider herself cured but may just be in remission. Smoldering cancerous stem cells may just be waiting to reignite.

The current battery of sophisticated chemo drugs and radiation regimens is based on animal models. Success of a given treatment is often measured by its ability to shrink tumors in rodents—but rats in laboratories only live for about two or three years in any case. Doctors may be shrinking tumors, but mutated stem cells may still be lurking, able to slowly rebuild new tumors over the ensuing years.[1756]

What we need to do is strike at the root of cancer. We need to devise treatments aimed not just at reducing tumor bulk but at targeting what has been called the "beating heart of the tumor":[1757] cancer stem cells.

That's where broccoli may come in.

Sulforaphane, a dietary component of cruciferous vegetables like broccoli, has been shown to suppress the ability of breast cancer stem cells to form tumors.[1758] This means that if you're currently in remission, eating lots of broccoli could theoretically help keep your cancer from returning. (I say theoretically because those results were from a petri dish.)

To be useful as a cancer fighter, sulforaphane would have to first be absorbed into our bloodstream when we eat broccoli. Then it would have to build up to the same concentration in breast tissue found to counter cancer stem cells in the lab. Is that possible? An innovative group at Johns Hopkins University sought to find out. The researchers asked women scheduled for breast reduction surgery to drink broccoli-sprout juice an hour before their procedure. Sure enough, after dissecting their breast tissue post-surgery, the researchers found evidence of significant sulforaphane buildup.[1759] In other words, we now know that the cancer-fighting nutrients in broccoli do find their way to the right place when we swallow them.

To reach the concentration of sulforaphane in the breast found to suppress breast cancer stem cells, however, we would have to eat at least 15 grams of broccoli sprouts a day.[1760] Broccoli sprouts are available in the produce aisle, but they are cheap and easy to grow at home. They have a bit of a radishy bite to them, so I like to mix them into a salad to dilute their intensity.

There have yet to be randomized clinical trials to see if breast cancer survivors who eat broccoli live longer than those who don't, but with no downside and only positive side effects, eating broccoli and other cruciferous vegetables is something I recommend for everyone.

Flaxseeds

Flaxseeds are one of the first items ever considered to be health foods, treasured for their purported healing properties since at least the times of ancient Greece, when the renowned physician Hippocrates wrote about using them to treat patients.[1761]

Better known as one of the richest plant sources of essential omega-3 fatty acids, flaxseeds are really set apart by their lignan content. Though lignans are found throughout the plant kingdom, flaxseeds have around one hundred times more lignans than most other foods.[1762] What are lignans?

Lignans are phytoestrogens that can dampen the effects of the body's own estrogen. This is why flaxseeds are considered a first-line medical therapy for menstrual breast pain.[1763] In terms of breast cancer risk, eating about a daily tablespoonful of ground flaxseeds can extend a woman's menstrual cycle by about a day.[1764] This means she'll have fewer periods over the course of a lifetime and, therefore, presumably less estrogen exposure and reduced breast cancer risk.[1765] Just as broccoli doesn't technically contain sulforaphane (only the precursors that turn into sulforaphane when chewed—see page 360), flaxseeds don't contain lignans, only lignan precursors, which need to be activated. This task is performed by the good bacteria in our gut.

The gut bacteria's role may help explain why women with frequent urinary tract infections may be at a higher risk of breast cancer: Every course of antibiotics we take can kill bacteria indiscriminately, meaning it may stymie the ability of the good bacteria in our gut to take full advantage of the lignans in our diet.[1766] (Yet another reason we should take antibiotics only when necessary.)

Lignan intake is associated with significantly reduced breast cancer risk in postmenopausal women.[1767] This effect is presumed to be due to lignans' further estrogen-dampening effects. But since lignans are found in healthy foods like berries, whole grains, and dark green leafy vegetables, could they just be an indicator of a healthy diet?

In a petri dish, lignans do directly suppress the proliferation of breast cancer cells.[1768] But the strongest evidence to date that there really is something special about this class of phytonutrients comes from interventional trials, starting with a 2010 study funded by the National Cancer Institute. Forty-five women at high risk of breast cancer—meaning they had suspicious breast biopsies or had previously suffered from breast cancer—were given the equivalent of about two teaspoons of ground flaxseeds every day. Needle biopsies of breast tissue were taken before and after the yearlong study. The results: On average, the women had fewer precancerous changes in their breasts after the year of flax lignans than before they started. Eighty percent (thirty-six of forty-five) had a drop in their levels of Ki-67, a biomarker (indicator) of increased cell proliferation. This finding suggests that sprinkling a few spoonsful of ground flaxseeds on our oatmeal or whatever we're eating throughout the day may reduce the risk of breast cancer.[1769]

What about women who already have breast cancer? Breast cancer survivors who have higher levels of lignans in their bloodstreams[1770,1771] and diets[1772] appear to survive significantly longer. This outcome may be due to the fact that women who eat flaxseeds may also see a rise in the levels of endostatin in their breasts.[1773] (Endostatin is a protein produced by our body to help starve tumors of their blood supply.)

The evidence from studies like these appeared so compelling that scientists performed a randomized, double-blind, placebo-controlled clinical trial of flaxseeds for breast cancer patients—one of the few times a food has ever been so rigorously put to the test for cancer. Researchers located women with breast cancer scheduled for surgery and divided them randomly into two groups: Every day, group one ate a muffin containing flaxseeds, while group two ate a muffin that looked and tasted the same, but had no flaxseeds in it. Biopsies of the tumors in the flax and no-flax groups were taken at the beginning of the study and then compared with the pathology of the tumor removed during surgery about five weeks later.

Was there any difference? Compared with the women who ate the placebo muffins, women consuming the muffins with flaxseeds, on average, witnessed their tumor-cell proliferation decrease, cancer-cell death rates increase, and their c-erB2 scores go down. C-erB2 is a marker of cancer aggressiveness; the higher the score, the higher the potential for breast cancer to metastasize and spread throughout the body. In other words, the flaxseeds appeared to make the participants' cancer less aggressive. The researchers concluded, "Dietary flaxseed has the potential to reduce tumor growth in patients with breast cancer . . . [F]laxseed, which is inexpensive and readily available, may be a potential dietary alternative or adjunct to currently used breast cancer drugs."[1774]

Soya and Breast Cancer

Soya beans naturally contain another class of phytoestrogens called *isoflavones*. People hear the word "estrogen" in the word "phytoestrogens" and assume that means soya has estrogen-like effects. Not necessarily. Phytoestrogens dock into the same receptors as our own estrogen but have a weaker effect, so they can act to block the effects of our more powerful animal estrogen.

There are two types of estrogen receptors in the body, alpha and beta. Our own estrogen prefers alpha receptors, while plant estrogens (phytoestrogens) have an affinity for the beta receptors.[1775] The effects of soya phytoestrogens on different tissues therefore depend on the ratio of alpha to beta receptors.[1776]

Estrogen has positive effects in some tissues and potentially negative effects in others. For example, high levels of estrogen can be good for the bones but can increase the likelihood of developing breast cancer. Ideally, we'd like what's called a "selective estrogen receptor modulator" in our body that would have pro-estrogenic effects in some tissues and anti-estrogenic effects in others.

Well, that's what soya phytoestrogens appear to be.[1777] Soya seems to lower breast cancer risk,[1778] an anti-estrogenic effect, but can also help reduce menopausal hot-flash symptoms,[1779] a pro-estrogenic effect. So, by eating soya, we may be able to enjoy the best of both worlds.

What about soya for women *with* breast cancer? There have been seven studies on soya consumption with a total of more than thirty thousand breast cancer survivors. Overall, researchers have found that women diagnosed with breast cancer who ate the most soya phytoestrogens lived significantly longer and had a significantly lower risk of breast cancer recurrence than those who ate less.[1780] The quantity of phytoestrogens found in just 250 ml of soya milk[1781] may reduce the risk of breast cancer returning by 25 percent.[1782] In perhaps the most dramatic study, 90 percent of the breast cancer patients who ate the most soya phytoestrogens after diagnosis were still alive five years later, while half of those who ate little to no soya were dead.[1783]

One way soya may decrease cancer risk and improve survival is by helping to reactivate BRCA genes.[1784] BRCA1 and BRCA2 are so-called caretaker genes, cancer-suppressing genes responsible for DNA repair. Mutations in this gene can cause a rare form of hereditary breast cancer. That was why Angelina Jolie famously decided to undergo a preventive double mastectomy. A National Breast Cancer Coalition survey found that the majority of women believe that most breast cancers occur among women with a family history or a genetic predisposition to the disease.[1785] The reality is that as few as 2.5 percent of breast cancer cases are attributable to breast cancer running in the family.[1786]

If the vast majority of breast cancer patients have fully functional BRCA genes, meaning that this DNA-repair mechanism is intact, how did their breast cancer form, grow, and spread? Breast tumors appear able to suppress the expression of the gene through an epigenetic process called *methylation*. While the gene itself is operational, the cancer has effectively turned it off or at least turned down its expression, potentially aiding the metastatic spread of a tumor.[1787] That's where soya may come in.

The isoflavones in soya appear to help turn BRCA protection back on, removing the methyl straitjacket the tumor tried to place on it.[1788] The dose breast cancer researchers used to achieve this result in vitro was the equivalent to eating about 200 grams of soya beans.

Soya may also help women with variations of other breast cancer susceptibility genes known as MDM2 and CYP1B1. Women at increased genetic risk of breast cancer may therefore especially benefit from high soya intake.[1789] The bottom line is that no matter which genes we inherit, changes in our diet may be able to affect DNA expression at a genetic level, potentially boosting our ability to fight disease.

Why Do Women in Asia Have Less Breast Cancer?

Though breast cancer is the most common cancer specific to women globally, Asian women are about three times less likely to develop breast cancer than North American women.[1790] Why?

One possibility is their intake of green tea, a common staple in many Asian diets. Green tea has been associated with about a 30 percent reduction in breast cancer risk.[1791] Another strong possibility is a relatively high intake of soya, which, if consumed consistently during childhood, may cut the risk of breast cancer later in life by half. If women consume soya primarily as an adult, though, their risk reduction may only be closer to 25 percent.[1792]

While intake of green tea and soya might account for a twofold reduction in Asian women's breast cancer risk, it doesn't fully account for the disparity between Eastern and Western breast cancer rates.

Asian populations also eat more mushrooms.[1793] As noted in the box on red wine on page 233, white mushrooms have also been shown to block the estrogen synthase enzyme, at least in a petri dish. So researchers decided to investigate if there was a link between mushroom intake and breast cancer. They compared the mushroom consumption of one thousand breast cancer patients to one thousand healthy subjects of similar age, weight, and smoking and exercise status. The women whose mushroom consumption averaged just about half a mushroom or more per day had 64 percent lower odds of breast cancer compared with women who didn't eat mushrooms at all. Eating mushrooms *and* sipping at least half a tea bag's worth of green tea each day was associated with nearly *90 percent* lower breast cancer odds.[1794]

Oncologists, doctors who treat cancer, can take pride in the strides they've made. Thanks to improvements in cancer treatment, cancer patients are living longer and healthier, as has been celebrated in oncology journal editorials with such titles as "Cancer Survivors, 10 Million Strong and Growing!" Yes, more than 10 million cancer patients are still alive today, with "perhaps as many as 1 million new individuals in the United States joining those ranks each year."[1795] That is an accomplishment, but wouldn't it be even better to prevent those million cases in the first place?

In medicine, a cancer diagnosis is considered a "teachable moment" when we can motivate a patient to improve his or her lifestyle.[1796] By then, though, it may already be too late.

How Not to Die from Parkinson's Disease

Back in the 1960s at the height of the civil rights movement, my dad was dodging bullets during the Brooklyn riots and setting up shots at just the right angle to best capture images of my mother being arrested at protests and dragged away again and again. His most famous work—one of *Esquire*'s 1963 Photos of the Year—depicted family friend Mineral Bramletter suspended in a Christlike pose between two white police officers as another cop clutched his throat.

What a cruel twist of fate that a celebrated photojournalist got a disease that caused his hands to shake. For years, my dad suffered with Parkinson's. Slowly and all too painfully, he lost the ability to take care of himself, to live his life in any semblance of the way he had before. He became bedridden and compromised in every way imaginable.

After sixteen years of fighting, he went to the hospital one last time. As so often happens with chronic disease, one complication led to another. He got pneumonia and spent his last few weeks on a ventilator, suffering through a painful, prolonged death. The weeks he spent in that hospital bed before he passed were the worst weeks of both his and my life.

Hospitals are terrible places to be and terrible places to die. That is why each of us needs to take care of ourselves.

As my father's story shows, Parkinson's can end badly. It is the second most common neurodegenerative disease after Alzheimer's. Parkinson's is a disabling disorder affecting the speed, quality, and ease of movement. Its hallmark symptoms, which worsen as the disease progresses, include hand tremors, limb stiffness, impaired balance, and difficulty walking. It can also affect mood, thinking, and sleep. Parkinson's is not currently curable.

The disease is caused by the die-off of specialized nerve cells in a region of the brain that controls movement. It typically presents after age fifty. A history of head trauma can increase risk,[1797] which may be why heavyweight boxers, including Muhammad Ali, and NFL players, including Hall of Famer Brett Favre, have fallen victim to the condition. However, most people may be more likely to develop the disease from toxic pollutants in our environment that can build up in the food supply and eventually affect the brain.

One of the National Cancer Institute's U.S. Presidential Cancer Panel reports discussed the degree to which we're being inundated with industrial chemicals. It concluded:

> *The American people—even before they are born—are bombarded continually with myriad combinations of these dangerous exposures. The Panel urges you [Mr. President] most strongly to use the power of your office to remove the carcinogens and other toxins from our food, water, and air that needlessly increase health care costs, cripple our Nation's productivity, and devastate American lives.*[1798]

In addition to increasing our risk of developing many cancers, industrial pollutants may also play a role in the onset of such brain-deteriorating (neurodegenerative) diseases as Parkinson's.[1799] And those toxins are residing in most of our bodies.

Every few years, the CDC measures the levels of chemical pollutants in the bodies of thousands of Americans from across the country.[1800] According to the agency's findings, the bodies of most women in the United States are contaminated with heavy metals, along with a number of toxic solvents, endocrine-disrupting chemicals, fire retardants, chemicals from plastics, polychlorinated biphenyls (PCBs), and banned pesticides such as DDT[1801] (publicized by American biologist Rachel Carson in her 1962 bestseller *Silent Spring*).

In many cases, 99 to 100 percent of the hundreds of women tested were found to have detectable levels of these pollutants circulating in their bloodstreams. Pregnant women were found to harbor, on average, up to fifty different chemicals.[1802] Could the presence of these potential toxicants in their bodies mean that they're also being passed on to their children? Researchers decided to put that question to the test by measuring pollutant levels right at delivery in the babies' umbilical cord blood. (As soon as the cord is cut, a little blood can be squirted into a vial.) After studying more than three hundred women who had recently given birth, researchers found that 95 percent of umbilical cord samples showed detectable DDT residues.[1803] And this is now decades after the pesticide was banned.

And men tend to have even higher levels of certain pollutants than women. A clue to solving this mystery was found when breast-feeding history was taken into account. Women who never breast-fed had about the same level of certain toxicants in their bodies as men, but the longer they breast-fed their children, the lower their levels fell, suggesting that they were detoxing themselves by passing the pollution down to their children.[1804]

It appears that blood levels of some pollutants in women may drop by nearly half during pregnancy,[1805] in part because their bodies pass them off through the placenta.[1806] That may be why breast milk concentrations of pollutants appear higher after the first pregnancy than in subsequent ones.[1807] This could also explain why birth order was found to be a significant predictor of pollutant levels in young people. Basically, firstborn kids may take one for the team when it comes to mom's store of toxic waste and leave less for their baby brothers and sisters.[1808]

Even mothers who were breast-fed as infants themselves tend to have higher levels of pollutants in their own breast milk when they grow up, suggesting a multigenerational passing down of these chemicals.[1809] In other words, what we eat now may affect the levels of toxic chemicals in our grandchildren. When it comes to feeding babies, breast is still best—absolutely[1810]—but rather than detoxing into our children, we should strive not to "tox" ourselves in the first place.

In 2012, researchers from the University of California–Davis, published an analysis of the diets of California kids aged two to seven. (Children are thought to be especially vulnerable to chemicals in the diet because they are still growing, and thus they have a comparatively greater intake of food and fluids relative to their weight.) Chemicals and heavy metals in children's bodies from the foods they ate were indeed found to exceed safety levels by a larger margin than in adults. Cancer risk ratios, for instance, were exceeded by a factor of up to one hundred or more. For every child studied, benchmark levels were surpassed for arsenic, the banned pesticide dieldrin, and potentially highly toxic industrial by-products called dioxins. They were also too high for DDE, a by-product of DDT.[1811]

Which foods contributed the most heavy metals? The number one food source of arsenic was poultry among preschoolers and, for their parents, tuna.[1812] The top source for lead? Dairy. For mercury? Seafood.[1813]

Those concerned about exposing their children to mercury-containing vaccines should know that eating just a single serving of fish each week during pregnancy can lead to more mercury in their infant's body than injecting them directly with about a dozen mercury-containing vaccines.[1814] (Today, the only childhood vaccines with mercury are certain formulations of the flu vaccine.[1815]) We should strive to minimize mercury exposure, but the benefits of childhood vaccination far exceed the risks. The same cannot be said for tuna.[1816]

Where in the food supply are these pollutants found? Most DDT comes from meat, particularly fish.[1817] The oceans are essentially humanity's sewer; everything eventually flows into the sea. The same is true when it comes to dietary exposure to PCBs—another set of banned chemicals, once widely used as insulating fluid in electrical equipment. A study of more than twelve thousand food and feed samples across eighteen countries found that the highest PCB contamination was found in fish and fish oil, followed by eggs, dairy, and then other meats. Salmon may be the most contaminated, followed by canned tuna.[1818] The lowest contamination was found at the bottom of the food chain, in plants.[1819]

Hexachlorobenzene, another pesticide banned in the United States sixty years ago, today may be found mainly in dairy and meat, including fish.[1820] Perfluorochemicals, or PFCs? Overwhelmingly found in fish and other meats.[1821] As for dioxins, in the United States, the most concentrated sources may be butter, followed by eggs, and then processed meat.[1822] The levels in eggs may help explain why one study found that eating more than half an egg a day was associated with about two to three times higher odds for cancers of the mouth, colon, bladder, prostate, and breast, compared to those who didn't eat eggs at all.[1823]

If women want to clean up their diets before conception, how long does it take for these pollutants to leave their systems? To find out, researchers asked people to eat one large serving of tuna or another high-mercury fish each week for fourteen weeks to boost their levels of the heavy metal, then stop. By measuring how fast the study participants' mercury levels dropped, the scientists were able to calculate the half-life of mercury in the body.[1824] The participants appeared to be able to clear about half the mercury from their bodies within two months. This result suggests that within a year of stopping fish consumption, the body can detox nearly 99 percent of it. Unfortunately, other industrial pollutants in fish can take longer for our bodies to get rid of; the half-lives for certain dioxins, PCBs, and DDT by-products found in fish are as long as ten years.[1825] So to get that same 99 percent drop, it could take more than a century—a long time to delay having your first child.

How do these chemicals get into our food in the first place? One reason is that we've so thoroughly polluted our planet that the chemicals can just come down in the rain. For example, scientists have reported eight different pesticides contaminating the snow-packed peaks of Rocky Mountain National Park in Colorado.[1826] Once pollutants get into the soil, they can work their way up the food chain at increasing concentrations. Consider that before she's slaughtered for meat, a dairy cow may eat thirty-four thousand kilos' worth of plants. The chemicals in the plants can get stored in her fat and build up in her body. So when it comes to many of the fat-soluble pesticides and pollutants, every time we eat a hamburger, we are, in effect, eating everything that cow ate. The best way to minimize our exposure to industrial toxins may be to eat as low as possible on the food chain, a plant-based diet.

Reducing Dioxin Intake

Dioxins are highly toxic pollutants that accumulate in the fat of animal tissue, such that about 95 percent of human exposure comes from eating animal products.[1827] Sometimes that's because of contaminated animal feed. In the 1990s, for example, a supermarket survey found that the highest concentration of dioxins was found in farm-raised catfish.[1828] Apparently, the catfish were provided feed mixed with an anticaking agent laced with dioxins that may have originated from sewage sludge.[1829]

That same feed was given to chickens, affecting approximately 5 percent of U.S. poultry production at the time.[1830] That would mean that people ate hundreds of millions of contaminated chickens.[1831] Of course, if it was in the chickens, then it was also in their eggs. Indeed, elevated dioxin levels were found in U.S. eggs too.[1832] The U.S. Department of Agriculture estimated that less than 1 percent of feed was contaminated, but 1 percent of egg production would mean more than a million tainted eggs *per day*. But the catfish contamination was even more widespread: More than one-third of all U.S. farm-raised catfish tested were found to be contaminated with dioxins.[1833]

In 1997, the U.S. Food and Drug Administration called on feed manufacturers to stop using these dioxin-tainted ingredients, stating that "[c]ontinued exposure to elevated dioxin levels in animal feed increases the risk of adverse health effects in animals and to humans consuming animal-derived food products."[1834] So did the feed industry clean up their act? Up to half a billion pounds of catfish continued to be churned out of U.S. fish farms every year,[1835] but it wasn't until more than a decade later that our government went back and checked for compliance. Researchers from the USDA tested samples of catfish from all over the country and in 2013 reported that *96 percent* of tested samples still contained dioxins or dioxin-like compounds. And when they checked the feed used to raise these fish? More than half the samples came back as contaminated.[1836]

In other words, the feed industry has known for decades that what they were feeding to animals (and, ultimately, to most of us[1837]) may contain dioxins, but they apparently continue this practice unabated. In 2024, dioxin-like PCBs in a sample of U.S. catfish were found to be nearly one hundred times higher than the World Health Organization's safety limits.[1838]

The Institute of Medicine has made suggestions for reducing dioxin exposure, such as trimming fat from meat, including from poultry and fish, and avoiding the recycling of animal fat into gravy.[1839] Wouldn't it be more prudent just to trim the amount of animal foods from our diet instead? Researchers have estimated that a plant-based diet could eliminate about 98 percent of our dioxin intake.[1840]

Smoking and Parkinson's Disease

The CDC recently celebrated the sixty-year anniversary of the landmark 1964 surgeon general's report on smoking, considered one of the great public health achievements of our time.[1841] It's interesting to go back and read the reactions of the tobacco industry to such reports. For example, an industry insider maintained that contrary to the surgeon general's argument that smoking costs our nation billions, "smoking *saves* the country money by increasing the number of people dying soon after retirement."[1842] In other words, just think how much we're saving on Medicare and Social Security thanks to cigarettes.

The tobacco industry also criticized the surgeon general's "lack of balance regarding benefits of smoking."[1843] As industry representatives testified before Congress, these "positive health benefits" include "the feeling of well-being, satisfaction, and happiness and everything else." Beyond all that happiness the surgeon general was trying to extinguish, the Tobacco Institute argued, "everything else" included protection against Parkinson's disease.[1844]

As it happens, quite unexpectedly, more than five dozen studies over the past half century have collectively shown that smoking tobacco is indeed associated with significantly lower incidence of Parkinson's disease.[1845] Valiant attempts have failed to explain away these findings. Maybe, public health scientists countered, it's because smokers are dying before they get Parkinson's. No, smoking appears protective at all ages.[1846] Maybe it's because smokers drink more coffee, which we know to be protective.[1847] No, the protective effect remained even after researchers controlled studies for coffee intake.[1848] Identical-twin studies helped rule out genetic factors in the link.[1849] Even simply growing up in a home where our parents smoked appears protective when it comes to developing Parkinson's.[1850] So was the tobacco industry right?

Since the surgeon general's groundbreaking 1964 report, more than twenty million Americans have died as a result of smoking.[1851] Even if we don't care about dying from lung cancer or emphysema, even if we care only about protecting our brain, we *still* shouldn't smoke, because smoking is a significant risk factor for stroke.[1852] But what if we could get the benefits of smoking without the risks?

Maybe we can. The neuroprotective agent in tobacco appears to be nicotine.[1853] Tobacco is part of the nightshade family, the group of plants that includes tomatoes, potatoes, aubergines, and peppers. It turns out they all contain nicotine too, but in such trace amounts—hundreds of times less than what's found in a single cigarette—that the protective potential of vegetables was dismissed as inconsequential.[1854] But then it was discovered that just one to two puffs of a cigarette can saturate half of our brain's nicotine receptors.[1855] Then we learned that just being *exposed* to secondhand smoke may lower the risk of Parkinson's[1856] and that the amount of nicotine exposure sitting in a smoky restaurant is on the same order as what we might get from eating a healthy meal in a smoke-free restaurant.[1857] So might eating lots of nightshade vegetables protect us from Parkinson's after all?

Researchers at the University of Washington decided to find out. When they tested for nicotine, they found none in aubergines, just a little in potatoes, some in tomatoes, and more significant amounts in bell peppers/capsicum. These results were consistent with what researchers found when they studied nearly five hundred newly diagnosed Parkinson's patients compared to controls. Eating nicotine-rich vegetables, especially peppers, was associated with significantly lower risk of Parkinson's disease.[1858] (This effect was found only in the nonsmokers, which makes sense because the flood of nicotine from cigarettes would likely overwhelm any dietary effect.) This study may help explain previous protective associations in terms of Parkinson's risk that had been tenuously found for tomato and potato consumption, as well as for the nightshade-rich Mediterranean diet.[1859] And in 2020, Harvard researchers confirmed that frequent dietary nicotine intake may indeed be associated with a lower risk of developing Parkinson's disease.[1860]

The University of Washington researchers concluded that more research is needed before individuals should consider dietary interventions to prevent Parkinson's disease, but when that intervention is simply enjoying more healthy dishes like stuffed peppers with tomato sauce, I don't see a reason why we should wait.

Essential Tremor

As documented in the book *The Case of the Frozen Addicts*,[1861] a bad batch of so-called synthetic heroin caused, within days, what appeared to be advanced-stage Parkinson's disease. Thanks to a chemical contaminant called MPTP, young men and women were left trapped inside their bodies, with near-complete immobility—in some cases, only able to move their eyes. The seminal paper describing the phenomenon ended with the silver lining that this may be able to help us find the culprit in Parkinson's.[1862]

Attention turned to a class of chemicals called *beta-carboline alkaloids*, due to their structural similarity to MPTP. Indeed, higher levels of these toxins were found in the brain fluid of Parkinson's patients.[1863] As we know, Parkinson's is one of our leading killers, but the most common movement disorder is what's called "essential tremor"—affecting one in twenty-five adults over the age of forty, up to one in five of those in their nineties.[1864] In addition to the potentially debilitating hand tremor, there can be other neurological manifestations, including cognitive impairment, depression, and sleeping problems.[1865]

In medical lingo, "essential" can mean "of unknown cause," like essential hypertension, the rise in blood pressure as we age.[1866] Just as there have been calls for decades to rename that phenomenon once it became clear that lifestyle behaviors played a critical role,[1867] there are those suggesting we rename essential tremor as we come to understand it better.[1868] Identical twin studies suggest it may be 60 percent genetic.[1869] Though there have been studies linking the development of essential tremor to lead exposure,[1870,1871] most attention has focused on beta-carboline alkaloids.[1872]

Beta-carboline alkaloids induce a tremor in a wide variety of animals,[1873] from mice[1874] to monkeys, that's similar to essential tremor in humans both clinically and in the type of brain damage they cause.[1875] As such, beta-carboline alkaloid administration produces the main animal model for essential tremor upon which to try out new drugs.[1876] Harmane is the most potent of the tremor-producing beta-carboline alkaloids.[1877] When people are exposed to a high dose of harmane, they develop tremors; when it is taken away, the tremors disappear.[1878] What if we're exposed to small doses over time?

Four out of five studies found that those with essential tremor have significantly higher levels of this toxin in their bloodstream compared to those without tremor.[1879,1880,1881,1882,1883] Furthermore, the higher the harmane levels, the worse the tremor.[1884] The highest levels are found in those who have both essential tremor *and* cancer, suggesting harmane may be playing a role in both diseases.[1885]

Elevated harmane levels have also been found directly in the brains of essential tremor patients on autopsy.[1886] Due to its high fat solubility, harmane accumulates in brain tissue.[1887] Using a high-tech brain scan called proton magnetic resonance spectroscopic imaging, higher harmane levels were found to be a significant predictor of signs of nerve degeneration in the cerebellum, the part of the brain that controls movement.[1888]

How do we get exposed to these chemicals? Small amounts of harmane are produced endogenously, but the main source is meat.[1889] Beta-carboline alkaloids are a type of heterocyclic amine, the class of carcinogens that are formed in a high-temperature chemical reaction between some of the components of muscle tissue. Under the same cooking conditions, chicken may produce the most harmane—more than twice as much as steak, for example—but the highest, single, per serving levels have been found in fried pork,[1890,1891] flame grilled steak, flame grilled chicken,[1892] and grilled salmon.[1893]

Researchers gave people a slice of fried turkey and saw a bump in harmane blood levels within five minutes. *Five minutes?* It isn't even digested in five minutes. The researchers suspect the rapid uptake is indicative of significant absorption directly through the mouth, straight into the bloodstream, bypassing the stomach, and, most important, bypassing the detoxifying enzymes of the liver before it makes it to the brain.[1894] So, if this "potent, tremor-producing neurotoxin"[1895] is concentrated in "cooked muscle foods," is meat consumption associated with a higher risk of essential tremor? A study out of Columbia University found that men who ate the most meat, about one and a half servings a day, had a staggering twenty-one times the odds of essential tremor compared to men who ate closer to half a serving a day.[1896] To put that in context, if we go back to the original studies on smoking and lung cancer,[1897] we see that smoking was only linked to about fourteen times the odds.[1898]

Arguing against a role of meat in essential tremor through harmane exposure is the fact that a similar relationship was not found in women, and there appeared to be no difference in tremor rates between those who preferred their meat rare versus well-cooked.[1899,1900] A reverse causation explanation was also proposed: Perhaps instead of greater meat consumption leading to essential tremor, the essential tremor led to greater meat consumption, as a solid stable food that may be more easily handled with a tremulous hand.[1901] A subsequent study found the consumption of bacon and pork chops was associated with essential tremor, but since so many different types of meat were studied, those links may have just been statistical flukes.[1902] Perhaps the elevated harmane levels in tremor victims are due to a reduced capacity to detoxify it or a combination of greater intake and lesser excretion.[1903]

For those reluctant to reduce their meat consumption, different marinades have been tested to reduce harmane production. Hibiscus extracts failed to alter harmane levels.[1904] Red wine made things worse, increasing harmane formation by up to nearly 1,000 percent.[1905] A Caribbean marinade[1906] and a variety of berry extracts worked, however. For example, marinating camel meat in strawberry juice for 24 hours before frying can reduce the formation of harmane as much as 40 percent.[1907]

> Are there any dietary treatments once you already have the disease? Vanillin—the primary fragrant compound in vanilla extract—was found to be beneficial against harmaline-induced tremors in rats, but there have yet to be any clinical studies.[1908]

Dairy

Individuals with Parkinson's have been found to have elevated levels of an organochlorine pesticide in their bloodstreams, the class of largely banned pesticides that includes DDT.[1909] Autopsy studies have also found elevated levels of pesticides in the brain tissue of those with Parkinson's.[1910] Elevated levels of other pollutants like PCBs were found in their brains too, and the higher the concentrations of certain PCBs, the higher the degree of damage found specifically in the brain region thought to be responsible for the disease, called the *substantia nigra*.[1911] As noted earlier, though many of these chemicals were banned decades ago, they may persist in the environment. We can continue to be exposed to them through the consumption of contaminated animal products in our diet, including dairy.[1912] Indeed, people who eat plant-based diets free of dairy were found to have significantly lower blood levels of the PCBs implicated in the development of Parkinson's disease.[1913]

A meta-analysis of studies involving more than three hundred thousand participants found that overall dairy consumption was associated with significantly increased risk of Parkinson's disease. They estimated that Parkinson's risk may increase by 17 percent for every 195 ml of cow's milk consumed per day.[1914] "Contamination of milk with neurotoxins may be of critical importance," researchers offered by way of explanation.[1915] For example, neurotoxic chemicals like tetrahydroisoquinoline, a compound used to induce parkinsonism in primates in laboratory studies,[1916] appears to be found predominantly in cheese.[1917] The concentrations found were low, but the concern is that they may accumulate over a lifetime of consumption,[1918] resulting in the elevated levels found in the brains of people with Parkinson's.[1919] There have been calls on the dairy industry to require screening of milk for such toxins,[1920] but they have so far gone unanswered.

Concluded one nutrition journal editorial: "The only possible explanation for this effect is the evidence of the contamination of milk by neurotoxins."[1921]

But there are alternate explanations for the "clear-cut" link between dairy and Parkinson's.[1922] For example, pollutant levels wouldn't explain why Parkinson's appears more closely tied to the consumption of the milk sugar lactose than to milk fat[1923] and more closely tied to milk than to butter.[1924] So maybe the culprit is galactose, the sugar in milk I will describe in chapter 14, blamed for an increased risk of bone fractures, cancer, and death.[1925] Those with an inability to detoxify the galactose in milk not only suffer damage to their bones but also to their brains.[1926] This may help explain the link between milk intake and Parkinson's, as well as the link between milk and another neurodegenerative disease called Huntington's disease. Indeed, higher consumption of dairy products appears to double the risk of earlier-onset Huntington's.[1927]

Another explanation is that milk consumption lowers blood levels of uric acid, an important brain antioxidant[1928] shown to protect nerve cells against the oxidative stress caused by pesticides.[1929] Uric acid may slow the progression of Huntington's[1930] and Parkinson's,[1931] and, most importantly, may lower the risk of getting Parkinson's in the first place.[1932] Too much uric acid, however, can crystallize in our joints and cause a painful disease called gout, so uric acid can be thought of as a double-edged sword.[1933] Too much uric acid is also associated with heart disease and kidney disease; too little, with Alzheimer's, Huntington's, Parkinson's, multiple sclerosis, and stroke.[1934] Those on plant-based diets devoid of dairy appear to hit the sweet spot[1935] in terms of most optimal uric acid levels for longevity.[1936]

Milk may *not* do a body good, at least when it comes to our bones and brain.

Plant-Based Diets and Pollutants

As we've discussed, organochlorines are a group of chemicals that includes dioxins, PCBs, and such insecticides as DDT. Although most were banned decades ago, they persist in the environment and creep up the food chain into the fat of the animals people eat.

What if you don't eat any animal products at all? Researchers have "found that vegans were significantly less polluted than omnivores" when measuring levels of organochlorines in their blood, including a variety of PCBs and one of Monsanto's long-banned Aroclor compounds.[1937] This finding is consistent with studies showing higher levels of organochlorine pesticides in the body fat[1938] and breast milk[1939] of those who eat meat.

People eating completely plant-based diets have also been found to have markedly lower levels of dioxins in their bodies[1940] as well as decreased contamination with PBDEs,[1941] the flame-retardant chemical pollutants also linked to neurological problems.[1942] No surprise: The highest levels of flame retardants in the U.S. food supply have been found in fish, though the primary source of intake for most Americans is poultry, followed by processed meat.[1943] This discovery helps explain the significantly lower levels of PBDEs in those eating meat-free diets.[1944] It appears that the more plant-based foods we eat and the longer we go without eating animal products, the lower our levels fall.[1945] No regulatory limits have been set for PBDEs in food, but as U.S. Department of Agriculture researchers noted in a survey of flame-retardant chemicals in domestic meat and poultry, "reducing the levels of unnecessary, persistent, toxic compounds in food and your diet is certainly desirable."[1946]

Eating healthier can also reduce the concentrations of heavy metals in our body. The levels of mercury in the hair of those eating plant-based diets were found to be up to ten times lower than of those who ate fish.[1947] Within three months of switching to a plant-based diet, the levels of mercury, lead, and cadmium growing out in our hair appear to drop significantly (but build back up when meat and eggs are added back into the diet).[1948] Unlike heavy metals, though, some organochlorine pollutants can stick around for decades.[1949] Any DDT in our KFC may stay with us for the rest of our life.

Berries

Dr. James Parkinson, in his original, centuries-old description of the disease that bears his name, described a characteristic feature: "torpid" bowels, or constipation that may precede the diagnosis by many years.[1950] We've since learned that bowel-movement frequency may even be predictive of Parkinson's. Men with less than daily bowel movements, for instance, were found to be four times more likely to develop the disease years later.[1951] Reverse causation has been suggested: Maybe constipation didn't lead to Parkinson's.

Maybe Parkinson's—even decades before it was diagnosed—led to constipation. This idea was supported by anecdotal evidence suggesting that throughout their lives, many who would go on to develop Parkinson's reported never feeling very thirsty and, perhaps, decreased water intake contributed to their constipation.[1952]

Alternatively, given the link between dietary pollutants and Parkinson's, constipation may be contributing directly to the disease: The longer feces stay in the bowel, the more neurotoxic chemicals in the diet may be absorbed.[1953] There are now more than one hundred studies linking pesticides to an increased risk for Parkinson's disease,[1954] but many of them are based on participants' occupational or ambient exposure. Approximately one billion pounds of pesticides are applied annually in the United States,[1955] and simply living or working in high-spray areas may increase our risk.[1956] The use of common household pesticides like bug sprays is also associated with significantly increased risk.[1957]

How exactly do pesticides increase our risk for Parkinson's? Scientists think they may cause DNA mutations that increase our susceptibility[1958] or affect the way certain proteins fold in our brain. For proteins to function effectively, they have to be the right shape. As we make new proteins in our cells, if they come out folded incorrectly, they are simply recycled, and our body tries again. Certain misfolded proteins, however, can take a shape that our body has difficulty breaking down. Should this glitch happen continuously, the malformed proteins can accumulate and result in the death of the brain's nerve cells. Misfolded beta amyloid proteins, for example, are implicated in Alzheimer's disease (see chapter 3); misfolded prion proteins cause mad cow disease; a different malformed protein causes Huntington's; and misfolded alpha-synuclein proteins can lead to Parkinson's disease.[1959]

As I've said, Parkinson's disease is caused by the die-off of specialized nerve cells in a region of the brain that controls movement. By the time the first symptoms arise, 70 percent of these critical cells may already be dead.[1960] Pesticides are so good at killing these neurons that scientists often use pesticides in the laboratory to try to re-create Parkinson's in animals to test new treatments.[1961]

If pesticides are killing off our brain cells, is there anything we can do to stop the process other than lowering our exposure to them? There are no known drugs that can prevent these misfolded proteins from accumulating, but certain phytonutrients called *flavonoids*—which are found in fruits and vegetables—may have protective effects. Researchers tested forty-eight different plant compounds able to cross the blood-brain barrier to see if any were able to stop alpha-synuclein proteins from clumping together. To their surprise, not only did a variety of flavonoids inhibit these proteins from accumulating, but they could also break up existing deposits.[1962]

This study suggests that by eating healthfully, we can reduce our exposure to pollutants while countering their effects at the same time. And when it comes to countering the effects of pesticides, berries may be particularly useful. In a head-to-head battle between pesticides and berries, researchers found that preincubating nerve cells with a blueberry extract allowed them to better withstand the debilitating effects of a common pesticide.[1963] But most such studies were performed on cells in a petri dish. Is there any evidence in people that eating berries could make a difference?

A small study published decades ago suggested that the consumption of blueberries and strawberries might protect against Parkinson's,[1964] but the question remained largely unanswered until a Harvard University study of about 130,000 people found that people who eat more berries do indeed appear to have a significantly lower risk of developing the disease.[1965] For those already diagnosed with Parkinson's, eating berries three or more times a week may also reduce the risk of dying with the disease.[1966]

The editorial that accompanied the study in the journal *Neurology* concluded that more research is necessary, but "until then, an apple a day might be a good idea."[1967] Apples did appear protective against Parkinson's, but only for men. Everyone, however, appeared to benefit from the consumption of blueberries and strawberries, the only berries included in the study.[1968]

If you do decide to follow my recommendation to eat berries every day, I would advise not serving them with cream. Not only has dairy been shown to block some of the beneficial effects of berries,[1969] but, as we saw earlier, dairy products may contain compounds that cause the very damage the berries may be trying to undo.

Cannibalistic Feed Biomagnification

If people just eat from the bottom two levels of the food chain, only plants and plant eaters—that is, cows, pigs, and chickens fed grain and soya beans—why is the American populace so contaminated? Those of you who remember the mad cow disease story may know the answer. In modern agribusiness, there are essentially no more herbivores.

Millions of tons of slaughter plant by-products continue to be fed to farm animals in the United States every year.[1970] Not only have we turned these animals into meat eaters but virtual cannibals as well. When we feed farm animals millions of tons of meat and bonemeal, we're also feeding them any pollutants this feed may contain. Then, after those animals are slaughtered, their trimmings go to feed the next generation of farm animals, potentially concentrating the pollutant levels higher and higher.[1971] So we can end up like polar bears or eagles at the top of the food chain and suffer the biomagnified pollutant consequences. When we eat these farmed animals, it's almost as if we're also eating every animal they ate.

The use of slaughter plant by-products in animal feed can recycle both toxic heavy metals and industrial chemicals back into the food supply. Lead accumulates in animal bones and mercury in animal protein[1972] (which is why egg whites contain up to twenty times more mercury than do yolks[1973]). Persistent lipophilic organic pollutants (known as PLOPs[1974]—really!) build up in animal fat. Reducing meat consumption can help reduce exposure, but these contaminants can come back to us in a variety of animal products. "Although a vegetarian lifestyle can lower the body burden of PLOP, MMHg [mercury], and lead," one toxicologist noted, "such benefits can be undermined by the consumption of contaminated milk and egg products. Farm animals that have been fed contaminated animal products produce contaminated milk and egg products."[1975]

If we want to drop our PLOP, we should eat as low as possible on the food chain.

There are a number of simple things we can do that may decrease our risk of dying from Parkinson's disease. We can wear seat belts and bicycle helmets to avoid getting hit in the head; we can exercise regularly,[1976] avoid becoming overweight,[1977] consume peppers and berries, and minimize our exposure to pesticides, heavy metals, and dairy and other animal products. It's worth it. Trust me when I say that no family should have to endure the tragedy of Parkinson's.

14

How Not to Die from Prostate Cancer

The prostate is a walnut-sized gland located between the bladder and base of the penis, just in front of the rectum. It surrounds the urethra, the outlet from the bladder, and secretes the fluid portion of semen. Just as glandular tissue in the breast can become cancerous, so can glandular tissue in the prostate.

Autopsy studies show that most older men develop prostate cancer.[1978] Most men die with prostate cancer without ever knowing they had it. That's the problem with the emphasis on screenings—many prostate cancers that are detected may never have led to harm even if they'd gone undiscovered.[1979] Unfortunately, not all men are so lucky. Around thirty-three thousand die each year in the United States from prostate cancer.[1980]

The Risks and Benefits of PSA Prostate Cancer Screening

While 64 percent of men may develop hidden prostate cancers by their sixties,[1981] the lifetime risk of being *diagnosed* with prostate cancer is only about 11 percent, and the risk of dying from it is 2.5 percent.[1982] So, most men die *with* their prostate tumors rather than *from* them. Indeed, most men with prostate cancer spend their whole lives never even knowing they had it. So, should we get a PSA prostate screening test or not?

The U.S. Preventive Services Task Force (USPSTF) recommends against routine PSA screening,[1983] as do the American College of Preventive Medicine,[1984] the American Academy of Family Physicians,[1985] and the majority of professional medical societies in developed countries around the world (thirty-six out of forty-two).[1986] In 2018, though, the USPSTF shifted from a summary judgment against routine screening to stating that "the decision about whether to be screened for prostate cancer should be an individual one" for men aged fifty-five to sixty-nine,[1987] which is more in line with the "shared decision making" stance of the American Urological Association,[1988] American College of Physicians,[1989] and American Cancer Society.[1990] In other words, men should be informed about the risks and benefits and decide for themselves. However, men who are on the fence and don't express a clear preference in favor of screening should not be screened, according to the latest USPSTF recommendations.[1991]

More recently, an international panel of experts concluded that clinicians need not feel obligated to even systematically bring it up, judging that most men would decide to decline PSA screening given the clear harms and small and uncertain benefits.[1992] That, however, is up to each individual. Let's run the numbers.

Similar to the 92 percent of women who either overestimated the mortality reduction from mammograms by tenfold or more or simply didn't know, 89 percent of men vastly overestimated the benefits of prostate cancer screening or had no idea. Most thought fifty prostate cancer deaths could be prevented out of one thousand men regularly screened,[1993] when in reality it's more like one.[1994] But doesn't even a one-in-a-thousand chance of not dying from cancer make a few blood tests worth it? The downsides are more than inconvenience.

About one in seven men who undergo PSA screening will test positive, yet in two-thirds of the cases the subsequent biopsy results will be normal.[1995] So, out of a thousand regularly screened men, about one hundred and fifty will have a false alarm and be biopsied unnecessarily, which can cause minor complications like pain and bloody ejaculate, or, in approximately 1 percent of cases, more serious complications, like bloodborne infections that require hospitalization.[1996] The greatest harm, however, is overdiagnosis. Unnecessary biopsies are bad enough but are nothing compared to unnecessary cancer treatment.

Large-scale randomized trials suggest that 20 to 50 percent of men diagnosed with prostate cancer would have never become symptomatic in their lifetime. They never would have been the wiser had they not been screened, but now they may be needlessly heading to the operating table. About three in a thousand men die during radical prostatectomy or soon after the surgery. That may help explain why there appears to be no overall mortality benefit to prostate cancer screening.[1997] For every life saved, another one may be extinguished for a cancer they would never have even known about.[1998]

Another fifty in a thousand end up with serious surgical complications. Even if the surgery goes smoothly, about one in five men develop long-term urinary incontinence requiring the use of pads, and most—two out of three—will experience long-term erectile dysfunction. Most men who receive radiation therapy also experience long-term sexual erectile dysfunction, and up to one in six experience long-term bowel issues, such as fecal incontinence. If this treatment was saving your life, it would be worth it, but it may be fifty times more likely that you were instead overdiagnosed with a cancer that would never have bothered you. In that much more likely case, you would be suffering all harms, no benefit.[1999] Yet it's like with mammograms—the people who have been harmed the most feel as though they've been helped the most.

Milk and Prostate Cancer

Since the U.S. National Dairy Board was first created by the Dairy and Tobacco Adjustment Act of 1983, it has spent more than $1 billion on advertising. By now, we're all familiar with its various slogans, such as "Milk is a natural." But is it? Humans are the only species who drink milk after weaning. It also does seem a bit *unnatural* to drink the milk of another species.

What about "Milk: It Does a Body Good"? All foods of animal origin contain sex steroid hormones, such as estrogen, but today's genetically "improved" dairy cows are milked throughout their pregnancies when their reproductive hormones are particularly high.[2000] These hormones naturally found even in organic cow's milk may play a role in the various associations identified between milk and other dairy products and hormone-related conditions, including acne,[2001] diminished male reproductive potential,[2002] and premature puberty.[2003] The hormone content in milk may explain why women who drink it appear to have five times the rate of twin births compared with women who do not drink it.[2004] When it comes to cancer, though, the greater concern may have to do with growth hormones.[2005]

Mother Nature designed cow's milk to put a few hundred pounds on a baby calf within a few months. A lifetime of human exposure to these growth factors in milk may help explain the connections found between dairy consumption and certain cancers.[2006] Leading Harvard University nutrition experts have expressed concern that the hormones in dairy products and other growth factors could stimulate the growth of hormone-sensitive tumors.[2007] Experimental evidence suggests that dairy could also promote the conversion of precancerous lesions or mutated cells into invasive cancers.[2008]

Concerns about milk and other dairy products first arose from population-scale data, such as the twenty-five-fold increase in prostate cancer in Japanese men since World War II, which coincided with a sevenfold increase in egg consumption, a ninefold increase in meat consumption, and a twentyfold increase in dairy consumption.[2009] Though the rest of their diets remained comparatively stable and similar trends have been noted in other countries,[2010] there were myriad changes in Japanese society beyond eating more animal products that could have contributed to these rising cancer rates. So scientists took a closer look.

To control for as many variables as possible, researchers devised an experiment in which they dripped milk on human prostate cancer cells in a petri dish. The researchers chose organic cow's milk to exclude any effect of added hormones, such as the bovine growth hormone, which is commonly injected into conventionally raised cows in the United States so they produce more milk.[2011] The researchers found that cow's milk stimulated the growth of human prostate cancer cells in each of fourteen separate experiments, producing an average increase in cancer growth rate of more than 30 percent. In contrast, almond milk *suppressed* the growth of the cancer cells by more than 30 percent.[2012]

What happens in a petri dish, though, doesn't necessarily happen in people. Nevertheless, a compilation of case-control studies did conclude that cow's milk consumption is a risk factor for prostate cancer,[2013] and the same outcome was found for cohort studies.[2014] Higher milk consumption is associated with a 23 percent higher risk of dying from prostate cancer.[2015]

But, you may be wondering, if you don't drink milk, what will happen to your bones? Doesn't milk help prevent osteoporosis? It turns out that the promised benefit may be just another empty marketing ploy. A recent meta-analysis of prospective cohort studies involving nearly half a million people found that greater milk intake is associated with an *elevated* risk of hip fracture.[2016] Even if we were to start drinking milk during adolescence in an attempt to bolster peak bone mass, it probably wouldn't reduce our chances of fracture later in life.[2017]

Some babies are born with a rare birth defect called *galactosemia*, in which they lack the enzymes needed to detoxify galactose, a type of sugar found in milk. This means they end up with elevated levels of galactose in their blood, which can cause bone loss.[2018] A group of Swedish researchers figured that even among people who can normally detoxify galactose, it might not be good for their bones to be drinking all that milk sugar every day.[2019] And galactose may not just hurt bones. Scientists actually use galactose to induce premature aging in lab animals. When researchers slipped lab animals some galactose, the "life-shortened animals showed neurodegeneration, mental retardation and cognitive dysfunction . . . diminished immune responses and reduction of reproductive ability."[2020] And it doesn't take much, just the human equivalent of one to two glasses' worth of milk a day.[2021]

However, since humans aren't rodents, researchers investigated the connection between milk intake and mortality, as well as fracture risk in large populations of milk drinkers.[2022] In addition to significantly *more* bone and hip fractures, researchers found higher rates of premature death, more heart disease, and significantly more cancer for each daily glass of milk women drank. Three glasses a day was associated with nearly twice the risk of dying early.[2023] Men with higher milk consumption also had a higher rate of death, although they didn't have higher fracture rates.[2024]

Overall, the study showed a dose-dependent higher rate of mortality (in both men and women) and fracture (in women), but the opposite was found for other dairy products, such as soured milk and yogurt, which would go along with the galactose theory, because the bacteria in these foods can ferment away some of the lactose.[2025]

The medical journal editorial accompanying the published study emphasized that, given the rise in milk consumption around the world, the "role of milk in mortality needs to be established definitively now."[2026]

With the then largest-ever study on milk intake and mortality showing such adverse effects, Harvard researchers stepped in with three of their cohorts to form a study twice as big to see whether the Swedish findings were just a fluke. After following more than two hundred thousand men and women for up to three decades, they confirmed the bad news in 2019. Those who consumed more dairy lived significantly shorter lives.[2027] Every additional half-serving of regular milk a day was associated with a 9 percent increased risk of dying from cardiovascular disease, an 11 percent increased risk of dying from cancer, and an 11 percent increased risk of dying from all causes put together. A meta-analysis of all such prospective cohort studies found that high intake of whole milk was indeed associated with a higher risk of dying from cancer, cardiovascular disease, and all causes put together.[2028]

Eggs, Choline, and Cancer

More than three million men are currently living with prostate cancer, but living with prostate cancer is better than dying from it. If the cancer is caught while still localized within the prostate, the chances of it killing us within the next five years are practically nil. However, if the cancer spreads far enough, our chances of surviving five years may be as low as one in three.[2029] For this reason, scientists have been desperate to identify factors involved in the spread of prostate cancer once it has emerged.

Hoping to identify possible culprits, Harvard University researchers recruited more than one thousand men with early-stage prostate cancer and followed them for several years. Compared with men who rarely ate eggs, men who ate even less than a single egg a day appeared to have twice the risk of prostate cancer progression, such as metastasizing into the bones. The only thing potentially worse for prostate cancer than eggs was poultry: Men with more aggressive cancer who regularly ate chicken and turkey had up to four times the risk of prostate cancer progression.[2030]

The researchers suggested that the link between consuming poultry and advancing cancer may be due to cooked-meat carcinogens (such as heterocyclic amines as discussed in chapter 12). For unknown reasons, these carcinogens build up more in the muscles of chickens and turkeys than in those of other animals.[2031]

But what cancer-promoting substance is there in eggs? How could eating less than an egg a day double the risk of cancer invasion? The answer may be choline, a compound found concentrated in eggs.[2032]

Higher levels of choline in the blood have been associated with increased risk of developing prostate cancer in the first place.[2033] This may explain the link between eggs and cancer progression.[2034] But what about cancer mortality? In a paper entitled "Choline Intake and Risk of Lethal Prostate Cancer," the same Harvard team found that men who consumed the most choline from food also had an increased risk of cancer death.[2035] Men who consume two and a half or more eggs per week—basically an egg every three days—may have an 81 percent increased risk of dying from prostate cancer.[2036] The choline in eggs, like the carnitine in red meat, is converted into a toxin called *trimethylamine*[2037] by bacteria that exist in the guts of those who eat meat.[2038] And trimethylamine, once oxidized in the liver, appears to increase the risk of heart attack, stroke, and premature death.[2039]

Ironically, the presence of choline in eggs is something the egg industry boasts about even though most Americans get more than enough choline.[2040] Mind you, the industry executives are aware of the cancer connection. Through the Freedom of Information Act, I was able to get my hands on an email from the executive director of the Egg Nutrition Board directed to another egg industry executive that discussed the Harvard study suggesting that choline is a culprit in promoting cancer progression. "Certainly worth keeping in mind," he wrote, "as we continue to promote choline as another good reason to consume eggs."[2041]

Diet vs. Exercise

Nathan Pritikin, the man who helped launch a lifestyle medicine revolution—and saved my grandma's life—wasn't a nutritionist or a dietitian. He wasn't even a doctor. He was an engineer. When he was diagnosed with heart disease in his forties, Pritikin reviewed all the available research himself and decided to try eating the type of diet followed by populations in places like rural Africa, where heart disease was rare. He figured that if he stopped eating a heart-disease-promoting diet, he could stop the advancement of the disease. What he found was even more remarkable. He didn't just stop the disease from getting worse, he reversed his condition.[2042] He then went on to help thousands of others do the same.

After attempting to vanquish our number one killer, heart disease, Dr. Dean Ornish and Pritikin Research Foundation researchers moved on to killer number two: cancer. They developed an elegant series of experiments, placing people on different diets and then dripping their blood on human cancer cells growing in a petri dish. Whose bloodstream would be better at suppressing cancer growth?

The research showed that the blood of people randomized to a plant-based-diet group was dramatically less hospitable to cancer-cell growth than the blood of people in the control group who continued to eat their typical diet. The blood of those eating the standard American diet does fight cancer—if it didn't, many of us right now would be dead!—but the blood of people eating plant-based diets was shown to fight cancer about eight times better.[2043]

The blood of men on the standard American diet slowed down the rate of prostate cancer cell growth by 9 percent. Place men on a plant-based diet for a year, though, and the blood circulating within their bodies can suppress cancer cell growth by 70 percent—that's nearly eight times the stopping power compared to a meat-centered menu.[2044] Similar studies have shown that women eating plant-based diets appear to strengthen their bodies' defenses against breast cancer in just fourteen days (as detailed in chapter 12).[2045] It's as if we're a totally different person inside after eating and living healthfully for just a couple weeks.

It should be noted that the strengthening of cancer defenses in all these studies involved eating a plant-based diet *and* exercising. In the breast cancer study, for example, the women were asked to walk thirty to sixty minutes a day. How, then, do we know it was the diet that made their blood more effective at suppressing cancer growth? To tease out the effects of diet and exercise, a UCLA research team compared three groups of men: a plant-based diet-and-exercise group, an exercise-only group, and a control group of sedentary people eating standard fare.[2046]

The diet-and-exercise group had been following a plant-based diet for fourteen years, along with participating in moderate exercise, such as a daily walk. The exercise-only group eating the standard American diet, on the other hand, had spent about fifteen years exercising strenuously for an hour a day at the gym at least five times a week. The researchers wanted to know if people who exercise hard enough for long enough develop cancer-fighting abilities that rival that of strolling plant eaters.[2047]

To find out, blood from each of the three groups was dripped onto human prostate cancer cells growing in a petri dish to see whose blood kicked more cancer butt. The blood of the control group wasn't completely defenseless. Even if you're a french fry-eating couch potato, your blood may still be able to kill off 1 to 2 percent of cancer cells. But the blood of those who exercised strenuously every weekday for fifteen years killed 2,000 percent more cancer cells than the control group's. Fantastic results, but the blood of those in the plant-based diet-and-exercise group wiped out an astounding 4,000 percent more cancer cells than that of the first group. Clearly exercise alone had a dramatic effect, but at the end of the day, thousands of hours in the gym appeared to be no match for a plant-based diet.[2048]

Reversing the Progression of Prostate Cancer with Diet?

If a healthy diet can turn our bloodstream into a cancer-fighting machine, what about using it not just to prevent cancer but also to treat it? The progression of other leading killers, including heart disease, type 2 diabetes, and hypertension, can be prevented, arrested, and even reversed, so why not cancer?

To test this question, Dr. Ornish and his colleagues recruited ninety-three men with prostate cancer who had chosen not to undergo any conventional treatment. Prostate cancer can be so slow growing and the side effects of treatment so onerous that men diagnosed with it often choose to be placed in a medical holding pattern called "watchful waiting" or "expectant management." Because the next step is often chemotherapy, radiation, and/or radical surgery that may leave men incontinent and impotent, doctors try to delay treatment as long as possible. And since these patients aren't actively doing anything to treat the disease, they represent an ideal population in whom to investigate the power of diet and lifestyle interventions.

The prostate cancer patients were randomized into two groups: a control group who wasn't given any diet or lifestyle advice beyond whatever their personal doctors told them to do, and a healthy-living group prescribed a strict plant-based diet centered around fruits, vegetables, whole grains, and beans, along with other healthy lifestyle changes, such as walking for thirty minutes, six days a week.[2049]

Cancer progression was tracked using PSA levels, a marker of prostate cancer growth inside the body. After a year, the control group's PSA levels increased by 6 percent. That's what cancer tends to do: grow over time. But among the healthy-living group, PSA levels *decreased* by 4 percent, suggesting an average shrinkage of their tumors.[2050] No surgery, no chemotherapy, no radiation—just eating and living healthfully.

Biopsies taken before and after the diet and lifestyle intervention showed that the expression of more than five hundred genes was affected. This was one of the first demonstrations that changing what we eat and how we live can affect us at a genetic level, in terms of which genes are switched on and off.[2051] Within a year after the study ended, the cancers in the patients in the control group grew so much that 10 percent of them were forced to undergo a radical prostatectomy,[2052] a surgery that involves the removal of the entire prostate gland and surrounding tissues. This treatment can lead not only to urinary incontinence (urine leakage) and impotence but to alterations in orgasmic function in approximately 80 percent of men undergoing the procedure.[2053] In contrast, none in the plant-based diet and lifestyle group ended up on the operating table.

How were the researchers able to convince a group of older men to basically eat a low-fat vegan diet for a year? They evidently delivered prepared meals to their homes.[2054] I guess the researchers figured the men would just eat whatever is put in front of them—and it worked!

Now, how about in the real world? Realizing that doctors apparently can't get most men with cancer to eat even just five servings of fruits and veggies daily,[2055] a group of researchers at the University of Massachusetts settled on just trying to change their A:V ratio, or the ratio of animal to vegetable proteins in their diets.[2056] Would just a reduction in meat and dairy and an increase in plant foods be enough to put cancer into remission?

To test this, the researchers randomized prostate cancer patients into two groups, one group who attended classes on eating a more plant-based diet and a conventional-care group who received no dietary instruction. The healthy-eating advice group was able to drop their A:V ratio down to about 1:1, getting half their protein from plant sources. In contrast, the control group's ratio stayed up around 3:1 animal-to-plant protein.[2057]

Those on the half-vegan diet did appear to slow down the growth of their cancer. Their average PSA doubling time—an estimate of how fast their tumors may have been doubling in size—slowed from twenty-one months to fifty-eight months.[2058] In other words, the cancer kept growing, but even a part-time plant-based diet appeared to be able to significantly slow down their tumors' expansion. It is worth noting, though, that Dr. Ornish and colleagues were able to demonstrate that a full-time plant-based diet allowed for an apparent *reversal* in cancer growth: Their study participants' PSA levels didn't just rise more slowly; they trended downward. Thus, the ideal animal-to-plant protein ratio may be closer to zero to one.

The Worst A and the Best V

What if there's just no way Grandpa's going vegan? What would be on the short list of foods for him to avoid, or to include, in his diet?

Based on the Harvard University prostate cancer progression and mortality data detailed above, eggs and poultry may be the worst offenders: Patients may face twice the cancer progression risk from eating less than a single egg per day and up to quadruple the risk from eating less than a single serving of chicken or turkey daily.[2059]

On the other hand, if we were to add only one thing to our diet, consider cruciferous vegetables. Less than a single serving a day of broccoli, brussels sprouts, cabbage, cauliflower, or kale may cut the risk of cancer progression by more than half.[2060]

Watching our animal-to-plant protein ratio might be useful for cancer prevention in general. For example, the largest study ever performed on diet and bladder cancer—comprising nearly five hundred thousand people—found that an increase in animal protein consumption of just 3 percent was associated with a 15 percent increased risk of bladder cancer. On the other hand, an increase in plant protein intake of only 2 percent was associated with a 23 percent *decreased* cancer risk.[2061]

Flaxseeds

Prostate cancer rates vary tremendously around the world. African Americans, for example, may have an incidence of clinically apparent prostate cancer that is some 30 times greater than that of Japanese men and 120 times greater than that of Chinese men. This discrepancy has been attributed in part to the higher amounts of animal protein and fat in Western diets.[2062] Another factor, though, may be the soya common in many Asian diets, which contains protective phytoestrogens called *isoflavones*.[2063]

As detailed in chapter 12, the other major class of phytoestrogens is lignans, found throughout the plant kingdom but especially concentrated in flaxseeds. Higher levels of lignans tend to be found in the prostate fluids of populations of men with relatively low rates of prostate cancer,[2064] and lignans have also been shown to slow the growth of prostate cancer cells in a petri dish.[2065]

Researchers decided to put lignans to the test by asking men with prostate cancer scheduled for prostate-removal surgery the following month to consume three tablespoons a day of flaxseeds. After surgery, their tumors were examined. Within just those few weeks, the flaxseed consumption appeared to have lowered their cancer-cell proliferation rates, while at the same time increasing their rate of cancer-cell clearance.[2066]

Even better, flaxseeds may also be able to prevent prostate cancer from advancing to that stage in the first place. Prostatic intraepithelial neoplasia (PIN) is a precancerous prostate lesion found during a biopsy; it is analogous to ductal carcinoma in situ of the breast. Those with PIN have a high risk for cancer to appear during subsequent biopsies—25 to 79 percent.[2067] Because men are repeatedly biopsied to monitor their condition, the procedures provide a perfect opportunity to see if a dietary intervention can keep these lesions from progressing to cancer.

After the first biopsies of their prostates came back PIN positive, fifteen men were asked to eat three tablespoons of flaxseeds a day for the six months until their next biopsy. After that time, they showed a significant drop in PSA levels and biopsy cell-proliferation rates, suggesting that flaxseeds may indeed thwart the progression of prostate cancer. Two of the men saw their PSA levels drop to normal and didn't even need a second biopsy.[2068]

Bottom line: The evidence suggests that flaxseeds are a safe, low-cost source of nutrition and may reduce tumor-proliferation rates.[2069] Why not give them a try? Just make sure to grind the flaxseeds first if you don't buy them pre-ground—otherwise, the seeds may pass right through your body undigested.

Enlarged Prostate

If a healthy diet can slow down the abnormal growth of prostate cancer cells, can it also slow down the abnormal growth of normal prostate cells? Benign prostatic hyperplasia (BPH) is a condition characterized by enlargement of the prostate gland. In the United States, BPH affects millions of men[2070]—as many as half of men by their fifties and 80 percent of men by their eighties.[2071] Because the male prostate surrounds the outlet from the bladder, it can obstruct the normal flow of urine if it grows too large. This obstruction can cause a weak or hesitant stream and inadequate emptying of the bladder, requiring frequent trips to the bathroom. The stagnant urine retained in the bladder can also become a breeding ground for infection.

Unfortunately, the problem only seems to worsen as the gland continues to grow. Billions of dollars have been spent on drugs and supplements, and millions of American men have undergone surgery for BPH.[2072] Surgical procedures involve a variety of Roto-Rooter techniques with innocent-sounding acronyms, such as TUMT, TUNA, and TURP. The *T*s stand for *transurethral*—meaning going up the penis with an instrument called a resectoscope. TUMT stands for *transurethral microwave thermotherapy*, in which doctors basically tunnel up the penis using an antenna-like tool and burn out a shaft with microwaves.[2073] TUNA stands for *transurethral needle ablation*; here, a column is burned out with a pair of heated needles. And these are so-called minimally invasive techniques![2074] The gold standard procedure is the TURP, wherein surgeons essentially use a loop of wire to core out the prostate. Side effects include "postoperative discomfort."[2075]

There has to be a better way.

BPH is so common that most doctors may assume that it's just an inevitable consequence of aging. But it wasn't always so. In China in the 1920s and 1930s, for example, a medical college in Beijing reported that BPH affected not 80 percent of male patients but about eighty cases *total* over fifteen years. Both the historic rarity of BPH and prostate cancer in Japan and China have been attributed to the countries' traditional plant-based diets.[2076]

This idea was studied by the same Pritikin Foundation researchers who pitted the blood of individuals before and after a plant-based diet against the growth of prostate cancer cells. This time, they performed the same experiment on the type of normal prostate cells that grow to obstruct urine flow. Within just two weeks, those eating plant-based diets saw their blood acquire the ability to suppress the abnormal growth of noncancerous prostate cells too—and the effect didn't seem to dissipate with time. The blood of those eating plant-based diets over the long term had the same beneficial effect for up to twenty-eight consecutive years. So it appears that as long as we continue to eat healthfully, prostate cell-growth rates could continue to go down and stay down.[2077]

Some plants may be particularly prostate friendly. Research has found that flaxseeds can be used to treat BPH. Men given the equivalent of about three tablespoons of flaxseeds a day experienced relief comparable to that provided by commonly prescribed such drugs as Flomax or Proscar[2078]—without the drugs' side effects, such as lightheadedness or sexual dysfunction.

Is it possible to prevent BPH in the first place? Eating garlic and onions has been associated with significantly lower risk of BPH.[2079] In general, cooked vegetables may work better than raw ones, and legumes—beans, chickpeas, split peas, and lentils—have also been associated with lower risk.[2080] TVP, short for textured vegetable protein, is the soya bean product often used in pasta sauces and veggie chili I mentioned in chapter 10. I would recommend that type of TVP over the one used in urology, which stands for *transurethral vaporization of the prostate*.[2081]

Wee Hours of the Night

One of the most burdensome symptoms of BPH is nocturia, frequently having to get up in the middle of the night to pee.[2082] Common sense might tell us to just try to drink less before bed, but, remarkably, there is not a clear association between fluid intake and nocturia.[2083] One study of about 150 men did find a correlation between the frequency of nocturia and nighttime water intake, as well as how much water you drink in the four hours before bedtime,[2084] but another study with more than a thousand older adults found no relationship between the amount of bedtime fluids and having to repeatedly get up to urinate.[2085] I was surprised to learn that fluid restriction has never been properly put to the test. There was a study in which a group of older men averaging four pees a night was told to reduce their daily fluid intake from about seven cups to around five cups, and they were able to shave nightly bathroom trips down to three,[2086] but it and other similar studies[2087,2088] failed to include a control group to really nail down cause and effect.

It's even harder to get people to restrict sodium. Nocturia reviews with titles asking the question "Which Matters Most, the Water or the Salt?"[2089] note that salt intake has been associated with nocturia frequency,[2090] presumably due to increased thirst-driven fluid intake. This has led to recommendations to cut down on salt to control nocturia severity, but sodium restriction is hard to study because compliance is notoriously poor.[2091] You can, however, compare the change in nocturia episodes of those who successfully cut down on salt intake versus those who didn't. Based on that, it appears even cutting back on as little as a half teaspoon of salt a day may reduce nightly episodes by 40 to 60 percent.[2092,2093]

Evening protein intake may also contribute to nocturia. The main determinant of urine concentration is not sodium, but urea, which is a breakdown product of protein excretion. Protein-rich suppers were found to correlate with excess overnight urine production, leading to the as-of-yet-untested conclusion that a "reduction of evening protein consumption may be an effective lifestyle intervention in the management of nocturia. . . ."[2094]

IGF-1

Why do people who live to be one hundred or older seem to escape cancer? As we age, our risk of developing and dying from cancer grows every year—until we reach eighty-five or ninety, when, interestingly, our cancer risk begins to drop.[2095] Indeed, if we don't get cancer by a certain age, we may never get it. What accounts for this relative resistance to cancer among centenarians? It may have to do with a cancer-promoting growth hormone called insulin-like growth factor 1 (IGF-1).[2096]

Each year, we are reborn. We create and destroy nearly our entire body weight in new cells every year. Every day, about fifty billion of our cells die, and about fifty billion new cells are born to keep us in balance.[2097] Of course, sometimes we need to grow, as when we're a baby or during puberty. Our cells don't become larger when we grow up; they simply become more numerous. An adult may have around forty trillion cells in their body, four times more than a child.

Once we've gotten through puberty, we no longer need to produce many more cells than we retire. We still need our cells to grow and divide, of course—out with the old, in with the new. We just don't want to make more cells than we're putting out to pasture. In adults, extra cell growth can mean the development of tumors.

How does our body keep itself in balance? By sending chemical signals called hormones to all the cells. A key signal is a growth hormone called IGF-1. It sounds like a droid from *Star Wars*, but IGF-1 is actually a crucial factor in regulating cell growth. Levels go up when we're a kid in order to power our development, but when we reach adulthood, IGF-1 levels diminish. It's our body's cue to stop producing more cells than it kills off.

Should our levels of IGF-1 remain too high when we reach adulthood, however, our cells will constantly receive a message to grow, divide, and keep going and growing. Not surprisingly, the more IGF-1 we have in our bloodstream, the higher our risk for developing cancers, such as prostate cancer.[2098]

There is a rare form of dwarfism called Laron syndrome that is caused by the body's inability to produce sufficient amounts of IGF-1. Affected individuals grow to be only a few feet tall, but they also almost never get cancer.[2099] Laron syndrome is a sort of cancer-proofing mutation, which led scientists to wonder: What if we could get all the IGF-1 we needed as a child to grow to a normal height but then down-regulate this hormone as adults and thereby turn off excess growth signals? It turns out we can do just that—not with surgery or medication but through simple dietary choices.

The release of IGF-1 appears to be triggered by the consumption of animal protein.[2100] This may explain why we can so dramatically bolster the cancer-fighting power of our bloodstream within weeks of eating a plant-based diet. Remember the experiments in which dripping the blood from people eating healthy diets onto cancer cells wiped more of them out? Well, if we add back to the cancer cells the amount of IGF-1 that left the plant eaters' systems, guess what happens? The diet-and-exercise effect disappears. The cancer cell growth comes surging back. This is one of the ways we suspect plant-based eating boosts our blood defenses: By reducing animal protein intake, we reduce our levels of IGF-1.[2101]

After just eleven days of cutting back on animal protein, our IGF-1 levels can drop by 20 percent, and our levels of IGF-1 *binding protein* can jump by 50 percent.[2102] One of the ways our body tries to protect itself from cancer—that is, excessive growth—is by releasing a binding protein into our bloodstream to tie up any excess IGF-1. Think of it as the body's emergency brake. Even if we've managed to down-regulate production of new IGF-1 through diet, what about all that excess IGF-1 still circulating from the bacon and eggs eaten at breakfast two weeks before? No problem: The liver releases a snatch squad of binding proteins to help take it out of circulation.

How plant-focused does a diet have to be to lower IGF-1 levels? Animal protein stimulates IGF-1 production whether it's the muscle proteins in meat, the egg-white protein in eggs, or the milk proteins in dairy. Vegetarians who include eggs and dairy in their diets don't seem to achieve a significant reduction in IGF-1. Only men[2103] and women[2104] who limit their intake of all animal proteins appear able to significantly drop their levels of the cancer-promoting hormone and raise their levels of the protective binding proteins.

Prostate cancer isn't inevitable. A healthy diet and lifestyle changes can presumably only help. That's the nice thing about lifestyle interventions—they can be implemented in addition to whatever other treatment options are chosen. In a research setting, that can complicate matters, as we don't know which action may be responsible for any improvement. But when facing a cancer diagnosis, we may want to opt for all the help we can get. Regardless of whether cancer patients elect chemo, surgery, or radiation, they can always improve their diets. A prostate-healthy diet is a breast-healthy diet is a heart-healthy diet is a body-healthy diet.

15

How Not to Die from Iatrogenic Causes (Or, How Not to Die from Doctors)

As the saying goes, an ounce of prevention is worth a pound of cure. That's quaint, but a pound isn't all that heavy. Why should we bother changing our diet and lifestyle when modern medicine can just fix us up?

Unfortunately, modern medicine isn't nearly as effective as most people think.[2105] Doctors excel at treating acute conditions, such as mending broken bones and curing infections, but for chronic diseases, which, as we know, are the leading causes of death and disability, conventional medicine doesn't have much to offer and, in fact, can sometimes do more harm than good.

For example, side effects from medications given in hospitals kill an estimated 106,000 Americans every year.[2106] That statistic alone effectively makes medical care the sixth-leading cause of death in the United States. And this number reflects only the number of deaths from taking the drugs as prescribed. An additional 7,000 people die every year from receiving the wrong medication by mistake, and 20,000 more die from other hospital errors.[2107] A more recent estimate places the number of individuals killed by hospital errors at closer to 200,000 a year.[2108] Hospitals are dangerous places, and that's not even counting the estimated 72,000 deaths each year due to hospital-acquired infections.[2109] But can deaths from infections be blamed on doctors? They can if doctors won't even wash their hands.

We've known since the 1840s that handwashing is the best way to prevent hospital-acquired infections, yet compliance among health care workers rarely exceeds 50 percent. And doctors are the worst offenders.[2110] One study found that even in a medical intensive care unit, displaying a "contact precautions" sign (signaling particularly high risk of infection) leads less than a quarter of doctors to properly wash their hands or use a hand sanitizer when treating patients.[2111] That's right. Not even one doctor out of four washed their hands before laying them on the ill. Many physicians are concerned that should it become widely known how many people doctors inadvertently kill every year, it could "undermine public trust."[2112] But if doctors can't even be bothered to wash their hands, how much trust do we deserve?

This unfortunate (and gross!) situation means that we could go into the hospital for a simple operation and leave with a life-threatening infection—if we leave at all. Every year, 12,000 Americans die from complications due to surgeries that weren't even necessary in the first place. For those keeping score, that's more than 200,000 Americans dead from so-called *iatrogenic causes* (from the Ancient Greek *iatrós*, meaning "doctor"). And that figure is based only on the data on hospitalized patients. In outpatient settings—at the doctor's office, for instance—prescription drug side effects may result in 199,000 additional deaths in the United States alone.[2113]

The Institute of Medicine estimates that medical errors may kill even more Americans, up to 98,000,[2114] bringing the total annual death count closer to 300,000. That's more than the entire population of cities like Newark, Buffalo, or Orlando. Even using more conservative estimates of deaths due to medical errors, health care comes in as the *real* third-leading cause of death in America.[2115]

How did the medical community respond to such damning conclusions? Deafening silence in both word and deed.[2116] The first such report, which appeared in 1978, suggested that about 120,000 deaths occurring in hospitals could be prevented.[2117] Then, sixteen years later, another scathing reminder was published in the *Journal of the American Medical Association*, suggesting the iatrogenic death toll may be "the equivalent of three jumbo-jet crashes every 2 days."[2118] In the years between these two reports, as many as nearly two million Americans may have died due to medical errors, yet the medical community refused to comment on this tragedy and made no substantial effort to reduce the number of deaths.[2119] Another estimated 600,000 deaths later, the prestigious Institute of Medicine released its own landmark report on the catastrophic consequences of medical error[2120]—but again, little was done as a result.[2121]

Eventually, a few changes were implemented. For instance, interns and residents could no longer be made to work for more than eighty hours a week (at least on paper), and shifts couldn't be more than thirty consecutive hours long. That may not sound like a big step, but when I started my internship after graduating from medical school, we worked thirty-six-hour shifts every three days. Combined with our other days of work, that added up to a 117-hour work week. When interns and residents are forced to pull all-nighters, studies suggest they may make 36 percent more serious medical errors, five times more diagnostic errors, and have twice as many "attentional failures" (such as nodding off during surgery).[2122] The patient is supposed to be asleep during surgery, not the surgeon. It's no surprise, then, that overworked doctors may cause 300 percent more fatigue-related medical errors that lead to patient death.[2123]

If every single day airliners crashed and killed hundreds of people, we would expect the Federal Aviation Administration to step in and do something. Why doesn't anyone confront the medical profession? Instead of just releasing reports, entities like the Institute of Medicine could have demanded that doctors and hospitals adopt at least a minimum set of preventive practices, such as barcoding drugs to avoid mix-ups[2124]—something that's even done with a packet of biscuits at the supermarket.

Only people on medications are killed by medication errors or the drugs' side effects, though. We have to actually be in the hospital to be killed by a hospital error or get an infection there. The good news is that most visits to doctors are for diseases that can be prevented with a healthy diet and lifestyle.[2125]

The best way to avoid the adverse effects of medical tests and treatments is not to avoid doctors but to avoid getting sick in the first place.

Ignaz Philipp Semmelweis

From the *Proceedings of the Royal Society of Medicine*:

Many men have been endowed with clear intellects and hearts full of love for their fellow men, with the enthusiasm of humanity, and they have been enabled to achieve some signal service for the human race in their day and

> *generation; but in the whole history of medicine there is only one Semmelweis in the magnitude of his services to Mankind, and in the depths of his sufferings from contemporary jealous stupidity and ingratitude.*[2126]

The year is 1846. The scene is the Vienna General Hospital, the largest of its kind in the world. Semmelweis gets a job as obstetrical assistant.[2127]

Semmelweis notices that three times as many women are dying at the hands of the medical students than at the hands of the midwifery students from puerperal fever, commonly known at the time as "the black death of the childbed."[2128] "In the medical school division the mortality from puerperal fever was so terrifying that this division became notorious," Semmelweis describes. "There were heart rendering scenes when [pregnant] patients knelt down, wringing their hands, to beg for a transfer [to the midwifery division] . . ."

Why the discrepancy? The food and ventilation were the same in both divisions. If anything, surgical skill was better in the medical school and overcrowding less. The idea at the time was that the excess mortality was due to the emotional strain of being examined by male students; the midwives were all female. The elders of the medical school met in council and proceeded to exclude the foreign students from the hospital on the ground that they were "rougher in their examination than the Viennese." Death rates didn't change.

Before Lister, before Pasteur, Semmelweis made the connection between the autopsies the medical students were performing and the "examining finger which introduces the cadaveric particles." In May 1847, he required every medical student to wash his hands with a chlorine solution before making an examination, and the death rate plummeted. For the first time in the history of the Vienna hospital, the mortality rate at the medical school fell below that of the school of midwives.[2129]

Knighted, no doubt, for the discovery of the century? Hardly. Historians believe his doctrine was unpalatable to colleagues since it implied that the obstetricians were the cause of death. He shared this knowledge with his superiors. From the *Proceedings of the Royal Society of Medicine*: "The suggestion was unheard of! Indeed, it was sheer impertinence to suggest that the Accoucheur to the Imperial household should carry contagion upon his hands." Semmelweis was summarily dismissed.[2130]

So, he lectured, he wrote papers, and he continued to be ridiculed. Doctors regarded antisepsis as a poor joke. His successor in Vienna publicly stated that the doctrine was "discredited and universally rejected." Semmelweis wrote a book, *The Cause, Nature, and Prevention of Puerperal Fever*, expecting it to save thousands of lives, but it was ignored.[2131]

He then turned from academics to polemics. He started to publish open letters to midwifery professors. "Your teaching . . . is based on the dead bodies of . . . women slaughtered through ignorance. If . . . you continue to teach your students and midwives that puerperal fever is an ordinary epidemic disease, I proclaim you before God and the world to be an assassin . . ."[2132]

By the summer of 1865, he had taken to the streets of Budapest, thrusting circulars into the hands of startled pedestrians. "The peril of childbed fever menaces your life! Beware of doctors for they will kill you . . . Unless everything that touches you is washed with soap and water and then chlorine solution, you will die and your child with you!"[2133]

Semmelweis, at the age of forty-seven, the father of three young children, was committed to an insane asylum in Vienna. He attempted to escape but was forcibly restrained by several guards, secured in a straitjacket, and confined to a darkened cell. The asylum guards beat him severely.

Quoting from the *Bulletin of the History of Medicine*: "He was not in the asylum for long. Thirteen days after admission he was dead." From the autopsy report: "It is obvious that these horrible injuries were . . . the consequences of brutal beating, tying down, trampling underfoot."[2134]

Radiation

There are risks associated not only with medical treatment but also sometimes with diagnosis. A paper entitled "Estimated Risks of Radiation-Induced Fatal Cancer from Pediatric CT" out of Columbia University in 2001 reignited long-standing concerns about the risks associated with medical diagnostic radiation exposure. CT, or CAT, scans use multiple x-rays from different angles to create cross-sectional images, exposing the body to hundreds of times more radiation than a simple x-ray.[2135] Based on the excess cancer risk of Hiroshima survivors exposed to similar doses of radiation,[2136] it was estimated that out of all children who undergo abdominal or head CT scans every year, five hundred "might ultimately die from cancer attributable to the CT radiation."[2137] In response to this revelation, the editor-in-chief of a leading radiology journal conceded, "We radiologists may be as guilty as others when it comes to not watching out for children."[2138]

The risk of developing cancer after a single CT scan may be as high as 1 in 150 for a baby girl.[2139] In general, the diagnostic medical radiation dealt out in one year is estimated to cause 2,800 breast cancers among American women, as well as 25,000 other cancers.[2140] In other words, doctors may be causing tens of thousands of cancers every year.

Patients undergoing these scans are rarely informed of these risks. For example, did you know that getting a chest CT scan is estimated to inflict the same cancer risk as smoking seven hundred cigarettes?[2141] One in every 270 middle-aged women may develop cancer due to a single angiogram.[2142] CT scans and x-rays can be lifesaving, but good evidence suggests that one-fifth to one-half of all CT scans aren't necessary at all and could be replaced with a safer type of imaging or simply not performed at all.[2143]

Many people expressed concern about the radiation exposure from the full-body scanners at airports using backscatter x-rays,[2144] but those machines have since been phased out. The airplane itself, however, is a different story. Because we're exposed to more cosmic rays from outer space at higher altitudes, just one round-trip flight across the United States may subject us to about the same level of radiation as a chest x-ray.[2145] (Given my speaking schedule, I should be glowing in the dark by now!)

Is there anything we can do to mediate the radiation risk? As with so many other health questions, the answer is that we can eat healthfully.

In an investigation funded by the National Cancer Institute, researchers studied the diets and chromosome integrity of airline pilots, who get zapped with extra radiation every time they go to work, to see which foods might be protective. They found that pilots who consumed the most dietary antioxidants suffered the least amount of DNA damage to their bodies. Note the word *dietary*. Antioxidant supplements, such as vitamins C and E, didn't seem to help. Pilots who consumed the most vitamin C through fruits and vegetables, though, appeared to be protected.[2146] Taking antioxidant supplements may be more than just a waste of money. People given 500 mg of vitamin C a day were found to end up with *more* oxidative DNA damage.[2147]

Remember that natural antioxidants in food work synergistically; it's the combination of many different compounds working together that tends to protect us, not high doses of single antioxidants found in supplements. Indeed, those pilots eating a mix of phytonutrients, concentrated in a variety of such plant foods as citrus, nuts, seeds, pumpkins, and peppers, had the lowest levels of DNA damage in response to the radiation they were bombarded with from the galaxy.[2148]

The research team found that dark green leafy vegetables like spinach and kale appear to have an edge over other vegetables and fruits when it comes to radiation protection.[2149] All this time I've been packing kale chips on flights just because they're so lightweight, but it turns out they may also be protecting my DNA.

The same plant-based protection enjoyed by pilots was also found among atomic bomb survivors. For several decades, researchers have followed thirty-six thousand survivors of the nuclear attacks on Hiroshima and Nagasaki. Those who ate vegetable- or fruit-rich diets appeared to cut their cancer risk by about 36 percent.[2150] We saw the same in the aftermath of the accident at the Chernobyl nuclear reactor in Ukraine, where consumption of fresh fruits and vegetables apparently protected children's immune systems, while egg and fish consumption was associated with a significantly increased risk of DNA damage. The researchers suggest this result could have been due to the possibility that the animal foods they ate were contaminated with radioactive elements or the role of animal fats in free-radical formation.[2151]

Nuclear events offer a rare opportunity to study these effects on humans since, obviously, it is unethical to intentionally expose people to radiation. However, as we've learned from declassified documents about U.S. Cold War radiation experiments, this didn't stop our government from injecting "colored" people with plutonium[2152] or feeding "retarded" children radioactive isotopes in their breakfast cereal.[2153] Despite the Pentagon's insistence that these methods were the "only feasible means" of developing ways to protect people from radiation,[2154] researchers have since come up with a few methods that don't violate the Nuremburg Code.

One is to study human cells in a test tube. Research has found, for example, that white blood cells blasted with gamma rays suffered less DNA damage when the cells had been pretreated with phytonutrients from ginger root. The ginger compounds protected DNA nearly as well as the leading radiation sickness drug[2155] at 150 times lower the dose.[2156] Those taking ginger in order to prevent motion sickness during air travel may be protecting themselves against more than just nausea.

Other common foods that may be protective against radiation damage include garlic, turmeric, goji berries, and mint leaves,[2157] but only turmeric has been tested in a clinical study. Taking a daily half teaspoon of a 50:1 ratio of turmeric to powdered black pepper for five days before radiation therapy reduced a measure of oxidative damage by about 50 percent compared to control.[2158] How else can we test the protective power of foods in people rather than petri dishes? To study how diet may protect against cosmic rays, airline pilots were studied. Guess who they studied to see if foods could be protective against x-rays? X-ray technicians.

Hospital workers who routinely operate x-ray machines have been found to suffer more chromosomal damage and to have higher levels of oxidative stress compared with other hospital workers.[2159] For this reason, researchers recruited a group of x-ray techs and asked them to drink two cups of lemon balm tea each day for a month. (Lemon balm is an herb in the mint family.) Even in that short time frame, the lemon balm tea appeared able to boost the level of antioxidant enzymes in the subjects' bloodstreams while also reducing the amount of DNA damage they suffered.[2160]

The Actual Benefit of Diet vs. Drugs

Based on a study of more than one hundred thousand Minnesotans, it appears that seven out of ten people may be prescribed at least one prescription drug in any given year. More than half are prescribed two or more drugs, and 20 percent are prescribed *five* or more medications.[2161] All told, physicians dispense more than *six billion* prescriptions for drugs every year in the United States.[2162] That comes out to twenty prescriptions a year for every man, woman, and child. How is that even possible?

The prescription drugs most often brought up in doctor visits are a cholesterol-lowering medication and blood-pressure pills.[2163] So, a lot of drugs are being doled out in an attempt to prevent disease, but how well are these billions of pills working?

An overconfidence in the power of pills and procedures for disease prevention may be one of the reasons doctors and patients alike may undervalue diet and lifestyle interventions. As we've discussed, when surveyed, people tend to wildly overestimate the ability of mammograms and colonoscopies to prevent cancer deaths, or the power of drugs like Fosamax to prevent hip fractures or drugs like Lipitor to prevent fatal heart attacks.[2164] Patients believe cholesterol-lowering statin drugs are about twenty times more effective than they actually are in preventing heart attacks.[2165] No wonder most people continue to rely on drugs to save them. But the dirty little secret is that most people surveyed said they wouldn't be willing to take many of these pharmaceuticals if they knew how little benefit these products actually offered.[2166]

How ineffectual are some of the most commonly prescribed drugs? When it comes to cholesterol, blood pressure, and blood-thinning drugs, the chance of even high-risk patients benefiting from them is typically less than 5 percent over a period of five years.[2167] When asked, most patients say they want to be told the truth.[2168] However, as doctors, we know that if we divulged this information, few of our patients would agree to take these drugs every day for the rest of their lives, which would be detrimental for the small percentage of people who do truly benefit from them. That's why some doctors in the know as well as drug companies oversell the benefits by conveniently not mentioning how tiny these benefits actually are. When it comes to chronic disease management, practicing conventional medicine can be thought of as practicing deceptive medicine.

For the hundreds of millions of people on these drugs who don't benefit, it's not simply a matter of all the money spent and all the side effects endured. To me, the true tragedy is all the lost opportunity to address the root causes of patients' conditions. When people dramatically overestimate how much their prescription pills protect them, they may be less likely to make the dietary changes necessary to dramatically lower their risk.

Take cholesterol-lowering statin drugs, for example. On average, they reduce the risk of having a heart attack, stroke, or death in the subsequent decade from 5.7 percent down to 3.9 percent, for an absolute risk reduction of about 2 percent.[2169] Meanwhile, a whole food, plant-based diet may work thirty times better, potentially offering an absolute risk reduction of 60 percent after fewer than four years.[2170] In 2014, Dr. Caldwell Esselstyn Jr. published a case series of about two hundred people with significant heart disease showing that a healthy enough plant-based diet may prevent further major cardiac episodes in 99.4 percent of patients who follow it.[2171]

We don't really have the luxury of choosing between following a healthy diet or taking a pill to prevent a heart attack because pills may not work in the near term in 97 percent of the cases. Of course, diet and drugs are not mutually exclusive, and many under Dr. Esselstyn's care wisely continued to take their cardiac meds. We just need to have a realistic understanding of how limited a role the contents of our medicine cabinets play compared to the contents of our refrigerator. Heart disease may continue to be the number one killer of men, women, and eventually our children if doctors continue to rely on drugs and stents. However, if we eat a healthy enough diet, we may be able to reverse the stranglehold it has on our heart. That is something doctors can be proud to divulge to our patients.

Aspirin

How well do over-the-counter drugs perform? Take aspirin, for example. Perhaps the most commonly used medication in the world,[2172] it's been around in pill form for more than a century. Its active anti-inflammatory ingredient, salicylic acid, has been used in its natural form (as an extract of willow tree bark) to ease pain and fever for thousands of years.[2173] One of the reasons it remains so popular—despite the fact that more potent anti-inflammatory painkillers exist now—is that it's used by millions of people on a daily basis as a blood thinner to reduce the risk of a heart attack. As we saw in chapter 1, heart attacks often occur when a blood clot forms in response to a ruptured atherosclerotic plaque in one of our coronary arteries. Taking aspirin may help stop this from happening.

Aspirin may also lower the risk of cancer.[2174] It works by suppressing an enzyme within our body that creates pro-clotting factors, thereby thinning our blood. At the same time, aspirin suppresses pro-inflammatory compounds called *prostaglandins*, which in turn reduces pain, swelling, and fever. Prostaglandins may also dilate the lymph vessels inside tumors, potentially allowing cancer cells to spread. One of the ways scientists think aspirin helps prevent cancer deaths is by counteracting a tumor's attempts to pry open the lymphatic bars on its cage and spread throughout the body.[2175]

So, should everyone take a "baby"-strength aspirin a day? (Note that aspirin should never actually be given to infants or children.[2176]) No. The problem is that aspirin can cause side effects. The same blood-thinning benefit that can prevent a heart attack can also cause a hemorrhagic stroke, in which we bleed into our brain. Aspirin can also damage the lining of the digestive tract.

For those who've already had a heart attack and continue to eat the same diet that led to the first one (and are therefore at exceedingly high risk of having another one), the risk-benefit analysis seems clear: Taking aspirin would probably prevent about six times more serious problems than it causes. But among the general population who have yet to have their first heart attack, the risks and benefits are more closely matched.[2177] Thus, taking an aspirin a day is generally not recommended.[2178] Throw in even a 10 percent reduction in cancer mortality, though, and it could tip the risk-benefit balance in favor of aspirin.[2179] Given that regular, low-dose aspirin use may reduce the risk of cancer mortality by one third,[2180] it is tempting to recommend it for nearly everyone. If only we could get the anti-inflammatory effects without the bleeding risk.

Aspirin is actually two drugs in one. It's technically *acetylsalicylic acid*. Within minutes of swallowing aspirin, enzymes in our gut split it apart into an acetyl group and salicylic acid.[2181] The acetyl group is what inactivates our platelets and thins our blood. If we could consume salicylic acid directly, we could combat inflammation without the risk of bleeding. And that's exactly what we can do with diet.

The willow tree isn't the only plant that contains salicylic acid. It's widely found in many of the fruits and vegetables in the plant kingdom.[2182] That's why we often find the active anti-inflammatory ingredient of aspirin in the bloodstreams of people who aren't taking it.[2183] The more fruits and vegetables we eat, the higher our blood level of salicylic acid may rise.[2184] In fact, the levels of people eating plant-based diets actually overlap with those of some people taking low-dose aspirin.[2185]

With all that salicylic acid flowing through their systems, one might think plant eaters would have higher ulcer rates, because aspirin is known to chew away at the gut. But those following plant-based diets actually appear to have a significantly *lower* risk of ulcers.[2186] How is that possible? Because in plants, the salicylic acid may come naturally prepackaged with gut-protective nutrients. For example, nitric oxide from dietary nitrates exerts stomach-protective effects by boosting blood flow and protective mucus production in the lining of the stomach, effects which demonstrably oppose the pro-ulcerative impact of aspirin.[2187] So, for the general population, by eating plants instead of taking aspirin, individuals may not only get some of aspirin's benefits without its risks but also get the benefits—with even more benefits.

People who have had a heart attack should follow their physician's advice, which probably includes taking aspirin every day. But what about everyone else? I think everyone should take aspirin—but in the form of produce, not a pill.

The salicylic acid content in plants may help explain why traditional, plant-based diets were so protective. For instance, before their diets were Westernized, animal products made up only about 5 percent of the average Japanese diet.[2188] During this period in the 1950s, age-adjusted death rates from colon, prostate, breast, and ovarian cancers were five to ten times lower in Japan than in the United States, while incidences of pancreatic cancer, leukemia, and lymphoma were three to four times lower. This phenomenon was not unique to the Japanese. As we've seen throughout this book, Western rates of cancers and heart disease have been found to be dramatically lower among populations whose diets are centered around plant foods.[2189]

If part of this protection arises from the aspirin phytonutrients, which plants in particular are packed with them? While salicylic acid is ubiquitously present in fruits and vegetables, herbs and spices contain the highest concentrations.[2190] Chili powder, paprika, and turmeric are rich in the compound, but cumin has the most per serving. Indeed, just one teaspoon of ground cumin may be about the anti-inflammatory equivalent of a baby aspirin. This may help explain why India, with its spice-rich diets, has among the lowest worldwide rates of colorectal cancer[2191]—the cancer that appears most sensitive to the effects of aspirin.[2192]

And the spicier, the better. A spicy vegetable vindaloo has been calculated to contain four times the salicylic acid content of a milder madras-style veggie dish. Eat a single meal, and we can get the same spike in salicylic acid in our bloodstream as if we had taken an aspirin.[2193]

The benefits of salicylic acid are one reason we should strive to choose organic produce. Because the plant uses the compound as a defense hormone, its concentration may be increased when that plant is bitten by bugs. Pesticide-laden plants aren't nibbled as much and, perhaps as a result, appear to produce less salicylic acid. For example, in one study, soup made from organic vegetables was found to contain nearly six times more salicylic acid than soup prepared from conventional, nonorganically grown ingredients.[2194]

Another way to get more salicylic acid bang for our buck is by opting for whole foods. Whole-grain breads, for example, not only offer more salicylic acid but reportedly contain one hundred times more phytonutrients in general than white bread.[2195]

Attention has been focused on salicylic acid because of the voluminous data on aspirin, but hundreds of the other phytonutrients have been found to have anti-inflammatory and antioxidant activity as well. Still, given the strength of the aspirin evidence, there are those in the public health community who talk of a widespread "salicylic acid deficiency," proposing that the compound be classed as an essential vitamin: "Vitamin S."[2196] Whether it's the salicylic acid or a combination of other phytonutrients that account for the benefits of whole plant foods, the solution is the same: Eat more of them.

Colonoscopies

The colonoscopy. You'll be hard pressed to find a more dreaded routine procedure. Every year, U.S. doctors may perform more than fifteen million colonoscopies,[2197] an exam used to detect abnormal changes in the large intestine (colon) and rectum. During the procedure, doctors insert a five-foot-long flexible tube fitted with a tiny video camera and inflate the colon with air to visualize the colon lining. Any suspicious polyps or other abnormal tissue can be biopsied during the procedure. Colonoscopies can help doctors diagnose causes of rectal bleeding or chronic diarrhea, but routine colon cancer screenings may be the most common reason they are performed.

The reasons doctors often find it difficult to convince their patients to keep coming back for colonoscopies include the necessary bowel prep, during which you have to drink quarts of a powerful liquid laxative before the procedure to completely clean yourself out. There's also the pain and discomfort of the procedure itself[2198] (though you're purposefully given drugs with amnesiac effects so you won't remember how it felt),[2199] feelings of embarrassment and vulnerability, and the fear of complications.[2200] These fears are not unfounded. Despite how routinely colonoscopies are performed, serious complications occur in about one out of every three hundred cases, including such issues as perforations and severe bleeding.[2201] Perforations can occur when the tip of the colonoscope punctures the wall of the colon, when the colon is overinflated, or when a doctor cauterizes a bleeding biopsy site. In extremely rare cases, this cautery can ignite some residual gas and cause the colon to literally explode.[2202]

Death from colonoscopy is rare, ranging anywhere from 1 in 1,400 procedures to 1 in 14,000.[2203] Yet this means colonoscopies may be killing thousands of Americans every year, raising the question: Do the benefits outweigh the risks?

Colonoscopies are not the only screening technique for colon cancer. The

U.S. Preventive Services Task Force (USPSTF), the preeminent prevention guidelines body, considers colonoscopies just one of six acceptable coloncancer screening strategies. Starting at age forty-five, everyone should at least get a colonoscopy once a decade, have their stool tested for hidden blood every year or for DNA cancer markers every one to three years (both of which involve no scoping at all), a "virtual" colonoscopy (CT colonography) once every five years (which is also noninvasive), a sigmoidoscopy every five years, or a sigmoidoscopy every ten years along with stool testing every year.[2204] Though routine screenings are no longer recommended at age seventy-five, this assumes we've been testing negative for decades. If you're now seventy-five and have never been screened, then it's probably a good idea to get screened at least into your eighties.[2205]

Sigmoidoscopy uses a much smaller scope than in a colonoscopy and has ten times fewer complications.[2206] However, because the scope may only go about two feet inside our body, it might miss tumors farther inside. So, which is better overall? We won't know until four randomized controlled colonoscopy trials are published.[2207] Only one has been published so far, and, to date, sigmoidoscopies would be expected to have the best chance of extending life.[2208] Most other developed countries do not recommend either scoping procedure, though. For routine colon cancer screening, they endorse the noninvasive stool blood testing.[2209]

Which of the six options is best for you? The USPSTF recommends that the decision should be made on an individualized basis after weighing the benefits and risks with your doctor.

To what extent, though, do doctors inform patients of their options? Researchers audiotaped clinic visits to find out. They were looking for the nine essential elements of informed decision making, which include explaining the pros and cons of each option, describing the alternatives, and making sure the patient understands these options.[2210]

Unfortunately, when it came to colon cancer screening, in most cases, the doctors and nurse practitioners studied communicated *none* of this vital information, zero out of nine elements.[2211] As an editorial in the *Journal of the American Medical Association* put it: "There are too many probabilities and uncertainties for patients to consider and too little time for clinicians to discuss them with patients."[2212] So doctors tend to just make up patients' minds for them. What do they choose? A National Cancer Institute-funded survey of more than one thousand physicians found that nearly all doctors (94.8 percent) recommended a colonoscopy.[2213] Why do doctors push colonoscopies in the United States when most of the rest of the world appears to prefer noninvasive alternatives?[2214] It may be because most doctors in the rest of the world don't get paid by procedure.[2215] As one U.S. gastroenterologist put it, "Colonoscopy . . . is the goose that has laid the golden egg."[2216]

An exposé in *The New York Times* on spiraling health care costs noted that in many other developed countries, colonoscopies cost just a few hundred dollars. In the United States? The procedure may cost thousands, which the journalists concluded has less to do with providing top-notch medical care and more with business plans aimed at maximizing revenue, marketing, and lobbying.[2217] Who's in charge of setting the prices? The American Medical Association. A *Washington Post* investigation exposed that each year, a secretive AMA committee determines billing standards for common procedures. The result is gross overestimates for the time it takes to perform common services like colonoscopies. As the *Post* pointed out, if AMA standards are to be believed, some doctors would have to work more than twenty-four hours a day to perform all the procedures they report to Medicare and private insurers. Is it any wonder that gastroenterologists in the United States bank nearly $500,000 per year?[2218]

But why would our family doctor or internist push the procedure if they're not the ones doing it? Many doctors who refer their patients to gastroenterologists receive what are essentially financial kickbacks. The U.S. Government Accountability Office (GAO) reported on this practice of so-called self-referrals, a scheme where providers refer patients to entities in which they have a financial interest. The GAO estimated that doctors make nearly a million more referrals every year than they would have if they were not personally profiting.[2219]

What to Take Before a Colonoscopy

Ever popped one of those breath mints into your mouth after a big meal at a restaurant? Peppermint doesn't just make our breath smell better; it also helps to reduce the gastrocolic reflex—the urge to defecate following a meal. Nerves in our stomach stretch after eating, which triggers spasms in the colon to enable our body to make room for more incoming food. Peppermint can reduce these spasms by relaxing the muscles that line our colon.[2220]

What does this have to do with colonoscopies? If you take circular strips of human colons removed during surgery and lay them on a table, they spontaneously contract about three times per minute. Kind of creepy. But if you drip menthol (found in peppermint) onto the colon strips, the strength of the contractions diminishes significantly.[2221] During a colonoscopy, such spasms can hinder the progress of the scope and cause the patient discomfort. By relaxing colon muscles, peppermint can make the procedure easier for both doctor and patient.

Doctors have experimented with spraying peppermint oil from the tip of the colonoscope,[2222] as well as using a hand pump to flood the colon with a peppermint solution prior to the procedure.[2223] The simplest solution might be the best, though: asking the patient to swallow peppermint oil capsules. Premedicating with eight drops' worth of peppermint essential oil four hours before a colonoscopy was found to significantly reduce colon spasms, patient pain, and make the scope easier to insert and withdraw compared with a placebo.[2224]

If you do need a colonoscopy, ask your doctor about using this simple plant remedy. It might make it easier on both of you.

Clearly, patients in the United States may be getting more medical care than they really need. So said Dr. Barbara Starfield, who literally wrote the book on primary care.[2225] One of our nation's most prestigious physicians, she composed the scathing commentary in the *Journal of the American Medical Association* naming medical care as the third-leading cause of death in the United States.[2226]

Her primary-care work has been widely embraced, but her findings on the potentially ineffective and even harmful nature of U.S. health care received almost no attention. "The American public appears to have been hoodwinked into believing that more interventions lead to better health," she later said in an interview.[2227] As one health care quality advisor noted, the widespread disregard of Dr. Starfield's evidence "recalls the dark dystopia of George Orwell's *1984*, where awkward facts swallowed up by the 'memory hole' become as if they had never existed at all."[2228]

Sadly, Dr. Starfield is no longer with us. Ironically, she may have died from one of the adverse drug reactions she so vociferously warned us about. After she was placed on two blood thinners to prevent a stent in her heart from clogging up, she told her cardiologist she was bruising more and bleeding longer—that's the drug risk you hope doesn't outweigh the benefits. Then Dr. Starfield died after apparently hitting her head while swimming and bleeding into her brain.[2229]

The question I ask myself is not whether she should have been put on two blood thinners for as long as she was, or whether she should have had the stent inserted to begin with. Rather, I wonder if she could have avoided the medication and the surgery both by avoiding the heart disease in the first place. Heart attacks are considered 96 percent avoidable in women who eat a wholesome diet and engage in other healthy lifestyle behaviors.[2230] The number one killer of women need almost never happen.

PART 2

Introduction

In Part 1 of this book, I explored the science that demonstrates the role a plant-based diet rich in certain foods may play in helping to prevent, treat, and even reverse the progression of some of the fifteen leading causes of death. For those who may have already been diagnosed with one or more of these diseases, the information in Part 1 can be lifesaving. But for everyone else—perhaps those worried about inheriting their family history of illness or those who simply want their diet to promote health and longevity—the primary question might concern the food choices to make day in and day out. I have given thousands of presentations, and one of the most common questions I get is, "What do *you* eat every day, Dr. Greger?"

This, Part 2 of *How Not to Die*, is my response to that question.

I've never had so much a sweet tooth as a grease tooth. Pepperoni pizza. Chicken wings by the basket. Sour cream and onion crisps. A Hardee's bacon cheeseburger nearly every day during high school. Anything oily and fatty—and all washed down with an ice-cold Dr Pepper. Okay, so maybe a little bit of a sweet tooth. I also really liked donuts with strawberry icing.

Even though my grandma's miraculous recovery from heart disease inspired me to pursue a career in medicine, I didn't clean up my own diet until the publication of Dr. Ornish's landmark Lifestyle Heart Trial in 1990.[2231] I was such a nerd in high school that I would spend my summer holidays hanging out in the science library at the local university. And there it was, published in the most prestigious medical journal in the world—proof that my family's story was not a fluke: Heart disease could potentially be reversed. Dr. Ornish and his team had taken before-and-after x-rays of people's arteries and demonstrated how they could sometimes be opened up without angioplasty. A subsequent study proved this translated into a significant improvement in blood flow to the heart.[2232] No surgery. No miracle drug. Just a plant-based diet and other healthy lifestyle changes. That's what motivated me to change my own diet and ignited my thirty-five-year love affair with nutritional science, a love that's still burning bright. From that point forward, I have been determined to spread the word about food's power to make us healthy, keep us healthy, and, if necessary, return us to health.

For the purposes of this book, I've created two simple tools to help you integrate what I've learned into your own daily life:

1. a Traffic Light system to quickly identify the healthiest options, and
2. a Daily Dozen checklist that will help you incorporate the foods that I consider essential to the optimal diet. (Check out the free Dr. Greger's Daily Dozen app on iPhone and Android.)

So which foods are good for you, and which are bad?

This sounds like a simple enough question. In truth, it can be difficult to answer. Whenever I'm asked at a lecture whether a certain food is healthy or not, I have to invariably reply, "Compared to what?" For example, are eggs healthy? Compared to oatmeal, no. But compared to the sausage links next to them on the breakfast platter? Yes.

What about white potatoes? They're vegetables, so they must be healthy, right? Someone asked me this after a group of Harvard University researchers raised concerns about baked and mashed potatoes.[2233] So are they healthy? Compared to french fries, yes. Compared to a baked or mashed *sweet* potato? No, they're not.

I realize these may not be satisfying answers for people who just want to know whether or not to eat the darned potato, but the only way to answer the question meaningfully is to ask what the other options are. In a fast-food restaurant, for example, a baked potato may very well be the healthiest option.

Compared to what? is not just a Socratic learning exercise. Eating is essentially a zero-sum game: When we choose to eat one thing, we are generally choosing not to eat another. Sure, we could just go hungry, but eventually our body tends to balance things out by eating more later.

So, anything we choose to eat has an opportunity cost.

Every time we put something in our mouth, it's a lost opportunity to put something even healthier in there. Think of it as having $2,000 in your daily caloric bank. How do you want to spend it? For the same number of calories, you can eat one Big Mac, one hundred strawberries, or a nineteen-liter bucket of salad. Of course, these three options don't exactly fill the same culinary niche—if you want a burger, you want a burger, and I don't expect kilos of strawberries to make it on the Value Menu anytime soon—but this is an illustration of how mountainous a nutritional bang we can get for the same caloric buck.

The opportunity costs exacted are not only the nutrients we could otherwise be getting but the unhealthy components we could otherwise be avoiding. After all, when was the last time you had a friend diagnosed with kwashiorkor, scurvy, or pellagra? These are some of the traditional nutrient-deficiency diseases upon which the foundation of the field of nutrition was built. To this day, the nutrition and dietetic professions remain focused on what nutrients we may be lacking, but most of our chronic diseases may have more to do with what we're getting too much of. Know anyone suffering from obesity, heart disease, type 2 diabetes, or high blood pressure?

Isn't It Expensive to Eat Healthfully?

Researchers at Harvard University compared the cost and healthfulness of various foods across the country, hunting for the best bargains. They found that, to get the greatest nutrition for our dollars, we should buy more nuts, soya foods, beans, and whole grains, and less meat and dairy. A meat-free diet, for example, could save individuals about an estimated $750 a year.[2234] The researchers concluded: "The purchase of plant-based foods may offer the best investment for dietary health."[2235]

Less healthy foods only beat out healthier foods on a cost-per-calorie basis, which is a way we measured food cost back in the nineteenth century. Back then, the emphasis was on cheap calories, no matter how we got them. So while beans and sugar both cost the same at that time (five cents a pound), the U.S. Department of Agriculture promoted sugar as more cost effective for pure "fuel value."[2236]

The USDA can be excused for discounting the nutritional difference between beans and pure sugar. After all, vitamins hadn't even been discovered yet. Nowadays, we know better and can compare the cost of foods based on their nutritional content. An average serving of vegetables may cost roughly four times more than the average serving of junk food, but those veggies have been calculated to average twenty-four times more nutrition. So on a cost-per-nutrition basis, vegetables offer six times more nutrition per dollar compared to highly processed foods. Meat costs about three times more than vegetables yet yields sixteen times less nutrition based on an aggregate of nutrients. Because meat is less nutritious *and* costs more, vegetables net us *forty-eight times* more nutrition per dollar than meat.[2237]

If our intent is to get as many calories as possible for the least amount of money, then healthier foods lose out, but if we want to get the most *nutrition* as cheaply as possible, we need to look no further than the produce aisle. Spending just fifty cents more per day on fruits and vegetables may buy us a 10 percent drop in mortality.[2238] Now that's a bargain! Imagine if there were a pill that could reduce our chance of dying by 10 percent over the next decade and only had good side effects. How much do you think the drug company would charge? Probably more than fifty cents.

Dining by Traffic Light

Historically, the U.S. government's official Dietary Guidelines for Americans has had a "Food Components to Reduce" chapter, which specifically lists added sugars, calories, cholesterol, saturated fat, sodium, and trans fat.[2239] At the same time, there are nine so-called shortfall nutrients, of which at least a quarter of the American population isn't reaching an adequate intake. These are fiber; the minerals calcium, magnesium, and potassium; and vitamins A, C, D, E, and K.[2240] But we don't eat food "components." We eat food. There's no magnesium aisle in the supermarket. So which foods tend to have the most of the good stuff and the least of the bad? I've simplified it into a traffic light illustration. (See figure 5.)

Just as on the road, *green* means go, *yellow* means caution, and *red* means stop. (In this case, stop and think before you put it into your mouth.) Ideally, green-light foods should be maximized, yellow-light ones minimized, and red-light foods avoided.

Is *avoid* too strong a word? After all, the Dietary Guidelines for Americans

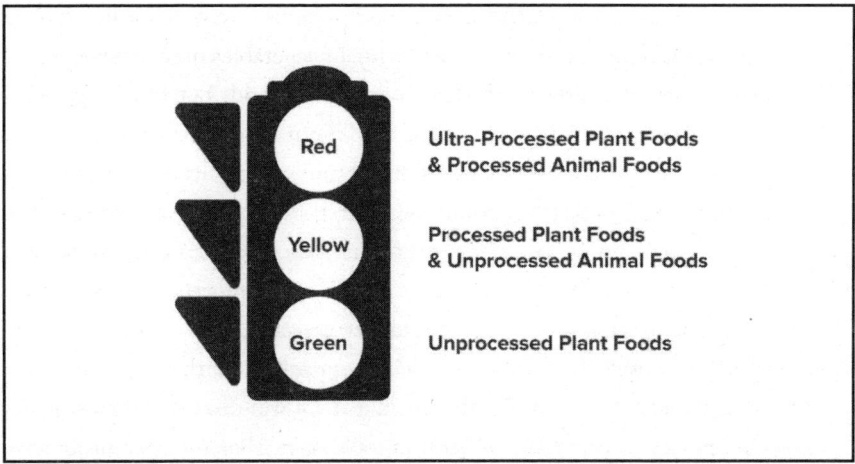

Figure 5

merely encourage us to "moderate" our intake of unhealthy foods.[2241] For example: "Eat less . . . candy."[2242] From a health standpoint, though, shouldn't we generally try to *avoid* candy? Public health authorities don't just advise us to smoke *less* tobacco. They tell us to quit. They know only a small fraction of smokers will actually heed this advice, but it's the job of public health authorities to say what's best and let us make up our own minds.

That's why I appreciate the American Institute for Cancer Research (AICR) recommendations. Not beholden to the USDA, the AICR simply lays out the science. When it comes to the worst of the worst, the institute doesn't pull any punches. The Dietary Guidelines for Americans has given advice like "Consume fewer . . . sodas [fizzy drinks],"[2243] while the AICR cancer prevention guidelines instead advise: "Avoid sugary drinks." Similarly, the AICR doesn't just say to cut back on bacon, ham, hot dogs, sausage, and lunch meats. The cancer guidelines tell us to "avoid processed meat." Period. Why? Because "data do not show any level of intake that can confidently be shown not to be associated with risk."[2244]

The healthiest diet is one that maximizes the intake of whole plant foods and minimizes the intake of animal-based foods and processed junk. Simply put, eat more green-light foods. Eat fewer yellow-light foods. And, especially, eat even fewer red-light foods. Just like running red lights in the real world, we may be able to get away with it once in a while, but we shouldn't make a habit out of it.

Given this, what we've seen in the previous chapters makes a lot of sense.

Unprocessed plant foods tend to have more of the protective nutrients that too many of us are lacking and fewer disease-promoting factors. No wonder the eating habit apparently best able to control our epidemics of dietary disease is a whole food, plant-based diet. After all, food is a package deal.

This is one of the most important concepts in all of nutrition. Yes, there is calcium in cheese, protein in pork, and iron in beef, but what about all the baggage that comes along with these nutrients—the dose of dairy hormones, the lard, the saturated fat? As much as Burger King proclaims you can "Have It Your Way," you can't go up to the counter and ask for a burger, hold the saturated fat and cholesterol. Food is, indeed, a package deal.

Dairy is a leading source of calcium in the United States, and it's also a leading source of saturated fat. What kind of "baggage" do we get along with the calcium in leafy green vegetables? Fiber, folate, iron, and antioxidants—some of the very nutrients lacking in milk. By getting most of our nutrition from whole plant foods, we get a bonus instead of baggage.

When the National Pork Board promotes ham as an "excellent source of protein,"[2245] I can't help but think of the famous quote from a McDonald's senior vice president for marketing who, under oath in a court of law, described Coca-Cola as nutritious because it is "providing water."[2246]

Why Don't the Dietary Guidelines Just Say No?

The green-light message shines brightly in pronouncements telling us to "eat more fruits and vegetables," but the yellow and red lights can be dim and cloudy thanks to politics. In other words, the guidelines are clear when there is eat-more messaging, but eat-less messaging is obscured into biochemical components. "Eat more fresh produce" versus "Eat less saturated and trans fatty acids." National health authorities rarely just say to "eat less meat and dairy." That's why my green-light message will sound familiar, but the yellow- and red-light messages may sound controversial to you. You've certainly heard we should "eat fruits and veggies," but maybe not "minimize meat."

Part of the USDA's mission is "expanding markets for agricultural products."[2247] At the same time, the federal agency is tasked with protecting public health by helping to develop the Dietary Guidelines for Americans. That's why, when those two directives are in sync, its eat-more language is clear:

"Increase fruit intake." "Increase vegetable intake."[2248] But when its dual mandates are in conflict—when "improving nutrition and health" is at odds with promoting "agriculture production"[2249]—the eat-less messaging of the Dietary Guidelines gets repackaged and ends up referring to biochemical components: "Reduce intake of solid fats (major sources of saturated and trans fatty acids)."

What's the average person supposed to do with that obscure little nugget?

When the guidelines tell us to eat less added sugar, calories, cholesterol, saturated fat, sodium, and trans fat, that's code for eat less junk food, less meat, less dairy, fewer eggs, and fewer processed foods. But they can't actually say that. When they did in the past, all heck broke loose. For example, when a USDA employee newsletter even suggested trying a meat-free lunch once a week as part of Johns Hopkins University's School of Public Health's "Meatless Mondays" initiative,[2250] the resulting political firestorm from the meat industry led the USDA to retract the advice just hours later.[2251] "As a result of these conflicts [of interest]," concluded an analysis in the *Food and Drug Law Journal*, "the Guidelines sometimes favor the interests of the food and drug industries over the public's interest in accurate and impartial dietary advice."[2252]

This reminds me of the landmark report on trans fat from the National Academy of Sciences' Institute of Medicine (IOM), one of our most prestigious institutions.[2253] It concluded that no amount of trans fat is safe "because any incremental increase in trans fatty acid intake increases C[oronary] H[eart] D[isease] risk."[2254] Since trans fats are found naturally in meat and dairy products,[2255] this placed the IOM in a quandary: "Because trans fats are unavoidable in ordinary, nonvegan diets, consuming 0 percent of energy would require significant changes in patterns of dietary intake."[2256]

So if trans fats are found in meat and dairy and the only safe intake of trans fats is zero, that means the Institute of Medicine went on to encourage everyone to start eating a plant-based diet, right? No, it did not. The director of Harvard's Cardiovascular Epidemiology Program famously explained why: "We can't tell people to stop eating all meat and all dairy products," he said. "Well, we could tell people to become vegetarians," he added. "If we were truly basing this only on science, we would, but it is a bit extreme."[2257]

We certainly wouldn't want scientists to base anything on science!

How Sad Is the Standard American Diet?

As cynical as I've become about diet and nutrition, particularly in the United States, I was still surprised by a report from the National Cancer Institute on the status of the American diet. For example, three out of four Americans don't eat a single piece of fruit in a given day, and nearly nine out of ten don't reach the minimum recommended daily intake of vegetables. On a weekly basis, 96 percent of Americans don't reach the minimum for greens or beans (three servings a week for adults), 98 percent don't reach the minimum for orange vegetables (two servings a week), and 99 percent don't reach the minimum for whole grains (about 85–115 grams a day).[2258]

Then there's junk food. The federal guidelines have been so lax that up to 25 percent of our diet could be made up of "discretionary calories," meaning junk. A quarter of our calories could come from candy floss washed down with Mountain Dew, and we'd still be within the guidelines. Yet we failed. Astoundingly, 95 percent of Americans exceeded their discretionary calorie allowance. The researchers found that only *one in a thousand* American children between the ages of two and eight made the cutoff, consuming less than the equivalent of about a dozen spoonsful of sugar a day.[2259]

And we wonder why there is an obesity epidemic?

"In conclusion," the researchers wrote, "nearly the entire U.S. population consumes a diet that is not on par with recommendations. These findings add another piece to the rather disturbing picture that is emerging of a nation's diet in crisis."[2260]

Producers of unhealthy commodities aren't out to make us sick. They're just trying to make a buck. Coca-Cola's profit margin, for example, is about one quarter of the drink's retail price, making soft-drink production, alongside tobacco, among the most profitable industries.[2261] What's harder to understand is why the public health community isn't doing more about it.

"When the history of the world's attempt to address obesity is written," wrote the head of Yale University's Rudd Center for Food Policy & Obesity, "the greatest failure may be collaboration with and appeasement of the food industry."[2262] For instance, Susan G. Komen, a leading U.S. breast cancer charity, linked up with fast-food giant KFC to sell pink buckets of fried chicken.[2263]

Save the Children used to be a leader in the push for taxes on fizzy drinks to offset some of the costs of childhood obesity. Then the organization did an abrupt 180-degree turn, withdrawing its support, saying that such campaigns no longer "fit with the way that Save the Children works." Perhaps it is only a coincidence that it was seeking a grant from Coca-Cola and had already accepted a $5 million grant from Pepsi.[2264]

Even though our eating habits are now killing more Americans than our smoking habits,[2265] I often hear the refrain in public health circles that we have to work with, rather than against, these companies, because unlike with tobacco, we don't have to smoke, but we do have to eat.[2266] Well, yes, we need to breathe—but we don't need to breathe smoke. And yes, we need to eat, but we don't need to eat junk.

How I Define "Processed"

My Traffic Light model stresses two important general concepts: Plant foods, with their greater protective nutritional factors and fewer disease-promoting ones, are healthier than animal foods, and unprocessed foods are healthier than processed foods. Is that always true? No. Am I saying that all plant foods are better than all animal foods? No. In fact, one of the worst items on store shelves is partially hydrogenated vegetable fat—a product that has *vegetable* right in its name. Even some unprocessed plants—such as blue-green algae—can be toxic.[2267] Anyone who's had a bad case of poison ivy knows plants don't always like to be messed with. In general, though, choose plant foods over animal foods, and unprocessed over processed. Michael Pollan, bestselling author of *The Omnivore's Dilemma*, said, "If it came from a plant, eat it. If it was made in a plant, don't."[2268]

What do I mean by *processed*? The classic example is the milling of grains from whole wheat to white flour. Isn't it ironic that these are called "refined" grains, a word meaning improved or made more elegant? The elegance was not felt by the millions who died in the nineteenth century from beriberi, a vitamin B-deficiency disease that resulted from polishing rice from brown to white.[2269] (White rice is now fortified with vitamins to compensate for the "refinement.") A Nobel Prize was awarded for the discovery of the cause of beriberi and its cure—rice bran, the brown part of rice that was removed. Beriberi can cause damage to the heart muscle, resulting in death from heart failure. Surely such a thing could never happen in modern times—an epidemic of heart disease that could be prevented and cured with a change in diet? (Please reread chapter 1.)

Sometimes, however, processing can make foods healthier. For example, tomato juice appears to be the one common juice that may actually be healthier than the whole fruit. The processing of tomato products boosts the availability of the antioxidant red pigment lycopene by as much as fivefold.[2270] Similarly, the removal of fat from cacao beans to make cocoa powder improves the nutritional profile because cocoa butter is one of the rare saturated plant fats (along with coconut and palm kernel oils) that can raise our cholesterol.[2271]

So for the purposes of the Traffic Light model, I like to think of "unprocessed" as *nothing bad added, nothing good taken away*. Through this lens, tomato juice could be seen as relatively unprocessed because even much of the fiber is retained—unless salt is added, which would make it a processed food in my book and bump it right out of the green zone. Similarly, I would consider chocolate—but not cocoa powder—processed because sugar is added.

Using my definition of *nothing bad added, nothing good taken away*, steel-cut oats, rolled oats, and even (plain) instant oatmeal can all be considered unprocessed. Almonds are obviously a whole plant food. I would also consider no-salt-added almond butter to be a green-light food, but even unsweetened almond milk is a processed food, a food from which nutrition has been stolen. Am I saying almond milk is bad for you? As we've discussed, foods are not so much good or bad as they are better or worse. All I'm saying is that unprocessed foods tend to be healthier than processed ones. Think of it this way: Eating almonds is healthier than drinking almond milk.

The limited role I see for yellow-light foods in a healthy diet is to promote the consumption of green-light foods. For instance, if the only way you'll eat oatmeal in the morning is if you make it creamy with almond milk, then go right ahead. The same could be said for red-light foods. Without hot sauce, my intake of dark green leafy vegetables would plummet. Yes, I know there are all sorts of sodium-free, exotically flavored vinegars out there that I could use, and maybe one day I'll completely wean myself off Tabasco. But given my current tastes, the green ends justify the red means. If the *only* way you're going to eat a big salad is to sprinkle Bac-Os (bacon-flavored bits) on top, then sprinkle away.

Bac-Os are what are referred to as an *ultra-processed* food, bearing few redeeming nutritional qualities or resemblance to anything that grew out of the ground, plus containing added garbage. Bac-Os, for example, had added trans fats and Red 40, a food dye banned in a number of European countries.[2272] As a red-light food, it ideally should be avoided, but if the alternative to your big spinach salad with Bac-Os is KFC, then it's better to have the salad with the Bac-Os. They can be the spoonful of sugar that makes the medicine go down. The same goes for real bacon bits, for that matter.

I realize some people have religious or ethical objections to even trivial amounts of animal products. (Growing up Jewish near the largest pig factory farm west of the Mississippi, I can relate to both sentiments.) But from a human health standpoint, when it comes to animal products and processed foods, it's the overall diet that matters.

What Does "Whole Food, Plant-Based" Mean, Exactly?

Sometimes people's diets take on a religiosity of their own. I remember a man once telling me that he could never "go plant-based" because he could never give up his grandma's chicken soup. Then don't! After I asked him to say hello to his bubbe for me, I told him that enjoying her soup shouldn't keep him from making healthier choices the rest of the time. The problem with all-or-nothing thinking is that it keeps people from even taking the first steps. The thought of *never* having pepperoni pizza again somehow turns into an excuse to keep ordering it every week. Why not scale down to once a month or reserve it for special occasions? We cannot let the "perfect" be the enemy of the good.

It's really the day-to-day choices we make that matter most. What we eat on special occasions is insignificant compared to what we eat day in and day out. So don't beat yourself up if you really want to put edible bacon-flavored candles on your birthday cake. (I'm not making those up![2273]) Our body has a remarkable ability to recover from sporadic insults as long as we aren't habitually poking it with a fork.

This book is not about vegetarianism, veganism, or any other "-ism." There are people who completely eliminate any and all animal products as part of a religious or moral stance and may indeed end up better off as a side benefit.[2274] But strictly from a human health standpoint, we would be hard pressed to argue, for example, that the traditional Okinawan diet, which is 96 percent plant-based,[2275] is inferior to a typical Western, 100 percent vegan diet. In Kaiser Permanente's guide "The Plant-Based Diet: A Healthier Way to Eat," the authors define a plant-based diet as one that excludes animal products completely, but they make sure to note: "If you find you cannot do a plant-based diet 100 percent of the time, then aim for 80 percent. Any movement toward more plants and fewer animal products can improve your health!"[2276]

From a nutrition standpoint, the reason I don't like the terms *vegetarian* and *vegan* is that they are only defined by what you *don't* eat. When I used to speak regularly on college campuses, I would meet vegans who appeared to be living off french fries and beer. Vegan, technically, but not exactly health promoting. That's why I prefer the term *whole food, plant-based nutrition*. As far as I can discern, the best available balance of evidence suggests that the healthiest diet is one centered on unprocessed plant foods. On a day-to-day basis, the more whole plant foods and the fewer processed and animal products, the better.[2277]

Preparing Yourself for Healthier Habits

First, you need to know your own psychology. There are certain personality types that do better when they go all in. If you tend to have an "addictive" personality, or if you are the kind of person who takes things to extremes—for instance, you either don't drink at all or you drink in excess—it's probably best for you to try to stick with the program. But some individuals can get away with "social smoking," for example; they can light up a few times a year and escape nicotine dependence.[2278] The reason we as physicians advocate for smokers to quit completely is not because we think that one cigarette every once in a while is going to do irreversible damage but because we're afraid that one cigarette may lead to two, and, before long, the unhealthy habit has taken hold. Similarly, one (well-cooked) hamburger is not going to kill anyone. It's what we eat day-to-day that adds up. We have to take stock of our own disposition to know if we can overcome the risk of sliding down the slippery slope.

There's a concept in psychology called "decision fatigue" that marketers use to exploit consumers. It appears we humans have a limited capacity to make many decisions in one short stretch of time, and the quality of our decisions will deteriorate to the extent that we eventually begin making downright irrational choices. Ever wonder why supermarkets stock junk food right by the checkout counter? After wading through the thirty thousand items in the average supermarket,[2279] we end up with less willpower to resist impulse purchases.[2280] So making rules for ourself and sticking to them may help us make more sensible choices over the long run. For instance, making a strict decision to never cook with oil, to avoid meat entirely, or to eat only whole grains may paradoxically make for sturdier life changes. By not having junk food in the house, we remove the temptation by removing the choice. I know if I get hungry enough, I'll eat an apple.

There may also be a *physiological* argument for not wildly deviating from a well-planned diet. After a holiday cruise during which we indulged in all manner of rich foods, our palate may get dulled to the point where the natural foods we enjoyed just the week before no longer deliver the same taste satisfaction. For some, this may simply require a period of readjustment. But for others, this departure from an otherwise healthy diet may lead back to a dietary glut involving added salt, sugar, and fat.

For those of us who grew up eating SAD (the standard American diet), starting to eat healthfully can be a big shift. I know it was for me. Though my mom tried to keep us eating good-for-us foods at home, when I was hanging out with friends, we'd go through boxes of Little Debbie snack cakes and indulge in greasy meals at the local Chinese restaurant, where I'd order spareribs or any dish with chunks of sugary deep-fried meat. One of my favorite snacks was nacho cheese-flavored Slim Jims (dried-meat sticks).

Thankfully, I was able to escape SAD's clutches before any overt health problems arose. That was thirty-five years ago. Looking back, I view that as one of the best decisions of my life.

Some go cold turkey, if you will, while others transition more slowly using a variety of approaches. One I've personally recommended is Kaiser Permanente's three-step method. Realizing that most American families tend to rotate through the same eight or nine meals, step one suggests that you think of three meals you already enjoy that are plant-based, like pasta and marinara sauce that could be easily tweaked to whole-grain pasta with some added veggies. Step two asks you to think of three meals you already eat that could be *adapted* to become a green-light meal, like switching from beef chili to five-bean chili. Step three is my favorite: Discover new healthy options.[2281]

Ironically, many people following healthy diets report eating an even greater variety of foods than when they ate their former "unrestricted" diet. I used to tell people to go to their public libraries and borrow cookbooks. (I've written three—*The How Not to Die Cookbook*, *The How Not to Diet Cookbook*, and *The How Not to Age Cookbook*—and I donate all the money I receive from them to charity.) But that was my advice before widespread use of the internet. Now, if you google *whole food, plant-based recipes*, a hundred million hits pop up. If you're feeling overwhelmed, good places to start include:

- **ForksOverKnives.com:** This site of the popular documentary and book of the same name offers hundreds of recipes.
- **StraightUpFood.com:** Cooking instructor Cathy Fisher shares some of the best recipes online.
- **HappyHealthyLongLife.com:** This site's tagline reads: "A [Cleveland Clinic] medical librarian's adventures in evidence-based living." She used the *e* word—I think I'm in love!
- **NutritionFacts.org/recipes:** My nonprofit organization's website has an ever-expanding recipe section with some of my favorites.

Once you've found three new meals you enjoy and can prepare with ease, step three is complete. Just like that, you have a nine-meal rotation, and moving on to breakfast and lunch is easy.

If you hate to cook and just want the cheapest, easiest way to make healthy meals, I recommend dietitian Jeff Novick's *Fast Food* video series. Using common staples like canned beans, frozen vegetables, quick-cook whole grains, and spice mixes, Jeff shows you how you can feed your friends and family healthfully in no time for about four dollars a day per person. The videos also include supermarket walk-throughs, shopping tips, and information on how to decipher nutrition labels. Check out his *Fast Food* series on YouTube.

If you crave more structure and social support, the Physicians Committee for Responsible Medicine (PCRM), a nonprofit nutrition research and policy advocacy organization in Washington, D.C., created an app for a three-week kick-start program for plant-based eating. You can find the download links at 21DayKickstart.org. This free app offers a full meal plan, recipes, tips, and other resources available in English and Spanish. Hundreds of thousands of people have already benefited from the program, so consider giving it a try.

In my experience, the best way to think of healthy eating is as an experiment. It can be overwhelming to think of such a sweeping change as permanent. That's why I ask for just three weeks. We can do just about anything for only three weeks, and we're more likely to go whole hog (whole grain?) and realize the maximum benefits. I suspect (because research has shown us) that once those three weeks are up, if you really gave it your all, you'll be feeling so much better, your lab values will be looking so much better, and your palate will have started to change. Healthy eating tastes better and better the longer you stick with it.

I remember talking about this with Dr. Neal Barnard, founding president of PCRM, which publishes a great deal of research pitting a healthy diet against a variety of common ailments—everything from acne and arthritis to menstrual cramps and migraines. He often uses what's called an "A-B-A" study design. Participants' health is assessed at baseline on their regular diets, and then they're switched to a therapeutic diet. In an effort to make sure any health changes participants experience on the new diet aren't merely a coincidence, they are then switched back to their regular diet to see if the changes disappear.

This kind of rigorous study design improves the validity of the results, but the problem, Dr. Barnard related, is that sometimes people improve *too* much. After a few weeks on a plant-based diet, sometimes people feel so much better that they refuse to go back on their baseline diet[2282]—even though it's required by the study protocol. Since they didn't complete the study as planned, their data have to be effectively thrown out and may never make it into the final paper. Ironically, healthy eating can be so effective that it undermines its own studies of effectiveness!

WWDGE: What Would Dr. Greger Eat?

I'm regularly asked what I eat every day. I've always been hesitant to answer for a number of reasons. First, it shouldn't matter what I or anyone else eats, says, or does. The science is the science. Too much of the nutrition world is split into camps, each following their respective guru. What other field of serious scientific inquiry is like that? After all, 2 + 2 = 4 regardless of what our favorite mathematician thinks. This is because there isn't a trillion-dollar industry that profits from confusing people about arithmetic. If we were getting conflicting messages from all sides about basic maths, in desperation, we might have to choose one authority to stick with, hoping that person will accurately represent the available research. Who has time to read and decipher all the original source material?

Early on in my career, I decided that I didn't want to rely on anyone else's interpretation for what could ultimately be life-or-death decisions for individuals in my care. I had the access, the resources, and the background to interpret the science on my own. When I initially began my annual reviews of the nutrition literature, it was really just to make myself a better doctor. But when I discovered such a treasure trove of information, I knew I couldn't keep it to myself. My hope is to disseminate it in a way that removes me as much as possible from the equation. I don't want to present the trademarked Dr. Greger Diet; I want to present the best-available-evidence diet. That's why I show the original papers, charts, graphs, and quotes with links to all the primary sources in my NutritionFacts.org videos. I try to keep my own interpretation to a minimum—though admittedly, I sometimes can't help myself.

What a person chooses to do with information is highly personalized and often depends on such factors as their current life situation and how risk averse they are. Given the same information, two people can make two entirely different but legitimate decisions. For this reason, I've been hesitant to share my own personal choices because I'm afraid they'll unduly sway people to make decisions that might not be right for them. I'd rather just present the science and let others decide for themselves. It's your body, your choice.

In addition, everyone's taste buds are different. I can imagine someone thinking, *He puts hot sauce on what?* When people hear me talk about the wonders of hummus (a Middle Eastern chickpea spread) but not baba ghanoush (a Middle Eastern roasted aubergine spread), they might come away with the impression that I think one is healthier than the other. This may be (and probably is, actually), but my real reason is simple: I don't like the taste of aubergine.

Conversely, just because I eat something doesn't mean it's healthy. For example, people are surprised to hear I used to use dutched (alkali-processed) cocoa. In that process, more than half of the antioxidants and flavanol phytonutrients are wiped out.[2283] Why would I use it, then? Because it tastes so much better to me than unprocessed cocoa. While I encourage people to use natural cocoa, I don't always take my own advice in that regard. In some cases, it would be better if people would do as I say, not as I do. (After researching the latest literature for *How Not to Age*, I was compelled to at least switch to half non-dutched natural cocoa.)

And what if I shared a recipe that someone found utterly repulsive? I would hate for them to think, *If this is healthy eating, count me out.* As I've said, as we eat more healthfully, our palate actually changes. It's an amazing phenomenon. Our taste buds are constantly adapting—minute to minute, in fact. If we drank some orange juice right now, it would taste sweet. But if we first ate some candy and then drank the same OJ, it could taste unpleasantly bitter. Over the long term, the more we eat healthfully, the better healthy foods taste.

I remember the first time I sipped a green smoothie. I was speaking somewhere in Michigan, hosted by a darling physician couple. They told me that they drank "blended salads" for breakfast. Intellectually, I loved the idea. Greens, the healthiest food on the planet, in convenient liquid form? I envisioned myself drinking a salad on my way to work every day. But then I tasted it. It felt like I was drinking someone's lawn. I gagged and almost threw up over my hosts' kitchen table.

Green smoothies are something you may have to build up to. Everyone loves fruit smoothies. Some frozen mango, strawberries—delicious! And surprisingly, you can throw a handful of baby spinach in there and may hardly even taste it. Give it a try! You'll be surprised. So if one handful is good, how about two? Slowly, your taste buds can adapt to increasing quantities of greens. This happens with all our senses. Walk into a dark room, and your eyes will slowly adapt. Stick your foot into a hot bath, and though at first it may be too hot, your body equilibrates to a new normal. Likewise, in just a couple of weeks, you can be drinking—and enjoying—concoctions you'd might initially consider absolutely unpalatable.

Having said all that, I will now proceed to tell you what I eat, what I drink, what I do, and how I do it. In each subsequent chapter, I will dive deeper into each of the entries on my Daily Dozen checklist to describe which types of these green-light foods are my favorites, as well as the tricks and techniques I use to prepare them. I will not be detailing every type of bean, fruit, vegetable, nut, or spice that I eat. Rather, my goal here is to explore some of the interesting science behind a few of my favorite options in each category.

Please understand that my strategy is *a* way to do it rather than *the* way to do it. If it happens to work for you too, great. If not, I hope you'll explore the myriad other ways you could use this same body of evidence to help improve and prolong your life.

Dr. Greger's Daily Dozen

Whole food, plant-based nutrition—pretty self-explanatory, right? But aren't some green-light foods better than others? For example, we can apparently live extended periods eating practically nothing but potatoes.[2284] That would, by definition, be a whole food, plant-based diet—but not a very healthy one. All plant foods are not created equal.

The more I've researched over the years, the more I've come to realize that healthy foods aren't necessarily interchangeable. Some foods and food groups have special nutrients not found in abundance elsewhere. For example, sulforaphane, the amazing liver-enzyme detox-boosting compound I profiled in chapters 2 and 12, is derived nearly exclusively from cruciferous vegetables. We could eat tons of different greens and other vegetables on a given day and get no appreciable sulforaphane if we didn't eat something cruciferous. It's the same with flaxseeds and the anticancer lignan compounds. As I mentioned in chapters 12 and 14, flax may average one hundred times more lignans than other foods. And mushrooms aren't even plants at all; they belong to an entirely different biological classification and may contain nutrients (like ergothioneine) not made anywhere in the plant kingdom.[2285] (So technically, maybe I should be referring to a whole food, plant- and fungus-based diet, but that doesn't have the best ring to it.)

It seems like every time I jump off my treadmill desk, buzzing with some exciting new data, my family rolls their eyes, sighs, and asks, "What can't we eat now?" Or they'll say, "Wait a second. Why does everything seem to have parsley in it all of a sudden?" My poor family. They've been very tolerant.

As the list of foods I tried to fit into my daily diet grew, I made a checklist and had it on a little dry-erase board on the fridge. My family would make a game out of ticking off the boxes. This evolved into the Daily Dozen. (See figure 6.)

By beans, I mean legumes, which comprise all the different kinds of beans,

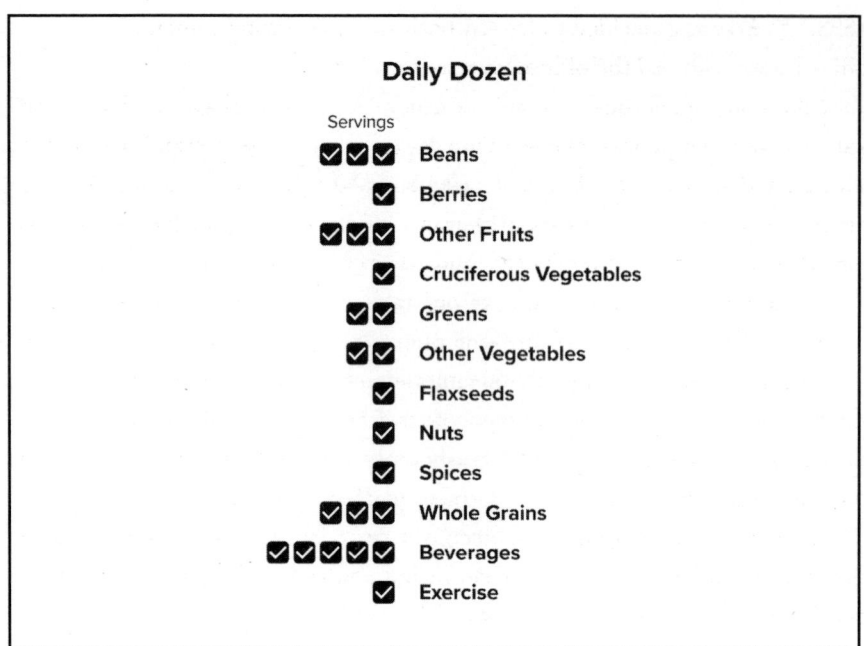

Figure 6

including soya beans, split peas, chickpeas, and lentils. While eating a bowl of pea soup or dipping carrots into hummus may not seem like eating beans, it is. We should try to get three servings a day. A serving is defined as 70 grams of hummus or bean dip; 100 grams of cooked beans, split peas, lentils, tofu, or tempeh; or 100 grams of fresh peas or sprouted lentils. Though peanuts are technically legumes, nutritionally, I've grouped them in the Nuts category, just as I would consider green (snap or string) beans to be better placed in the Other Vegetables category.

A serving of berries is 70 grams of fresh or frozen, or 40 grams of dried. Biologically speaking, avocados, bananas, and even watermelons are technically berries, but I'm using the colloquial term for any small edible fruit, which is why I include kumquats and grapes (and raisins) in this category, as well as fruits that are typically thought of as berries but aren't technically, such as blackberries, cherries, mulberries, raspberries, and strawberries.

For Other Fruits, a serving is a medium-sized fruit, 150 grams of cut-up fruit, or 40 grams of dried fruit. Again, I'm using the colloquial rather than the botanical definition, so I place tomatoes in the Other Vegetables group. (Interestingly, this is something the U.S. Supreme Court actually ruled on in

1893.[2286] Arkansas decided to have it both ways, declaring tomatoes both the official state fruit *and* the official state vegetable.[2287])

Common cruciferous vegetables include broccoli, cabbage, collards, and kale. I recommend at least one serving a day (typically 90 grams) and at least two additional daily servings of greens, cruciferous or otherwise. Serving sizes for other greens and vegetables are 100 grams for raw leafy vegetables, 90 grams for other raw or cooked vegetables, and 10 grams for dried mushrooms.

We should all try to incorporate one tablespoon of ground flaxseeds into our daily diet, in addition to a serving of nuts or other seeds. Thirty grams of nuts is considered a serving, or two tablespoons of nut or seed butters, including peanut butter. (Chestnuts and coconuts don't nutritionally count as nuts.)

I also recommend one-quarter teaspoon a day of the spice turmeric, along with any other (salt-free) herbs and spices you may enjoy.

A serving of whole grains can be considered a 100 grams of hot cereal such as oatmeal, cooked grain such as rice (including the "pseudograins" amaranth, buckwheat, and quinoa), cooked pasta, or sweetcorn; 30 grams of ready-to-eat (cold) cereal; one tortilla or slice of bread; half a bagel or English muffin; or 30 grams of popped popcorn.

The serving size in the beverage category is one glass (12 fluid ounces or about 350 ml), and the recommended five glasses a day is in addition to the water you get naturally from the foods in your diet.

Finally, I advise one daily "serving" of exercise, which can be split up over the day. I recommend ninety minutes of moderate-intensity activity, such as brisk (four miles per hour) walking or forty minutes of vigorous activity (such as jogging or active sports) each day. Why so much? I'll explain my reasoning in the Exercise chapter.

This may sound like a lot of boxes to check, but it's not difficult to tick a bunch at one time. Enjoy one simple peanut butter and banana sandwich, and you can check off four boxes. Or imagine sitting down to a big salad. One hundred and twenty grams of spinach, a handful of rocket, a handful of walnuts, 50 grams of chickpeas, 45 grams of red bell pepper/capsicum, and a small tomato. You just knocked out *seven* boxes in one dish. Sprinkle on your flax, add a handful of goji berries, and enjoy it with a glass of water and fruit for dessert, and you've ticked nearly half your daily check boxes in a single meal. And then if you ate it on a treadmill . . . just kidding!

Do I check off each glass of water I drink? No. In fact, I don't even use the checklist anymore; I just used it initially as a tool to get me into a routine.

Whenever I sat down to a meal, I would ask myself, *Could I add greens to this? Could I add beans to that? Can I sprinkle on some flax or pumpkin seeds, or maybe some dried fruit?* The checklist just got me into the habit of thinking, *How can I make this meal even healthier?*

I also found the checklist helped with grocery shopping. Although I always keep bags of frozen berries and greens in the freezer, if I'm at the store and want to buy fresh produce for the week, it helps me figure out how much kale or blueberries I need.

The checklist also helps me picture what a meal might look like. Looking over the checklist, you'll see there are three servings each of beans, fruits, and whole grains, and about twice as many veggies in total than any other food component. Glancing at my plate, I can imagine one quarter of it filled with whole grains, one quarter with legumes, and a half plate filled with vegetables, along with maybe a side salad and fruit for dessert. I prefer one-bowl meals where everything's mixed together, but the checklist still helps me to visualize. Instead of a big bowl of spaghetti with some veggies and lentils on top, I think of a big bowl of vegetables with some pasta and lentils mixed in. Instead of a big plate of brown rice with some stir-fried vegetables on top, I picture a meal that's mostly veggies with some rice and beans in there too.

But there is no need to be obsessive about the Daily Dozen. On hectic travel days when I've burned through my snacks and I'm trying to piece together some semblance of a healthy meal at the airport food court, sometimes I'm lucky if I hit even a quarter of my goals. If you eat poorly on one day, just try to eat better the next. My hope is that the checklist will serve you as a helpful reminder to try to eat a variety of the healthiest of healthy foods every day.

But should you eat your veggies raw or cooked? Do you need to choose organic or is conventional okay? What about GMOs? Gluten? All these questions and more will be answered as I go through each of the Daily Dozen in detail in the following chapters.

Beans

My Favorite Beans

Black beans, black soya beans, black-eyed peas, butter beans, cannellini beans, chickpeas (also known as garbanzo beans), edamame, garden peas, great northern beans, haricot beans, kidney beans, lentils (beluga, green, and red varieties), miso, pinto beans, small red beans, split peas (yellow or green), and tempeh

Serving Sizes:
¼ cup (70 g) of hummus or bean dip
½ cup (100 g) cooked beans, split peas, lentils
⅓ cup (85 g) tofu or tempeh
1 cup (100 g) of fresh peas or sprouted lentils

Daily Recommendation:
3 servings per day

The U.S. federal government's MyPlate campaign was developed to prompt Americans to think about building healthy meals. Most of our plate should be covered with vegetables and grains, preferably whole grains, with the rest of the plate split between fruits and the protein group. Legumes were given special treatment, straddling both the protein and the vegetable groups. They're loaded with protein, iron, and zinc, as you might expect from other protein sources like meat, but legumes also contain nutrients that are concentrated in the vegetable kingdom, including fiber, folate, and potassium. We get the best of both worlds with beans, all while enjoying foods that are naturally low in saturated fat and sodium and free of cholesterol. The Scientific Report of the 2025 Dietary Guidelines Advisory Committee suggested Beans, Peas, and Lentils (formerly "Legumes") be listed first in the Protein Foods to emphasize their consumption, followed by Nuts, Seeds, and Soya Products.[2288]

One of the most comprehensive analyses of diet and cancer ever performed was published by the American Institute for Cancer Research and World Cancer Research Fund. Sifting through some half a million studies, nine independent research teams from around the globe created a landmark scientific consensus report reviewed by twenty-one of the top cancer researchers in the world. One of their summary cancer-prevention recommendations was to eat whole grains and/or legumes (beans, split peas, chickpeas, or lentils) with every meal.[2289] Not every week or every day. *Every meal!*

Having some oatmeal in the morning makes it easy enough to fulfill the whole grains recommendation, but legumes? Who eats beans for breakfast? Well, lots of people around the world do. A traditional English breakfast includes savory combinations of baked beans on toast, mushrooms, and grilled tomatoes. Japanese breakfasts traditionally include miso soup, and many children in India start their days with idli, a type of steamed lentil cake. More familiar ways for American palates to meet the cancer prevention guidelines might be a whole-grain bagel schmeared with hummus. My friend Paul mashes cannellini beans into his oatmeal and swears you can't even see or taste them. Why not?

Soya

Soya beans are probably the beans Americans are most comfortable incorporating into their breakfasts in the form of soya milk, which has grown into a billion-dollar business. But soya milk and even tofu are processed foods. When it comes to the nutrients we tend to associate with legumes—fiber, iron, magnesium, potassium, protein, and zinc—about half are lost when soya beans are converted into tofu. However, beans are so healthy that we can throw away half the nutrition and *still* have a really healthy food. If you do eat tofu, choose varieties made with calcium (you'll see it in the ingredients list), which can weigh in at an impressive 550 mg of calcium per (3 oz or about 85 g) slice.[2290]

Even better than tofu, though, would be a *whole* Soya food like tempeh, which is a type of fermented soya bean patty. If you look closely at tempeh, you can actually see all the little soya beans. I don't usually eat tempeh for breakfast, but I do like to slice it thin, dip it into a thick flax "egg" mixture (see page 397 for my recipe), dredge it through some rosemary-seasoned whole-grain bread crumbs or coarse blue cornmeal, and air fry it until it's golden brown. (You can also just bake it in a toaster oven.) Then I dip it in buffalo hot sauce for a healthier approximation of the chicken wings I enjoyed in my youth.

I've recently gotten into black soya beans after I read a remarkable study in which people were randomized to the berrylike pigments found in the equivalent[2291] of just a few spoonsful a day of black soya beans. Compared to placebo, LDL cholesterol lowered by 14 points on the black soya beans.[2292] You can buy them canned or cook them from scratch from dried beans in 45 minutes in a pressure cooker like an Instant Pot.

What About GMO Soya?

A prominent scientific journal editorialized that although we are now swimming in information about genetically modified crops, much of what we're being told is wrong—from both sides of the debate. "But a lot of this incorrect information is sophisticated, backed by legitimate-sounding research and written with certitude," the editorial read, quipping that when it comes to GMOs, a good gauge of a statement's fallacy may be "the conviction with which it is delivered."[2293]

Monsanto's Roundup Ready soya beans are the number one genetically modified crop, engineered to be resistant to the herbicide Roundup (also sold by Monsanto), which allows farmers to spray the crops to kill weeds while leaving the soya standing.[2294]

Though much debate continues to swarm around the hypothetical risks of GMO crops, the greater concern for human health may be the potential for GMO crops to contain elevated pesticide residues.[2295] This fear was realized in 2014 when high levels of Roundup pesticides were reported on GMO soya beans (but not on non-GMO or organic soya beans).[2296] The pesticide levels were considered high compared to maximum allowable residue levels at the time, but were they high enough to have adverse effects on consumers?

Anti-GMO activists point to studies showing Roundup may interfere with embryonic development and disrupt hormones. These studies were, respectively, on sea urchin embryos[2297] and cells from mouse testicles.[2298]

Blogs screamed headlines like "Men! Save Your Testicles," citing articles with concerning names like "Prepubertal Exposure to Commercial Formulation of the Herbicide Glyphosate Alters Testosterone Levels and Testicular Morphology."[2299] But that study was about puberty in rats. I doubt the blog would have gotten as many hits if it had been titled "Men! Save Prepubescent Rats' Testicles!"[2300]

Am I being too harsh? After all, where could scientists find live human tissue to experiment on? A research team came up with a brilliant solution—study placentas. Millions of women in the United States give birth each year, and the placenta, the temporary organ formed in the uterus to nourish the fetus during pregnancy, is typically incinerated after delivery. Why not test Roundup on human placental tissue? The researchers did and found that at the concentration that's sprayed on crops in the fields, the pesticides did indeed have toxic effects on human tissue.[2301]

That finding may help explain studies suggesting adverse effects on pesticide workers[2302,2303] and their children,[2304] but by the time the pesticides enter the food supply, they are highly diluted. Concentrations of Roundup pesticides may only reach a few parts per million in food and a few parts per billion in our body. Researchers, however, discovered the pesticide may still have effects at a few parts per *trillion*. Even at that minuscule dose, Roundup pesticides were found to have estrogenic effects in vitro, stimulating the growth of estrogen-receptor-positive human breast cancer cells.[2305] The ante was raised in 2017 when the Roundup herbicide glyphosate was officially designated "probably carcinogenic" in humans.[2306]

As we saw in chapter 12, though, soya consumption is associated with *lower* breast cancer risk and improved breast cancer survival. That may be because most GMO soya in the United States is used as feed for chickens, pigs, and cattle, whereas many of the major soya *food* manufacturers use non-GMO soya. It could also be because the benefits of eating any kind of soya far outweigh the risks. Regardless, why accept any risk at all when we can choose organic soya products, which at least by U.S. law exclude GMOs?

The bottom line is that there are no direct human data suggesting any harm from eating GMO crops, though such studies haven't been done (which critics say is exactly the point).[2307] As of 2022, it is mandatory in the United States for bioengineered products or foods containing bioengineered ingredients to be labeled, although this labeling can be as vague as listing a phone number to call to determine the food's designation.[2308] Ultimately, this could be helpful for public health researchers to track whether GMOs are having any adverse effects.

I believe it is important to put the GMO issue in perspective. As I've tried to show, there are dietary and lifestyle changes we can make that could eliminate most heart disease, strokes, diabetes, and cancer. *Millions* of lives could be saved. For this reason, I'm sympathetic to the biotech industry's exasperation about GMO concerns when we still have people dying from everything else they're eating.[2309] As one review concluded: "Consumption of genetically modified food entails risk of undesirable effects similar to the consumption of traditional food."[2310] In other words, buying the non-GMO cookie isn't doing our body much good.

Miso is another fermented whole soya food. This thick paste is commonly mixed with hot water to make a delicious soup that's a staple in Japanese cuisine. If you want to give it a try, I suggest white miso, which has a mellower flavor than red miso. Making miso soup can be as easy as mixing one tablespoon of miso with a few cups of hot water and adding whatever vegetables you prefer. That's it!

Because miso may contain probiotic bacteria,[2311] it's probably best not to actually cook the miso, lest the good bugs be eliminated. When I prepare it, I boil dried mushrooms, a pinch of arame seaweed, a few dried tomatoes, and greens in a pot and ladle off about 60 ml of hot broth into a large bowl, add the miso, and mash it with a fork until only a thin paste remains. I then pour the rest of the soup into the bowl and stir to combine it with the miso. And, because I'm a bit of a hot-sauce freak, I add some sriracha for a little kick. Then I sprinkle some black sesame seeds on top.

Miso Soup: Soya vs. Sodium

The process of producing miso involves adding salt—lots of salt. A single bowl of miso soup could contain half the American Heart Association's recommended daily limit, which is why I always reflexively avoided it when I'd see it on a menu. But when I actually looked into it, I was surprised by what I found.

There are two principal reasons to avoid salt: stomach cancer and high blood pressure. Considered a "probable cause" of stomach cancer,[2312] excess salt intake may cause thousands of cases every year in the United States alone.[2313] The elevated stomach cancer risk associated with higher salt intake appears on par with that of smoking or heavy alcohol use but may only be half as bad as opium use[2314] or a daily serving of meat. A study of nearly half a million people found that a daily portion of meat (about the size of a deck of cards) was associated with up to five times the odds of stomach cancer.[2315]

This may explain why people eating plant-based diets appear to be at significantly lower risk.[2316] But it's not just sodium-rich animal products like processed meats and salted fish that are associated with higher stomach cancer risk; salt-preserved plant foods are as well.[2317,2318] Kimchi, a spicy pickled vegetable side dish, is a staple in Korean cuisine and could help explain why that country may have the highest stomach cancer rates in the world.[2319]

Miso, however, was *not* associated with increased cancer risk.[2320] The carcinogenic effects of the salt may be counteracted by the anticarcinogenic effects of the soya. For example, tofu intake has been associated with about 50 percent less stomach cancer risk[2321] and salt with about 50 percent more risk,[2322] which explains how they may effectively cancel each other out. Further protection apparently offered by allium (onion) family vegetables[2323] may tip the cancer-fighting scale in favor of miso soup that's garlicky or has some scallions thrown in.

Cancer isn't the primary reason people are told to avoid salt, though. What about miso soup and high blood pressure? There may be a similar relationship. The salt in miso may push up our blood pressure while the soya protein in miso may lower it back down.[2324] If we compare the effects of soya milk to skimmed milk (to make a fairer comparison by removing the saturated butterfat factor), soya milk lowers blood pressure about nine times more effectively than skimmed dairy milk, for instance.[2325] Would the benefits of soya be enough to counter the effects of the salt in miso?

Over a four-year period, Japanese researchers tracked men and women in their sixties who started out with normal blood pressures to see who was more likely to be diagnosed with high blood pressure: those who had two or more bowls of miso soup a day or those who had one or less. Two bowls a day would be like adding half a teaspoon of salt to our daily diet, yet those who consumed at least that much miso were found to have five times *lower* risk of becoming hypertensive. The researchers concluded: "Our results on miso-soup have shown that [the] anti-hypertensive effect of miso is possibly above [the] hypertensive effect of salt."[2326] So miso soup may actually be protective overall.

But what if you are already hypertensive? Men and women with stage 1 or 2 hypertension (blood pressures ranging from 130 to 159 over 85 to 99) were randomized to eat either two bowls a day of miso soup, which alone exceeded the recommended daily sodium limit, or soya beans with no added salt for two months. Surprisingly, the miso group ended up with *lower* nighttime blood pressures than the soya bean control group. The mechanism is unclear.[2327] Given a slight drop in body weight in the miso group, the miso may have a diuretic effect by increasing sodium excretion through the kidneys, a phenomenon that has been demonstrated in rats.[2328,2329] Regardless, miso is now a staple in my kitchen and in my cookbooks.

Edamame is about as whole a soya food as we can get. After all, these are soya beans still in their pods. You can buy them frozen and just throw a handful into some boiling water anytime you want a healthy snack. They cook in just two or three minutes. Then, all you need to do is strain them and, if you're like me, crack lots of fresh pepper onto the pods, sprinkle on garlic powder and nutritional yeast (and potassium salt if you like them salty), and nibble the beans right out. (You can also buy them pre-shelled, but then they're not as fun to eat.)

On the opposite end of the processing spectrum are plant-based meat alternatives like veggie burgers, which are healthy only insofar as they replace the real thing. Beyond Chicken, for example, was a product with fiber, zero saturated fat, zero cholesterol, and equal protein to and fewer calories than an actual chicken breast (plus presumably less food-poisoning risk). But Beyond Chicken paled in comparison to the nutrition found in the soya beans, yellow peas, and amaranth grain from which it was made. Of course, most people choosing these meat alternatives are not standing in the supermarket agonizing between Beyond Chicken Grilled Strips and a bowl of legumes and whole grains. So if fajitas are the foregone conclusion, then it would certainly be healthier to choose the plant-based meat. I see the value of these meat-alternative products as healthier transition foods to wean people off the standard American diet. Even if you just stopped there, you'd be better off, but the more you can move toward whole food nutrition, the better. You don't want to get stuck at the yellow light.

Peas

Like edamame, raw garden peas can be a great au naturel snack. I fell in love with peas in the pod when I first picked them off the vine at a farm my brother and I spent time on one summer as kids. They were like candy. Every year, I look forward to the few weeks I can find them fresh.

Green peas are not included in the federal MyPlate recommendations for beans, peas, and lentils since they are not as nutritious as cooked dried peas, like chickpeas and black-eyed peas,[2330] but they're more comparable at double the dose. (Note their serving size is 100 grams.)

Lentils

Lentils are little lens-shaped legumes. (Lenses were actually named after lentils; *lens* is lentil in Latin.) They gained fame in 1982 upon the discovery of the "lentil effect," or the ability of lentil consumption to blunt the sugar spike of foods consumed hours later at a subsequent meal.[2331] Lentils are so rich in prebiotics that they create a feast for our friendly flora, which in turn feed us right back with beneficial compounds, such as propionate, that relax our stomach and slow the rate at which sugars are absorbed into our system.[2332] Chickpeas and other legumes were found to have a similar influence, so this phenomenon was later renamed the "second-meal effect."[2333]

Lentils are already one of the most nutrient-dense legumes. But when sprouted, their antioxidant power doubles (and even quintuples for chickpeas).[2334] Lentils can be easily sprouted into one of the healthiest possible snacks. I was amazed when I first tried making them. What started out looking like hard little pebbles transformed into tender morsels in just a couple of days. Why add protein powder to your smoothies when you can add sprouted lentils? In a sprouting jar, or simply a mason jar covered with cheesecloth secured with a rubber band, soak lentils overnight in water, drain, and then rinse and drain twice daily for another couple of days. Sprouting to me is like gardening on steroids. I can create fresh produce in three days right on my kitchen counter. (Of course, if you open a can of lentils, you can enjoy them in about three seconds.)

Are Canned Beans as Healthy as Home Cooked?

Canned beans are convenient, but are they as nutritious as home cooked? Yes—with one exception: sodium. Salt is often added to canned beans, resulting in sodium levels up to one hundred times more than if you cooked them without any salt.[2335] Draining and rinsing your canned beans can remove about half the added salt, but then you'd also be rinsing away some of the nutrition. I recommend purchasing the no-salt-added varieties and cooking with the bean liquid in whatever dish you're whipping up.

Home-cooked beans may come out tastier, particularly texture-wise. Canned beans can sometimes be a bit mushy, whereas when properly soaked and cooked, beans can come out nice and firm yet tender. Using dried beans is also cheaper. Some bean-counting researchers found that canned beans can be about three times as expensive as home cooked, but the difference only came out to about twenty cents per serving.[2336] I used to spend that extra twenty cents to save the hours beans can take to cook until I discovered the Instant Pot, an electronic pressure cooker that can cook legumes from scratch in 10 to 45 minutes depending on the bean.

The only legumes I have the patience to cook on the stove are lentils. You can just simmer them as you would pasta, in a pot with an abundance of water, for about half an hour. In fact, if you're making pasta and have the time, why not let some lentils boil in the water for twenty minutes before adding in the pasta? Lentils are great in spaghetti sauce. Similarly, when I make rice or quinoa, I throw a handful of dried lentils into the rice cooker, and they're done when the grain is cooked. Mashed and seasoned cooked lentils also make a great veggie dip. Double Daily Dozen check marks!

Intimidated by the thought of cooking lentils or other legumes? Don't be. See Cooking Legumes in the appendix.

Dipping veggies in hummus is a double-check-box snack. And don't forget other bean blends, from garlicky white bean spreads and pinto pâtés to spicy black bean dip. Another fantastic snack—can you tell I love snacking?—is roasted chickpeas. Google it. My favorite, not surprisingly, is a buffalo ranch flavor (featured on the *Rachael Ray Show*[2337]), using a silicone baking mat.

Mealtime options can include dishes like bean burritos; chili; pasta e fagioli; red beans and rice; minestrone; Tuscan white bean stew; and black bean, lentil, or split pea soup. My mom turned me on to dehydrated precooked pea soup mixes. (Look for no- or low-sodium brands, like Dr. John McDougall's.) You simply add the mix to boiling water with some frozen greens and stir. (Most grocers sell inexpensive frozen bags of prechopped kale. If you're lucky, you may even find blends of kale, collards, and mustard greens in the freezer section. Couldn't be easier!) I pack pea soup mix when I travel. It's lightweight, and I can prepare it in the hotel room coffeemaker.

Big Bucks on Beans' Benefits

For more than two decades, soya foods have enjoyed the rare privilege of an "FDA-approved" food-label health claim about soya's ability to protect against heart disease. A billion-dollar industry, Big Soya has a lot of money to fund research touting the benefits of their bean. But is soya really the top bean, or are other legumes just as powerful? It turns out that *non*-soya beans, including lentils, lima beans, haricot beans, and pinto beans, lower bad cholesterol levels[2338] as effectively as soya.[2339] One study, for example, found that eating 140 grams a day of cooked pinto beans for two months may drop cholesterol by nineteen points.[2340]

One of my favorite go-to quickie meals starts with toasting some corn tortillas. (Food for Life, the same company that makes Ezekiel bread, makes a sprouted yellow corn tortilla usually sold in the frozen section.) Then I mash some beans on them with a fork and add a spoonful or two of salsa. All the better if I have fresh coriander, salad greens, or avocado to top it all off. If I'm lucky enough to have fresh collard greens, I'll steam a few leaves and use them as burrito wraps to replace the tortillas. We call them *collarditos* in our house. Greens and beans—can't get healthier than that!

Any leguminous dessert options? Three words: black-bean brownies. I have a recipe in *The How Not to Die Cookbook* that you can see at <u>nutritionfacts .org/recipe/fudgy-no-bake-brownies/</u>, and if you want to poke around online, you'll find many other good ones, including the one Dr. Joel Fuhrman shared on national television, which uses almond butter as the green-light source of fat and dates as the green-light source of sugar.[2341]

Mostly, I just add beans to whatever I happen to be making. I used to always keep an open can front and center in the fridge as a reminder, but now I just batch cook beans weekly to always have them on hand.

Clearing the Air About Beans and Gas

Beans, beans. Good for your heart. The more you eat 'em, the . . . longer you live? Legumes have been found to be "the most important predictor of survival in older people"[2342] around the globe. Whether it was the Japanese eating soya products, the Swedes eating brown beans and peas, or those in the Mediterranean region eating lentils, chickpeas, and white beans, legume intake was consistently associated with a longer lifespan. Researchers found an 8 percent reduction in risk of premature death for every twenty-gram increase in daily legume intake—that's barely two tablespoons' worth![2343]

So why aren't more people taking advantage of this dietary "fountain of youth"? Fear of flatulence.[2344] Is that really the choice we're left with, then? Breaking wind or breaking down? Passing gas or passing on?

Are the concerns about the gassiness of beans just a bunch of hot air?

When researchers added a half cup (about 100 grams) of beans to people's diets, the majority experienced no symptoms at all. Even among people who did get gassy, 70 percent or more reported that it diminished by the second or third week of the study. The researchers concluded: "People's concerns about excessive flatulence from eating beans may be exaggerated."[2345]

Flatulence may be more common than we think. Americans report passing gas an average of fourteen times a day,[2346] with the normal range extending up to twenty-three times daily.[2347] Flatulence comes from two places: swallowed air and fermentation in the bowel. Factors that might cause us to swallow extra air include chewing gum, wearing ill-fitting dentures, sucking on hard candies, drinking through a straw, eating too fast, talking while we eat, and smoking cigarettes. So, if the fear of lung cancer doesn't get you to quit smoking, maybe fear of flatulence will.

The main source of gas, though, is the normal bacterial fermentation in the colon of undigested sugars. Dairy products are a leading cause of excessive flatulence,[2348] which is due to poor digestion of the milk sugar lactose.[2349] One of the most flatulent patients ever reported in the medical literature was effectively cured once all dairy products were removed from his diet. The case, reported in *The New England Journal of Medicine* and submitted to the *Guinness Book of World Records*, involved a man who, after consuming dairy, experienced "70 passages in one four-hour period."[2350] Cutting the cheese, indeed.

It turns out that much of beans' bad rap may have grown out of short-term studies in the 1960s that did not account for our body's ability to adapt.[2351] Long term, most people bulking up on high-fiber plant foods do not appear to have significantly increased problems with gas.[2352] The indigestible sugars in beans that make it down to our colon may even function as prebiotics to feed our good bacteria and make for a healthier colon.

Even if at first they make you gassy, beans are so health-promoting that you should experiment with ways to keep them in your diet at all costs. Lentils, split peas, and canned beans tend to produce less gas, and tofu isn't usually an offender. Repeated soakings of dried beans in water containing a quarter teaspoon of bicarbonate of soda per four liters[2353] and tossing out the cooking water may help if you boil your own beans. Of the spices that have been tested, cloves, cinnamon, and garlic seem to be the most gas-reducing, followed by turmeric (but only if uncooked), pepper, and ginger.[2354] If worse comes to worst, there are cheap supplements that contain alpha-galactosidase, an enzyme shown to break up the bean sugars and take the sail out of your wind.[2355]

Odor is a separate issue. The smell appears to come primarily from the digestion of sulfur-rich foods. So to cut down on the stench, experts have recommended cutting back on such foods as meat and eggs.[2356] (Hydrogen sulfide is called "rotten egg gas" for a reason.) This may be why people who eat meat regularly were found to generate as much as fifteen times the sulfides as those eating plant-based diets.[2357]

There *are* healthy sulfur-rich foods, such as garlic and cauliflower. If you're about to embark on a long trip in a confined space after a big meal of aloo gobi, Pepto-Bismol and generic equivalents can act as a windbreaker by binding up the sulfur in your gut to eliminate odors. But this should be used only as a short-term solution due to the potential for bismuth toxicity with chronic use.[2358]

Then there are the high-tech solutions, such as carbon-fiber, odor-eating underwear (cost: $65), which were put to the test in a series of studies that included such gems as "Utilizing gas-tight Mylar pantaloons, the ability of a charcoal-lined cushion to absorb sulfur-containing gases instilled at the anus of eight subjects was assessed."[2359] The name of the charcoal-lined cushion? The "Toot Trapper."

The bottom line: Intestinal gas is normal and healthy. No less an expert than Hippocrates himself was attributed as saying, "Passing gas is necessary to well-being."[2360] In a review of degassing drugs and devices, Dr. John Fardy, a chair of gastroenterology, wrote: "Perhaps increased tolerance of flatus would be a better solution, for we tamper with harmless natural phenomena at our peril."[2361] And, yes, Dr. Fardy is his real name.

Legume consumption is associated with a slimmer waist and lower blood pressure, and randomized trials have shown it can match or beat out calorie cutting for slimming belly fat as well as improving the regulation of blood sugar, insulin levels, and cholesterol. Beans are packed with fiber, folate, and phytates, which may help reduce the risk of stroke, depression, and colon cancer. The phytoestrogens in soya in particular appear to both help prevent breast cancer and improve breast cancer survival. No wonder the cancer guidelines suggest we try to fit beans into our meals—and it's so easy. They can be added to nearly any meal, easily incorporated into snack times, or served as the star attraction. The possibilities are endless.

Berries

My Favorite Berries

Açai berries, barberries, blackberries, blueberries, cherries (sweet or tart), Concord grapes, cranberries, goji berries, kumquats, mulberries, raspberries (black or red), and strawberries

Serving Sizes:
½ cup (70 g) fresh or frozen
¼ cup (40 g) dried

Daily Recommendation:
1 serving per day

The case for berries has been made throughout this book. Berries offer potential protection against cancer (chapters 7 and 12), a boost to the immune system (chapter 5), and a guard for the liver (chapter 9) and brain (chapters 3 and 14). An American Cancer Society study of nearly one hundred thousand men and women found that those who ate the most berries appeared significantly less likely to die of cardiovascular disease.[2362]

Tastes great *and* may help us live longer—that's what plant-based eating is all about.

Greens are the healthiest vegetables, and berries are the healthiest fruits—in part due to their respective plant pigments. Leaves contain the green pigment chlorophyll, which sets off the firestorm of photosynthesis, so greens have to be packed with antioxidants to deal with the charged high-energy electrons that are formed. (Remember superoxide from chapter 3?) Meanwhile, berries evolved to have bright, contrasting colors to attract fruit-eating critters to help disperse their seeds. And the same molecular characteristics that give berries such vibrant colors may account for some of their antioxidant abilities.[2363]

Too many of us eat a lot of pale and beige foods: white bread, white pasta, white potatoes, white rice. Colorful foods are often healthier because they contain antioxidant pigments, whether it's the beta-carotene that makes carrots and sweet potatoes orange, the lycopene antioxidant pigment that makes tomatoes red, or the anthocyanin pigments that make blueberries blue. The colors *are* the antioxidants. That knowledge alone should revolutionize your stroll down the produce aisle.

Guess which have more antioxidants—red onions or white onions? You don't need to look up the answer. You can see the difference with your own eyes. (Indeed, red onions have 76 percent more antioxidant capacity than white, with brown onions in between.[2364]) So, given the choice, why buy another white onion ever again?

Red cabbage may contain eight times more antioxidants than green cabbage,[2365] which is why you'll never find a green cabbage in my house.

Which eliminates more free radicals—pink grapefruit or regular grapefruit? Granny Smith or Red Delicious? Iceberg lettuce or romaine? Red grapes or green? Yellow sweetcorn or white sweetcorn? You don't need me to go to the supermarket with you. You don't even need to take a cheat sheet. You can make all these calls yourself.

What about a purple-skinned aubergine or a white-skinned aubergine? Trick question! Remember, the pigment is the antioxidant, so the color of the skin doesn't matter if you peel it off. As we learned in chapter 12, that's why we shouldn't peel our apples. It's for this same reason kumquats may be the healthiest citrus fruit, since we can eat them rind and all.

Shop for the reddest of strawberries, the blackest of blackberries, the most scarlet tomato, the darkest green broccoli you can find. The colors *are* the antiaging, anticancer antioxidants.

Antioxidant content is one of the reasons I've singled out berries for special treatment. They are second only to herbs and spices as the most antioxidant-packed food category. As a group, they average nearly ten times more antioxidants than other fruits and vegetables (and exceed fifty times more than animal-based foods).[2366]

The Antioxidant Power of Berries

As with other green-light foods, the healthiest variety is the one you'll eat most often, but if you have no particular preference, why not put the berry with the most antioxidants in your morning oatmeal? Thanks to a study that compared more than a hundred different berries and berry products, we now know which one that is.[2367]

America's favorite fruits are apples and bananas, with antioxidant power of about 60 units and 40 units, respectively. Mangos, the preferred fruit around the world outside of the United States, have even more antioxidant punch at around 110 units. (It makes sense when you consider how much more colorful they are on the inside.) But none of these fruits is a match for berries. Strawberries weigh in at about 310 units per 140 grams, cranberries at 330, raspberries at 350, blueberries at 380 (and wild blueberries may have twice as much[2368]), and blackberries at a staggering 650 units. Above even those are exotic types you can pick wild in the Arctic tundra, like red whortleberries, which sound like something from a Dr. Seuss book. But in terms of what you can find readily in the store, it's wild blueberries and blackberries for the win. (I share my whole-fruit cocktail recipe for using one of the runners-up, cranberries, on page 179.) I'm happy as long as you're eating a serving of any type of berry every day, but in terms of antioxidant content, choosing blackberries over strawberries appears to give you twice the bang for your berry.[2369] In *How Not to Age*, I discuss the limitations of this approach, as strawberries offer a concentrated source of the potentially anti-aging compound *fisetin*, which is why I end up recommending eating fresh, frozen, or freeze-dried strawberries on a daily basis.

What About All the Sugar in Fruit?

There are a few popular diets out there that urge people to stop eating fruits because their natural sugars (fructose) are thought to contribute to weight gain. The truth is, only fructose from *added* sugars appears to be associated with declining liver function,[2370] high blood pressure, and weight gain.[2371] How could the fructose in sugar be bad but the same fructose in fruit be harmless? Think about the difference between a sugar cube and a sugar beet. (Beets are the primary source of sugar in the United States.[2372])

In nature, fructose comes prepackaged with the fiber, antioxidants, and phytonutrients that appear to nullify adverse fructose effects.[2373]

Studies show that if we drink a glass of water with three tablespoons of sugar (similar to what would be in a can of fizzy drink), we'll have a big spike in our blood sugar levels within the first hour. That causes our body to release so much insulin to mop up the excess sugar that we actually overshoot and become hypoglycemic by the second hour, meaning our blood sugar drops even lower than it would if we were fasting. Our body detects this low blood sugar, thinks we might be in some sort of famine situation, and responds by dumping fat into our bloodstream as an energy source to keep us alive.[2374] This excess fat in the blood can then go on to cause further problems. (See chapter 8.)

But what if we eat 140 grams of blended berries in *addition* to the sugar? The berries, of course, have sugars of their own—an additional tablespoon's worth—so the blood sugar spike should be even worse, right? Actually, no. Study participants who ate berries with their glass of sugar water showed no additional blood sugar spike and no hypoglycemic dip afterward; their blood sugar levels merely went up and down, and there was no surge of fat into the blood.[2375]

Consuming sugar in fruit form is not only harmless but actually helpful. Eating berries can blunt the insulin spike from high-glycemic foods like white bread, for example.[2376] This may be because the fiber in fruits has a gelling effect in our stomach and small intestine that slows the release of sugars[2377] or because of certain phytonutrients in fruits that appear to block the absorption of sugar through the gut wall and into our bloodstream.[2378] So eating fructose the way nature intended carries benefits rather than risks.

In fact, low-dose fructose may actually benefit blood sugar control. Eating a piece of fruit with each meal could be expected to lower, rather than raise, the blood sugar response.[2379] What about people with type 2 diabetes? When they were randomized into a group restricted to no more than two daily pieces of fruits, they had no better blood sugar control than those randomized into a group told to eat a *minimum* of two pieces of fruits per day. The researchers concluded that "the intake of fruit should not be restricted in patients with type 2 diabetes."[2380]

Surely there must be *some* level of fructose consumption that's harmful even when served in its natural green-light form, right? Apparently not.

> Seventeen people were asked to eat *twenty* servings of fruits per day for months. Despite the extraordinarily high fructose content of this fruit-based diet—the sugar equivalent of about eight cans of fizzy drink a day—the investigators reported beneficial outcomes with no overall adverse effects for body weight, blood pressure,[2381] insulin, cholesterol, and triglyceride levels.[2382] More recently, the research group who invented the glycemic index found that feeding subjects a fruit-, vegetable-, and nut-based diet that included about twenty servings of fruits per day for a couple of weeks had no adverse effects on weight, blood pressure, or triglycerides—all while lowering LDL ("bad") cholesterol by an astounding thirty-eight points.[2383]
>
> Cholesterol lowering was not the only record broken: Participants were asked to eat forty-three servings of vegetables a day in addition to the fruits, the result of which was that the researchers recorded the largest-ever bowel movements documented in a dietary intervention.[2384]

Are frozen berries as nutritious as fresh ones? Studies on cherries,[2385] raspberries,[2386] and strawberries[2387] suggest that most of their nutrition is retained even when frozen. I usually opt for frozen berries since they last longer, are available year-round, and tend to be cheaper. If you looked in our freezer right now, you'd see it's about half frozen greens and half frozen berries. What do I do with those berries? Make ice cream, of course.

The favored dessert in our home is soft-serve "ice cream" made by blending frozen fruit. Simply whip up frozen fruit in a blender, food processor, or juicer, and voilà! Instant all-fruit *nice* cream. You have to taste it to believe it. The simplest recipe has one ingredient: frozen bananas. Peel and freeze some ripe bananas (the riper, the better—I'm talking brown). Once frozen, throw them in a food processor and blend. They transform into a smooth, light, fluffy dessert cheaper, healthier, and tastier than anything you might get in a trendy gelato shop.

Of course making *berry* ice cream or at least a berry-banana mix is even healthier. My favorite is chocolate. To make it, blend dark, sweet cherries or strawberries mixed with a tablespoon of cocoa powder, a splash of a milk of your choice (more if you want a milkshake), a capful of vanilla extract, and some pitted dates. If you didn't yet get your nuts for the day, you can add some almond butter. Either way, you get an instant, decadent, chocolate dessert so nutritious that the more you eat, the healthier you are. Let me repeat that: The more you eat, the healthier you are. That's my kind of ice cream!

Tart Cherries

Research dating back half a century suggests tart cherries are so anti-inflammatory that they can be used to successfully treat a painful type of arthritis called gout.[2388] Delicious dietary treatments are much welcomed, as some gout drugs can cost $2,000 a dose,[2389] carry no clear-cut distinction between nontoxic, toxic, and lethal doses,[2390] or can cause a rare side effect in which our skin detaches from our body.[2391] (Of course, the best way to deal with gout is to try to prevent it in the first place with a more plant-based diet.[2392])

Cherries can reduce the level of inflammation among healthy people too (as measured by a drop in C-reactive protein levels),[2393] so I was excited to find a green-light source available year-round—a canned product with only two ingredients: cherries and water. I drain off the liquid (which then goes into my hibiscus punch recipe on page 452) and mix the cherries in a bowl of cooked oatmeal along with cocoa powder and pumpkin seeds. If you sweeten it with date powder or chocolate-flavored balsamic vinegar (see page 373), it's like eating chocolate-covered cherries for breakfast.

A note of caution: For the same reason that high doses of anti-inflammatory drugs such as aspirin should be avoided during the third trimester of pregnancy, cocoa, berries, and other foods high in anti-inflammatory polyphenols should only be eaten in moderation in late pregnancy.[2394]

Goji Berries

Tart cherries naturally contain melatonin and have been used to improve sleep without any side effects.[2395] Goji berries, however, have the highest concentrations of melatonin.[2396] Gojis have the third-highest antioxidant capacity of any common dried fruit—five times more than raisins and second only to dried pomegranate seeds and barberries (a fruit commonly found in Middle Eastern markets and spice stores).[2397] Gojis also have a specific antioxidant pigment that makes corn yellow—zeaxanthin. When eaten, zeaxanthin is shuttled into our retinas (the back of our eyes) and appears to protect against macular degeneration, a leading cause of vision loss.[2398]

The egg industry boasts about the zeaxanthin content in yolks, but goji berries have about fifty times more than eggs.[2399] A double-blind, randomized, placebo-controlled trial found that gojis may even help people already suffering from macular degeneration.[2400] The researchers used milk to improve the absorption of zeaxanthin (which, like all carotenoids, is fat-soluble), but a healthier way would be to use green-light sources of fat, such as nuts and seeds. In other words, goji trail mix!

Aren't goji berries expensive, though? In natural foods stores, they can go for twenty dollars a pound, but in Asian supermarkets, you can buy them as "Lycium" berries, and they're even cheaper than raisins. So, however you used to eat raisins—as a snack, in baked goods, in your breakfast cereal or oatmeal, whatever—I recommend you make the switch to gojis.

Black Currants and Bilberries

Speaking of berries and eyesight, a double-blind, placebo-controlled, crossover trial of black currants found they can improve the symptoms of computer eye strain (known in doctor-speak as "video display terminal work-induced transient refractive alteration").[2401] What passes for currants in the United States are usually champagne grape raisins, not actual black currants, which were banned in the country a century ago at the behest of the lumber industry. (The industry feared they might spread a plant disease that affects white pines, a tree we hardly harvest anymore, so the ban has since been lifted in many states.) Real black currants are currently making a comeback, but if—as the researchers suspected—the benefits have to do with the anthocyanin pigments, other berries like bilberries, blueberries, or blackberries may help as well. Anthocyanin pigments are responsible for many of the intense blue, black, purple, and red colors of berries and other fruits and vegetables. The highest concentrations are found in aronia berries and elderberries, followed by black raspberries, blueberries (especially the smaller "wild" varieties), and blackberries. The cheapest source, though, is probably red cabbage.[2402]

Bilberries gained notoriety during World War II when it was said that pilots in the British Royal Air Force "were eating bilberry jam to improve their night vision."[2403] It turns out this may have been a story concocted to fool the Germans. The more likely reason the Brits were able to suddenly target Nazi bombers in the middle of the night wasn't because of bilberries but thanks to a top-secret new invention: radar.

Unfortunately, these anthocyanin pigments take a hit when berries are processed into jam. As much as 97 percent of anthocyanins are lost when strawberries are turned into strawberry jam.[2404] Freeze-drying, however, appears to be remarkably nutrient preserving.[2405] I remember trying "astronaut ice cream" as a kid when I visited the Smithsonian's Air and Space Museum in Washington, D.C. That's what freeze-dried strawberries taste like to me. They just melt in your mouth. Delicious, nutritious, but a bit pricey.

Fresh berries, of course, are divine. My family enjoys pick-your-own outings and then freezes the abundance. In my old neighborhood, I would lay a sheet under branches of mulberry trees that grew in a nearby park and gently knock down a ripe bounty with a broom handle. Evidently, nearly all wild "aggregate" berries (meaning berries that look like clusters of little balls, like blackberries, raspberries, and mulberries) in North America are edible,[2406] but please be sure you make an ironclad identification before foraging.

Berries in all their colorful, sweet, and flavorful glory are protective little antioxidant powerhouses. The issue shouldn't be how you are going to get your one minimum daily serving but rather how you are going to pry yourself away from them. In your smoothie, as a dessert, on your salad, or just popped right into your mouth—they are nature's candy.

Other Fruits

> ### My Favorite Other Fruits
>
> Apples, dried apricots, avocados, bananas, cantaloupe, clementines, dates, dried figs, grapefruit, honeydew, kiwifruit, lemons, limes, lychees, mangos, nectarines, oranges, papaya, passion fruit, peaches, pears, pineapple, plums (especially black plums), pluots, pomegranates, prunes, tangerines, and watermelon
>
> **Serving Sizes:**
> 1 medium-sized fruit
> 1 cup (150 g) cut-up fruit
> ¼ cup (40 g) dried fruit
>
> **Daily Recommendation:**
> 3 servings per day

It took years for nearly five hundred researchers from more than three hundred institutions in fifty countries to develop the Global Burden of Disease Study. Funded by the Gates Foundation, it is the largest analysis of risk factors for death and disease in history.[2407] In the United States, the massive study determined that the American diet was a leading cause of both death and disability.[2408] What did the researchers determine to be the worst aspect about our diet in terms of years of healthy life lost? Not eating enough fruits.[2409]

Don't limit yourself to eating fruits just the way they come plucked off the tree. Although they make for a perfect, quick snack, don't forget that they can be cooked as well. Think baked apples, poached pears, and grilled pineapple.

If you like drinking your fruit, blending is better than juicing to preserve nutrition. Juicing removes more than just fiber. Most of the polyphenol phytonutrients (see chapter 3) in fruits and vegetables appear to be bound to the fiber and are only liberated for absorption by the friendly flora in our gut. When we merely drink the juice, we lose out on the fiber and all the nutrition that was attached to it.[2410] Even just cloudy apple juice, which retains a bit of the fruit fiber, appears to have nearly triple the phenolics compared to clear apple juice.[2411]

Whereas greater consumption of whole fruits has been associated with a lower likelihood of developing type 2 diabetes, Harvard University researchers found that greater juice consumption was associated with higher diabetes risk. So, by choosing yellow-light sources of fruits, like juice or jam, we may not only be missing out on nutrients but actively working against our health.[2412]

An Apple a Day

Anyone who says they don't have time to eat healthfully has never met an apple. Talk about a convenience food! For those who grew up in a world dominated by Red Delicious and Granny Smith, I'm happy to report there are thousands of varieties. Health-wise, crab apples probably top the charts (but I'll pass, thank you),[2413] and taste-wise, my personal favorite is SweeTango—or any pick-your-own variety I can find locally. If you've never tried an apple you picked right off a tree, you don't know what you're missing. Failing that, farmers markets can offer good deals on great produce. My family buys apples by the half bushel.

Dates

My favorite fruit snack in the autumn and winter is apple slices with dates, for the perfect mix of tart and sweet. Growing up, I never liked dates. They tasted dry and kind of waxy. But then I discovered there were soft, plump, moist varieties that didn't taste like the chalky ones that haunted my childhood. Barhi and honey dates, for example, are wet and sticky, but when frozen, they acquire the taste and chew of caramel candy. Seriously. Paired with my SweeTango, it's like eating a butterscotch-flavored caramel apple.

Locally, you should be able to find decent Medjool dates in Middle Eastern food shops and many natural foods markets, but for the too-moist-to-be-sold-commercially varieties, you'll probably have to shop online. I have tried dates from most of the major online retailers and always go back to ordering from the Date People, a small farm in California. I am averse to commercial endorsements, but I've never tasted consistently better dates from any other source (although Black Sphinx dates from Phoenix, Arizona, come close). The Date People's annual harvest comes in around my birthday in October, and I always splurge as a present to myself and get a big box to put in our freezer.

Olives and Olive Oil

Olives and extra-virgin olive oil are yellow-light foods. Olive consumption should be minimized because they're soaked in brine—a dozen large olives could take up nearly half our recommended sodium limit for an entire day. Olive oil is sodium-free, but most of its nutrition has been removed. You can think of extra-virgin olive oil a little like fruit juice: It has nutrients, but the calories we get are relatively empty compared to those from the whole fruit. (Olives are, after all, fruits.)

Freshly squeezed olive juice already has less nutrition than the whole fruit, but then olive-oil producers also throw away the olive wastewater, which contains the water-soluble nutrients. As a result, we end up getting just a small fraction of the nutrition of the whole fruit by the time extra-virgin olive oil is bottled. Refined olive oil (nonvirgin) is even worse. I would classify it, along with other vegetable oils, as red-light foods, as they offer such scant nutrition for their heavy caloric loads. One tablespoon of oil can contain more than one hundred calories without filling us up. (Compare that single tablespoon to the one-hundred-calorie serving sizes of other foods on page 157.)

I think of oil as the table sugar of the fat kingdom. Similar to the way manufacturers take healthy foods like beets and throw out all their nutrition to make sugar, they take wholesome corn and scorch-earth it down to corn oil. Like sugar, corn oil calories may be worse than just empty. In chapter 1, I touched on the impairment of artery function that can occur within hours of eating red-light fare like fast food and cheesecake. The same detrimental effect happens after the consumption of olive oil[2414] and other oils[2415] (but not after eating green-light sources of fat like nuts).[2416] Even extra-virgin olive oil may impair our arteries' ability to relax and dilate normally.[2417] So, like any yellow-light food, its use should be curtailed.

Cooking without oil is surprisingly easy. To keep foods from sticking, sauté in wine, sherry, broth, vinegar, or just plain water. For baking, I've successfully used green-light ingredients such as mashed bananas or avocado, soaked prunes, and even canned pumpkin to substitute for oil to provide a similar moistness.

The reduction of yellow-light foods is all about frequency and quantity. If you are going to trek outside the green zone, my advice is simple: Make it count. Don't waste precious indulgences on crappy food. I don't want to sound like a food snob, but if you're going to eat something less than maximally healthy, I say pamper yourself and truly relish it. When I eat olives, there's no way I'm going to eat those waxy black abominations in a can. I'm going to slice up some purple kalamatas that actually have some flavor. If you're going to spoil yourself once in a while, I say do it right!

Mangos

Mangos make fantastic fruit treats during spring and summer, but you have to know where to look to get good ones. Check out Hispanic markets and Indian food shops. The difference between a mango from Walmart and one from an Indian spice store is like the difference between a hard, pale, tasteless, pink tomato and a ripe, flavorful, farm-stand heirloom. You should be able to smell the mango at arm's length.

My favorite way to eat a mango is like sipping a Capri Sun drink pouch. When the fruit gets soft and ripe, I roll it between my palms, kneading it with my fingers until it becomes essentially liquid pulp in a pouch. Then I nip off the tip with my teeth, gently squeeze, and suck the mango right out of its peel.

Why I No Longer Eat My Favorite Fruit

The pawpaw is the largest fruit native to North America, weighing up to two pounds.[2418] It's like a tropical custard you can scoop right out of its peel. Pawpaws taste like a mixture of bananas, mangos, and pineapples,[2419] but they're found in temperate forests across the eastern United States.[2420] They've been nourishing humankind for thousands of years and now have their own pawpaw festivals.[2421] Papayas are sometimes called pawpaws, but they're completely different fruits. The real pawpaw is also known as the dog banana, false-banana, Indian banana,[2422] prairie banana, poor man's banana, Ozark banana, Kentucky banana, and Banango.[2423] I like that one. Indiana banana has a nice ring to it too.

Pawpaws are my favorite fruit, or should I say *were* my favorite fruit. One of the reasons I moved to rural Virginia was because the property had a whole grove of pawpaw trees. I was going to be set for life! Then, I ate a few too many on the first harvest, became quite ill, and *then* looked them up. Pro tip: In the future, find out if a food is toxic *before* you eat it. Little did I know the pawpaw belonged to an infamous family of fruits that contain three different types of neurotoxins.[2424] Neurotoxins! I had actually done a video years earlier warning people not to eat soursop, also known as graviola, but didn't realize pawpaws were related.

In addition to soursop, the family also includes guanabana, sweetsop, sugar apple, cherimoya, and custard apple, which are all linked to a neurodegenerative disease called *progressive supranuclear palsy*, which is like a treatment-resistant Parkinson's, with hallucinations, widespread brain atrophy, and dementia. And consumption of these fruits is associated with about twenty times the odds of having this kind of atypical Parkinson's syndrome.[2425] Expose rats to even a fraction of the dose the people were exposed to, and they develop the same kind of brain lesions you see on autopsy in human victims.[2426] Thankfully, in several patients who stopped consuming these fruits, the progression of their condition ceased, and in one patient, the symptoms even disappeared after a change of diet.[2427] There is an urgent need to raise public awareness about the neurotoxicity of this family of fruits, which are often praised for their taste and medicinal values.[2428]

You can even find dietary supplements containing these plants, promoted for their purported anticancer effects. A soursop extract, for example, can inhibit cancer cell growth in a petri dish but only at concentrations much higher than the amount that kills off brain cells.[2429] Even a low cumulative consumption may worsen disease severity and cognitive deficits in degenerative Parkinson's-type disease. How low? As in just 0.2 fruit-years, so that's only about one-fifth of a fruit a day for a year, a single fruit a month for six years, or a single fruit a year throughout your entire life. The bottom line is that these fruits could contribute to the development of degenerative parkinsonism in humans, so, as a precaution, more restrictive public health preventive recommendations should be made regarding their consumption.[2430]

But what about pawpaws?[2431] Pawpaws have about ten times more of the primary neurotoxin found in soursop.[2432] So why aren't pawpaw eaters getting sick? Well, it's only ripe for a few weeks a year.[2433] So, unlike tropical fruits that can be eaten year-round, people may not have a lot of exposure to pawpaws. What's more, fresh pawpaws aren't typically sold commercially because they bruise so easily. But, the fruit is now available in any season, sold as frozen pulp or jam, and there are supplements out there too.[2434]

When the U.S. Food and Drug Administration was asked about them, it noted that pawpaw has a long history of food use, and it didn't have any evidence that the fruit was unsafe to eat.[2435] You'll hear things like: "Currently, there have been no reports of neurogenerative diseases linked to the consumption of the pawpaw fruit"[2436]—until, of course, there were. A case report entitled "Progressive Supranuclear Palsy and Pawpaw" described a man who had trouble speaking and walking, as his brain was atrophying in his skull. Tragically, he actually died before the cause was figured out. His wife, however, disclosed that they owned pawpaw trees and he had been eating dozens of the fruits each year.[2437] When researchers started investigating, they indeed seemed to find a link between this neurodegenerative disease and pawpaw consumption in the United States.[2438]

Watermelon

Are some whole fruits better than others? Berries contain the most antioxidants, whereas melons wallow down around iceberg lettuce levels. Watermelon *seeds*, on the other hand, have pretty respectable antioxidant levels, so I try to avoid seedless varieties. A spoonful of watermelon seeds may have as many antioxidants as a whole cup of melon balls.[2439] Seedless or not, watermelon contains a compound called *citrulline* that can boost the activity of the enzyme responsible for dilating the blood vessels in the penis that result in erections. A group of Italian researchers found that citrulline supplementation at the level of five servings of red watermelon a day improved erection hardness in men with mild erectile dysfunction, allowing for a 68 percent increase in monthly intercourse frequency.[2440] Yellow watermelon has four times more citrulline,[2441] though, so just about one wedge a day (one-sixteenth of a modest melon) may have the same effect. If this information is new to you, perhaps it's because the advertising budgets of drug companies like Pfizer, which bring in billions of dollars each year from the sale of erectile dysfunction drugs, are about a thousand times[2442] that of the entire budget of the National Watermelon Promotion Board.[2443]

Dried Fruit

I love dried mangos, but they are hard to find without added sugar. I remember naïvely asking a friend in the food business why the industry felt the need to sugar-up an already sweet fruit. "Added weight," he explained. Just as poultry processors inject salt water into chickens to add water weight, processed food companies often use sugar as a cheap way to bulk up products sold by the pound.

This made me determined to make my own. I bought an inexpensive dehydrator from eBay, and I'm so glad I did. Fruit is about 90 percent water, so imagine intensifying the flavor of a fresh, ripe mango tenfold. Mind-blowing! Mangos can be a messy pain to peel (and dangerously slippery too—I recommend wearing a steel-mesh glove), but once that's done, I slice them about a centimeter thick and sprinkle them with chia seeds before putting them in the dehydrator. If I'm taking them on a plane or a hike, I'll dry them completely. Otherwise, I only wait until just the outside is dry. The outer layer, encrusted with chia, gets a crispy texture while the core remains moist and ready to burst.

I also like drying thin apple slices. I either sprinkle them with cinnamon or rub them with freshly grated ginger. They can be just dried until chewy or completely dehydrated into crunchy apple chips. Eating a dozen dried apple rings a day may drop LDL cholesterol levels by 16 percent within three months and by 24 percent within six months.[2444]

If you buy dried fruit, I recommend choosing unsulfured varieties. Sulfur-containing preservatives, such as sulfur dioxide in dried fruit and sulfites in wine, can form hydrogen sulfide in our gut. That's the rotten egg gas implicated in the development of the inflammatory bowel disease, ulcerative colitis. The main source of hydrogen sulfide in our diets is the metabolism of animal protein,[2445] but we can lower our exposure even further by avoiding sulfur additives (either by reading labels or choosing organic, in which such preservatives are forbidden). The sulfur naturally contained in cruciferous vegetables does not appear to elevate colitis risk,[2446] so feel free to add kale chips to your healthy snacking menu.

Prescribing Kiwifruit

There appear to be a disproportionate number of articles in the medical literature about the clinical benefits of kiwifruit. Is that because they're better than other fruits? Or is it because the kiwi industry has more research dollars? One country, New Zealand, holds a substantial share of the global kiwi market, so it's in its best interest to underwrite research on the fruit. As a result, there is no shortage of papers touting the benefits of kiwifruit.

Kiwi is one of the fruits I recommend for insomnia. (Eating two of them an hour before bedtime appears to significantly improve sleep onset, duration, and efficiency.[2447]) It also helps with constipation-type irritable bowel syndrome. (Two kiwifruit a day also seems to significantly improve bowel function.) Kiwi certainly seems like a better option than the leading IBS drug, which was pulled from the market for apparently killing too many people.[2448]

Kiwifruits appear to benefit immune function too. Preschoolers randomized to eat gold kiwifruits every day appeared to cut in half their risk of contracting a cold or flu-like illness, compared to those randomly selected to eat bananas instead.[2449] A similar experiment was tried on older individuals, another high-risk group. Those in the banana control group who got an upper-respiratory-tract infection suffered for about five days with a sore throat and congestion, compared to the kiwifruit eaters, who felt better after just a day or two.[2450] About 1 in 130 children may be allergic to kiwifruit, though.[2451] Kiwis may rank as the third-most-common childhood food allergen (second only to milk and eggs),[2452] so they are not for everyone.

Citrus

Adding citrus zest to our meals not only adds color, flavor, aroma, and a bit of culinary flair but also nutrition. Citrus zest lives up to its name in terms of enlivening dishes, and it may do the same to our DNA-repair capabilities. On average, humans appear to suffer eight hundred hits to our DNA per hour. If not fixed, this can cause mutations that give rise to cancer.[2453] Comparing identical and fraternal twins, researchers have established that only part of our DNA-repair function is determined genetically. The rest may be under our control.[2454]

The dietary factor found best able to boost DNA repair was citrus fruits.[2455] Within two hours of consuming citrus, our DNA becomes significantly more resistant to damage,[2456] which may help explain why citrus consumption is associated with lower risk of breast cancer.[2457] Some of the citrus compounds thought responsible—which concentrate in the breast[2458] and enhance DNA repair[2459]—are found in the peel, though. This may be why people who eat at least some citrus peel appear to have lower skin cancer rates than those who don't.[2460]

Stick with the whole fruit, because supplements don't appear to boost DNA repair,[2461] and citrus juice doesn't appear to help, either. In fact, drinking orange juice every morning may even increase skin cancer risk.[2462] Green-light forms of foods always seem to be the best, and we can eat citrus in an even *less* processed way by slipping some of the rind into our diet through zesting. I like to freeze whole lemons, limes, and oranges so we always have them on hand to grate onto meals that could use a little zing.

My only whole-citrus caveat: Inform your physician if you eat grapefruit.

This fruit can suppress the enzymes that help clear more than half of commonly prescribed drugs, and less drug clearance means higher drug levels in the body.[2463] This may actually be good if you want a better caffeine buzz from your morning coffee[2464] or if your doctor wants to help you save money by boosting the effects of expensive drugs instead of just peeing them away.[2465] But higher drug levels may also mean higher risk of side effects, so if you regularly eat grapefruits, your physician may want to change your prescription or alter the dosing.

Exotic (to Me) Fruits

The medical school I attended sits in the middle of Boston's Chinatown. I remember the first time I perused the produce aisle at a large Asian supermarket. With options from bizarre-looking dragon fruit to tribble-like rambutans, I felt like I was on another planet. Every week I tried something new. Some stuck with me—I still sneak lychees into the movies—but others were onetime affairs. Let me share with you the Durian Incident.

Durians are the most badass of all fruits. Imagine a two-kilo football covered in sharp spikes like some medieval mace. What other fruit could be described in the medical literature as causing "severe body injury" in papers with titles like "Penetrating Ocular Injury by Durian Fruit"?[2466] And I haven't even gotten to its most distinctive quality: its smell. With an odor perhaps best described as "pig-shit, turpentine and onions, garnished with a gym sock,"[2467] durian fruits are banned from many public spaces, like subways and airports, in Southeast Asia, where they are grown.

I had to try eating one of these wild things!

Durian fruits are sold frozen. (I would soon come to understand why.) I took one back to campus and managed to hack off a piece without impaling myself on a spike. The fruit tasted like a caramelized onion popsicle. I left the rest in my locker. Big mistake! I arrived the next day to find an entire floor of the medical center—including the dean's office—cordoned off. They were going locker to locker, cutting off all the locks, searching in vain for the cause of a stench so overpowering you couldn't even locate it. It was like a fog of stink. Hospital staff seriously thought someone had stolen body parts from the cadaver lab. And then it struck me. The durian had thawed in my locker. When I realized it was all my fault, I crawled to the dean to beg forgiveness. I already had a history of run-ins with the administration over issues I had raised about the curriculum, and now this. I'll never forget what he said to me that day: "Why am I not surprised you had something to do with this?"

When adding as much fruit as possible to your diet, you certainly don't have to seek out weapons-grade stinky fruit, but you also don't have to stick with the same old, same old. Treat yourself! Have fun sampling the many varieties of the many different fruits around. How lovely it can be to stroll through your farmers market on a weekend and pick up locally grown fruits that you can zest onto your meals, blend into smoothies, chew when dried, incorporate into your favorite dishes, or best of all, bite right into. The opportunities are ripe for the picking.

Cruciferous Vegetables

> ## My Favorite Cruciferous Vegetables
>
> Broccoli, brussels sprouts, cabbage, cauliflower, collard greens, horseradish, kale (black, green, and red), mustard greens, pak choi, radishes, rocket, turnip greens, and watercress
>
> **Serving Sizes:**
> ½ cup (90 g) cooked leafy vegetables
> 1 cup (60 g) raw leafy vegetables
> ½ cup (90 g) raw or cooked non-leafy vegetables
> ¼ cup (20 g) broccoli sprouts
> 1 tablespoon horseradish
>
> **Daily Recommendation:**
> 1 serving per day

When I used to teach medical students at Tufts, I gave a lecture about this amazing new therapeutic called *iloccorB*. I'd talk about all the evidence supporting it, the great things it could do, and its excellent safety profile. Just as I imagined the students scheming to buy stock in the company and prescribing it to their future patients, I'd do the big reveal. Apologizing for my "dyslexia," I would admit that I'd gotten it backward. All that time, I had been talking about broccoli.

I've mentioned broccoli more than any other food in this book, and for good reason. We've seen how cruciferous vegetables like broccoli can potentially prevent DNA damage and metastatic cancer spread in chapter 2, activate defenses against pathogens and pollutants in chapter 4, potentially help prevent lymphoma in chapter 9, boost our liver detox enzymes and target breast cancer stem cells in chapter 12, and reduce the risk of prostate cancer progression in chapter 14. The component responsible for these benefits, as we've discussed, is thought to be sulforaphane, which is formed almost exclusively in cruciferous vegetables. This is why they get their own spot on the Daily Dozen.

Beyond being a promising anticancer agent,[2468] sulforaphane may also help protect our brain[2469] and our eyesight,[2470] reduce nasal allergy inflammation,[2471] and manage type 2 diabetes,[2472] and it was recently found to successfully help treat autism. A placebo-controlled, double-blind, randomized trial of boys with autism found that about two to three cruciferous vegetable servings' worth[2473] of sulforaphane a day improved social interaction, abnormal behavior, and verbal communication within a matter of weeks. The researchers, primarily from Harvard University and Johns Hopkins University, suggest that the effect might be due to sulforaphane's role as a "detoxicant."[2474]

Ways to Enhance Sulforaphane Formation

The formation of sulforaphane in cruciferous vegetables is like a chemical flare reaction. It requires the mixing of a precursor compound with an enzyme called *myrosinase*, which is inactivated by cooking (though microwaved broccoli appears to retain some cancer-fighting capacity).[2475] This may explain why we see dramatic suppression of test-tube cancer-cell growth by raw broccoli, cauliflower, and brussels sprouts, but hardly any reaction when they're cooked.[2476] But who wants to eat raw brussels sprouts? Thankfully, we can get the benefits of raw vegetables in cooked form.

Biting into broccoli is like snapping that chemical flare. When raw broccoli (or any other cruciferous vegetable) is chopped or chewed, the sulforaphane precursor mixes with the myrosinase enzyme, and sulforaphane is created as the vegetable sits on the cutting board or lies in our upper stomach waiting to be digested.[2477] Though the enzyme is destroyed by cooking, both the precursor and the final product are relatively resistant to heat. So here's my trick, the "Hack and Hold" (aka the "Whack and Wait") technique.

If you chop the broccoli, brussels sprouts, kale, collards, cauliflower, or any other cruciferous vegetable, and then wait thirty minutes,[2478] you can then cook it. At that point, the sulforaphane has already been made, so the enzyme is no longer needed to achieve maximum benefit. It's already done its job. (You can also buy bags of fresh greens and other crucifers that are prechopped or shredded, which can presumably be cooked immediately.)

Given this understanding, can you see how broccoli soup is often prepared incorrectly? Typically, broccoli is cooked, then blended. But, when it's blended, the precursor is just being mixed with an enzyme that's already been inactivated by cooking. Do it in the opposite order: First blend the veggies and then wait thirty minutes before cooking them. This way, we can maximize sulforaphane production.

What about *frozen* broccoli and other crucifers? Commercially produced frozen broccoli lacks the ability to form sulforaphane because the vegetables are blanched (flash-cooked) before they're frozen for the very purpose of deactivating enzymes.[2479] This process prolongs shelf life, but when we take the veggies out of our freezer, the enzyme is inert. At that point, it doesn't matter how much we chop or how long we wait—no sulforaphane is going to be made. This may be why fresh kale has been shown to suppress cancer cell growth in vitro up to ten times better than frozen kale.[2480]

The frozen crucifer is still packed with the precursor, though—remember, it's heat resistant. We could make lots of sulforaphane from it by adding back some enzyme.[2481] But where can you get myrosinase? Scientists buy theirs from chemical companies, but we can just walk into any supermarket.

Mustard greens are also cruciferous vegetables. They grow from mustard seeds, which we can buy ground up in the spice aisle as mustard powder. If we sprinkled some mustard powder on frozen broccoli that's been cooked, would it start producing sulforaphane? Yes!

Boiling broccoli prevents the formation of any significant levels of sulforaphane due to inactivation of the enzyme. However, the addition of powdered mustard seeds to cooked broccoli significantly increases sulforaphane formation.[2482] Then it's almost as good as eating it raw! So, if you don't have thirty minutes to spare between chopping and cooking, or if you're using frozen greens, just sprinkle the crucifers with some mustard powder before you eat them, and you'll be all set. Daikon radishes, regular radishes, horseradish, and wasabi are cruciferous vegetables too, and may have the same effect. All it appears to take is a pinch to revitalize sulforaphane production.[2483] We can also add a small amount of fresh greens to our cooked greens. So when I add shreds of red cabbage to my finished dishes, it not only adds a beautiful garnish with a delightful crunch, but it's also filled with the sulforaphane-producing enzyme.

One of my first tasks every morning is chopping greens for the day, using my Hack and Hold technique. But any day I run out of time, I know I have the backup Mustard Powder Plan.

Horseradish

The serving sizes I offer on page 359 correspond roughly to the daily intake required to achieve cancer-preventive levels according to the innovative breast-surgery study I detailed in chapter 12. As you can see, horseradish has the smallest serving size, which means it's the most concentrated of the cruciferous vegetables. One tablespoon and your Daily Dozen is down to an Everyday Eleven. Horseradish can be made into a sauce, relish, or dressing to score an extra check mark with a kick. It's great in mashed potatoes or, for a healthier option still, mashed cauliflower. Just boil cauliflower for about ten minutes until tender and then mash with a fork or potato masher or purée in a food processor with some of the reserved cooking liquid until smooth. I season it with pepper, roasted garlic, and a dollop of horseradish and then pour mushroom gravy on it. Delicious!

Roasting Cruciferous Vegetables

As much as I love mashed cauliflower, roasted cauliflower (or broccoli, for that matter) is a favorite. Roasting brings out a nutty, caramelized flavor. I slice raw cauliflower into "steaks," roast at 400°F (204°C) for about half an hour, then smother it in a lemon-tahini sauce. Sometimes I go minimalist and just sprinkle on lemon juice, zest, capers, and garlic. (This chapter is making me hungry!)

Kale Chips

I'll talk about some of the more traditional ways I prepare greens in the next section, but kale chips deserve a special mention. You can use a dehydrator if you have one, but I often don't have the patience. When I'm in the mood for kale chips, I want them *now*. They can be as simple as one ingredient: kale. Pull the leaves off the stems and tear into large pieces. Make sure that they are dry, or they'll steam rather than crisp. Air fry them for a few minutes at 350°F (177°C), shaking the basket about halfway through, or, if you don't have an air fryer, lay out the torn leaves in a single layer on a cookie tray lined with parchment paper or a silicone mat to prevent sticking, and bake at a low temperature (about 250°F or 120°C) and check often to make sure they don't burn. Within about twenty minutes, they transform into light, crispy snacks. Preseason the leaves before you roast them, or add your spices after they're done. There are thousands of recipes online. With kale chips, the more you snack, the healthier you are.

Cruciferous Garnishes

Similar to the way I used to use an open can of beans in the fridge as a reminder to try to bean-up any dish, we always have a red cabbage in the crisper to help us cruciferize our meals. I slice off shreds and garnish nearly anything with them. Red cabbage averages about a dollar and a quarter per 500 grams,[2484] is found at pretty much any supermarket or market, can last weeks in the fridge (though if it does, that means you're not eating enough of it!), and has more antioxidants per dollar than anything else found in the produce aisle. There are healthier foods we can buy, but not for the same amount of money. For example, red cabbage may have nearly three times the antioxidant power per dollar that blueberries do.[2485] In terms of eating healthfully on a budget, red cabbage can't be beat. Or can it?

After chopping and discarding the waste, red cabbage averages 53 cents per 180 grams.[2486] But broccoli sprouts—if you make them yourself—may be even cheaper. Broccoli sprout seeds can be purchased online or at natural foods stores for about twenty dollars per 500 grams, but that makes about 6 kilos of sprouts. In terms of sulforaphane content, that may be around 54 kilos of mature broccoli. So DIY broccoli sprouts provide a green-light sulforaphane source for about a nickel a day.

Sprouting broccoli sprouts is as easy as sprouting lentils. Start with a mason jar with a sprouting (screen) lid. Add a tablespoon of seeds, let them soak overnight in water, drain in the morning, and then after that, just rinse and drain twice a day. Most people wait for about five days, until the seeds fully sprout (taking on the look of alfalfa sprouts), but newer science suggests sulforaphane content peaks at forty-eight hours after the seeds are initially drained.[2487] This makes them even quicker and easier to grow and eat. When I'm not traveling, I usually have a few jars in rotation. It can be the middle of winter, and I'm growing my own salad on my kitchen counter! Every day, you can get portions of fresh produce without ever having to go to the store.

Cruciferous Supplements?

If you don't like the taste of cruciferous vegetables but still want the benefits of the sulforaphane, what about the broccoli supplements currently on the market? Researchers put a commercial supplement to the test. BroccoMax boasts the equivalent of 225 grams of broccoli in every capsule. Study subjects were given either six capsules a day or 80 grams of broccoli sprouts. The supplement hardly worked at all, whereas the sprouts boosted blood levels about eight times higher for eight times less cost. The researchers concluded that "our data provide further evidence that bioavailability of [sulforaphane] is dramatically lower when subjects consume broccoli supplements compared to fresh broccoli sprouts."[2488]

Too Much of a Good Thing?

If broccoli sprouts are so cheap and effective, why not eat bowls of them? A formal safety analysis found no significant adverse effects to about 120 grams a day,[2489] but we didn't have data on a potential upper limit until a team of Italian researchers tried to push the envelope. They were attempting to come up with an intravenous infusion dose to use as chemotherapy, so they wanted to know how high they could go. The researchers discovered that blood levels achieved by 320 grams or more of broccoli sprouts may indeed be detrimental.[2490] They concluded, however, that no harm was found at "nutritionally attainable concentrations." But that's not really true. Broccoli sprouts do have a radishy bite, but someone *could* theoretically eat 320 grams of sprouts a day. (They don't know health nuts like I know some health nuts.)

Let me tell you a story. Someone came up to me after a lecture in Miami and told me he had heard that wheatgrass juice was good for you. "It cleans you out," he had read. So he thought, *Why not?* He told me how he calculated the volume of the human digestive tract (all nine meters or so) and proceeded to drink that amount continuously, liter after liter, until it started coming out the other end. Intrigued, I asked him what happened. He looked up at me with an expression that I can only describe as rapturous and said, "It was *volcanic*."

It would be hard for me to say too many good things about crucifers. These vegetables do wonders for our health, from fighting cancer progression and boosting defenses against pathogens and pollutants to helping protect our brain and vision and more. And we can use this family of veggies as an excuse to play Mad Scientist in the kitchen, manipulating enzyme chemistry to maximize the health benefits.

Greens

My Favorite Greens

Assorted young salad greens, beetroot greens, collard greens, kale (black, green, and red), mustard greens, rocket, sorrel, spinach, Swiss chard, and turnip greens

Serving Sizes:
1 cup (60 g) raw
½ cup (90 g) cooked

Daily Recommendation:
2 servings per day

Popeye was right when he bragged that he was strong to the finish because he ate his spinach. Dark green leafy vegetables are the healthiest foods on the planet. As whole foods go, they offer the most nutrition per calorie. Just to emphasize the point, there was a study published in the journal *Nutrition and Cancer* entitled "Antioxidant, Antimutagenic, and Antitumor Effects of Pine Needles."[2491] Edible leaves, in all their shapes and sizes, it seems, can be healthy foods.

In 1777, General George Washington issued a general order that American troops should forage for wild greens growing around their camps "as these vegetables are very conducive to health, and tend to prevent . . . all putrid disorders."[2492] Since then, however, Americans have declared their independence from greens. Today, only about one in twenty-five of us even reach a dozen servings throughout the course of an entire month.[2493] I advise getting more than a dozen servings per week.

Important Caveat: Greens and Warfarin

In 1984, the tragic case of a thirty-five-year-old woman unfolded when she failed to inform her physician about her change in diet. Because of her mechanical heart valve, the woman was on a blood-thinning drug called warfarin. But because she wanted to lose weight, she started eating a diet composed almost entirely of salad, broccoli, turnip greens, and mustard greens. Five weeks later, she suffered a blood clot and died.[2494]

If you are on the drug warfarin (also known as Coumadin), talk with your physician before you increase your greens intake. The drug works (both as a rat poison and a human blood-thinner) by crippling the enzyme that recycles vitamin K, which is involved in clotting your blood. If your system gets an influx of fresh vitamin K, which is concentrated in greens, you can thereby undermine the effectiveness of the drug. You should still be able to eat your greens, but your physician will have to titrate the dose of the drug to match your regular greens intake.

Eating greens nearly every day may be one of the most powerful steps we can take to prolong our lives.[2495] Of all the food groups analyzed by a team of Harvard University researchers, greens turned out to be associated with the strongest protection against major chronic diseases,[2496] including up to about a 20 percent reduction in risk for both heart attacks[2497] and strokes[2498] for every additional daily serving.

Imagine if there were a pill that could prolong life and only had good side effects. Everyone would be taking it. It would be making billions of dollars for the lucky drug company that created it. All health plans by law would have to cover it. People from every walk of life and every corner of the globe would be clamoring for it. But when that "pill" is just eat-your-greens, people lose interest.

Drug companies have yet to patent broccoli (though Monsanto tried[2499]). Doctors, however, don't have to wait for perky pharmaceutical sales reps to wine, dine, and cajole them into prescribing Pfizer-brand spinach or GlaxoSmithKline-brand collards. Here's my prescription for you:

If the full spectrum of colorful plant pigments are good for you, why are greens the healthiest? When autumn in New England becomes aflame with

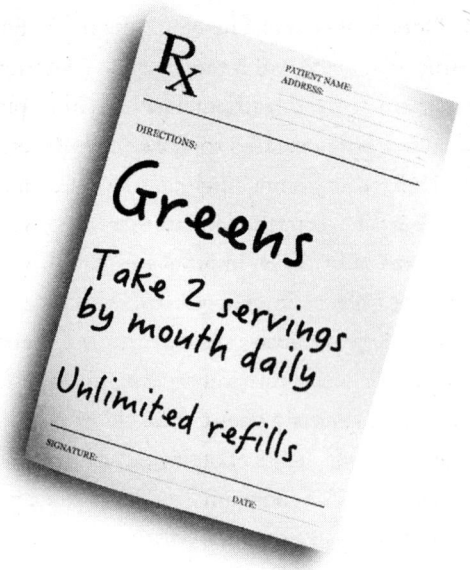

brilliant hues, where do those oranges and yellows come from? They were there all along—just masked by the green pigment chlorophyll that starts to break down in the autumn.[2500] Similarly, the dark green leaves of vegetables contain many of the other plant pigments all wrapped up in one package. As I mentioned, these colorful compounds are often the very same antioxidants implicated in many of the benefits of fruit and vegetable consumption. So, in essence, when we eat our greens, we are eating the rainbow.

Regenerating Coenzyme Q10, Naturally

One of the reasons greens are some of the healthiest green-light foods may be due to their green color. Decades ago, a search began for "interceptor" molecules that could serve as the body's first line of defense against cancer. The theory was that if we could find something that could tightly bind to carcinogens and prevent them from slipping into our DNA, we might be able to prevent some of the mutations that lead to cancer. After years of combing for the existence of such carcinogen-binding molecules, an interceptor was found: chlorophyll, the most ubiquitous plant pigment in the world. It was right under our noses all along.[2501]

In a petri dish, certain DNA damage in human cells exposed to a carcinogen could be "totally abolished" by chlorophyll.[2502] But what about in people? In the name of science, volunteers drank a solution of radioactive aflatoxin (a carcinogen) with or without spinach chlorophyll. Six cups of spinach worth of chlorophyll appeared to block about 40 percent of the carcinogen.[2503] Amazing! But that's not all chlorophyll can do.

In college, we learn that pretty much everything we were taught in high school biology isn't true. Then in graduate school, we unlearn all the oversimplifications we learned in college. Just when we think we understand something in biology, it always seems a little more complicated than we thought. For example, until relatively recently, we assumed plants and plantlike organisms were the only ones that could directly capture and utilize the energy from the sun. Plants photosynthesize. Animals don't. That's because plants have chlorophyll and animals do not. Well, technically, we *do* have chlorophyll in our body—temporarily, at least—after we eat greens. But it would seem there's no way the chlorophyll that enters our bloodstream after we eat that salad could react with sunlight. After all, light can't penetrate through our skin, right?

Wrong. Any kid who's ever shined a flashlight through their fingers could have told you that.

The red wavelengths of sunlight do penetrate our body.[2504] In fact, if we step outside on a sunny day, there's enough light reaching our brain that we could actually read this page inside our skull.[2505] Our internal organs are bathed in sunlight, along with any chlorophyll circulating in our bloodstream. Although any energy produced by the chlorophyll would be negligible,[2506] it turns out that light-activated chlorophyll in our body may help regenerate a critical molecule called coenzyme Q10.[2507]

CoQ10, also known as *ubiquinol*, is an antioxidant. When ubiquin*ol* extinguishes a free radical, it is oxidized to ubiquin*one*. To act as an effective antioxidant again, the body must regenerate ubiquinol from ubiquinone. Think of it like an electrical fuse: Ubiquinol can only be used once before having to be reset. That's where sunlight and chlorophyll may come in.

Researchers exposed some ubiquinone and dietary chlorophyll metabolites to the kind of light that reaches our bloodstream, and CoQ10 was reborn. However, without the chlorophyll, or without the light, nothing happened. All along, we've been thinking that the main benefit of sunlight was only the formation of vitamin D and that the main benefit of greens was the antioxidants they contain. But now we suspect the combination of the two may actually help the body create and maintain its own internal stock of antioxidants.

Eating a plant-based, chlorophyll-rich diet may be especially important for those on cholesterol-lowering statin drugs, as these medications can interfere with CoQ10 production.[2508]

Green Can Taste Great

I hope I've been able to convince you to eat greens as often as possible. The problem for many people is getting them to *taste* good. I'm afraid too many of us still suffer flashbacks from overcooked, slimy green lumps on school cafeteria trays.

Take kale, for example. Fibrous and grassy tasting, right? Kind of bitter too? Some varieties are more palatable than others. In a good supermarket produce section, you may be able to find three types: green, black, and red. Nutritionally, the differences among them appear to be insignificant compared to how much of each you may be willing to eat.[2509,2510] The healthiest kale is the one you'll eat the most of.

I would suggest using black kale (also called Cavolo nero, lacinato, or Tuscan kale), red kale (also found as red Russian kale), or baby kale, since these varieties are all milder and more tender than the more common mature green (curly) kale.

Start by rinsing the leaves thoroughly under running water. Then rip off the stems and tear the leaves into bite-sized pieces. Alternatively, after the leaves are removed from their stems, roll them up and slice into thin ribbons. If you want to make it even easier on yourself, just use whatever type you can find frozen. Frozen greens are cheaper, last longer, and come prewashed and prechopped.

There's a phenomenon called flavor-flavor conditioning in which we can change our palate by linking a less pleasant flavor (for instance, sour or bitter) with a more pleasant one (say, sweet). For example, when researchers tried adding sugar to sour grapefruit juice, people liked it better. No surprise. But within a few days, the study subjects began to like even *unsweetened* grapefruit juice more than they did before the experiment started. In fact, this reconditioning of the palate lasted for at least weeks after the sugar was removed.[2511]

The same happens when researchers dip or spritz broccoli with sugar water or aspartame.[2512] I know that sounds gross, but they're not actually making the broccoli taste sweet. The added sweetness merely masks the bitterness by fooling our taste buds.[2513] This is why the so-called secret ingredient in many collard greens recipes is a spoonful of sugar. Certainly, if there were ever a food to justify the use of a yellow- or red-light condiment to boost consumption, it would be the single healthiest of all foods: greens. I use a variety of savory flavored balsamic vinegars on my greens, like hickory smoke or black garlic. It would be even healthier, though, to add green-light sweetness in the form of something like figs or grated apples.

The sweetness trick is why green smoothies can be so delicious. Smoothies can be a great way to introduce greens into diets of the uninitiated, especially children. The basic triad is a liquid, ripe fruit, and fresh greens. I'd start with a two-to-one ratio of fruits to greens before tipping heavier toward greens on the scale. So, for example, a classic starter green smoothie is 250 ml of water, a frozen banana, 140 grams of frozen berries, and 60 grams of packed baby spinach. Mango or sweet potato would be even healthier than the banana, though, since there's an enzyme in raw bananas that can potentially cut down on the bioavailability of some other smoothie components.[2514] See my video series that starts with see.nf/bananaswap for more information.

I like to add fresh mint leaves as well for a boost of flavor (and even more greens). Fresh herbs can be expensive at the store, but mint can grow like a weed in your yard or in a pot on your windowsill. Eating greens for breakfast can be as delicious as mint chocolate oatmeal—cooked oatmeal, chopped mint leaves, cocoa powder, and a healthy sweetener. (See page 345.)

When you're thinking about ways to pair your greens with something you already love to make the greens more palatable, consider mixing them with a green-light source of fat: nuts, seeds, nut or seed butters, or avocados. Many of the nutrients greens are famous for are fat-soluble, including beta-carotene, lutein, vitamin K, and zeaxanthin. So pairing greens with a green-light source of fat may not only make them taste better but will maximize nutrient absorption. This can mean enjoying a creamy tahini-based dressing on your salad, putting walnuts in your pesto, or sprinkling some sesame seeds on your sautéed kale.

The jump in nutrient absorption is no small effect. When researchers tried feeding people a healthy salad of spinach, romaine, carrots, and tomatoes along with a source of fat, there was an impressive spike in carotenoid phytonutrients in their bloodstream over the next eight hours. With a fat-free dressing, carotenoid absorption flatlined down to negligible amounts; it was as if they'd never eaten the salad at all.[2515] Similarly, adding some avocado to your salsa may triple the amount of fat-soluble nutrients that make it into your bloodstream (in this case, the lycopene in the tomatoes).[2516] It doesn't take much. Just three grams of fat in an entire hot meal may be sufficient to boost absorption.[2517] That's just a single walnut or a spoonful of avocado or shredded coconut. Snack on a few pistachios after a meal, and you're all set. The greens and the source of fat just have to end up in your stomach at the same time.

Another way to remove bitterness from greens is to blanch or boil them, but unfortunately this works by leaching some of the healthy compounds into the cooking water.[2518] If you're making soup, that's not a problem, because the nutrients aren't destroyed as much as they are displaced. If the cooking liquid is poured off, however, you could be losing some nutrition. But even if 50 percent of these healthy compounds go down the drain, if the decreased bitterness motivates you to eat twice as many greens, problem solved! When I'm boiling pasta, for example, I'll sometimes add a bunch of fresh greens to the pot a few minutes before I'm ready to drain the pasta. I know I'll lose some nutrients when I pour off the cooking water, but it's worth it to me for the convenience of throwing everything into one pot and getting my family to eat even more greens.

Try to incorporate greens into as many meals as possible. I put just about everything I eat on a bed of greens. That way, the greens take on the flavor of the rest of the dish. However, if you want to eat cooked greens "straight," you can try adding lemon juice, flavored vinegars, red pepper flakes, garlic, ginger, low-sodium soya sauce, or caramelized onions. I personally like mine hot, sweet, smoky, and salty. I use hot sauce for heat, flavored balsamics for sweetness, and smoked paprika. For saltiness, I used to be fond of a soya sauce substitute called Bragg Liquid Aminos until I got more serious about cutting down my sodium intake and switched to potassium-based salt substitutes.

There are whole grocery aisles full of prepared sauces with which you can experiment. Most have added salt, oil, or sugar, so I try to reserve them for exceptionally healthy foods. Mixing yellow- and red-light foods together (like dipping your fries or McNuggets in barbecue sauce) may just add insult to injury, but I wouldn't eat half as many baked rosemary sweet-potato fries if I weren't dipping them in hot-sauce-spiked ketchup (salt-free, but with added sugar). And if there were ever an excuse to dip out of the green-light zone, it would be for green leafy vegetables.

During my medical school days, I would regularly order Chinese food for delivery—usually broccoli and garlic sauce (hold the white rice). Then I'd throw brown rice or quinoa along with dried lentils into my rice cooker and steam or microwave a pound of greens. By the time the delivery arrived, everything was ready and I would just mix it all together and have a few meals' worth of leftovers.

You can also find prepackaged pouches of Indian food online or at Indian or natural foods markets. Again, I'd use them as sauces rather than eat them as a meal in themselves. My favorite is spinach dal—that way, I'm eating greens in a greens sauce! That's like the kale-pesto principle: Use one green (basil) to make the other green (kale) taste better.

The Health Benefits of Vinegar

Vinegar, like salt-free mustard, may be one condiment that's good for us. Randomized, controlled trials involving people with diabetes and without suggest that adding two teaspoons of vinegar to a meal may improve blood sugar control, effectively blunting the blood sugar spike after a meal by about 20 percent.[2519] So adding vinegar to potato salad or to rice (like the Japanese do to make sushi rice) or dipping bread in balsamic vinegar may blunt the effects of these high-glycemic foods.

We've known about the anti-glycemic effect of vinegar for more than thirty-five years, but we're still not sure of the mechanism.[2520] Originally, it was thought that vinegar slowed stomach emptying, but even consuming vinegar outside of meals appears to help. Individuals with type 2 diabetes consuming two tablespoons of apple cider vinegar at bedtime, for example, were found to wake up with better blood sugar in the morning.[2521] Consuming pickles or vinegar *pills* does not seem to have the same effect.[2522] Do not, however, drink vinegar straight, as it can burn your esophagus,[2523] and don't drink it in excess— 250 ml a day for six years (547.5 liters!) was discovered to be a bad idea.[2524]

Vinegar may also help with polycystic ovary syndrome (PCOS), improve arterial function, and help reduce body fat. A daily tablespoon of apple cider vinegar restored ovarian function within a few months in four out of seven women with PCOS.[2525] A tablespoon of rice vinegar was found to acutely improve artery function in postmenopausal women. We're not sure why, but the acetate from the acetic acid in vinegar may lead to improved nitric oxide production.[2526] (See page 120.) Such an effect would be expected to help with hypertension, and indeed there is a study purporting to show blood pressure benefits from a tablespoon of vinegar a day.[2527]

Despite folk wisdom to the contrary, vinegar does not appear to be an effective treatment for head lice,[2528] but it may help with weight loss. A double-blind, placebo-controlled (but vinegar company-funded) study was performed in which obese participants consumed daily vinegar drinks with either one or two tablespoons of apple cider vinegar or a placebo drink that tasted like vinegar but contained no acetic acid. Both vinegar groups lost significantly more weight than the control group. Though the effect was modest—about 1–2 kilos over a three-month period—CT scans showed the participants in the vinegar groups lost a significant amount of their "visceral" fat, the abdominal fat that is particularly associated with chronic disease risk.[2529]

In *How Not to Diet*, I get into the specifics for using vinegar for weight loss and in *How Not to Age* discuss its role in boosting an anti-aging enzyme called AMPK. There are all sorts of flavorful, exotic vinegars to explore these days, including fig, peach, and pomegranate. I encourage you to experiment and find ways to incorporate some into your diet.

Salad Days

Having a big salad every day is a great way to tick off boxes in the Daily Dozen. To a base of mixed salad leaves and rocket, I add tomato, red bell pepper/capsicum, beans, and barberries, along with walnuts or pumpkin seeds if I'm using a fat-free dressing. My favorite dressing recipe is a take on a Caesar spin-off shared by Dr. Michael Klaper from the TrueNorth Health Center:

2 tablespoons almond meal or ground flaxseeds
1 tablespoon walnuts
3 cloves crushed garlic
3 tablespoons dijon mustard
3 tablespoons nutritional yeast flakes
2 tablespoons white miso
3 tablespoons lemon juice
125 ml water

Blend and enjoy! (If you have a high-speed blender, you could probably use whole almonds instead of almond meal.)

Baby spinach may have higher levels of phytonutrients than mature spinach leaves,[2530] but what about *real* baby spinach—so-called microgreens, the seedlings of vegetables and herbs? A nutritional analysis of twenty-five commercially available microgreens found they did have significantly higher nutrient densities. For example, red cabbage microgreens have a sixfold higher vitamin C concentration than mature red cabbage and nearly seventy times the vitamin K.[2531] But they tend to be eaten in such microquantities that even the healthiest upscale restaurant garnish probably isn't going to do much for you.

If, however, you want to grow your own, you could have rotating trays of microgreens that you snip off with scissors for probably the healthiest salad out there. (On a lecture tour, I once stayed with someone who did just that, and I've been jealous ever since.) Microgreens are the perfect plants for the impatient gardener—fully grown in just one to two weeks.

The One Green to Avoid

Although greens are the healthiest of foods, there's one green I caution against eating: alfalfa sprouts. Over a dozen years, twenty-eight outbreaks of *Salmonella* food poisoning linked to sprouts have been documented in the United States, affecting 1,275 people.[2532] Of course, *Salmonella*-tainted eggs sicken an estimated 142,000 Americans every year,[2533] but that doesn't make it any less tragic for those hospitalized and killed in "sproutbreaks." Alfalfa sprout seeds have all sorts of microscopic nooks and crannies where bacteria from manure-contaminated irrigation water can hide. So even home-sprouted alfalfa seeds should not be considered safe.

I will never forget a presentation I gave in Boston. It was in a game show-style format in which contestants from the audience tried to rank, from healthiest to unhealthiest, the foods I'd brought with me. There was a lively cacophony of conflicting advice shouted from the crowd. You can imagine the groans when I revealed that alfalfa sprouts—a quintessential health food—belonged way at the top on the foods-to-avoid list.

Later that night, I was stuck with the sprouts after all the healthier and yummier items had been given away as prizes. I had just told my audience not to eat them—but I hate wasting food. In a do-as-I-say-not-as-I-do moment, I added them to my salad that night. Yes, they had been sitting in the car all day and on stage for hours more. Yes, they were at the top of my game show's list of foods you should not eat. But, what were the odds that that one particular package was contaminated? I went back to my place of work the next day at the New England Medical Center emergency room—not as a physician but as a patient with *Salmonella* food poisoning.

So other than the dreaded alfalfa sprout, greens truly are the healthiest foods on the planet. You simply can't do better in terms of nutrition per calorie. Explore, innovate, taste test, play, and teach your palate to enjoy them. Whether you sneak them into a refreshing smoothie, incorporate them into sauces and dressings, use them as a base for main dishes, or eat them straight in a big, vibrant salad—just do it. Your body will thank you with every bite of greens you take.

Other Vegetables

My Other Favorite Vegetables

Artichokes, asparagus, beetroot, bell peppers/capsicum, carrots, courgette, garlic, mushrooms (button, oyster, porcini, portobello, and shiitake), okra, onions, pumpkin, sea vegetables (arame, dulse, and nori), snap peas, squash (delicata, spaghetti, and summer squash varieties), purple sweet potatoes, sweetcorn and tomatoes

Serving Sizes:
1 cup (60 g) raw leafy vegetables
½ cup (90 g) raw or cooked non-leafy vegetables
½ cup (120 ml) vegetable juice
¼ cup (10 g) dried mushrooms

Daily Recommendation:
2 servings per day

The mammoth Global Burden of Disease Study identified the typical American diet as a primary cause of Americans' death and disability[2534] and inadequate vegetable intake as our fourth-leading dietary risk factor for death, nearly as bad as our consumption of processed meat.[2535] The Union of Concerned Scientists estimates that if the nation increased its consumption of fruits and veggies to meet the dietary guidelines, we might save the lives of more than one hundred thousand people a year.[2536]

We should eat more fruits and vegetables as if our life depended on it, because it very well may.

Garden Variety: Diversifying Our Vegetable Portfolio

Perhaps the least controversial advice in all of nutrition is to eat more fruits and vegetables, which is to say *eat more plants*, since the term *vegetable* basically just means all parts of the plant that aren't fruit. There are root vegetables like sweet potatoes, stem vegetables like rhubarb, pod vegetables like peas, and even flower vegetables like broccoli. (It isn't called cauli*flower* for nothing.) We've already talked about the leafy vegetables in the greens section. If dark green leafy vegetables are the healthiest foods around, then why branch out to other parts of the plant? (Pun intended!) Yes, we're supposed to eat the rainbow, but didn't we just learn that green leaves have an entire spectrum of colors hidden inside?

Unlike more generic compounds like vitamin C, which is broadly available in various fruits and vegetables, other nutrients are not so evenly distributed. Just as certain fruits like citrus offer unique nonpigment phytonutrients not found in other fruits, different vegetables contribute different compounds. White cauliflower, lacking antioxidant pigments, doesn't appear to have much to offer at first glance, but because it belongs to the cruciferous family, it's one of our healthiest options. Similarly, white mushrooms may look pretty drab, but they can provide *myco*nutrients not made anywhere in the plant kingdom.

We now know that certain phytonutrients bind to specific receptors and other proteins in the body. I talked about the Ah "broccoli receptors" in chapter 4. There are also effectively green-tea receptors in our body—that is, receptors for EGCG, a key component of green tea. There are binding proteins for the phytonutrients in grapes, onions, and capers. A cell surface receptor has even been identified for a nutrient concentrated in apple peels. These specific proteins may not be activated, though, unless we eat specific foods.[2537]

The different phytonutrient profiles may then result in different clinical effects. For example, drinking tomato juice can rescue the immune function of study participants crippled by two weeks of fruit and vegetable deficiency, but carrot juice apparently cannot.[2538] Even different parts of the same vegetable can have different effects. One of the reasons certain tomato products appear to be protective against heart attacks[2539] is because the yellow fluid surrounding the seeds concentrates a compound that suppresses platelet activation.[2540] (Platelets are what help trigger the blood clots that cause heart attacks and most strokes.) Aspirin has a similar effect, but it doesn't work in everyone and can increase bleeding risk—two limitations that the tomato compound may be able to overcome.[2541,2542] But if you only consume tomato sauce, juice, or ketchup, you may be missing out[2543] since the seeds are removed during processing. So when picking out canned tomato products, choose whole, crushed, or diced tomatoes instead of tomato sauce, purée, or paste.

Different plants may also affect the same part of the body in different ways. Consider mental function, for instance. In a study of dozens of fruits and vegetables, from strawberries to swede, certain plants appear to shore up specific cognitive domains. For example, the consumption of some plant foods was associated with better executive function, perceptual speed, and semantic (fact-based) memory, while the consumption of others was more consistently associated with visual-spatial skills and autobiographical memory.[2544] In other words, we should build up a portfolio of many fruits and vegetables to cover all our bases.

One of the reasons studies may underestimate the protective effects of plant foods is that they tend to measure *quantity* of fruit and vegetable consumption rather than *quality* of fruit and vegetable consumption. People are more likely to eat bananas and cucumbers than blueberries and kale. But variety is important too. Half the fruit servings in the United States are taken up by just five fruits—apples and apple juice, bananas, grapes, orange juice, and watermelon—and most vegetable servings are from canned tomatoes, potatoes, and iceberg lettuce.[2545]

In one of the few studies that looked specifically at the diversity of fruit and vegetable consumption, the variety of intake was an even better predictor of decreased inflammation in the bodies of middle-aged adults than the absolute quantity of consumption.[2546] Even after removing the effects of quantity, the addition of two different types of fruits and vegetables per week has been associated with an 8 percent reduction in the incidence of type 2 diabetes.[2547] These kinds of data led the American Heart Association to add a recommendation to its dietary guidelines to also eat a *variety* of fruits and vegetables.[2548] It's an important addition; otherwise, a big bag of crisps or one head of iceberg lettuce could technically fulfill or exceed the recommended nine servings a day.

It's better to eat a whole orange rather than take a vitamin C pill, since the pill deprives us of all the other wonderful nutrients in the oranges themselves. The same principle applies when we don't diversify our fruit and vegetable consumption. By only eating apples, we also miss out on oranges' nutrients. We don't get the limonoids in citrus, like limonin, limonol, or tangeretin, though we may get more malic acid (from the Latin *malum*, meaning apple). When it comes to the unique phytonutrient profile of each fruit and vegetable, it's like comparing apples to oranges! That's why we should mix it up.

In a sense, though, all fruits are just fruits, whereas vegetables can be any other part of the plant. Roots may harbor different nutrients than shoots. For this reason, it may be even more important to get a variety of vegetables, so we can benefit from all parts of the plant, as one large cancer study of nearly half a million people did indeed find.[2549] "Because each vegetable contains a unique combination," a review concluded, "a great diversity of vegetables should be eaten . . . to get all the health benefits."[2550] Variety is not only the spice of life; it may prolong it as well.

Eating Better to Look Better

We've all heard of the proverbial golden glow that's often equated with health, vitality, and youth. But instead of using a tanning bed to achieve a more golden hue, you can do it with a bed of greens.

There are certain animals who use diet to increase their sexual attractiveness. Great tits, distinctive olive-and-black songbirds ubiquitous throughout Europe and Asia, tend to prefer carotenoid-rich caterpillars, which make their breast plumage a brighter yellow, to become more attractive to potential mates.[2551] Can a similar phenomenon be found in humans?

Researchers took digital photographs of African, Asian, and Caucasian men and women and asked others to manipulate the skin tone of their faces with a dial until they reached what they perceived to be the healthiest-looking color.[2552] Sure enough, both men and women preferred the yellow "golden glow" that can be achieved through "dietary carotenoid deposition in the skin."[2553] In other words, by eating the yellow and red pigments in fruits and vegetables, like beta-carotene in sweet potatoes and lycopene in tomatoes, men and women may be able to naturally acquire more of a golden and rosy glow. Researchers decided to put it to the test.

Based on a six-week study of college students, the complexion achieved by eating my Daily Dozen recommendation of nine servings of fruits and vegetables a day was found to be significantly healthier and more attractive looking than that achieved by eating three daily servings.[2554] The healthier we eat, the healthier we look. Indeed, studies find that "individuals with the lowest fruit and vegetable intake may enjoy the most improvement in appearance."[2555]

What about wrinkles? A study out of Japan used the six-point Daniell scale to rate the extent of crow's-feet wrinkles around the eyes of more than seven hundred women, with a score of one being the least severe and a score of six being the most severe. The researchers found that "a higher intake of green and yellow vegetables was associated with decreased facial wrinkling." Women who ate less than one daily serving of green and yellow veggies averaged about a three on the Daniell scale, while women who ate more than two servings a day averaged closer to a two. The researchers celebrated "the potential for these studies to promote a healthy diet . . ."[2556] In *How Not to Age*, I detail some healthy foods that have even been shown in interventional trials to improve wrinkles.

I am certainly not above appealing to vanity, especially for younger people who have seemed more interested in which dietary changes will clear their acne than which will clear their future risk of chronic disease. So I'm happy to see articles embrace these types of studies with headlines like "Greens to Be Gorgeous."[2557] Still, although looking great on the outside is fine, looking great on the inside is even better.

Mushrooming Benefits

Ergothioneine is an unusual amino acid. Although it was discovered more than a century ago, it was ignored until recently, when researchers found that humans have a transporter protein in their bodies specifically designed to pull ergothioneine out of food and into body tissue. This suggests that this amino acid plays some important physiological role. But what? Our first clue was the tissue distribution. Ergothioneine concentrates in parts of our body where there is a lot of oxidative stress—our liver and the lenses of our eyes, for example, as well as such sensitive tissues as bone marrow and semen. Researchers guessed, then, that it might act as a so-called cytoprotectant, a cell protector, and that's indeed what was subsequently found.[2558]

Ergothioneine appears to function as a potent intramitochondrial antioxidant, meaning it can get inside the mitochondria—the microscopic power plants within our cells. The DNA inside the mitochondria is especially vulnerable to free-radical damage, since many other antioxidants are unable to penetrate the mitochondrial membrane. This is one reason ergothioneine may be so important. Depriving human cells of this amino acid increases risk of accelerated DNA damage and cell death. Unfortunately, the human body cannot make ergothioneine; we can only get it through food. "Because of its dietary origin and the toxicity associated with its depletion," Johns Hopkins University researchers concluded, "ET [ergothioneine] may represent a new vitamin . . ."[2559] If it were classified as such, that would make it the first new vitamin since vitamin B12 was isolated back in 1948.[2560]

What are the best dietary sources of ergothioneine? The highest levels by far have been reported in mushrooms. For example, oyster mushrooms, which you can grow yourself in only two weeks from a just-add-water kit, have more than one thousand units (μg/dag) of ergothioneine, about nine times more than their closest competitor, black beans. And a serving of black beans has about eight times more than a serving of the third-leading source, chicken liver. Chicken meat, along with beef and pork, only has about ten units, one hundred times less than oyster mushrooms. Kidney beans have about four times more than meat, but even at forty-five units, they pale in comparison to some of the mushrooms.[2561]

Ergothioneine is heat stable, which means it's not destroyed when mushrooms are cooked.[2562] This is good news because it's best not to eat many mushrooms raw; there's a toxin called *agaritine* in white, crimini, and portobello mushrooms to which we should minimize our exposure. Thankfully, the toxin is destroyed by cooking. Just thirty seconds in the microwave wipes out most agaritine in mushrooms. Freezing also gets rid of most of it, but drying does not. If you put dried mushrooms in your soup, it's best to boil them for at least five minutes.[2563] Morel mushrooms are a special case. The toxin levels appear higher and may react with alcohol even after cooking.[2564] Raw morel mushrooms, cooked morels served with alcohol, and all wild-foraged mushrooms should be considered red-light foods, in my opinion.

Do you have to eat mushrooms to be healthy? No. (Otherwise, it would be the Daily *Baker's* Dozen.) Famously in our family, my mom has never eaten a mushroom in her life and never will, because they "look funny." But given the potential immune and anticancer benefits documented in chapters 6 and 11, I would encourage you to try to find ways to incorporate them into your diet.

My favorite way to enjoy mushrooms is to grill portobellos. Ages ago, I picked up a George Foreman Grill from my local charity shop, and my family has officially renamed it the Portobello Mushroom Grill. I know people tend to marinate portobellos first, but I just drizzle them with balsamic vinegar, grill until the juice starts dripping, and then add cracked pepper. They're so good, we eat them just like that.

Which is healthier? Plain white mushrooms or portobellos? Trick question! They're the same mushroom. The little white button mushrooms grow up to be portobellos. White mushrooms are just baby 'bellos.

Mushrooms can be stuffed, enjoyed in soups like mushroom barley, featured as the star of a creamy risotto or pâté, served as the base of a great gravy or as a flavorful addition to any pasta sauce, or simply braised with crushed garlic in red wine.

Even More Vegetables!

My favorite way to eat raw veggies is to dip bell pepper/capsicum strips, carrots, or snap peas in a hummus or bean dip, and my favorite way to eat them cooked is by roasting them. Roasting can transform vegetables into otherworldly creations. If you don't believe me, try roasting red bell peppers/capsicum, brussels sprouts, beetroot, or squash. Never thought you liked okra because it's too slimy? Try it roasted.

One of my favorite springtime dishes is roasted asparagus dipped in guacamole. (Here's an interesting asparagus fact: Did you know there are four types of people in the world? Those whose pee turns stinky after eating asparagus, those whose doesn't, those who are apparently genetically incapable of smelling the asparagus pee odor, and, finally, those who can. So some people may not think they get stinky pee from asparagus, but they actually do and just can't smell it![2565])

Sweet potatoes are one of my favorite snacks. During harsh Boston winters while I was in medical school, I would take two freshly microwaved sweet potatoes and pop them in my coat pockets as natural hand warmers. When they cooled down, my hand warmers became instant healthy snacks! It's actually better to boil them, though, to best preserve their nutritional content.[2566] Regardless of your cooking method, be sure to keep on the skin. The peel of the sweet potato has nearly ten times the antioxidant power as the inner flesh (on a per-weight basis), giving it an antioxidant capacity approaching that of blueberries.[2567]

Sweet potatoes themselves can be considered a superfood.[2568] They are ranked as one of the healthiest foods on the planet[2569] and one day, perhaps, even off the planet—NASA has chosen them for future space missions.[2570] In fact, they're among the healthiest *and* cheapest, with one of the highest nutrient-rich food scores per dollar.[2571] When picking out varieties at the supermarket, remember that a sweet potato's nutritional content is tied directly to the intensity of its color. The more yellow or orange its flesh, the healthier it may be.[2572]

Sweet potatoes are healthier than plain potatoes, but if you're going to choose the latter, seek out those with blue or purple flesh. The consumption of one boiled purple potato a day for six weeks was found to significantly decrease inflammation, something neither white nor yellow potatoes were able to accomplish.[2573] The same was found for oxidation, but much faster. Within hours of consumption, purple potatoes increased the antioxidant capacity of study participants' bloodstream, whereas white potato starch appeared to actually have a pro-oxidant effect.[2574] Blue potatoes may have ten times more antioxidant power than regular white ones.[2575] The most exciting purple potato study to date had people with hypertension eat six to eight microwaved small purple potatoes a day, and they were able to significantly bring down their blood pressure levels within a month.[2576]

Purple *sweet* potatoes may offer the best of both worlds.[2577] I was so excited to discover them that I bought them as holiday gifts for everyone in my family one year—stocking stuffers they could stuff themselves with!

Getting Kids (and Parents) to Eat Their Veggies

Published strategies for getting kids (of all ages) to eat their vegetables include cutting them into slices, sticks, or stars—the most popular shape.[2578] Supposedly, putting an Elmo sticker on veggies swayed 50 percent of children to choose broccoli over a chocolate bar.[2579] If they're still not biting, though, apply the same trick I use to get our dog to take her pills: Dip the veggies in peanut butter. A study found that pairing vegetables with peanut butter successfully increases intake "even in vegetable-resistant children."[2580] Offering a salad dressing dip has also been found to help.[2581]

Simply having healthy foods out and available can boost intake. Guess what happened when researchers put out bowls of cut-up fresh fruits in addition to the regular party fare brought by parents for kindergarten or preschool celebrations? No special effort was made to encourage students to choose the fruits—the researchers just put it out on the table with all the other food. Would kids actually eat fruits when such foods as birthday cake, ice cream, and cheese puffs were available? Yes! On average, each kid ate a full fruit serving.[2582] Take that, cheese puffs!

Let's not forget the hide-the-veggies strategy. Studies have shown that broccoli, cauliflower, tomatoes, squash, and courgette can be added covertly to familiar entrées such that the appearance, flavor, and texture of the original recipes are maintained (like puréeing vegetables into a pasta sauce).[2583] Studies found the trick works for adults too. Researchers were able to slip in up to a 450 grams of clandestine vegetables a day (resulting in 350 fewer calories eaten overall).[2584] Surreptitiously incorporating vegetables into foods shouldn't be the only way that vegetables are served to children, though. Since the appetite for an initially unappetizing vegetable can be increased through repeated exposure, it is important to use several strategies to ensure that kids experience whole vegetables. After all, they're not always going to be eating at home. One of the most important predictors of children's fruit and vegetable consumption has been found to be parents' consumption,[2585] so if you want your kids to eat healthfully, it helps to be a healthy role model.

The Top Cancer-Fighting Vegetables

According to a landmark American Institute for Cancer Research report, any effect of plant-based diets is "likely to be due not only to the exclusion of meat, but also to the inclusion of a larger number and of wider range of plant foods, containing an extensive variety of potential cancer-preventive substances."[2586] In other words, it may not be enough to cut down on meat; we need to eat as many whole, healthy plant foods as possible. Meatless Mondays are great, but even more so when followed by Tomato Tuesdays, Watercress Wednesdays, and so on.

Different vegetables may target different cancers—sometimes even in the same organ. For example, cabbage, cauliflower, broccoli, and brussels sprouts are associated with lower risk of colon cancer in the middle and right side of our body, whereas risk of colon cancer farther down on the left side appears to be lowered more by carrots, pumpkins, and apples.[2587]

An extraordinary study published in the journal *Food Chemistry* pitted thirty-four common vegetables in vitro against eight different types of human cancer cells: breast cancer, brain tumors, kidney cancer, lung cancer, childhood brain tumors, pancreatic cancer, prostate cancer, and stomach cancer. Take breast cancer, for example. Seven vegetables (aubergine, pak choi, carrot, tomato, endive, fennel bulb, and romaine lettuce) appeared useless, suppressing breast cancer cell growth no more than the control. Six vegetables (orange bell pepper/capsicum, cucumber, radicchio, jalapeño, potato, and beetroot) nearly halved cancer growth, but five veggies (cauliflower, brussels sprouts, green onion, leek, and garlic) "abolished" cancer growth completely, stopping breast tumor cells dead in their tracks.[2588]

There were two take-home messages to come out of this remarkable study. The first is that we should eat a portfolio of vegetables. Radishes, for example, are completely unable to stop pancreatic cancer cell growth. However, radishes were 100 percent effective at halting the growth of stomach cancer cells. Orange bell peppers/capsicum were useless against stomach cancer, but they were able to suppress prostate cancer cell growth by more than 75 percent. In the words of the researchers, "a diversified diet, containing several distinct classes of vegetables (and hence of phytochemicals) is essential for effective prevention of cancer."[2589]

How to Make a Cancer-Fighting Salad

Imagine you're standing in a queue at one of those made-to-order salad places where you get to choose your lettuce, your toppings, and your dressing. You start with the greens. For the sake of this example, let's say you are offered a choice between the five covered in the *Food Chemistry* study: Butterhead lettuce, endive, radicchio, romaine lettuce, and spinach. Which should you choose? Based on the study findings: spinach. Out of the five options, spinach beat out the others against breast cancer, brain tumors, kidney cancer, lung cancer, pediatric brain tumors, pancreatic cancer, prostate cancer, and stomach cancer. The runner up? Radicchio.[2590]

Which toppings should you add to your spinach salad? You only get five to choose from and, after consulting the Daily Dozen app on your smartphone, you can tick three check boxes immediately: beans, berries, and nuts. Now you only have two toppings left. Out of the thirty-two remaining vegetables included in the study, which two of the following should you pick? Choose carefully:

Acorn squash	Celery	Leek
Asparagus	Cucumber	Orange bell pepper/
Aubergine	Curly cabbage	capsicum
Beetroot	Endive	Pak choi
Broccoli	Fennel bulb	Potato
Brown onion	Fiddleheads	Radicchio
Brussels sprouts	Garlic	Radish
Butterhead lettuce	Green beans	Red cabbage
Cabbage	Green onions	Romaine lettuce
Carrot	Jalapeño	Swede
Cauliflower	Kale	Tomato

Which two did you choose? If one of your choices was brussels sprouts, cabbage, curly cabbage, or kale, *and* the other choice was garlic, green onions, or leek, you get a gold star! Of all the vegetables tested, those had the most cancer-preventing potential. Notice anything they have in common? All the top choices belong to one of only two superfood families: cruciferous vegetables and the allium veggie family, which includes garlic and onions. As the researchers put it, "the inclusion of cruciferous and Allium vegetables in the diet is essential for effective dietary-based chemopreventive [cancer-preventing] strategies."[2591]

Note that the most common vegetables didn't make the cut. "The majority of the vegetable extracts tested in this study, including vegetables that are commonly consumed in Western countries such as potato, carrot, lettuce and tomato," the researchers concluded, "had little effect on the proliferation of the tumour cell lines."[2592]

The single most effective vegetable was garlic, which came in first against breast cancer, both child and adult brain cancer, lung cancer, pancreatic cancer, prostate cancer, and stomach cancer, and second after leeks against kidney cancer. So might I suggest a garlicky salad dressing like the one on page 375?

Garlic and Onions

As the above salad example illustrates, garlic, onions, leeks, and other vegetables in the allium family appear to have special properties. But, like chemotherapy, maybe garlic isn't just toxic to cancer cells but toxic to *all* cells? That wouldn't be good. Researchers also wondered about this, so they decided to compare the effects of garlic and other vegetables on the growth of both cancer cells and normal cells. The same garlic dose that blocked nearly 80 percent of cancer cell proliferation appeared to have no effect whatsoever against normal cells, and similar results were found for the other allium and cruciferous vegetables. In other words, vegetables are selective; they destroy cancer cells but leave normal cells alone.

These results were seen in a petri dish, though, and while such studies may have direct relevance for digestive-tract cancers that come in close contact with these foods, for these foods to be protective against other cancers, the anticancer compounds would have to be absorbed into the bloodstream. And in the case of brain tumors, the anticancer compounds would additionally have to cross the blood-brain barrier. The findings do seem to sync with other studies, though, both among human populations and in other laboratories, that corroborate the potential cancer-fighting benefits of cruciferous vegetables,[2593] garlic, and onions.[2594] Regardless, this study illustrates the dramatic differences between the biological capacities of individual vegetables and families of veggies and underscores the importance of including a variety of vegetables in our diet.

Which Is the Best Cooking Method?

Is it better to eat our vegetables raw or cooked? If you're thinking raw, you're right. But if you guessed cooked, you're also right.[2595] Confused? Well, a number of nutrients, like vitamin C, are partially destroyed by cooking. For example, steamed broccoli may have about 10 percent less vitamin C than raw broccoli.[2596] If, however, you prefer cooked broccoli enough to eat seven florets of steamed rather than six florets of raw, then you just more than made up the difference.

Other nutrients, however, actually become *more* absorbable after cooking. For example, we end up with more than six times the vitamin A in our bloodstream from cooked carrots compared to raw ones.[2597] A study of long-term raw foodists found surprisingly low blood levels of the red antioxidant pigment lycopene.[2598] It's not what we eat but what we absorb, and cooked tomatoes appear able to better boost our lycopene levels.[2599] Steaming may also improve the bile acid-binding capacity of vegetables,[2600] which may help lower breast cancer risk.[2601]

Raw-food diets automatically eliminate most red- and yellow-light foods, which is not only an improvement over the standard American diet but also over many plant-based diets. There is no evidence to suggest, however, that eating raw foods largely or exclusively is healthier than eating a combination of cooked and raw whole plant foods.

Some cooking methods, though, are preferable to others. Deep-fried foods, whether of plant origin (like french fries) or from animals (like fried chicken), have been associated with higher cancer risk.[2602] Deep-frying leads to the production of dangerous heterocyclic amines in meat (as detailed in chapter 12) and to acrylamide in deep-fried plant foods. The excess lifetime cancer risk attributable to the consumption of french fries in young children, for example, may be as high as one or two in ten thousand—meaning about one in ten thousand boys and girls eating french fries may develop cancer that would have otherwise not occurred had they *not* eaten french fries. The researchers urge deep-fryer cooking times and temperatures be set as low as possible "while still maintaining a tasty quality."[2603] (They wouldn't want to reduce cancer so much that the deep-fried foods wouldn't be as tasty!) Blanching potatoes first can reduce acrylamide formation, but potato chip companies argue that this might have a negative impact on the "nutritional properties of the fried product," because it would leach away some of the vitamin C.[2604] But if we're relying on crisps to get our vitamin C, acrylamide is probably the least of our worries.

What is the best way to cook vegetables to preserve nutrition? I am often asked that question, and it's difficult to answer, as it varies for different vegetables. What we would need is a study that measures a variety of different cooking methods with a variety of different vegetables. Thankfully, we got exactly that in 2009. A Spanish research team pulled out all the stops, performing more than three hundred separate experiments with twenty vegetables and six cooking methods, all while considering three different measures of antioxidant activity. They tested baking, boiling, frying, griddling (cooking in a thick frying pan with no oil), microwaving, and pressure-cooking.[2605]

Let's start with the worst methods in terms of antioxidant loss: boiling and pressure-cooking. When we use these wet-cooking methods, some of the nutrition is lost into the cooking water, but less than I would have thought. For instance, the researchers found that boiling removes an average of 14 percent of the vegetables' antioxidant capacity. So, if you like your corn on the cob boiled, you could just add an extra quarter ear to the pot. (Six quarters boiled may have all the antioxidant power of five quarters raw, baked, or microwaved.[2606]) Of the six cooking methods studied, griddling and microwaving were the gentlest. Nuking your veggies appears to preserve, on average, more than 95 percent of antioxidant capacity.[2607]

Those are averages across twenty vegetables, however. Some vegetables are more resistant, and antioxidant power actually *increases* with cooking in some veggies. Which do you think was the most vulnerable vegetable—that is, the one probably best eaten raw? If you guessed bell peppers/capsicum, you're right. They've been shown to lose up to 70 percent of their antioxidant capacity when baked in an oven. I'm going to continue to roast my peppers because of how much I love the taste, but I realize I'm getting less nutritional bang for my buck. (Not a big deal, though, because I can just add an extra sprinkle of oregano to my roasted red pepper/capsicum pasta sauce.)

On the other hand, three vegetables hardly seem to be affected at all by cooking: artichokes, beetroot, and onions. You can even boil them, and they'll still retain 97.5 percent of their antioxidant power.

Finally, there are two vegetables that may actually become *healthier* through cooking: the humble carrot and the celery stalk. No matter how you prepare them—even by boiling—carrots and celery appear to gain in antioxidant power. Green beans get an honorable mention, because they increase in antioxidant power when cooked by all methods except boiling or pressure-cooking. Microwaved green beans, for example, have more antioxidants than raw. So go ahead and make a nice vegetable soup and boost the ingredients' antioxidant content at the same time.

DIY Fruit and Vegetable Wash

Buying organic foods reduces our exposure to pesticides, but it doesn't eliminate them entirely. Pesticide residues have been detected in 11 percent of organic crop samples due to accidental or fraudulent use, cross-contamination from neighboring nonorganic fields, or the lingering presence of persistent pollutants like DDT in the soil.[2608]

> There are many commercial fruit and vegetable wash products that purport to improve the removal of pesticides, but a variety have been tested and appear to be a complete waste of money.[2609] For example, Procter & Gamble had a product that claimed it was "proven to be 98% more effective than water in removing pesticides." When it was put to the test, though, it did no better than plain tap water.[2610] Rinsing produce under running water generally removes less than half of the pesticide residue.[2611] A fingernail-polish-remover acetone bath has been found to be more effective at removing pesticides,[2612] but of course I'm not advocating dunking your fruits and veggies in that! The goal is to make your tomato *less* toxic.
>
> One effective method is to use a 5 percent acetic-acid bath—in other words, plain white vinegar, which has been found to remove the bulk of certain pesticide residues.[2613] But 5 percent is full strength, and it would get expensive buying gallons of white vinegar just to wash your fruits and veggies. Unfortunately, a diluted white-vinegar bath only seems marginally more effective than tap water.[2614]
>
> Thankfully, there is a solution that is both cheap and effective: salt water. A 10 percent saltwater rinse has been found to work as well as full-strength vinegar.[2615] To make your own pesticide-reducing bath, add one part salt to nine parts water. Just make sure to rinse off all the salt before eating.

Is Buying Organic Worth It?

Stroll down the produce aisle of your supermarket. You'll see lots of foods labeled "organic," but what does that really mean?

According to the USDA, organic farming practices preserve the environment and avoid most synthetic materials, including pesticides and antibiotics. Among other requirements, organic farmers must receive annual on-site inspections, use only USDA-approved materials, and not use genetically modified crops. In order to be counted in the $64 billion U.S. organic retail market, products receive a USDA organic stamp.[2616,2617]

The fact is that being organic doesn't mean a food is healthy. The organic food industry didn't become so lucrative by selling carrots. For instance, you can now buy pesticide-free crisps and organic jelly beans.[2618] There are even organic Oreo cookies. Junk food is still junk food, even if it was produced organically. The organic label cannot turn red lights green.

Many are surprised to learn (I know I was!) that a review of hundreds of studies found that organic produce does not seem to have significantly more vitamins and minerals. Organic fruits and vegetables do, however, appear to have more nontraditional nutrients like polyphenol antioxidants,[2619] thought to be because conventionally grown plants given high-dose synthetic nitrogen fertilizers may divert more resources to growth rather than defense.[2620] This may be why, as we learned in chapter 6, organic berries appear to suppress cancer growth better than conventional berries in vitro.

Based on its elevated antioxidant levels, organic produce may be considered 20 to 40 percent healthier, the equivalent of adding one or two servings' worth to a five-a-day regimen. But organic produce may be 40 percent more expensive, so for the same money, we could just buy the extra servings' worth of conventional produce. From a purely nutrients-per-dollar standpoint, it's not clear that organic foods are any better.[2621] But people don't just buy organic foods because they're healthier—what about safety?

Conventional produce appears to have twice the levels of cadmium, one of the three toxic heavy metals in the food supply, along with mercury and lead.[2622] The cadmium is thought to come from the phosphate fertilizers that are added to conventional crops.[2623] The greatest concern most people have about conventionally grown produce, though, is the pesticide residues.

People not only tend to overestimate the nutritional benefit of organic food, they also overestimate the risks of pesticides.[2624] For example, surveys have found that many consumers erroneously believe that just as many people die from pesticide residues on conventional food as they do from automobile accidents,[2625] or that eating nonorganic produce is almost as bad as smoking a daily pack of cigarettes.[2626] This kind of thinking is dangerous, as it could lead to a decrease in overall fruit and vegetable consumption.

If just half the U.S. population were to increase their intake of fruits and vegetables by a single serving per day, an estimated twenty thousand cancer cases might be avoided each year. That's how powerful produce is. However, this estimate was calculated using conventional produce, so the additional pesticide burden might be expected to cause ten new cancer cases. On balance, the study suggested, if half of Americans ate just one more serving of produce per day, we'd prevent 19,990 people from becoming cancer patients *every year*!

Unfortunately, this paper was written by scientists-for-hire paid by conventional produce growers, so they had an incentive to exaggerate the benefits and downplay the risks.[2627] Nevertheless, I think the bottom line is sound. We receive tremendous benefit from eating conventional fruits and vegetables that far outweighs whatever little bump in risk we may get from the pesticides.[2628] But why accept any risk at all when we can choose organic? My own family buys organic whenever we can, but we never let concern about pesticides stop us from enjoying as many fruits and vegetables as possible.

At least half our plate should be filled with vegetables. Here's a simple rule: Include vegetables in everything, and the more the better. Bean burritos are better than carnitas, but better still is a bean burrito with lots of veggies wrapped inside. Instead of spaghetti with marinara sauce, make it spaghetti with marinara sauce . . . and loads of veggies. Marinara is certainly better than Alfredo, but it's even better still to go the extra veggie mile and heap on your favorite vegetables.

Flaxseeds

My Favorite Flaxseeds

Golden or brown

Serving Size:
1 tablespoon ground

Daily Recommendation:
1 serving per day

I have talked about the wonders of flaxseeds in a few of this book's earlier chapters, including those on high blood pressure (chapter 5), breast cancer (chapter 12), and prostate cancer (chapter 14). Remember how flaxseeds apparently offer "miraculous defense against some critical maladies"?

Okay, you're convinced. But just where do you get flaxseeds, and how do you best use them?

You can buy flaxseeds in bulk at natural foods stores for just a few dollars per half kilo. They come in nature's finest packaging: a hard natural hull that keeps them fresh. However, Mother Nature packs them a little too well. If you eat flaxseeds whole, they're likely to pass right through you without releasing any of their nutrients. So, for best results, first grind up the seeds with a blender or coffee or spice grinder, or buy them pre-ground or "milled." (The other option is to chew them really well.) Thanks to their antioxidant content, ground flaxseeds should last at least four months at room temperature in an airtight container.[26][29]

Ground flax is a light, nutty powder that can be sprinkled on oatmeal, salads, soups—frankly, just about anything you're eating. You can even bake with flax without damaging the lignans[2630] or omega-3 fatty acids[2631] (unlike flaxseed *oil*). During medical school, I used to make a few dozen flaxseed muffins at a time and put them in the freezer. Then I'd pop one in the microwave every morning before I ran out the door and get my daily flax fix while eating breakfast on the subway.

Are Fruit-and-Nut Bars Fattening?

There are a number of energy bars on the market containing only green-light ingredients, such as dried fruits, seeds, and nuts. They're so easy to throw into a briefcase, backpack, or bag and eat as a convenient snack on the go, but should we?

Dried fruits, seeds, and nuts are all nutrient-dense foods, but they're also calorie dense. Might concentrating so many calories into such a small energy bar contribute to weight gain? To find out, Yale University researchers split about one hundred overweight men and women into two groups. All the participants ate their normal diet, but half were told to add two fruit-and-nut bars daily. After two months, despite the extra 340 calories a day from the bars, the fruit-and-nut bar group did not gain any weight.[2632]

Dried fruits and nuts appear to be so satiating that people feel full and unintentionally offset the calories elsewhere throughout the day. Studies on apple rings,[2633] figs,[2634] prunes,[2635] and raisins[2636] have found similar results. In the apple study, postmenopausal women who added two apples' worth of apple rings to their daily diet for six months not only didn't gain weight but experienced an impressive 24 percent drop in their LDL ("bad") cholesterol.[2637] (That's nearly the effect we can get with some statin drugs!) In general, the 7 percent of Americans who average a tablespoon or more of dried fruit per day tend to be less overweight and less obese, and they have slimmer waistlines and less abdominal obesity than Americans who don't eat as much dried fruit.[2638]

Of course, when shopping for energy bars, it's imperative that you read their labels, as many brands have added sugars. Or you can just save yourself some money and choose good old-fashioned trail mix. Better yet, how about eating a piece of fresh fruit? Still, if the choice is between an energy bar and a candy bar as an afternoon snack, the choice is clear.

Other Ways to Eat Flaxseeds

When you're not sprinkling ground flax on your cereal, salads, or soups or baking it into your muffins, there are plenty of other ways to get your daily serving of flaxseeds. There are a lot of convenient flax bars, crackers, and snacks on the market these days, a few of which even have all green-light ingredients.

Honestly, it's pretty easy to make your own flax crackers. Mix 270 grams of ground flaxseeds with 250 ml of water, add whatever herbs and spices you want, and then spread the dough thinly on a parchment- or silicone-lined baking sheet. Score the dough into thirty-two crackers and bake at 400°F (204°C) for about twenty minutes. To flavor mine, I use a half teaspoon each of smoked paprika, garlic powder, and onion powder, but you should play around until you find a (salt-free) spice profile you prefer. When cut into thirty-two pieces, each cracker meets your Daily Dozen serving requirement.

I also use my trusty discount dehydrator to make raw flax crackers. All I do is mix 150 grams of whole flaxseeds with 250 ml of water along with flavorful ingredients like sun-dried tomatoes and basil. After it firms for about an hour and gets a jam-like consistency, I spread it out thinly and dehydrate away. Dip flax crackers in hummus or another bean dip for double Daily Dozen check marks. Since whole flaxseeds are used, though, make sure to chew thoroughly for maximum benefit.

Flaxseeds have a wonderful binding quality that makes them a great ingredient for thick milkshake-like smoothies. Toss a tablespoon of ground flax into a blender with some frozen berries, unsweetened soya milk, and half a ripe banana or mango or a few dates for sweetness, and you have a delicious drink containing both classes of protective phytoestrogens—lignans in flax and isoflavones in soya. (See chapter 12.) Blend in some cocoa powder for a chocolate milkshake that could help improve your chances of both preventing and surviving breast and prostate cancers.

This same binding quality makes flaxseeds a green-light thickener to replace cornstarch. I use flax to make my favorite quickie stir-fry sauce. I start with some pak choi and fresh mushrooms. The water clinging to the pak choi after it's rinsed, along with the liquid that gets released from the mushrooms while cooking, is enough to flash-steam the veggies in a hot pan without any added oil. Once the pak choi is tender-crisp, I add 250 ml of water mixed with a tablespoon each of tahini, ground flaxseeds, and Asian black-bean garlic sauce, a fermented yellow-light condiment you can find in a jar at most large supermarkets. Once the sauce thickens, it's ready for some fresh ground pepper (and hot sauce, if you've got that spicy tooth like I do) and . . . voilà!

One of my favorite ways to use ground flaxseeds is as a replacement for eggs in baking. For each egg in the recipe, whisk one tablespoon of ground flaxseeds with three tablespoons of water until the mixture becomes gooey. Unlike chicken eggs, "flax eggs" are not only cholesterol-free, but they're also packed with soluble fiber to bring down our cholesterol[2639] instead of pushing it up.

It never ceases to amaze me how these tiny little seeds can pack such a health-promoting punch. With just a single tablespoon a day and so many delicious, easy ways to incorporate ground flax into your sips and bites, there's no reason you shouldn't be able to tick this Daily Dozen check box every day.

Nuts and Seeds

> ### My Favorite Nuts and Seeds
>
> Almonds, Brazil nuts, cashews, chia seeds, hazelnuts/filberts, hemp seeds, macadamia nuts, pecans, pistachios, pumpkin seeds, sesame seeds, sunflower seeds, and walnuts
>
> **Serving Sizes:**
> ¼ cup (30 g) nuts or seeds
> 2 tablespoons nut or seed butter
>
> **Daily Recommendation:**
> 1 serving per day

Sometimes it feels like there just aren't enough hours in a day to get everything done. So instead of trying to make your day longer, why not make your life longer by an extra two years? That's about how long your lifespan may be increased by eating nuts regularly—one handful (or about 30 grams) five or more days a week.[2640] Just that one simple and delicious act alone may extend your life.

The Uses of Blended Nuts

Nuts make for quick and delicious snacks on their own, but my personal favorite use for them is as green-light sources of fat to make rich, creamy sauces. Whether in a cashew Alfredo, a ginger-peanut sauce, or a tahini-based green goddess dressing, nuts and seeds can maximize nutrient acquisition by both improving absorption and increasing our total intake of vegetables by adding some creamy cachet.

An often-overlooked use for nuts is as a key ingredient in soups, such as African-inspired peanut stew. When blended and heated, cashews thicken to make an amazingly creamy soup base. Nut and seed butters also pair well with veggies and fruits. Most everyone loves the classic childhood pairings of peanut butter with celery or apples. One of my favorite treats is dipping fresh strawberries into a decadent chocolate sauce. All you need is 125 ml of an unsweetened plant-based milk, one tablespoon of chia seeds, one tablespoon of cocoa, one teaspoon of almond butter, and date powder to taste. Mix all the ingredients and heat until the almond butter melts. Pour into a bowl, whisk until smooth, and put it in the fridge to cool. The chia and fiber from the cocoa powder help it thicken into an indulgent delight. (You can grind up the chia seeds first, but I like the tapioca-like texture the little chia balls form.)

Walnuts for the Win

Which nut is healthiest? Normally, my answer is whichever you're most willing and able to eat regularly, but walnuts really do seem to take the lead. Not only do they have some of the highest antioxidant[2641] and omega-3[2642] levels, but walnuts are the only nuts known to significantly improve artery function,[2643] and they beat out others in suppressing cancer cell growth in vitro.[2644] But how do walnuts do outside the laboratory in real life?

PREDIMED is one of the largest interventional dietary trials ever performed. Interventional studies, if you remember, include those in which participants are randomized to different diets to see who fares better. This helps researchers avoid the problem of confounding variables when trying to determine cause and effect in cohort studies. For example, in major study[2645] after study,[2646] after study,[2647] researchers found that people who eat nuts tend to live longer and suffer fewer deaths from cancer, heart disease, and respiratory disease. There was a lingering question, though: Did these findings show causation or merely correlation? It could be possible, after all, that nut eaters also tend to have other healthy lifestyle behaviors. Maybe those who eat nuts are more likely to be, well, health nuts. On the other hand, if scientists randomly assign thousands of people to various levels of nut consumption and the nuttier group ends up the healthiest, we could have more confidence that nuts aren't just *associated* with better health but actually *cause* better health. This is what PREDIMED ended up doing.[2648]

More than seven thousand men and women at high cardiovascular risk were randomized into different diet groups and followed for years. One of the groups received 210 grams of nuts every week for free. In addition to eating more nuts, they were told to improve their diets in other ways, such as eating more fruits and vegetables and less meat and dairy, but they weren't as successful at any of those other goals compared to the control group. Nevertheless, having free nuts sent to them every week for four consecutive years did indeed persuade them to start eating more nuts.[2649] (It's too bad the researchers couldn't have slipped in a little free broccoli too!)

At baseline, before the study even started, the thousands assigned to the nut group were already eating about 15 grams of nuts a day. Thanks to the ensuing freebies, they ended up bumping up their consumption to 30 grams (about a handful). As a result, the study was able to determine what happens when people at high risk for heart disease following a particular diet eat an extra 15 grams of nuts every day.

With no significant differences in meat and dairy intake, there were no significant differences in saturated fat or cholesterol intake. So, unsurprisingly, there were no significant differences in their blood cholesterol levels or the subsequent number of heart attacks. However, the added-nuts group did end up having significantly fewer strokes. In a sense, all the dietary groups were eating stroke-promoting diets. People in all the groups had strokes after eating each of the diets for years—so, ideally, they'd instead choose diets that can stop or reverse the disease process rather than encourage it. But for those not willing to make major shifts in their diet, just the minor tweak of adding nuts appeared to cut stroke risk in half.[2650] Those in the extra-nut-eating group still had strokes, but only about half as many. If this worked as well in the general population, hundreds of thousand strokes a year would be prevented in the United States alone.[2651] That could be dozens of strokes an hour, around the clock, prevented simply by adding about four walnuts, almonds, and hazelnuts to the nation's daily diet.

Regardless of which group participants were assigned to, those eating more nuts each day had a significantly lower risk of dying prematurely overall.[2652] Those who consumed more red- and yellow-light sources of fat—olive oil or extra virgin olive oil—failed to have any survival benefit.[2653]

This is consistent with the way Ancel Keys, the so-called father of the Mediterranean diet, viewed olive oil. He thought of its benefit more as a means of replacing animal fats—that is, anything to get people to eat less lard and butter.[2654]

Of all the nuts studied in PREDIMED, the researchers found the greatest benefits associated with walnuts, particularly for preventing cancer deaths.[2655] People who ate more than three servings of walnuts per week appeared to cut their risk of dying from cancer in half. A review of the scientific literature concluded that "the far-reaching positive effects of a plant-based diet that includes walnuts may be the most critical message for the public."[2656]

Nuts and Obesity: Weighing the Evidence

Nuts and nut butters are packed with nutrition—and calories. For example, just two tablespoons of a nut or seed butter might contain nearly two hundred calories. Nevertheless, it's probably better to eat two hundred calories of nut butter than two hundred calories of what most Americans would eat otherwise. Given how concentrated nut calories are—we'd have to eat nearly an entire head of cabbage to get the same amount—if we add a serving of nuts to our daily diet, won't we gain weight?

There have been about twenty clinical trials on nuts and weight, and not a single one showed the weight gain you might expect. All the studies showed less weight gain than predicted, no weight gain at all, or weight *loss*—even after study participants added a handful or two of nuts to their daily diets.[2657] However, these studies lasted just a few weeks or months. Perhaps prolonged nut consumption leads to weight gain? That question has been examined six different ways in studies lasting up to eight years. One found no significant change, and the other five measures found significantly *less* weight gain and reduced risk of abdominal obesity in those who ate more nuts.[2658]

The first law of thermodynamics states that energy can neither be created nor destroyed. If calories, which are units of energy, can't just disappear, then where are they all going? In one trial, for instance, participants who ate up to 120 pistachios as an afternoon snack every day for three months didn't appear to gain a pound.[2659] How could thirty thousand calories vanish into thin air?

One theory offered was dubbed the Pistachio Principle: Maybe nuts just take a lot of work to eat. Pistachios are typically bought in their shells, which slows consumption time, allowing our brain to better regulate our appetite.[2660] Sounds plausible, but what about shelled nuts like almonds and cashews? A study out of Japan did suggest that increasing "dietary hardness" (meaning chewing difficulty) is associated with a slimmer waist.[2661] Perhaps all that chewing simply tires us out?

Then there's the fecal-excretion theory. Many of the cell walls of chewed almonds, for example, remain intact in the gastrointestinal tract. In other words, it's possible a lot of the calories in nuts just never get digested and wind up in our waste because we didn't chew well enough. Both of these theories were put to the test by an international group of researchers who gave participants either half a cup of peanuts or half a cup of peanuts ground into peanut butter. If either the dietary hardness or the fecal-extraction theory were correct, the peanut-butter group would gain weight, since no calories would be left in undigested nuts, and no calories would be burned chewing. But after four weeks, neither group gained weight, so there must be another answer.[2662]

What about the dietary-compensation theory? The idea here is that nuts are so satiating and good at suppressing appetite that we end up eating less food overall. This could explain why some studies found that people lost weight after eating nuts. To test this idea, Harvard Medical School researchers gave two groups smoothies with the same number of calories, but one contained walnuts, and the other didn't. Despite drinking the same amount of calories, the placebo (nut-free) smoothie group reported feeling significantly less full than the walnut group.[2663] So, yes—it does seem that nuts can make us feel fuller faster than some other foods.

At this point, it looks as if 70 percent of nut calories are lost through dietary compensation and 10 percent are flushed as fat in our feces.[2664] But what about the last 20 percent? Unless all the calories are accounted for, we would still expect some weight gain. The answer appears to lie in the ability of nuts to boost metabolism. When we eat nuts, we burn more of our own fat. Researchers have found that while control-diet subjects were burning about twenty grams of fat within an eight-hour period, a group eating the same number of calories and fat, but with walnuts included in their diet, burned off more—about thirty-one grams of fat.[2665] If a pill could do that, drug companies would be raking it in!

The bottom line? Yes, nuts are high in calories, but through a combination of dietary compensation mechanisms, our body's failure to absorb some of the fat, and increased fat-burning metabolism, nuts can be a lifeline without expanding our waistline.

Pistachio Nuts for Sexual Dysfunction

Erectile dysfunction (ED) is the recurrent or persistent inability to attain or maintain an erection for satisfactory sexual performance. It is present in about thirty million men in the United States[2666] and approximately one hundred million men worldwide.[2667] Wait a second. The United States has less than 5 percent of the world's population yet up to 30 percent of the impotence?

The reason may be due to the standard American artery-clogging diet. Erectile dysfunction and our number one killer, coronary artery disease, may actually be two manifestations of the same disease—inflamed, clogged, and crippled arteries—regardless of which organs are affected.[2668] Not to worry, though, because Americans have red, white, and blue pills like Viagra . . . right? The problem is that these pills just cover up the symptoms of vascular disease and don't do anything for the underlying pathology.

Atherosclerosis is considered a systemic disorder that uniformly affects all major blood vessels in the body. Hardening of the arteries can lead to softening of the penis, since stiffened arteries can't relax open and let the blood flow. Thus, erectile dysfunction may just be the flaccid tip of the iceberg in terms of a systemic disorder.[2669] For two-thirds of men showing up at emergency rooms with crushing chest pain, their penises had been trying to warn them for years that something was wrong with their circulation.[2670]

Why does atherosclerosis tend to hit the penis first? The arteries in the penis are half the size of the "widow-maker" coronary artery in the heart. Therefore, the amount of plaque we wouldn't even feel in the heart could clog half the penile artery, causing symptomatic restriction in blood flow.[2671] This is why erectile dysfunction has been called "penile angina."[2672] In fact, by measuring blood flow in a man's penis with ultrasound, doctors can predict the results of his cardiac stress test with an accuracy of 80 percent.[2673] Male sexual function is like a penile stress test, a "window into the hearts of men."[2674]

In medical school, we were taught the forty-over-forty rule: 40 percent of men over age forty have erectile dysfunction. Men with erection difficulties in their forties have a fiftyfold increased risk of having a cardiac event (like sudden death).[2675]

We used to think of erectile dysfunction in younger men (those under age forty) as "psychogenic"—meaning it's all in their heads. But now we're realizing that ED is more likely an early sign of vascular disease. Some experts believe that a man with erectile dysfunction—even if he doesn't have cardiac symptoms—"should be considered a cardiac . . . patient until proved otherwise."[2676]

The reason even young men should care about their cholesterol levels is because they predict erectile dysfunction later in life,[2677] which in turn predicts heart attacks, strokes, and a shortened lifespan.[2678] As one medical journal put it, the take-home message is that "ED = Early Death."[2679]

What does this have to do with nuts? A clinical study found that men who ate three to four handfuls of pistachios a day for three weeks experienced a significant improvement in blood flow through the penis, accompanied by significantly firmer erections. The researchers concluded that three weeks of pistachios "resulted in a significant improvement in erectile function . . . without any side effects."[2680]

This is not just a male issue. Women with higher cholesterol levels report significantly lower arousal, orgasm, lubrication, and sexual satisfaction. Atherosclerosis of the pelvic arteries can lead to decreased vaginal engorgement and "clitoral erectile insufficiency syndrome," defined as "failure to achieve clitoral tumescence [engorgement]." This is thought to be an important factor in female sexual dysfunction.[2681] We learned from the Harvard Nurses' Health Study that eating just two handfuls of nuts weekly may extend a woman's life as much as jogging four hours a week.[2682] So eating more healthfully may not only extend our love life but also our entire life.

Why are beans, nuts, and whole grains so health promoting? Maybe it's because they are all seeds. Think about it: All it takes for an acorn to start to explode into an oak tree is water, air, and sunlight. Everything else is contained within the seed, which possesses the entire complex of protective nutrients required to mature its way into a plant or tree. Whether you're eating a black bean, a walnut, a grain of brown rice, or a sesame seed, in essence you're getting the makings of a whole plant in a tiny little package. As two noted nutrition experts concluded, "[D]ietary recommendations should embrace a wide array of seeds as part of a plant-based dietary pattern . . ."[2683]

Should People with Diverticulosis Avoid Nuts?

Diverticulosis involves abnormal outpouchings from the wall of our colon, affecting most people by the time they reach their sixties—whether they know it or not.[2684] In as many as 10 to 25 percent of individuals, these outpouchings can become inflamed and turn the diverticulosis into *diverticulitis*,[2685] resulting in hundreds of thousands of ER visits and hospitalizations. It can sometimes even lead to perforation of the colon, which may have a fatality rate as high as one in five.[2686] But it wasn't always like this.

Diverticulosis only became a problem in the twentieth century.[2687] What is now a massive epidemic didn't even start showing up in medical textbooks until 1920.[2688] Diverticulosis appeared to be a deficiency disease of Western civilization.[2689] Just like scurvy is a deficiency disease caused by a lack of vitamin C,[2690] diverticulosis may be a deficiency disease caused by a lack of fiber.[2691]

Bowel movements should be effortless, but when we don't get enough fiber-containing foods in our diet, like whole grains and beans, we have to strain to push along unnaturally firm stools. The pressure necessary to force along small hard stools may essentially blow pouches out of the wall, like when you squeeze a gel stress ball.[2692]

As we got better and better at refining grains and stripping away the fiber, diverticulosis rates shot up to epidemic levels.[2693] But what about populations like those in rural Africa where they were eating quantities of fiber up to the triple digits that we as a species were meant to be getting (based on paleolithic diet estimates and paleopoo fossilized feces)?[2694] Diverticulosis remained almost completely absent in areas where people continued to center their diets around whole plant foods, the *only* foods where fiber is found in abundance.[2695] So just like heart disease is the number one killer in the United States but has been virtually unknown in rural Africa, diverticulosis has been almost unknown there, whereas it's the most common disease of the colon here and around the rest of the Westernized world.[2696] Migration studies prove it's not due to some genetic racial difference either. The prevalence of diverticulosis was 1 percent in Japan at the same time it was fifty times higher in Japanese people who started eating and living like

Americans.[2697] Higher fiber intake may also explain why vegetarians may be up to nearly three times less likely to be affected.[2698]

Today, increasing fiber intake is accepted as the overriding dietary recommendation for people afflicted with the condition,[2699] but what about the common advice from doctors telling their patients with diverticulosis not to eat nuts, seeds, and sweetcorn?[2700]

The rationale for this was that those could get lodged in one of the blown-out pockets and trigger inflammation, but the myth of needing to avoid nuts, sweetcorn, popcorn, and seeds to prevent episodes of diverticulitis has been debunked with modern data.[2701] In fact, when Harvard researchers actually looked into this, they found *protective* associations between nut and popcorn consumption and the risk of diverticulitis.[2702] So doctors should tell patients with diverticulosis that they *can* eat nuts, sweetcorn, and popcorn without fear,[2703] advice echoed by Harvard[2704] and the Mayo Clinic.[2705] The Cleveland Clinic even identified this as the number one myth.[2706] A healthy, high-fiber diet is the best medicine for diverticulitis, and seeds and nuts certainly fit the bill. In fact, increasing dietary fiber intake should be seen as a major public health issue that may have a dramatic beneficial effect in diet-related diseases and deaths in general.[2707] In other words, eat more plants.

Nuts may be the easiest and tastiest Daily Dozen check box to tick. This one simple and delicious act has the potential to add years to your life without adding on pounds.

Herbs and Spices

> ## My Favorite Herbs and Spices
>
> Allspice, barberries, basil, bay leaves, cardamom, chili powder, cinnamon, cloves, coriander, cumin, curry powder, dill, fenugreek, garlic, ginger, horseradish, lemongrass, marjoram, mustard powder, nutmeg, oregano, parsley, pepper, peppermint, rosemary, saffron, sage, smoked paprika, thyme, turmeric, and vanilla
>
> ## Daily Recommendation:
> ¼ teaspoon of turmeric, along with any other (salt-free) herbs and spices you enjoy

Here's a simple tip: Use your senses to pick out healthy foods. As we've discussed, there is a good biological reason we should be so attracted to the vibrant colors found in the produce aisle: In many cases, the colors *are* the antioxidants. We can figure out which of two tomatoes has more antioxidants just by looking at which has a deeper red color. Of course, the food industry tries to hijack this natural instinct for colorful foods with abominations like Lucky Charms cereal, but if we stick to green-light foods, we can let color guide us. The same is true, we're now realizing, with flavor.

Just as many of the plant pigments are beneficial, scientists are discovering that many of the flavor compounds in herbs and spices are powerful antioxidants as well.[2708] Guess where the antioxidant rosmarinic acid is found? What about cuminal, thymol, and gingerols? The flavors *are* the antioxidants. We can use this knowledge to help us make decisions at the supermarket. We can see that red onions have more antioxidants than white, and we can taste that regular onions have more antioxidants than mellower, milder Vidalia-type onions.[2709]

The bitter and pungent compounds in the cruciferous and allium families are thought to be responsible for their health benefits. Intense colors and intense flavors can be signs of intense benefit. For optimum health, we should try to eat both colorful and flavorful foods. Indeed, the dietary guidelines for a number of countries now specifically encourage the consumption of herbs and spices, not only as a substitute for salt but for the healthy properties they have in their own right.[2710] And on the top of my list of healthful herbs and spices is turmeric—a spice that is both colorful *and* flavorful.

Why We Should Include Turmeric in Our Daily Diet

In recent years, more than twenty-five thousand articles have been published in the medical literature about curcumin, the pigment in turmeric that gives it that bright yellow color. Many of these papers sport impressive-looking diagrams suggesting that curcumin can benefit a multitude of conditions with a dizzying array of mechanisms.[2711] Curcumin was first isolated more than a century ago, yet out of the thousands of experiments, only a few in the twentieth century were clinical studies involving actual human participants. But since the turn of the century, more than five hundred clinical trials have tested curcumin against a variety of diseases.

We have seen how curcumin may play a role in preventing or treating lung disease, brain disease, and a variety of cancers, including multiple myeloma, colon cancer, and pancreatic cancer. But curcumin has also been shown to help speed recovery after surgery[2712] and effectively treat rheumatoid arthritis better than the leading drug of choice.[2713] It also may be effective in treating osteoarthritis[2714] and other inflammatory conditions, such as lupus[2715] and inflammatory bowel disease.[2716] In one trial for ulcerative colitis, a multicenter, randomized, placebo-controlled, double-blind study found that more than 50 percent of patients achieved remission within just one month on curcumin compared to *none* of the patients who received the placebo.[2717] A total of seven such studies found that curcumin, on average, doubled the chances of clinical remission.[2718] If you are as convinced as I am that you should include turmeric in your diet to benefit from its pigment curcumin, the next questions, then, are: How much do you eat, how do you eat it, and what are the risks?

A Quarter Teaspoon of Turmeric Every Day

Turmeric is potent stuff. If I took a sample of your blood and exposed it to an oxidizing chemical, researchers could quantify the damage it caused to the DNA in your blood cells with sophisticated technology that allows them to count the number of breaks in DNA strands. If I then gave you a single pinch of turmeric to eat once a day for a week, redrew your blood, and again exposed your blood cells to the same free radicals, you would see that with the tiny bit of turmeric on board, the number of cells with DNA damage could be cut in half.[2719] Not from mixing turmeric with cells in a petri dish, but from you ingesting the spice and then measuring its effects in your blood. And this was not some fancy curcumin supplement, not some turmeric *extract*. It was just the plain spice you can buy at any supermarket. And, the dose was tiny, about one-eighth of a teaspoon.

Now that's powerful!

The doses of turmeric that have been used in human studies range from less than one-sixteenth of a teaspoon up to nearly two tablespoons a day.[2720] Few adverse effects have been reported even at high doses, but the studies typically have lasted only a month or so. We don't know what long-term effects of high doses there may be. Because turmeric can have such powerful drug-like effects, until we have better safety data, I would not advise anyone to take more than the culinary doses that have a long-standing record of apparent safety. How much is that? Though traditional Indian diets can include up to about a teaspoon of turmeric daily, the average intake in India is closer to a quarter teaspoon a day.[2721] So that's how much I recommend you get as part of your Daily Dozen.

How to Eat Turmeric

Primitive peoples often used spices in sophisticated ways. For instance, quinine from cinchona bark was used to treat the symptoms of malaria long before the disease was even identified, and the raw ingredients of aspirin had been used as a popular painkiller long before Mr. Friedrich Bayer came along.[2722] Over the last few decades, about half of new drug discoveries have come from natural products.[2723]

There's a plant in South Asia called adhatoda (*adu*, meaning "goat," and *thoda*, meaning "not touch"—it's so bitter even the goats won't eat it). Its leaves are steeped with pepper to make a folk remedy effective for treating asthma. Somehow our ancestors figured out what scientists didn't discover until 1928: Adding pepper vastly boosted the plant's antiasthmatic properties. And now we know why. About 5 percent of black pepper by weight is composed of a compound called *piperine*, which accounts for pepper's pungent flavor and aroma. But piperine is also a potent inhibitor of drug metabolism.[2724] One of the ways our liver gets rid of foreign substances is by making them water soluble so we can pee them out. This black pepper molecule, however, inhibits that process, thereby boosting blood levels of the medicinal compounds in adhatoda—and it can do the same for curcumin in turmeric root.

Within an hour of eating turmeric, curcumin appears in our bloodstream, but only in small traces. Why only scant amounts? Presumably, our liver is actively working to get rid of it. But what if we suppress that elimination process by eating some black pepper? If we consume the same amount of curcumin but add a quarter teaspoon of black pepper, the level of curcumin in our blood shoots up by 2,000 percent.[2725] Even just the littlest pinch of pepper, just one-twentieth of a teaspoon, can significantly boost curcumin blood levels.[2726] And guess what is a common ingredient in many curry powders besides turmeric? Black pepper. Curry powder in India is also often served with a source of fat, which alone can enhance the bioavailability of curcumin seven- to eightfold.[2727] (Unfortunately, traditional knowledge appeared to fail here as to the best source of that fat. Indian cuisine employs a great deal of clarified butter, or ghee, which may explain the country's relatively high rates of heart disease despite its otherwise relatively healthy diet.[2728])

My favorite way to incorporate turmeric is to use fresh turmeric root. Any large Asian or natural foods market should carry it in the produce aisle. It looks like skinny fingers of gingerroot, but when you snap it open, you are greeted by the most unreal, Day-Glo, fluorescent-orange color. My quarter teaspoon of dried turmeric recommendation translates into about a half centimeter of fresh turmeric root. The roots are usually about 5 cm long, cost about ten cents each, and can last for weeks in the fridge or seemingly forever in the freezer. Every year, you can go to the store and buy a twelve-month supply of fresh turmeric for about five dollars.

There's evidence to suggest that the cooked and raw forms may have different properties. Cooked turmeric appears to offer better DNA protection, while raw turmeric may have greater anti-inflammatory effects.[2729] I enjoy it both ways. I use a grater to add my daily half centimeter into whatever I may be cooking (or right onto a cooked purple sweet potato), or I throw a raw slice into a smoothie (where I don't even taste it). Fresh turmeric has a much more subtle flavor than dried, so it may be an especially good option for those who don't like turmeric's taste. You will see it, though. Be careful—it can stain clothing and surfaces. Turmeric may not just make your health golden but your fingertips, as well.

Consuming turmeric with soya may offer a double benefit for osteoarthritis sufferers.[2730] Scrambled tofu is the classic turmeric soya combination, but let me share two of my favorites: one raw and one cooked. You can whip up a pumpkin pie smoothie in less than three minutes. Simply blend a can of pumpkin purée, a handful of frozen cranberries and pitted dates, pumpkin pie spice to taste, a half-centimeter turmeric slice (or a quarter teaspoon of powder), and unsweetened soya milk to reach your preferred consistency.

Another favorite is my pumpkin custard (aka crustless pie). All you need to do is blend one can of pumpkin purée with about 280 grams of silken tofu (the Mori-Nu brand is convenient because it stays fresh without refrigeration), as much pumpkin pie spice as you like, and one to two dozen pitted dates (depending on how much of a sweet tooth you have). Pour into a dish and bake at 350°F (177°C) until cracks appear on the surface. By skipping the piecrust and sticking with a custard, you're left with vegetables, tofu, spices, and fruit. The more of this dessert you eat, the healthier you may be.

Fresh or powdered, turmeric is a natural flavor fit for Indian and Moroccan cuisines, but I add it to most anything. I find it pairs particularly well with brown rice dishes, lentil soup, and roasted cauliflower. Prepared yellow mustard typically already has turmeric in it for color, but try to find a salt-free variety—one that's essentially just vinegar, a cruciferous vegetable (mustard seeds), and turmeric. I can't think of a healthier condiment.

What About Turmeric Supplements?

Wouldn't it be more convenient to just take a curcumin supplement every day? Added expense aside, I see three potential downsides. First, curcumin is not equivalent to turmeric. Supplement manufacturers often fall into the same reductionist trap as the drug companies do. Herbs are assumed to have only one main active ingredient, so the thinking goes that if we can isolate and purify it into a pill, we should be able to boost the effects. Well, curcumin is described as the active ingredient in turmeric,[2731] but is it *the* active ingredient or just *an* active ingredient? In fact, it's just one of many different components of the whole food spice.[2732]

Few studies have compared turmeric with curcumin, but some that have suggest that turmeric may work even better. For example, researchers at the MD Anderson Cancer Center in Texas pitted both turmeric and curcumin against seven different types of human cancer cells in vitro. Against breast cancer, for instance, curcumin kicked butt, but turmeric kicked even more butt. The same was true against pancreatic cancer, colon cancer, multiple myeloma, myelogenous leukemia, and others—turmeric came out on top, more effective than just its yellow pigment curcumin. These findings suggest that components other than curcumin can also contribute to anticancer activities.[2733]

Although curcumin is believed to account for most of turmeric's health-promoting activities, research published over the past decade has indicated that curcumin-*free* turmeric—turmeric with the so-called active ingredient removed—may be as effective as or even more effective than turmeric with curcumin. There are turmerones, for example, in turmeric (but processed out of curcumin supplements) that may exhibit both anticancer and anti-inflammatory activities. I naïvely assumed that the researchers who discovered this would advocate that people consume turmeric rather than take curcumin supplements, but instead, they suggested the production of all sorts of different turmeric-derived supplements.[2734] After all, who can make any money on a whole food that costs pennies a day?

My second concern involves dosing. While the turmeric trials have used modest amounts that could conceivably be achieved through diet, curcumin-only trials have tested the amount of curcumin found in 150 grams of turmeric spice—one hundred times more than what curry lovers have been eating for centuries.[2735] Some supplements add black pepper as well, potentially boosting levels to the equivalent of 4.3 kilos a day of turmeric, which might result in enough curcumin in the blood to potentially *cause* DNA damage based on in vitro data.[2736]

High supplemental doses may explain cases of liver injury tied to turmeric extracts.[2737] It's like green tea and green tea extract pills. Brewed green tea appears to be completely safe for the liver, but give people green tea extract supplements, and the liver of as many as one in seventeen people becomes inflamed.[2738] So we should consume our green tea in beverage form, not pill form, and, similarly, our turmeric in spice form at culinary doses, not capsules.

There is a mistaken assumption that if a little is good, then more must be better. We'd never make that assumption for drugs, so why is it made for supplements? For example, a review of nearly a hundred randomized, placebo-controlled trials of turmeric or curcumin supplements for fatty liver disease found that they successfully calmed liver inflammation, and guess which worked better? Low dose supplements worked about ten times better than high dose ones.[2739]

Finally, there is a concern about contamination with toxic metals. Lead chromate has been used to make turmeric appear yellower[2740] in Bangladesh, which exports much of the turmeric sold in the United States, leading to multiple recalls.[2741] The good news is, thanks to a country-wide food safety initiative, the proportion of turmeric market samples with detectable lead went from about 50 percent down to zero.[2742] Unfortunately, there is still more work to be done. In four South Asian countries where more than 80 percent of the world's turmeric is produced, 14 percent of samples had detectable lead above 2 micrograms per gram, which could easily exceed California's limit is of 0.5 mcg of lead per daily serving.[2743] Thankfully, none of the recently tested samples of powdered turmeric on the U.S. market has been found to be contaminated with heavy metals, but the same cannot be said of curcumin supplements.[2744]

None of these concerns (except cost) applies to supplements containing only whole ground turmeric powder. Nearly all turmeric supplements are extracts, however. How else could they get away with selling a small bottle of pills for twenty dollars when the bulk spice may be less than twenty dollars for 450 grams? A bottle might last two or three months. For the same price, bulk turmeric could offer two or three years' worth at Daily Dozen dosing.

One compromise between convenience and cost may be to make your own turmeric capsules. There are capsule-stuffing gadgets that allow you to fill your own. Given the cost discrepancy between bulk turmeric and supplements, such a gadget would probably pay for itself after your first batch. A "00"-sized capsule would fit a day's quarter-teaspoon dose. Making your own capsules might be a little time consuming, but if you won't otherwise consume turmeric in your daily diet, it might be time well spent. If there were ever such thing as a magic pill, single-ingredient, ground turmeric root would probably come closest.

Who Should Not Take Turmeric

If you suffer from gallstones, turmeric may trigger pain. Turmeric is a cholecystokinetic agent, meaning it facilitates the pumping action of the gallbladder to keep bile from stagnating.[2745] Ultrasound studies show that a quarter teaspoon of turmeric causes the gallbladder to contract, squeezing out half its contents.[2746] In this way, it may help *prevent* gallstones from forming in the first place. But what if you already have a stone obstructing your bile duct? That turmeric-induced squeeze could be painful.[2747] For everyone else, though, the effect of turmeric would be expected to reduce the risk of gallstone formation and ultimately even reduce the risk of gallbladder cancer.[2748]

Too much turmeric, however, may increase the risk of certain kidney stones. Turmeric is high in soluble oxalates, which can bind to calcium and develop into the most common form of kidney stone—insoluble calcium oxalate, which is responsible for about 75 percent of all cases. Those who have a tendency to form those stones should probably restrict consumption of total dietary oxalate to no more than 50 mg per day. This would mean no more than a teaspoon of turmeric daily at most.[2749] (Turmeric, by the way, is considered safe during pregnancy, but curcumin supplements may not be.[2750])

My recommended daily quarter teaspoon of turmeric is in addition to whatever other (salt-free) herbs and spices you enjoy. The reason the Daily Dozen encourages herb and spice consumption in general and not just turmeric is not because they're all interchangeable—turmeric appears to have unique benefits—but because there's evidence other herbs and spices have health benefits as well. I've talked about the role of saffron, for example, in the treatment of Alzheimer's (chapter 3) and depression (chapter 11). Spices don't just make food taste better; they make food better for you. I encourage you to keep a well-stocked spice cabinet and make it a habit to add whatever herbs and spices you find appealing to any dish you might be eating.

What follows here is a more in-depth examination of some of the herbs and spices for which we have the most scientific data. I will describe some of the fascinating studies that illustrate the benefits of these flavor boosters and explain some of the easiest ways to add them to your meals.

Black Cumin

Black cumin is not actually related to cumin; it's a member of the buttercup rather than carrot family. Also known as *Nigella sativa* or simply "nigella seeds," black cumin a common spice with a peppery flavor, prized for its purported medicinal benefits. Described as a "miracle herb,"[2751] black cumin was mentioned in the Old Testament (Isaiah 28:25, 27) and found cached in King Tut's tomb, and it's been said that Prophet Muhammad claimed it could "heal every disease except death."[2752] Only in the last fifty years or so has it been put to the test, though, culminating in more than a thousand papers published in the medical literature about the spice.

Typical doses used in studies are just one or two grams of black cumin a day, which is about a quarter teaspoon.[2753] Using such small amounts allows researchers to conduct randomized, double-blind, placebo-controlled trials by putting the whole food spice into capsules rather than extracting out just a few components.

Daily black cumin consumption has been found in systematic reviews and meta-analyses of randomized controlled trials to significantly improve cholesterol, triglycerides,[2754] blood pressure,[2755] and blood sugar control.[2756] Some of the results are extraordinary. One study, for example, found that menopausal women randomized to less than a daily quarter teaspoon of black cumin powder reduced their bad LDL cholesterol by 27 percent within two months.[2757] That's the kind of result you'd expect from a starting dose of a statin drug, but it was achieved with just a few sprinkles of a spice. Black cumin may also help with the symptoms of menopause.[2758]

Now, taking black cumin didn't actually *cure* anything. One month after stopping the spice, cholesterol levels crept back up.[2759] Nevertheless, it does appear to be an inexpensive, safe, effective, and tasty (if you like the flavor) treatment for some of our deadliest risk factors. One of the side-effects may even be weight loss.[2760]

A recent systematic review and meta-analysis of randomized, controlled, weight-loss trials found that about a quarter teaspoon of black cumin powder every day appears to reduce body mass index within a couple of months.[2761] The spice also lowers markers of inflammation, such as C-reactive protein,[2762] and has favorable effects on inflammatory conditions, such as asthma,[2763] rheumatoid arthritis,[2764] and a common cause of hypothyroidism called

Hashimoto's thyroiditis.[2765] Black cumin also appears to help get rid of kidney stones.[2766]

If it's truly so beneficial to so many facets of our health, why don't we hear more about it? Why wasn't I taught about black cumin in medical school? Perhaps because there's little profit motive. Black cumin is just a spice. I put it in a pepper grinder and mill it onto meals just like black pepper. The daily dose used in most of these studies would cost about three cents a day.

Fennel Seeds

Fennel seeds, which aren't actually seeds at all but the whole little fruits of the fennel plant, are a spice found commonly in Indian and Middle Eastern cuisines. You'll typically find a bowl of fennel seeds, sometimes candy-coated, as you walk out of Indian restaurants. Beyond mouth freshening, chewing them can lead to a significant bump in nitric oxide production due to their nitrate content, which has the predictable vasodilatory effect of opening up blood vessels. (See chapter 5.) They are an inexpensive and easy way to carry a lightweight, nonperishable source of nitrates for activities like hiking, where pocketing spinach and beetroot may be less convenient. Chewing fennel seeds could help maintain oxygen levels at high altitudes and help prevent HAPE—high altitude pulmonary edema, one of the leading killers of mountain climbers once you get more than a mile and a half or so above sea level.[2767] HAPE is not to be confused with HAFE, which is caused by the expansion of gas at high altitudes[2768]—a condition known as high altitude flatus expulsion or "Rocky Mountain barking spiders."[2769] Fennel seeds may help with that too, as they've been used traditionally as a carminative, meaning a remedy for intestinal gas, but they also have hormonal effects.[2770]

There have been cases reported of premature breast development among young girls drinking fennel seed tea a couple times a day for several months.[2771] Their estrogen levels were elevated, but, after stopping the tea, their chests and hormone levels went back to normal. Fennel seeds can also increase breast milk production,[2772] treat painful periods,[2773] and, when incorporated into a topical cream, decrease unwanted hair growth in women.[2774]

Fenugreek

The spice fenugreek is also a galactagogue. No, not another sci-fi reboot, a galactagogue is something that increases breast milk production in lactating women.[2775] One randomized, double-blind, placebo-controlled trial in which breastfeeding women took about a half teaspoon of both fenugreek and ground ginger, along with about a quarter of a teaspoon of turmeric every day, doubled their milk production within a month.[2776] Other hormonal effects include an improvement in menstrual pain using half a teaspoon of fenugreek powder three times a day, taken the first three days of your period.[2777] What about menopausal symptoms?

In a randomized, double-blind, placebo-controlled trial, the equivalent of one teaspoon[2778] of fenugreek twice a day significantly reduced the number of hot flashes and night sweats within four weeks compared to placebo, and symptoms of depression, insomnia, and vaginal dryness within seven weeks.[2779] Fenugreek can cut the frequency of hot flashes and night sweats in half within three months.[2780] These studies used proprietary fenugreek supplements, but just the plain powder seems to work as well at one and a half teaspoons a day.[2781]

While the estrogen hormone estradiol stimulates vaginal lubrication and blood flow, facilitating a woman's capacity for sexual arousal and orgasm, it's the testosterone that's linked with sexual desire in both men and women. Fenugreek raises the levels of both estradiol and testosterone, resulting in both an increase in sexual desire and function, translating into about a doubling of sexual activity compared to placebo.[2782] That was in premenopausal women, but the same dose was subsequently shown to improve sexual symptoms in postmenopausal women as well.[2783] However, it was not found to be as effective as estrogen cream in a head-to-head comparison.[2784]

In men, fenugreek seed is a spice used historically as an aphrodisiac and for male reproductive issues.[2785] It can increase the testicular weight and testosterone production in rats, but what about people?[2786] Clinical trials of fenugreek with dose equivalents as low as a quarter teaspoon[2787] to two-thirds of a teaspoon[2788] a day were found to raise testosterone levels[2789] by about 10 percent within three months, accompanied by a rise in sex drive and arousal.[2790] This was accompanied by improved sexual function in men, for example, a doubling of the frequency of morning erections.[2791]

Young men randomized to capsules containing fenugreek also got significant gains in body composition and upper (bench press) and lower (leg press) strength compared to placebo.²⁷⁹² Side benefits include an improvement in LDL cholesterol, triglycerides,²⁷⁹³ and short- and long-term blood sugar control (with actual fenugreek powder working better than fenugreek extract supplements).²⁷⁹⁴ It can also make your armpits smell like maple syrup.²⁷⁹⁵ (Really!)

Coriander

One sign of changing U.S. demographics is that salsa has replaced ketchup as America's top table condiment.²⁷⁹⁶ One popular salsa ingredient is coriander, one of the most polarizing and divisive food ingredients. Some people absolutely love it, and some people absolutely hate it. What's interesting is that the lovers and the haters appear to experience the taste differently. Individuals who like coriander may describe it as fresh, fragrant, or citrusy, whereas people who dislike the herb report that it tastes like soap, mold, dirt, or bugs.²⁷⁹⁷ I'm not sure how so many people know what bugs taste like, but rarely are polarizing opinions about flavors so extreme.

Different ethnic groups do seem to have different rates of coriander dislike, with Ashkenazi Jews scoring among the highest on the coriander hate-o-meter.²⁷⁹⁸ Another clue came from twin studies that show that identical twins tend to share coriander preferences, whereas fraternal twins do not have such a strong correlation.²⁷⁹⁹ The human genetic code contains about three billion letters, so we'd have to analyze the DNA of roughly ten thousand people to find a coriander gene. Obviously, genetic researchers have better things to do than undertake that challenge . . . right?

Thankfully for us, apparently not. Genetic studies of more than twenty-five thousand participants who reported their coriander preferences discovered an area on chromosome 11 that seemed to be a match. What's there? A gene called OR6A2 that enables us to smell certain chemicals like E-(2)-decenal, which is both a primary constituent of coriander and a defensive secretion of stink bugs. So maybe coriander does taste like bugs! Coriander lovers may just be genetic mutants who have an inability to smell the unpleasant compound.²⁸⁰⁰

This may actually be an advantage, though, because coriander is healthy stuff. Mother Nature has been described as the most comprehensive pharmacy of all time, and coriander is one of her oldest herbal prescriptions.²⁸⁰¹ About twenty sprigs of coriander daily for two months reduced inflammation levels in arthritis sufferers and cut uric-acid levels in half, suggesting that lots of coriander may be useful for people suffering from gout.[2802]

Cayenne Pepper

In a study published as "Secretion, Pain and Sneezing Induced by the Application of Capsaicin to the Nasal Mucosa in Man," researchers found that if we cut a hot pepper and rub it inside our nostrils, our nose will start running and hurting, and we'll start sneezing. (Capsaicin is the burning component of hot peppers.) Why would they perform such an experiment? People who have handled hot peppers know that if they get some up their nose, they can experience an intense burning sensation. (And it doesn't even have to get up your nose, which I was chagrined to learn after I once failed to wash my hands before using the restroom!) However, the researchers noted that "these phenomena have not been investigated." So they decided it "appeared worthwhile to study the effects produced by topical application of capsaicin in the human [nose] . . ."[2803]

The researchers enlisted a group of medical students and dripped some capsaicin in their noses. The students started sneezing, burning, and snotting, describing the pain at about eight or nine on a scale of one to ten. No surprise. But it gets a little more interesting. What happened when they repeated the experiment day after day? You'd think the students might be more sensitive to capsaicin, with their nose still irritated from the day before, causing even greater pain and discomfort, right? Actually, the capsaicin hurt less. By day five, in fact, it hardly hurt at all—they didn't even get a runny nose anymore.

Were the med students permanently numbed? No. After a month or so, the desensitization wore off, and they were back in agony whenever the researchers tried dripping capsaicin back in their noses. What was likely happening is that the pain fibers—the nerves that carry pain sensation—used up so much of the pain neurotransmitter (called *substance P*) that they ran out. Exposed day after day, the nerves exhausted their stores and could no longer transmit pain messages until they made more neurotransmitter from scratch, which takes a couple of weeks.

How could this be exploited for medical purposes? There's a rare headache syndrome called *cluster headache*, which has been described as one of the worst pains humans can experience. Few, if any, medical disorders are more painful.

It's nicknamed the "suicide headache" because patients have taken their lives because of it.[2804]

Cluster headaches are thought to be caused by pressure on the trigeminal nerve in the face. Treatments involve everything from nerve blocks to Botox to surgery. But that same nerve goes down to the nose. What if we cause the whole nerve to dump all its substance P? Researchers tried the daily capsaicin experiment with cluster headache sufferers. Unlike the medical students who rated the nose burning as an eight or nine on the ten-point pain scale, those used to the violence of cluster headache attacks rated the pain caused by capsaicin at only a three or four. By day five, they too became desensitized to the pain of the capsaicin. What happened to their headaches? Those who rubbed capsaicin in the nostril on the side of the head where the headaches occurred cut the average number of attacks in half. In fact, half the patients were apparently cured—their cluster headaches were gone completely. All in all, 80 percent responded, which is at least equal to, if not better than, all the current available therapies.[2805]

What about other pain syndromes? Irritable bowel syndrome is thought to be caused by a hypersensitivity of the lining of the colon. How do you determine if someone's gut is hypersensitive? Innovative Japanese researchers developed a device to deliver "repetitive painful rectal distention," which is basically a half liter balloon hooked up to a fancy bicycle pump that is inserted and inflated until you can't stand the pain anymore. Those with IBS had a significantly lower pain threshold, significantly less "rectal compliance."[2806]

So how about trying to desensitize the gut by depleting substance P stores? It's bad enough to have to rub hot peppers up your nose, but where would you have to stick them for irritable bowel? Thankfully, researchers chose the oral route. They found that the enteric-coated capsules of red pepper powder were able to significantly decrease the intensity of abdominal pain and bloating, suggesting "a way of dealing with this frequent and distressing functional disease . . ."[2807]

What about red pepper powder for the pain of chronic indigestion (dyspepsia)? Within a month of taking about one and a half teaspoons' worth of cayenne pepper a day, stomach pain and nausea improved.[2808] The frequently prescribed drug Propulsid (cisapride) worked almost as well as the red pepper powder and was considered generally well tolerated—until, that is, it started killing people. Propulsid was pulled from the market after causing fatal heart rhythms.[2809]

Ginger

Many successful natural treatments start like this: A doctor learns that a plant has been used in some ancient medical tradition and figures, "Why not try it in my practice?" Ginger has been used for centuries for headaches, so a group of Danish physicians advised one of their migraine patients to give it a go. At the first sign of a migraine coming on, the patient mixed a quarter teaspoon of powdered ginger in some water and drank it. Within thirty minutes, the migraine disappeared. And it worked every time for her, with no apparent side effects.[2810]

This is what's called a case report. Though they're really just glorified anecdotes, case reports have played an important role in the history of medicine, from the discovery of AIDS[2811] to a failed chest-pain drug with a billion-dollar side effect—Viagra.[2812] Case reports are considered the weakest form of evidence, but that's often where investigations begin.[2813] So the case report of successfully treating one migraine patient with ginger isn't so much helpful in itself, but it can inspire researchers to put it to the test.

Eventually, a double-blind, randomized, controlled clinical trial was performed comparing the efficacy of ginger for the treatment of migraine headaches to sumatriptan, one of the top-selling, billion-dollar drugs in the world. Just one-eighth of a teaspoon of powdered ginger worked about just as well and just as fast as the drug (and costs less than a penny). Most migraine sufferers started with moderate or severe pain, but after taking the drug or the ginger, ended up in mild pain or were entirely pain-free. The same proportion of migraine sufferers reported satisfaction with the results either way.

As far as I'm concerned, ginger won. Not only is ginger a billion dollars cheaper, but it caused significantly fewer side effects. While on the drug, people reported dizziness, a sedative effect, vertigo, and heartburn, but the only side effect reported for ginger was an upset stomach in about one out of twenty-five people.[2814] (A whole tablespoon of ginger powder at one time on an empty stomach could irritate anyone, though,[2815] so don't overdo it.) Sticking to one-eighth of a teaspoon is not only up to three thousand times cheaper than taking the drug, but you're also probably less likely to end up as a case report yourself, like the people who have had a heart attack after taking sumatriptan for a migraine,[2816] or have died.[2817]

Migraines are described as "one of the most common" pain syndromes, affecting as much as 12 percent of the population.[2818] That's common? How about menstrual cramps, which plague up to 90 percent of younger women?[2819]

Can ginger help? Even just one-eighth of a teaspoon of ginger powder three times a day dropped pain from an eight to a six on a scale of one to ten, and down further to a three in the second month.[2820] And these women hadn't been taking ginger all month; they started the day before their periods began, suggesting that even if it doesn't seem to help much the first month, women should try sticking with it.

What about the duration of pain? A quarter teaspoon of ginger powder three times a day was found to not only drop the severity of menstrual pain from about seven down to five but decrease the duration from a total of nineteen hours in pain down to about fifteen hours,[2821] significantly better than the placebo, which were capsules filled with powdered toast. But women don't take bread crumbs for their cramps. How does ginger compare to ibuprofen? Researchers pitted one-eighth of a teaspoon of powdered ginger head-to-head against 400 mg of ibuprofen, and the ginger worked just as effectively as this leading drug.[2822] Unlike the drug, ginger can also reduce the amount of menstrual bleeding, from around 125 ml per period down to 60 ml.[2823] What's more, ginger intake of one-eighth of a teaspoon twice daily started a week before your period can yield a significant drop in premenstrual mood, physical, and behavioral symptoms.[2824]

I like sprinkling powdered ginger on sweet potatoes or using it fresh to make lemon-ginger apple chews as an antinausea remedy. (Ever since I was a little kid, I've suffered from motion sickness.) There is an array of powerful antinausea drugs, but they come with a nausea-inducing list of side effects, so I've always striven to find natural remedies whenever possible for myself and for my patients.

Ginger has been used for thousands of years in traditional healing systems. In India, it's known as *maha-aushadhi*, meaning "the great medicine." However, it wasn't proven to reduce nausea until 1982, when it beat out Dramamine in a head-to-head test in blindfolded volunteers who were spun around in a tilted, rotating chair.[2825] Ginger is now considered a nontoxic, broad-spectrum antiemetic (antivomiting agent) effective in countering nausea during motion sickness, pregnancy, chemotherapy, and radiation, and after surgery.[2826]

Try making my lemon-ginger apple chews: In a blender, liquefy one peeled lemon with a palm-sized "hand" of fresh gingerroot. Use the mixture to coat thin slices of four apples, then place them in a dehydrator or on a tray and bake in the oven at the lowest setting until they reach desired chewiness. I like them a little moist, but you can dehydrate them further to make lemon-ginger apple chips, which store longer than the chews. For me, a few pieces eaten about twenty minutes before travel works wonders.

Note: Ginger is generally considered safe during pregnancy, but the maximum recommended daily dose of fresh ginger while pregnant is 20 grams (about four teaspoons of freshly grated gingerroot).[2827] Any more may have uterus-stimulating effects. Women using my apple chews recipe to combat morning sickness should spread out the four apples' worth of chews or chips over several days.

Peppermint

Which herbs have the most antioxidants? The most antioxidant-packed herb is dried Norwegian bearberry leaf. (Good luck finding that!) The most antioxidant-packed *common* herb is peppermint.[2828] That's why I add mint to my favorite hibiscus cocktail recipe (see page 452) and why I try to add it to food whenever possible. Mint is a traditional ingredient in Middle Eastern salads like tabbouleh, Indian chutneys, and Vietnamese soups and fresh summer rolls. I like to put it into anything chocolaty as well.

Oregano and Marjoram

Oregano is such an antioxidant-rich herb that researchers decided to test if it could reduce the DNA-damaging effects of radiation. Radioactive iodine is sometimes given to people with overactive thyroid glands or thyroid cancer to destroy part of the gland or mop up any remaining tumor cells after surgery. For days after the isotope injection, patients are so radioactive that they are advised not to kiss anyone or to sleep close to anyone (including their pets), and to maximize the distance between themselves and children or pregnant women.[2829] The treatment can be very effective, but all that radiation exposure appears to increase the risk of developing new cancers later on.[2830] Hoping to prevent the DNA damage associated with this treatment, researchers tested the ability of oregano to protect chromosomes of human blood cells in vitro from exposure to radioactive iodine. At the highest dose, chromosome damage was reduced by 70 percent. The researchers concluded that oregano may "act as a potent radioprotective agent."[2831]

Other petri-dish studies with oregano suggest anticancer and anti-inflammatory properties. In a comparison of the effects of various spice extracts—bay leaves, fennel, lavender, paprika, parsley, rosemary, and thyme—oregano beat out all but bay leaves in its ability to suppress cervical cancer cell growth in vitro while leaving normal cells alone.[2832] Of 115 different foods tested for anti-inflammatory properties in vitro, oregano made it into the top five, along with oyster mushrooms, onions, cinnamon, and tea leaves.[2833]

Marjoram is a closely related herb and also shows promise in laboratory studies. It appears to significantly inhibit the migration and invasion of breast cancer cells in vitro.[2834] Few studies on oregano family herbs have been done on people, though, so we have little idea how, if at all, these effects will translate to a clinical setting. One of the only randomized, controlled trials I'm aware of is a study of marjoram tea for polycystic ovary syndrome (PCOS). The tea was purportedly used in traditional herbal medicine to "restore hormonal balance," so researchers decided to put it to the test. They instructed women with PCOS to drink two cups of marjoram tea on an empty stomach every day for a month. Beneficial effects on hormone levels were observed, which, the researchers concluded, "may justify the improvement claimed by traditional medicine practitioners and patients."[2835]

In 2022, a study was published in which soldiers were randomized to about a third of a teaspoon a day of powdered oregano stuffed into capsules to pit them against placebo before their rigorous army combat readiness testing. Those in the oregano group appeared to experience significantly less muscle damage while getting boosts to the antioxidant capacity of their bloodstream. The researchers concluded: "Supplementation with oregano may serve as a dietary strategy to increase preparedness and promote recovery in military recruits."[2836]

The same dose of savory—a related herb and a common constituent of *herbes de Provence*—taken once a day for ten weeks reduced LDL cholesterol by 27 points over placebo in a double-blind trial.[2837] A drop that great over a lifetime could decrease the risk of heart disease by 40 percent[2838] at a cost of about three cents a day.

Cloves

The most antioxidant-packed common *spice* is the clove.[2839] It has an exceptionally strong flavor, so try adding just a teensy pinch to anything you'd normally put cinnamon or ginger on. Ground cloves are great on stewed pears and baked apples, giving them a pleasant mulled cider taste, and a mug of chai tea is a fantastic way to pack in a bunch of high-impact common spices at once.

Amla

The most antioxidant-packed *uncommon* spice is amla,[2840] which is powdered dried Indian gooseberry fruit. As a Western-trained physician, I had never heard of amla despite its common use in Ayurvedic herbal preparations. I was surprised to find more than a thousand articles on this lesser-known spice in the medical literature, and even more surprised to find papers with titles like "Amla . . . a Wonder Berry in the Treatment and Prevention of Cancer." Amla is arguably the most important plant in Ayurvedic medicine, used traditionally as everything from a neutralizer of snake venom to a hair tonic.[2841] I eat it because it's apparently the single most antioxidant-packed green-light food on Earth.[2842]

Using an argon laser, researchers can measure and track human carotenoid antioxidant levels in real time. The most important finding from this body of work is that antioxidant levels can plummet within two hours of an oxidatively stressful event. When we're stuck in traffic breathing diesel fumes, deprived of sleep, or suffering from a cold, for example, our body starts using up some of its antioxidant stores. What may only take two hours to lose can take up to three days to build back up.[2843]

Even ordinary body processes, such as turning food into energy, can produce free radicals. This is okay as long as the food we eat comes prepackaged with antioxidants. But if it doesn't—if we drink straight sugar water, for example—the level of free radicals and oxidized fat in our bloodstream rises over the next few hours, while vitamin E levels drop as our body's antioxidant stores are expended.[2844] If we were to eat the same amount of sugar in the form of an orange, though, we wouldn't get a spike in oxidation.[2845] Researchers concluded: "This argues strongly for the need to include high antioxidant foods in each and every meal in order to prevent this redox [free-radical versus antioxidant] imbalance."[2846]

The standard American diet (SAD) isn't exactly antioxidant packed. Here is the antioxidant content (in modified FRAP assay daµmol antioxidant units) of some typical American breakfast foods: bacon (7) and eggs (8), a bowl of corn flakes (25) with milk (10), an Egg McMuffin (11), pancakes (21) with maple syrup (9), and a bagel (20) with cream cheese (4). A typical breakfast may average about 25 antioxidant units.[2847]

Compare those to the smoothie I had for breakfast this morning. I started with 250 ml of water (0), 70 grams of frozen blueberries (323), and the pulp of a ripe mango (108). I added a tablespoon of ground flaxseeds (8), along with 15 grams of fresh mint leaves (33) and a palmful of bulk white tea leaves (103). (For more about tea leaves, see page 448.) While the typical SAD breakfast may give us only about 25 antioxidant units, my breakfast smoothie offered more than 500. And, when I add the final ingredient, a single teaspoon of amla, I get an additional 753 antioxidant units. That's about four cents' worth of amla, and it more than doubled the antioxidant content of my entire smoothie. Before I've even fully woken up, I've already consumed more than 1,000 antioxidant units. That's more than the average person may get in an entire week. I could drink my smoothie and eat nothing but donuts for the rest of the week, and most people *still* wouldn't catch up. Notice that even though I packed the blender with amazing foods like blueberries and tea leaves, fully half the antioxidant power came from that single four-cent teaspoon of powdered gooseberries.

You can buy amla online or at any Indian spice store. Ayurvedic herbal supplements are typically something you'd want to stay away from, as they have been found to be heavily contaminated with heavy metals,[2848] some of which are actually added intentionally.[2849] But none of the samples of powdered amla I've ever seen tested so far has been found to be contaminated beyond World Health Organization safety limits.[2850] You can find whole Indian gooseberries in the frozen section of Indian food shops, but frankly, I find them inedible—astringent, sour, bitter, and fibrous all at the same time. The powder isn't much tastier, but it can be disguised in something with a strong flavor, like a smoothie. Alternatively, you could pack amla into capsules like the turmeric.

Spice Mixes

While there has been a considerable number of studies done with individual spices, few have looked at increasing spice consumption in general. One group at Pennsylvania State University did compare the effects of a high-fat chicken meal with and without a mixture of nine herbs and spices. Herbs and spices were chosen because, ounce for ounce, they have more antioxidants than any other food group (and because the study was funded by the McCormick spice company).[2851]

Unsurprisingly, the people in the spice group experienced a doubling of the antioxidant power in their bloodstreams compared to participants in the spice-free group. Remarkably, though, the spice group ended up with 30 percent less fat (triglycerides) in their blood after the meal and improved insulin sensitivity. The researchers concluded that "the incorporation of spices into the daily diet may help normalize postprandial [after-meal] disturbances in glucose [sugar] and lipid [fat] homeostasis [control] while enhancing antioxidant defense."

But why experience such disturbances in the first place? The study reminds me of those that show eating greens may be particularly protective against cancer among smokers.[2852] That is, the take-home message shouldn't be telling smokers to eat greens—it should be telling smokers to quit smoking. Of course, they could do both, which in the context of the spice study would mean adopting an antioxidant-rich, green-light diet, offering the best of both worlds.

Some of my favorite spice mixes are pumpkin pie spice, curry powder, chili powder, Chinese five-spice powder, a savory Indian spice blend called garam masala, an Ethiopian blend called berbere, Italian seasoning, poultry seasoning, and a Middle Eastern blend called za'atar. Spice mixes are a convenient way to provide a balance of flavors while boosting the variety of your spice intake, but make sure to check that the mixes are salt-free.

Some Risks to Spicing Up Our Life

There are a few spices, however, of which you can have too much of a good thing. Take poppy seeds, for example.

The opium poppy used to make heroin is the same opium poppy that produces the poppy seeds in muffins and bagels. The idea that poppy seeds could serve as the source of appreciable amounts of narcotics was not given much credence despite the existence of an old European custom recommending a poppy seed-filled pacifier to quiet a noisy baby.[2853] It wasn't given much credence, that is, until a mother tried giving her six-month-old some strained milk in which she had boiled some poppy seeds with the very best intentions of helping the child sleep better. The baby stopped breathing—but luckily survived.[2854]

The cases of poppy seed overdose aren't limited to children. There's another case in the literature of an adult who felt "dim feelings in the head" after eating spaghetti with 70 grams of poppy seeds on top.[2855] So what's the upper limit of poppy seed consumption that's probably safe? Based on median morphine levels,[2856] about one teaspoon for every 4.5 kilos of body weight. This means that someone weighing about 67.5 kilos should probably eat no more than five tablespoons of raw poppy seeds at a time.[2857]

Cooking may wipe out half of the morphine and codeine contained naturally in poppy seeds, which gives us some more leeway when baking.[2858] Soaking the poppy seeds for five minutes and then discarding the water before adding the seeds to your recipe can eliminate half of that remaining, if you're making some poppy seed-filled pastry or other baked goods for children. Otherwise, there shouldn't be any risk at usual levels of intake—unless you're going in for a drug test, in which case you may want to avoid poppy seeds altogether.[2859] In 2023, a bill was introduced in the U.S. Congress to ban the sale of poppy seeds containing unsafe levels of opiate-type compounds.[2860]

Too much nutmeg can also be a problem. A paper entitled "Christmas Gingerbread . . . and Christmas Cheer: Review of the Potential Role of Mood Elevating Amphetamine-like Compounds . . ." suggested that certain natural constituents of spices like nutmeg may form amphetamine compounds within the body sufficient "to elevate the mood and to help provide some added Christmas cheer" during the holiday season.[2861]

This hypothetical risk was raised as far back as the 1960s in *The New England Journal of Medicine* in an article called "Nutmeg Intoxication."[2862] The paper pondered whether the age-old custom of adding nutmeg to eggnog arose from the "psychopharmacological effect" described in cases of nutmeg intoxication. Such cases evidently go back to the 1500s, when nutmeg was used as an abortifacient to induce a miscarriage.[2863] In the 1960s, the spice was used as a psychotropic drug.[2864] During that decade, mental health professionals concluded that while nutmeg "is much cheaper for use and probably less dangerous than the habit-forming heroin, it must be stated that it is not free from danger and may cause death."[2865]

The toxic dose of nutmeg is two to three teaspoons. I had assumed no one would ever come close to that amount unintentionally until I saw a report in which a married couple ate some pasta, collapsed, and were subsequently hospitalized. What had happened was a big mystery until the husband revealed that he had accidentally added one-third of a jar of nutmeg to the meal while cooking.[2866] That's about four teaspoons of the spice. I don't know how they could have eaten it! I imagine his partner was just trying to be polite.

Another popular and powerful spice is cinnamon, which has been prized for its ability to lower blood sugar levels.[2867] It works so well that you can even "cheat" on a diabetes test by consuming two teaspoons of cinnamon the night before. Twelve hours later, your blood sugar spike in response to meals will still be significantly dampened.[2868] Even just a teaspoon a day appears to make a significant difference.[2869] Unfortunately, cinnamon can no longer be considered a safe and effective treatment for diabetes.

There are two main types of cinnamon: Ceylon cinnamon and cassia cinnamon (also known as Chinese cinnamon). In the United States, anything simply labeled "cinnamon" is probably cassia, since it's cheaper. This is unfortunate, because cassia contains a compound called *coumarin*, which may be toxic to the liver at high doses. Unless it's specifically labeled Ceylon cinnamon, a quarter teaspoon of cinnamon even a few times a week may be too much for small children, and a daily teaspoon would exceed the tolerable upper safety limit for adults.[2870] Can't you just switch to Ceylon cinnamon and get the benefits without the risks? Without the risks, yes, but we're no longer so sure about the benefits.

Nearly all the studies showing blood sugar benefits of cinnamon have been performed with cassia. We've just assumed that the same would apply for the safer Ceylon cinnamon, but it was only recently put to the test. The nice blunting of blood sugars we see in response to cassia cinnamon disappeared when the researchers tried using Ceylon cinnamon instead.[2871] In fact, all along it may actually have been the toxic coumarin itself that was the active blood-sugar-lowering ingredient in the cassia cinnamon. Thus, sidestepping the toxin by switching to Ceylon cinnamon may sidestep the benefit. So, in a nutshell, when it comes to lowering blood sugars, cinnamon may not be safe (cassia), or it may be safe, but apparently not effective in reducing blood sugar (Ceylon).

I still encourage Ceylon cinnamon consumption, given that it is one of the cheapest common food sources of antioxidants, second only to red cabbage. But what's a person with type 2 diabetes to do? Even the cassia cinnamon only brought down blood sugars modestly—in other words, it was only as good as the leading diabetes drug in the world, metformin, sold as Glucophage.[2872] Yes, cassia cinnamon may work as effectively as the leading drug, but that's not saying much. The best way to treat type 2 diabetes is to attempt to cure it entirely with a healthy diet. (See chapter 7.)

Who knew that the herbs and spices we've been tossing into sauces and sprinkling onto dishes could have such impacts on our health? Work your creativity in the kitchen and spice up your meals and drinks to make them more flavorful and more healthful—but don't forget the quarter teaspoon of daily turmeric. I am sufficiently convinced by the available body of evidence to single turmeric out as something every one of us should add to our daily diet.

Whole Grains

My Favorite Whole Grains

Barley groats, buckwheat, yellow corn tortillas, millet, oat groats, popcorn, quinoa, rye groats, sorghum, teff, whole-wheat pasta, and wild rice

Serving Sizes:
½ cup (100 g) hot cereal or cooked grains, pasta, or sweetcorn
1 cup (30 g) cold cereal
1 tortilla or slice of bread
½ bagel or English muffin
3 cups (30 g) popped popcorn

Daily Recommendation:
3 servings per day

Consistent with recommendations from leading cancer[2873] and heart disease[2874] authorities, I recommend at least three servings of whole grains a day. Harvard University's preeminent twin nutrition studies—the Nurses' Health Study and the Health Professionals Follow-Up Study—have accumulated nearly six million person-years of data.[2875] They found that people who eat more whole grains tend to live significantly longer lives independent of other dietary and lifestyle factors.[2876] No surprise, given that whole grains appear to reduce the risk of heart disease,[2877] type 2 diabetes,[2878] obesity, and stroke.[2879] Eating more whole grains might save the lives of more than a million people around the world every year.[2880]

There are so many nutrition claims floating around the internet that lack scientific backing, but a few especially persistent memes directly contradict the available evidence. When I see books, websites, articles, and blogs parroting claims like "grains are inflammatory—even whole grains," I can't help but wonder what alternate dimension the authors call home.

Pick your indicator of inflammation. Take C-reactive protein (CRP), for instance. CRP levels rise within the body in response to inflammatory insults and are therefore used as a screening test for systemic inflammation. Each daily serving of whole grains is estimated to *reduce* CRP concentrations by approximately 7 percent.[2881] Furthermore, there's a whole alphabet soup of inflammation markers that appear to be improved by whole grains: ALT, GGT,[2882] IL-6,[2883] IL-8,[2884] IL-10,[2885] IL-18,[2886] PAI-1,[2887] TNF-α,[2888] TNF-R2,[2889] whole blood viscosity, and erythrocyte filtration.[2890] Or, as presented in less technical terms in *The American Journal of Clinical Nutrition*, "Whole-grain intake cools down inflammation."[2891] Even excluding heart disease and cancer, habitual whole-grain intake is linked to a significantly lower risk of dying from inflammatory diseases.[2892]

What About Gluten?

You've probably heard about an autoimmune disorder called celiac disease, in which the consumption of gluten causes adverse reactions, including gastrointestinal problems. Gluten is a group of proteins found in certain grains, including wheat, barley, and rye. Celiac disease is relatively rare, though, affecting less than 1 percent of the population.[2893] For the more than 99 percent of the rest of us who don't have the disorder, is gluten okay or, indeed, health-promoting like other plant proteins?

In 1980, researchers in England reported a series of women suffering from chronic diarrhea who were cured by a gluten-free diet, yet none of the women had evidence of celiac disease.[2894] They appeared to have some sort of *non-celiac gluten sensitivity*. At the time, the medical profession expressed skepticism that there was such a thing,[2895] and even now there are experts who question its existence.[2896] In fact, doctors commonly referred their patients claiming non-celiac gluten sensitivity to psychiatrists because they were believed to have an underlying mental illness.[2897]

The medical profession has a history of dismissing diseases as existing "just in your head." Examples of these include post-traumatic stress disorder (PTSD), ulcerative colitis, migraines, ulcers, asthma, Parkinson's, Lyme disease, and multiple sclerosis. Despite resistance from the prevailing medical community, each one of these conditions has subsequently been confirmed as a legitimate disorder.[2898] On the flip side, the internet is rife with unsubstantiated claims about gluten-free diets that have spilled over into the popular press, making gluten the diet villain du jour.[2899] And, of course, the gluten-free processed food industry, today worth billions, has a financial interest in the public's confusion.[2900] Whenever that much money is at stake, it's hard to trust anyone, so as always, stick to the science. And what sort of evidence is there for the existence of a condition presumed to be so widespread?

The first double-blind, randomized, placebo-controlled gluten challenge was published in 2011. Patients complaining of irritable bowel-type symptoms who claimed they felt better on a gluten-free diet—despite not having celiac disease—were tested to see if they could tell if bread and muffins they were given contained gluten or were gluten-free. All the subjects started out gluten-free and symptom-free for two weeks, then were challenged with one of the two types of bread and muffins. Even those who ate the gluten-free placebo products felt worse, meaning they started out on a gluten-free diet and continued on a gluten-free diet, yet they reported feeling crampy and bloated. This is what's called the *nocebo effect*. The placebo effect takes place when you give patients something useless and they feel better; the nocebo effect occurs when you give someone something harmless and they feel worse. Nevertheless, the participants who received actual gluten felt even worse. So the researchers concluded that non-celiac gluten intolerance may indeed exist.[2901]

However, this was a small study, and even though the researchers claimed the gluten-free products were indistinguishable from those containing gluten, it's possible that the patients were able to tell which foods were which. So, in 2012, Italian researchers created a double-blinded test with 920 patients diagnosed with non-celiac gluten sensitivity. Each was given capsules filled with either wheat flour or a placebo powder. More than two-thirds failed the test: Those on the placebo got worse, or those on the wheat felt better. But for those who passed, there was a clear benefit to staying on the wheat-free diet, confirming the "existence of non-celiac WS [wheat sensitivity]."[2902] Note that they said *wheat* sensitivity, though, not *gluten* sensitivity. In other words, gluten itself may not be causing gut symptoms at all.

Most people who are sensitive to wheat are sensitive to a variety of other foods too. For example, two-thirds of people with wheat sensitivity have also been found to be sensitive to cow's milk protein. Eggs appear to be the next leading culprit.[2903] If people are put on a diet low in common triggers of irritable bowel symptoms and *then* challenged with gluten, there's no effect, calling into question the existence of non-celiac gluten sensitivity.[2904]

Interestingly, despite being informed that avoiding gluten was apparently not helping their gut symptoms, many participants opted to continue following a gluten-free diet, as they subjectively described "feeling better." This led the researchers to wonder if avoiding gluten might improve the mood of those with wheat sensitivity and, indeed, short-term exposure to gluten appeared to induce feelings of depression in these patients.[2905] Regardless of whether non-celiac gluten sensitivity is a disease of the mind or the gut, it is no longer considered a condition that can be dismissed.[2906]

The next question, then, is what percentage of the population should avoid wheat and other gluten-containing grains? About one in a thousand may have an allergy to wheat,[2907] and nearly one in a hundred have celiac disease,[2908] which appears to be on the rise. Still, there's less than a one-in-ten-thousand chance that an American will be diagnosed with celiac disease in a given year.[2909] Our best estimate for the prevalence of wheat sensitivity is in the same general range of celiac disease: slightly higher than 1 percent.[2910] So only about 2 percent of the population appears to have a problem with wheat, but that's potentially millions of people who may have been suffering for years and could have been cured by simple dietary means, yet were unrecognized and not helped by the medical profession until recently.[2911]

For the 98 percent of people who don't have wheat issues, there is no evidence to suggest that following a gluten-free diet has any benefits.[2912] In fact, there is some evidence suggesting that a gluten-free diet may adversely affect gut health in people without celiac disease, wheat sensitivity, or wheat allergy. A month on a gluten-free diet was found to adversely affect gut flora and immune function, potentially setting up those on gluten-free diets for an overgrowth of harmful bacteria in their intestines.[2913] This is due, ironically, to the beneficial effects of the very components wheat-sensitive individuals have problems with, such as the "FODMAP" fructans that act as prebiotics and feed our good bacteria, or the gluten itself, which may boost immune function.[2914] Less than a week of added gluten protein may significantly increase natural killer cell activity,[2915] which could be expected to improve our body's ability to fight cancer and viral infections.

The greatest threat gluten-free diets may pose, though, is that they may undermine our ability to diagnose celiac disease, the much more serious form of wheat intolerance. Doctors diagnose celiac by looking for the inflammation caused by gluten in celiac sufferers, but if patients complaining of digestive problems go to the doctor having already eliminated much of the gluten in their diets, physicians might miss the disease.[2916] Why would getting a formal diagnosis matter if you're already on a gluten-free diet? First of all, it's a genetic disease, so you'll know to test your family. More significantly, though, many people on so-called gluten-free diets are not actually on truly gluten-free diets. Even twenty parts per million can be toxic to someone with celiac disease. Sometimes, even foods labeled "gluten-free" may not be safe for celiac sufferers.[2917]

What's the best course of action to take if you suspect you might be sensitive to gluten? First off, do *not* go on a gluten-free diet. If you suffer from chronic irritable bowel-type symptoms, such as bloating, abdominal pain, and irregular bowel habits, ask your doctor about getting a formal evaluation for celiac disease. If you have celiac, *then* go on a strict gluten-free diet. If you don't have the disease, the current recommendation is that you first try a healthier diet that includes more fruits, vegetables, whole grains, and beans, all the while avoiding processed foods.[2918] The reason people may feel better on a gluten-free diet—and therefore conclude they have a problem with gluten—is because they've suddenly stopped eating so much fast food and other processed junk. In other words, if you eat a deep-fried Twinkie and your stomach aches, it may not be the gluten.

If a healthier diet doesn't help, I suggest you try to rule out other causes of chronic gastrointestinal distress. When researchers have studied PWAWGs—that's what they're called in the medical literature: People Who Avoid Wheat and/or Gluten—they've found that about one-third of them didn't appear to have gluten sensitivity but instead had other conditions like an overgrowth of bacteria in their small intestines, were fructose or lactose intolerant, or had a neuromuscular disorder like gastroparesis or pelvic floor dysfunction.[2919] After each of these is ruled out as well, *then* I'd suggest people suffering from chronic, suspicious symptoms try a gluten-free diet.

No current data suggest that the general population should try to avoid gluten, but for those with celiac disease, a wheat allergy, or a wheat sensitivity *diagnosis*, gluten-free diets can be a lifesaver.[2920]

Eat Whole ... Within Minutes

Eating whole grains should be more than just replacing white bread with whole wheat and white rice with brown. There is a wonderful universe of whole grains out there. You may have tried quinoa, but what about kañiwa or fonio? Even wild rice (which is not actually even rice) may not sound as wild as the grain called *freekeh*. Have fun and try some amaranth, millet, sorghum, or teff to expand the amber waves of your horizon. Buckwheat is my mom's favorite.

As with vegetables, use color to make decisions at the supermarket. If you have a choice, pick red quinoa over white quinoa, blue sweetcorn over yellow, and yellow sweetcorn over white. Beyond just comparing antioxidant content, there's experimental evidence to suggest that pigmented rice—red, purple, or black—has benefits over brown. For example, in addition to having about five times more antioxidants,[2921] colored rice varieties have shown greater anti-allergy activity in vitro,[2922] as well as superior anticancer effects against breast cancer[2923] and leukemia cells.[2924]

For convenience's sake, there are a number of quick-cooking grains: Amaranth, millet, regular oats, quinoa, and teff can all be prepared in fifteen to thirty minutes. For grains that take longer, such as barley, rye, farro, or steel-cut oats, consider cooking a big pot in advance on the weekend so you can simply reheat for your meals throughout the week. Or get a rice cooker—you can buy one for less than twenty dollars. I use an electric pressure cooker to cook my weekly batch of groats in about a half hour. See Cooking Grains in the appendix for more guidance on preparing whole grains on the stove or in a multicooker.

Whole-wheat pasta cooks in about ten minutes. Improved production technologies have created a new generation of whole-grain pastas that no longer have the rough and mealy texture of yesteryear. Try it with one of my favorite sauces:

My Eight Check-Mark Pesto

40 g fresh basil leaves
30 g walnuts
2 cloves fresh garlic
¼ of a peeled lemon

¼ teaspoon lemon zest
½ cm fresh turmeric root (or ¼ teaspoon turmeric powder)
50 g pinto beans
60 ml water or liquid from bean can
1 tablespoon white miso
Pepper to taste

Combine all ingredients in a food processor. Blend until smooth. Scoop onto 200 grams of cooked whole-grain pasta.

Popcorn is a whole grain that takes less than five minutes to prepare. A hot-air popper is another inexpensive, useful appliance. There's an endless variety of savory, sweet, and spicy toppings to try. I used to use a combination of chlorella and nutritional yeast. (In my family, the green color earned it the name "zombie corn.") But due to evidence of contamination of chlorella with toxin-producing algae, I've since stopped using it. (See my video see.nf/chlorella for details.) I still use nutritional yeast, though. By lightly misting air-popped popcorn with a spray bottle, dry seasonings stick wonderfully. I like to spritz with malt vinegar, lime juice, or Tabasco. Be sure to stay away from artificial butter flavorings. Originally, we thought the artificial butter flavor chemical diacetyl was just an occupational health hazard, resulting in the deaths of workers who handled the chemical from a condition that became known as "popcorn lung."[2925] Now we know consumers are also at risk, given a case series of serious lung disease thought to be caused by butter-flavored microwave popcorn consumption.[2926]

There are even one-minute whole-grain options: fully precooked bowls and pouches of brown rice and quinoa that can be microwaved and don't even need to be refrigerated—just heat and eat.

Arsenic in Rice

You may have noticed brown rice was removed from my list of favorite grains. A few months after *How Not to Die* was originally published, the FDA released a risk assessment on how much cancer the arsenic in rice may be causing. I turned this concern into a thirteen-part video series on arsenic in food, released on NutritionFacts.org (starting with see.nf/arsenic), concluding that we should diversify our grains.

Arsenic is found naturally in the Earth's crust as well as unnaturally—from soil contaminated with historic use of arsenic-based pesticides[2927] or arsenic-containing drugs found in chicken manure used, in part, to pinken poultry.[2928] Rice plants accumulate arsenic up to ten times that of other grain crops.[2929] This is a concern since chronic consumption of arsenic can increase the risks of skin, bladder, liver, kidney, and lung cancers.[2930]

Conventionally, the "acceptable" risk of cancer-causing substances is an extra one-in-a-million chance of getting cancer. The FDA determined that eating a single serving of rice every day over a lifetime would cause an extra 136 cases of cancer per million people.[2931] I explain in the video series where to source lower-arsenic rice and how to cook rice (like pasta, in an abundance of water) to reduce the risk. Still, based on cancer risk, infants probably shouldn't regularly consume more than about a teaspoon of rice a day, children under three shouldn't regularly eat more than about a tablespoon a day, and adults should stick to under three tablespoons a day.[2932] I still eat rice on occasion, but day-to-day, I use other grains like sorghum or riced cauliflower as a substitute.

The Five-to-One Rule

If you buy packaged grain products, anything boasting labels like "multigrain," "stone-ground," "100% wheat," "cracked wheat," "seven-grain," or "bran" is likely *not* a whole-grain product. Those words are intended to distract you from the fact that the products are made from refined grains, not whole grains. Here, color may not help. Ingredients like "raisin juice concentrate" are used to darken white bread to make it look healthier. Even if the first word in the ingredients list is "whole," the rest of the ingredients could be junk.

I suggest using the Five-to-One Rule. When buying healthier, processed whole-grain products, look at the Nutrition Facts label on the package and see if the ratio of grams of carbohydrates to grams of dietary fiber is five or less. (See figure 8.) Does 100 percent whole-wheat Wonder Bread pass the test? Per serving, the package lists 30 grams of carbohydrates and 3 grams of fiber. Thirty divided by 3 is 10. Well, 10 is more than 5, so the 100 percent whole-wheat Wonder Bread goes back on the shelf even though, technically, it is a whole-grain product. Compare that to Ezekiel bread, a sprouted-grain bread. It has 15 grams of carbohydrates and 3 grams of fiber, and, just like that, passes the test. So do Ezekiel English muffins, which I love with fruit-only preserves and nut butter. Though the science on the potential benefits of sprouted grains is still in its infancy, available data look promising.[2933]

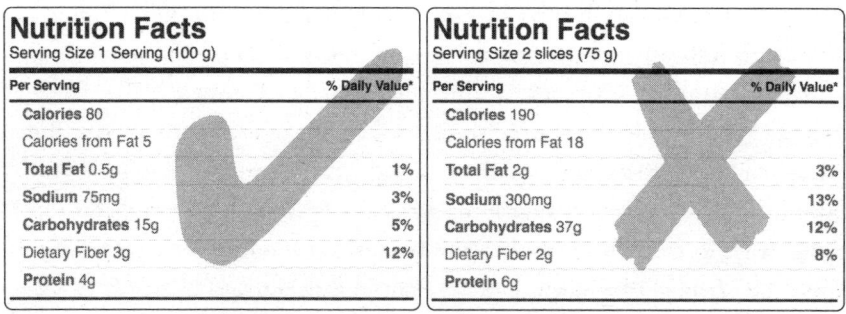

Figure 8

Apply the same Five-to-One Rule to breakfast cereals, another grocery category that can lull you into believing nearly everything is healthy. Multi-Grain Cheerios, for example, sounds good, but it has a ratio over 7. And then it just goes downhill from there with Frosted Cheerios and Fruity Cheerios, which have carbohydrate-to-fiber ratios that exceed 10. Compare that with Uncle Sam cereal, sliding in with a ratio under 4. Others that make the cut include some no-added-sugar puffed-grain cereals like puffed barley, but the healthiest whole grains are the least processed, the so-called intact grains.

Even though wheat berries, shredded wheat, whole-wheat flour, and puffed-wheat cereal may all be 100 percent whole wheat, they are handled by the body very differently. When grains are ground into flour or puffed, they are digested more rapidly and more completely. This increases their glycemic index and leaves fewer leftovers for the friendly flora down in our colon.

Researchers have experimented with this by splitting people into two groups. One group ate nuts, seeds, and beans that were more or less intact. The other group ate the same exact foods, but ground into flours and pastes. The first group ate nuts instead of nut butters, whole chickpeas instead of hummus, and muesli instead of muesli ground into a cream-of-wheat texture. Note that both groups were eating whole foods, just in different forms.

What happened? The intact-whole-grain group doubled their stool size, which was significantly greater than that of the ground-whole-grain group, even though they were eating the same foods in the same quantities.[2934] How is that possible? There is so much more left over for our gut flora to eat when we eat our grains intact. Few people realize that the bulk of stool is not undigested food but pure bacteria—trillions and trillions of bacteria.[2935] That may be why we get an increase of nearly 60 grams of stool for every 30 grams of fiber we eat. That's not just water weight—we're feeding our good bacteria so they can be fruitful and multiply.[2936]

As the study demonstrated, when we eat intact grains, even if we chew our food thoroughly, pieces of whole seeds and grains transport starch and other beneficial bits all the way down to our colon for our flora to feast on.[2937] But when grains are unnaturally processed into flour, almost all the starch is digested in the small intestine, and we end up starving our microbial self. When that happens regularly, it can result in *dysbiosis*, an imbalance in which bad bacteria can take over and increase our susceptibility to inflammatory diseases or colon cancer.[2938] The moral of the story: Whole grains are great, but intact whole grains may be even better.

Instead of a puffed barley cereal, how about just barley? Barley for breakfast may sound strange, but warm bowls of grains are traditional breakfast foods in many parts of the world. There are savory versions, or you can sweeten it up with fresh, frozen, dried, or freeze-dried berries. There are online sites where you can buy freeze-dried strawberries in bulk for less than a dollar per 20 grams.

Oats

Oatmeal, of course, is the classic whole-grain breakfast. Just as cruciferous vegetables and flaxseeds harbor beneficial compounds found in abundance nowhere else, oats contain a unique class of anti-inflammatory compounds called *avenanthramides*. They're thought to be responsible in part for the fresh odor and flavor of oats[2939] as well as the ability of oatmeal lotion to relieve skin itching and irritation.[2940] Studies on human skin fragments from plastic surgery that were subjected to inflammatory chemicals reveal that oatmeal extract can suppress inflammation[2941]—so much that oatmeal now appears to be the treatment of choice for certain serious chemotherapy-induced skin rashes.[2942] Ironically, two of the cancer cell lines found to be resistant to that type of chemotherapy[2943] were found to be sensitive to avenanthramides in vitro, suggesting that people should be applying oatmeal to their insides as well.[2944] Oatmeal is more than just a whole grain.[2945]

Oatmeal is my go-to breakfast when I travel. If there isn't a nearby Starbucks where I can pick up some oatmeal, I prepare instant oatmeal with dried fruit in the coffeemaker in my hotel room or a just-add-hot-water pouch of Leafside, a brand of whole food, plant-based, freeze-dried meals based on my Daily Dozen. (As always, I have never and will never accept money for product endorsements.) At home, if you want to spice up your oatmeal routine, google "savory oatmeal" for all sorts of interesting dishes involving sautéed mushrooms, herbs, spinach, curry, roasted vegetables—you name it!

The Daily Dozen calls on you to eat three servings of whole grains a day. This might seem like a lot, but when you look at the actual size of those recommended servings, it'll be a snap for you to succeed. Just one pasta dish at an Italian restaurant may average the equivalent of six servings, for instance.[2946] A morning oatmeal habit is a great way to kick-start your day, and then there are a variety of quick-cooking whole grains that serve as convenient, filling ways to fight chronic disease risk all day long.

Beverages

My Favorite Beverages

Black tea, chai tea, vanilla chamomile tea, coffee, earl grey tea, green tea, hibiscus tea, hot chocolate, jasmine tea, lemon balm tea, matcha tea, oolong tea, peppermint tea, rooibos tea, water, and white tea

Serving Size:
1 glass (12 ounces / 350 ml)

Daily Recommendation:
5 servings per day

There are plenty of dietary guidelines for eating, but what about for drinking? The Beverage Guidance Panel was assembled to provide "recommendations on the relative health and nutritional benefits and risks of various beverage categories." The panel included such heavyweights as Dr. Walter Willett, former chair of the nutrition department at Harvard University School of Public Health and professor of medicine at Harvard Medical School.

The panel's nutrition experts ranked beverage categories on a six-tier scale from best to worst. Unsurprisingly, fizzy drinks ranked last. Whole milk, meanwhile, was grouped with beer, with a recommendation for zero milliliters a day. Their justification included concerns about links between milk and prostate cancer, as well as aggressive ovarian cancer, perhaps "related to its well-documented effect on circulating concentrations of insulin-like growth factor 1." (See chapter 14.) Tea and coffee—preferably without creamer or sweetener—tied as the number two healthiest beverages, second only to water, the top-ranked drink.[2947]

Water

More than two thousand years ago, Hippocrates said, "If we could give every individual the right amount of nourishment and exercise, not too little and not too much, we would have found the safest way to health."[2948] Water is the healthiest beverage to drink—but how much is too little, and how much is too much? Water has been described as a "neglected, unappreciated and under researched" subject,[2949] but many of the studies extolling the need for proper hydration have been funded by the bottled water industry.[2950] It turns out the oft-quoted "drink at least eight glasses of water a day" recommendation actually has little underpinning scientific evidence.[2951]

The eight-a-day recommendation can be traced back to a 1921 paper in which the author measured his own urine and sweat output and determined he lost about 3 percent of his body weight in water a day, which comes out to about eight cups.[2952] Consequently, for the longest time, water requirement guidelines for humanity were based on just one person's urine and sweat measurements.

But now there's actually extensive evidence suggesting that not drinking enough water may be associated with a variety of problems, including falls and fractures, heat stroke, heart disease, lung disorders, kidney disease, kidney stones, bladder and colon cancer, urinary tract infections, constipation, dry-eye disease, cavities, decreased immune function, and cataract formation.[2953] The problem with many of these studies, though, is that low water intake is also associated with several unhealthy behaviors, including low fruit and vegetable intake, more fast-food consumption, and even less "shopping at farmers markets."[2954] And think about it—who drinks lots of water? People who exercise a lot. So perhaps it's no wonder that heavy water drinkers have lower disease rates.

Only large and expensive randomized trials could definitively settle these questions. But given that water cannot be patented, such trials seem unlikely.[2955] As a result, we're left with studies that just link disease with low water intake. But are people sick because they don't drink enough water, or are they not drinking enough because they're sick? There have been a few large prospective studies in which fluid intake was measured before disease developed. For example, a Harvard University study of nearly forty-eight thousand men found that the risk of bladder cancer decreased by 7 percent for every extra 240 ml of fluid consumed daily. A high intake of water—say, two liters a day—may reduce the risk of bladder cancer by about 50 percent, potentially saving thousands of lives.[2956]

Probably the best evidence we have for a specific recommendation for how much water we should be drinking comes from the Adventist Health Study. Twenty thousand men and women were studied. Those who drank five or more glasses of water a day had about half the risk of dying from heart disease compared to those who drank two glasses or less daily. About half of the cohort consisted of vegetarians, so they were also getting extra water by eating more fruits and vegetables. As in the Harvard study, this protection remained even after controlling for other factors, such as diet and exercise, suggesting that water indeed was the cause, perhaps by lowering blood "viscosity" (that is, by improving blood flow).[2957]

If protection against cancer and heart disease isn't enough motivation, perhaps the prospect of being a better kisser will be. Brushing artificial skin against the lips of young women, researchers found that hydrated lips showed greater sensitivity to light touch.[2958]

Based on the best evidence to date, authorities from Europe, the U.S. Institute of Medicine, and the World Health Organization recommend about 2.0–2.7 liters of water a day for women and 2.5–3.7 liters a day for men.[2959] These recommendations include water from all sources, though, not solely beverages. We get about a liter from the food we eat and the water our body actually produces on its own,[2960] so these guidelines roughly translate into a daily recommendation for drinking 1–1.75 liters of water for women and 1.5–2.75 liters for men (assuming only moderate physical activity at moderate ambient temperatures).[2961]

We can also get water from all the other drinks we consume, including caffeinated beverages, with the exception of stronger alcoholic drinks like wines and spirits. Coffee,[2962] tea,[2963] and beer can leave us with more water than we started with, but wine actively dehydrates us.[2964] Note, though, in the cancer and heart disease studies mentioned earlier, the health benefits were almost exclusively associated with increased consumption of water, not other beverages. I address the problems with alcoholic drinks in chapters 8 and 12.

Bottom line: Unless you have a condition like heart or kidney failure or your physician otherwise advises you to restrict your fluid intake, I recommend you drink five glasses of tap water a day. I prefer tap not only because it's less economically and environmentally costly but because it may have less chemical, microbial,[2965] and microplastics[2966] contamination than bottled water.

Can Drinking Water Make Us Smarter?

Our brain is 75 percent water.[2967] When we become dehydrated, our brain actually shrinks.[2968] How might this affect brain function?

Based on urine samples obtained from groups of nine- to eleven-year-old kids in Los Angeles and Manhattan, nearly two-thirds of children may arrive at school in a state of mild dehydration,[2969] which may in turn negatively affect scholastic performance. If a group of schoolkids is randomly assigned to drink either one or zero cups of water before taking a test, guess which group does significantly better? The group given the water. These results, the researchers concluded, suggest that "even children in a state of mild dehydration, not induced by intentional water deprivation or by heat stress and living in a cold climate, can benefit from drinking more water and improve their cognitive performance."[2970]

Our hydration status may also affect our mood. Restriction of fluid intake has been shown to increase sleepiness and fatigue, lower levels of vigor and alertness, and increase feelings of confusion. But as soon as study participants are allowed to drink again, the deleterious effects on alertness, happiness, and clarity of thought are almost immediately reversed.[2971] Water absorption begins very rapidly, within five minutes from mouth to bloodstream, peaking around minute twenty.[2972] Interestingly enough, cold water gets absorbed about 20 percent faster than body-temperature water.[2973]

How can you tell if you're dehydrated? Just ask your body. If you drink some water and pee most of it out soon after, this would be your body's way of saying it was all topped off. But if you drink a bunch of water and your body keeps most of it, then your tank was running low. Researchers used this concept to develop a formal dehydration assessment tool: Empty your bladder, drink three cups of water, and then see how much you pee an hour later. They determined that if you drink three cups and urinate less than one cup within that hour, there's a good chance you were dehydrated.[2974]

But water can be so *boring*. So try adding fresh fruits or veggies as they do in posh spas and upscale hotels. I like adding frozen strawberries in place of ice cubes. Sometimes I add a few drops of a potent juice concentrate, like tart cherry or pomegranate. Cucumber slices, ginger shavings, a cinnamon stick, lavender, and a mint leaf or two are also common refreshing additions. My latest favorite flavor fusions involve mixing tangerine slices and fresh basil or frozen blackberries and fresh sage.

Bubbles! One of my former work colleagues had a SodaStream on his desk, and he made his own sparkling water for about twenty-five cents a cup. In addition to making water more interesting, carbonation may also help relieve gastrointestinal symptoms. A randomized trial of the effects of sparkling versus still water found that drinking carbonated water may improve symptoms of constipation and dyspepsia, including bloating and nausea.[2975]

What if you took water and added beans or greens—that is, coffee beans or tea leaves? Wouldn't you get all the water you need plus a bonus of additional nutrients? A cup of black coffee, tea, or herbal tea only has two calories, potentially offering nutrition at little caloric cost. Think of healthy beverages as the opposite of junk food: Junk food offers calories with scarce nutrition, whereas healthy beverages offer nutrition with scarce calories. But just how healthy are coffee and tea?

Coffee

I have already discussed the benefits of coffee for the liver (chapter 8), mind (chapter 11), and brain (chapter 13). What about overall longevity? Do people who drink coffee live longer lives than people who don't?

Interventional studies on rats showing that coffee can improve lifespans go back to the 1940s.[2976] We only have observational research on coffee and mortality in humans, but, to date, more than twenty studies following more than ten million individuals over time have found that, overall, those drinking three cups of coffee a day had 13 percent lower risk of death from any cause.[2977] If practiced throughout adulthood, that would be expected to translate into approximately an extra year of life.[2978]

Three cups of decaf appeared to be just as protective, so it's not the caffeine.[2979] This is supported by data showing the longevity link extended similarly to those who were genetically slow caffeine metabolizers and others who metabolize caffeine more quickly.[2980]

Coffee is not for everyone, though. For example, be careful if you have gastroesophageal reflux disease (GERD). While a population study found no link between coffee consumption and subjective symptoms of GERD, such as heartburn and regurgitation,[2981] scientists who actually stuck tubes down people's throats to measure their pH found that coffee does seem to induce significant acid reflux, whereas tea does not. Caffeine does not appear to be the culprit, since caffeinated water doesn't cause a problem. However, the coffee decaffeination process seems to reduce the level of whichever compounds are responsible, since decaf coffee appeared to cause less reflux. The researchers advised that people who suffer from GERD should consider switching to decaf or—even better—drink tea instead.[2982]

People with glaucoma,[2983] or perhaps merely a family history of glaucoma,[2984] may also want to stay away from caffeinated coffee. And there are case reports of individuals with epilepsy having fewer seizures after laying off coffee, so avoiding it is certainly worth a try for people with seizure disorders.[2985] Finally, it almost goes without saying that people who have trouble sleeping might not want to drink too much coffee. Just a single cup at night can cause a significant deterioration in sleep quality.[2986]

The mystery as to why some studies showed that coffee consumption increased cholesterol and others did not was solved when it was discovered that the cholesterol-raising compound thought to be responsible was fat soluble. The culprit compound, cafestol, is found in the fines of coffee beans that become trapped in the paper filter, so drip coffee doesn't raise cholesterol as much as French press, boiled, or Turkish ("mud"-style) coffee. Neither the degree of roasting nor decaffeination appears to make a difference, though Robusta beans have less cafestol than Arabica beans. If you don't have optimal cholesterol levels, you should consider sticking to filtered coffee or using instant coffee, which also lacks these compounds.[2987] If these tweaks don't help, consider eliminating coffee completely, as even paper-filtered coffee may raise cholesterol levels a small amount.[2988]

We used to think caffeine might increase the risk of an irregular heart rhythm called *atrial fibrillation*, but this was based on anecdotal case reports involving the acute ingestion of very large quantities of caffeine[2989] (including a case blamed in part on a woman's "chocolate intake abuse"[2990]). As a result, the erroneous notion that caffeine ingestion may trigger abnormal heart rhythms became "common knowledge," an assumption that led to changes in medical practice. More recently, however, actual studies were performed that revealed caffeine intake does *not* appear to increase the risk of atrial fibrillation after all.[2991] If anything, regular coffee intake may have a protective effect on heart rhythm.[2992]

There are also consistent associations between drinking coffee and certain adverse outcomes during pregnancy, including miscarriage, early preterm birth, and low birth weight. Coffee consumption has not been linked to birth defects, but it may increase the risk of childhood leukemia.[2993]

Also, don't stick it up your butt. A recent review on the questionable safety of coffee enemas warned against their use, citing reports of colitis, electrolyte imbalance, rectal burns, and perforation.[2994]

Moderate caffeine consumption in healthy, nonpregnant adults is not only safe but has been found to increase energy and alertness and enhance physical, motor, and cognitive performance.[2995] Despite these benefits, one medical journal editorialized that doctors should "temper any message that suggests that caffeine is beneficial . . . given the proliferation of energy drinks that contain massive quantities of caffeine . . ."[2996] Indeed, drinking a dozen highly caffeinated energy drinks within a few hours could cause a lethal caffeine overdose.[2997]

Keep in mind that daily consumption of caffeinated beverages can lead to physical dependence. It's no coincidence that Americans alone spend nearly $75 billion annually on the stuff.[2998] Caffeine withdrawal symptoms can include days of headache, fatigue, difficulty concentrating, and mood disturbances.[2999] Ironically, coffee's tendency to be habit-forming could turn out to be a good thing. If coffee is indeed confirmed to induce a cellular rejuvenating process called autophagy and increase longevity as I detail in *How Not to Age*, then daily consumption may ultimately prove to be an advantage.[3000]

Coffee is health-promoting, but there may be an even healthier beverage. Every cup of coffee is a lost opportunity for a cup of green tea.

Tea

Black, green, and white teas are all made from the leaves of the same evergreen shrub. Herbal tea, on the other hand, involves pouring hot water over any plant in the world *other* than the tea plant.

What's so special about the tea bush? Phytonutrients exclusive to the tea plant appear so powerful that they can reverse disease even when merely applied to the skin. For example, the topical application of green tea in ointment form on genital warts results in an astounding 100 percent clearance in more than half the patients tested.[3001] It's no wonder that this wonder treatment has been officially incorporated into the Centers for Disease Control STD Treatment Guidelines.[3002] There was even a remarkable case report of a woman whose skin cancers were apparently stopped with topical green tea application.[3003] If green tea can do that on the outside of our body, what might it be able to do internally?

I already discussed the role green tea may play in breast cancer prevention in chapter 12. Drinking tea may protect against gynecological malignancies, such as ovarian cancer[3004] and endometrial cancer,[3005] as well as lower our cholesterol,[3006] blood pressure,[3007] blood sugar,[3008] and body fat.[3009] It may protect the brain from both cognitive decline[3010] and stroke.[3011] Tea consumption is also associated with decreased risk of diabetes,[3012] tooth loss,[3013] and up to half the risk of dying from pneumonia.[3014] Those who suffer from seasonal allergies may also benefit from drinking tea. Randomized trials have shown that drinking about three cups of Japanese Benifuuki green tea per day starting six[3015] to ten[3016] weeks before pollen season significantly reduces allergy symptoms. That's nothing to sneeze at!

Riding the Waves

The invention of the electroencephalogram (EEG) to measure brain-wave activity has been described as "one of the most surprising, remarkable, and momentous developments in the history of clinical neurology."[3017] Scientists discovered that humans have four main mental states—two while sleeping and two while awake. Delta waves, in which our brain is electrically pulsing slowly at about one wave per second, are typically only seen in deep sleep. Then there's theta-wave sleep. At about five cycles per second, this mental state occurs when we're dreaming. The two waking states are alpha and beta. The alpha state is relaxed, aware, and attentive, such as when we close our eyes and meditate. Beta, meanwhile, is the stimulated, hustle-and-bustle state in which most of us live our lives.

Alpha, however, is where we want to be—fully alert and focused, yet calm. How do we get there? If we relax in a pleasant, peaceful place, after

> about ninety minutes, we can start to generate some significant alpha activity (though such practicing meditators as Buddhist monks can achieve this state much earlier and maintain it even with their eyes open). To acquire this talent, we could meditate every day for a few years—or we could just drink some tea. Within minutes of tea consumption, anyone may be able to attain that same relaxed but alert brain-wave pattern.[3018] That dramatic alteration in brain activity may explain why tea is the world's single most popular beverage after water.

Both white and green teas are less processed than black tea and are probably preferable.[3019] White tea is made from young leaves and is named after the silvery-white hairs on the immature buds; green tea is made from more mature leaves. Which tea is healthier? The answer seems to depend on whether you add lemon. If you drink your tea without lemon, green tea appears preferable to white tea. But if you add lemon, white tea jumps ahead.[3020] The reason is that while there are more phytonutrients in white tea, they may only be released at a certain pH level.[3021]

In terms of cancer prevention potential, both green and white teas have been shown to protect against DNA damage in vitro against PhIP, the cooked-meat carcinogen I described in chapter 12. White tea won out, though, blocking upward of 100 percent of DNA damage compared to green tea, which at the same concentration only blocked about half. The "potent antimutagenic activity of white tea in comparison with green tea" was achieved at a brewing time of one minute. For most of the teas tested, steeping longer than a minute had no additional effect. In terms of antioxidant activity, though, it may be better not to brew at all.[3022]

Cold-steeping is a popular way to prepare tea in Taiwan, especially during the summer months. Cold-steeped tea is not like conventional iced tea, in which you brew your tea hot and then cool it down. Rather, cold-steeping involves tossing the tea in cold water and letting it sit at room temperature or in the fridge for at least two hours. This method has been found to reduce the caffeine content and is said to reduce bitterness and improve the aroma.[3023] But what does cold-steeping do to the nutrient content? You would think that cold water wouldn't draw out as many antioxidants. After all, nutrient extraction is presumably the whole point of brewing tea with hot water, right? A group of scientists took it upon themselves to compare the antioxidant activity of hot-versus cold-steeped tea. Essentially, they mixed LDL cholesterol with free radicals and timed how long it took the cholesterol to oxidize in the presence of both hot- and cold-steeped tea.

In a surprise upset, cold-steeped white tea was significantly better at slowing down oxidation.[3024] (No significant effect of brewing temperature on the antioxidant activity of green tea was found.) The researchers surmised that traditional tea water is so hot that it manages to destroy some of the more sensitive antioxidants in white tea. Cold-steeping saves prep time and energy, and may even be healthier.

We don't have to care how much nutrition is extracted from tea leaves, though, if we simply eat them. Matcha is powdered green tea, produced by milling whole tea leaves into a fine powder that can be added straight to water. Why waste nutrition by dumping a tea bag when we're done, when we can drink the leaves instead? Think of it this way: Drinking steeped tea is akin to boiling a pot of collard greens and then throwing away the veggies and just drinking the cooking water. Sure, some of the nutrition leached into the water, but wouldn't it be better to eat the leaves themselves? That's why I now just throw whole tea leaves straight into my smoothies. (See page 426.) This is also a great way to incorporate tea in our diet if drinking tea on an empty stomach causes discomfort. If you develop a taste for matcha (I find it a bit grassy), you can carry around little packets of it wherever you go and just put some in your water bottle and shake. For essentially zero calories, you can drink dark green leafy vegetables all day.

If you want to get into a matcha habit, I would suggest favoring matcha sourced from Japan rather than China to minimize your lead exposure.[3025] Very little lead leaches out of steeped green tea leaves, so the country of origin of steeped tea is less important than when you're actually *eating* the leaves.[3026] Also, because you're consuming the whole leaf when you drink matcha, just one cup can have nearly as much caffeine[3027] as a shot of espresso.[3028]

There is one tea beverage I'd stay away from. Based on a few cases of serious, life-threatening outcomes linked to kombucha, a type of fermented tea, the consumption of kombucha "should be discouraged," according to one case report of a person who ended up in a coma after drinking it.[3029]

Are there any caveats to regular tea consumption? The fluoride content of tea appears to be the limiting factor. The tea plant naturally concentrates fluoride from the soil, which is one of the reasons drinking tea may help fight cavities,[3030] but too much fluoride can be toxic. A case reported in *The New England Journal of Medicine* described a woman who started experiencing bone pain after seventeen years of habitually consuming a pitcher of tea made from 100 to 150 tea bags daily.[3031] That's too much.

To prevent skeletal fluorosis, adults should probably not drink more than about twenty tea bags' worth of black tea a day for twenty years straight, or thirty bags of green tea daily, or eighty bags of white tea a day.[3032] To prevent dental fluorosis, a harmless but unsightly mottled tooth discoloration, children should probably refrain from drinking more than about three bags of black tea a day (or around four bags of green tea or twelve of white)[3033] while their teeth are still developing, up until around age nine.[3034]

My Hibiscus Punch

In 2010, an antioxidant analysis of three hundred different beverages was published, examining everything from Red Bull to red wine.[3035] And the winner? Hibiscus tea! I documented its potent antihypertensive effects in chapter 5. I've always had "normal" blood pressure by U.S. standards, but I wanted to shoot for optimal, so hibiscus became a daily staple for me.

Give this recipe a try: To two liters of water, add a handful of bulk dried hibiscus or four bags of tea in which hibiscus is the first ingredient. Then add the juice of one lemon and three tablespoons of date powder, then leave it in your fridge to cold-steep overnight. In the morning, strain out the hibiscus or take out the tea bags, shake well, and drink throughout the day.

For extra credit, add green foam: Pour a cup of the tea into a blender with several fresh mint leaves, blend on high, and enjoy. You end up with dark green leafies blended into what may be the highest antioxidant beverage in the world, and it tastes like fruit punch. Delicious at any age!

As with any sour food or beverage, make sure to rinse your mouth with water after consumption to prevent the natural acids from dissolving your enamel.[3036] Do *not* brush your teeth within an hour after eating or drinking something sour, as your enamel may be in a softened state and be further damaged by brushing.[3037] If you sip continuously throughout the day, I suggest using a straw to bypass your teeth.[3038]

The Best Sweetener

In chapter 11, I shared research suggesting that adding sugar may negate some of the benefits of beverages, while adding artificial sweeteners like aspartame or sucralose may even make things worse. Are there any health-promoting sweeteners? The only two concentrated, green-light sweeteners may be blackstrap molasses and date sugar. Other natural caloric sweeteners, such as honey, less processed cane sugars, and maple, agave, and brown rice syrups don't appear to have much to offer nutritionally.[3039] Date sugar is a whole food—just dried dates ground up—as are date and prune pastes, which can be homemade or purchased. These are all good options for baking, but for sweetening drinks, the taste of molasses may be too strong, and granular date sugar doesn't fully dissolve. But you can also buy date powder, which is more finely ground and dissolves quite well. That's what I use in my coffee.

How about stevia? During the 1990s, research out of Japan found that steviosides, the "active" ingredient in stevia, appeared harmless. But in the guts of rats, intestinal bacteria transformed steviosides into a toxic substance called *steviol*, which can cause a big spike in mutagenic DNA damage in vitro.[3040] Unfortunately, it turns out that humans have the same bacterial activity in their guts.[3041] It's the dose that makes the poison, though. The World Health Organization considers up to 1.8 mg of stevia compounds per pound of body weight to be a safe amount. Given the American sweet tooth, if we sweetened everything with stevia, we could exceed that safety limit. But just drinking up to two stevia-sweetened beverages a day should be considered harmless from a steviol standpoint.[3042]

When people were randomized to drink beverages sweetened with aspartame, monk fruit, or stevia instead of sixteen spoonsful of sugar[3043] (the amount of added sugar in a 20 oz bottle of Coke[3044]), they were all found to be equally bad when it came to calorie intake, blood sugars, or insulin spikes throughout the day.[3045] Similar results were found for Splenda (sucralose).[3046] How is that possible? The mystery is solved in my video see.nf/sweeteners.

The sugar alcohols sorbitol and xylitol largely aren't absorbed by the body and end up in the colon, where they can draw in fluid and cause diarrhea. This is why they're only used commercially in small quantities, such as in mints or chewing gum, as opposed to beverages.

A related compound, however, erythritol, is absorbed and offered the potential for the harmlessness of xylitol without the laxative effect—until 2023, that is, when a prestigious lab out of the Cleveland Clinic raised the disturbing possibility that erythritol causes increased clotting susceptibility in human blood.[3047] I immediately stopped consuming anything with erythritol and encouraged everyone to do the same. Since then, the prothrombotic (blood-clot forming) concerns have been confirmed in human volunteers[3048] and extended to other sugar alcohols, such as xylitol.[3049]

Sugar-Free, but Not Risk-Free

Over the years, numerous large-scale studies have found a correlation between artificial-sweetener use and weight gain.[3050] The most common explanation for this counterintuitive finding is reverse causation: People aren't overweight because they drink diet fizzy drinks; they drink diet fizzy drinks because they're overweight.

But there are at least three other less benign alternative explanations. The first involves maintaining cravings for, and dependency on, all things sweet. By continuing to consume any sweeteners—with or without calories—we are unable to train our flavor preferences away from intensely sweet foods.[3051] This can lead to making less-than-healthy eating choices. With great sweetness comes great responsibility.

The second way diet fizzy drinks could counterintuitively lead to weight gain is called "overcompensation for expected caloric reduction." If people's fizzy drinks are covertly switched with diet versions without their knowledge, their caloric intake drops.[3052] This makes sense, since they're not drinking all that sugar anymore. But people who *knowingly* consume artificial sweeteners may actually end up eating *more* calories; they may figure after their zero-calorie drink, they can indulge in that second piece of pie. Indeed, that's what studies have shown. For example, when researchers gave participants an aspartame-sweetened cereal for breakfast, but only informed half that the sweetener was artificial, when lunchtime came, the aspartame-informed group ended up eating significantly more than the aspartame-naïve group.[3053] I think of this concept anytime I see someone at a fast-food restaurant ordering a diet fizzy drink with their meal.

A second explanation for gaining weight while using artificial sweeteners is based on how humankind evolved: When our brain registers the sensation of sweetness on our tongue, millions of years of evolution remind our brain to boost our appetite to eat as much as possible—after all, naturally sweet plant foods like fruits or sweet potatoes are among the healthiest. When we drink a can of diet fizzy drink, our brain thinks we just stumbled across something wonderful, like a wild blueberry bush, and it sends urgent signals to eat large and eat fast before someone else gets wind of our bounty. At the same time, our body knows that if we eat too many calories, we might get too heavy and not be able to outrun that saber-toothed tiger. So, when our gut senses that we've absorbed enough calories, it sends signals up to our brain to urge us to stop eating. When we ingest low-calorie sweeteners, however, we experience the familiar hunger-boosting effect due to the sensation of sweetness on our tongue, yet we may lack the hunger-suppressing effect of calories entering our gut. The result can be a revved-up appetite that can lead to eating more food than we otherwise would have.[3054]

Drink five glasses of water a day, be they plain tap water or flavored with fruits, tea leaves, or herbs. Keeping hydrated may elevate your mood (and vigor!), improve your thinking, and perhaps even help cut your risk for heart disease, bladder cancer, and other diseases. Cheers!

Exercise

Moderate-Intensity Activities

Bicycling; canoeing; dancing; doing housework, water aerobics, or gardening; downhill skiing; fencing; hiking; ice-skating; in-line skating; juggling; jumping on a trampoline; paddleboating; playing dodgeball, Frisbee, or tennis (doubles); practicing yoga; roller-skating; shooting baskets; shoveling light snow; skateboarding; snorkeling; surfing; swimming recreationally; treading water; walking briskly (4 mph or 6.5 km/h); and waterskiing

Vigorous Activities

Backpacking; bicycling uphill; circuit weight training; cross-country skiing; doing jumping jacks, pull-ups, push-ups, or step aerobics; jogging; jumping rope; playing basketball, football, hockey, lacrosse, racquetball, rugby, soccer, squash, or tennis (singles); rock climbing; running; scuba diving; speed skating; swimming laps; walking briskly uphill; and water jogging

Serving Sizes:
90 minutes of moderate-intensity activity
40 minutes of vigorous activity

Daily Recommendation:
1 serving per day

Nearly three-quarters (73.6 percent) of American adults are overweight.[3055] Think about that. Only about one in four maintain a healthy weight.

What's more, it's been predicted that by 2030, more than *half* the country's population will be clinically obese.[3056] (As of 2023, we were at 40.3 percent.[3057]) Since the 1970s, childhood obesity has quadrupled,[3058,3059] and most overweight kids will continue to be overweight into adulthood.[3060] As mentioned earlier, we may be in the process of raising the first generation of children in America with a shorter predicted lifespan than their parents.[3061]

The food industries like to blame inactivity as the prime cause of obesity, not the promotion and consumption of their calorie-rich products.[3062] On the contrary, however, research suggests that the level of physical activity may have actually *increased* in the United States over the past several decades.[3063] We know that obesity is rising even in areas where people are exercising more.[3064] This is likely explained by the fact that eating activity levels are outstripping physical activity levels.[3065]

Compared to eating habits in the 1970s, every day, children are consuming the caloric equivalent of an extra can of fizzy drink and small fries, and adults are eating an extra Big Mac's worth of calories. Just to make up for the extra calories Americans are taking in compared to a few decades ago, as a nation, we'd need to walk an extra two hours a day, every day of the week.[3066]

Surveys suggest that most people believe controlling diet and getting enough exercise are equally important for weight control.[3067] It's a lot easier to eat, however, than to move. To walk off the calories found in a single pat of butter or margarine, we'd have to add about an extra half mile to our evening stroll. For every additional sardine on our Caesar salad, that's another quarter-mile jog. If we eat two chicken legs, we'll need to get up on our own two legs and run three miles just to make up for it—and that's stewed chicken, skin removed.[3068]

Researchers who accepted grants from the Coca-Cola Company[3069] call physical inactivity "the biggest public health problem of the 21st century."[3070] Actually, physical inactivity ranks down at number fourteen in terms of risk factors for death in the United States and number thirteen in terms of risk factors for disability.[3071] And inactivity doesn't even make the top fifteen globally.[3072] A fridge kills more than ten times more than the couch.[3073]

Of course, that doesn't mean we should sit around all day. As we've seen in this book, in addition to helping us enjoy a healthy body weight, exercise can also ward off and possibly reverse mild cognitive decline, boost our immune system, prevent and treat high blood pressure, and improve our mood and quality of sleep, among many other benefits. If the U.S. population collectively exercised enough to shave just 1 percent off the national body mass index (BMI), 2 million cases of diabetes, 1.5 million cases of heart disease, and up to 127,000 cases of cancer might be prevented.[3074]

Stand Up for Our Health

It turns out your mom and dad were right about the hazards of watching too much television—although it may not rot the brain so much as the body. Based on a study of about nine thousand adults followed for seven years, researchers calculated that every additional hour spent watching TV per day may be associated with an 11 percent increased risk of death.[3075] Screen time in general—including playing video games—appears to be a risk factor for premature death.[3076] So does that mean we have to kill our TV and PlayStation before they kill us?

It's not the electronics themselves but the sedentary behavior associated with enjoying them. Of course, not all sedentary behaviors are bad.[3077] Consider sleeping—we can't be more sedentary than that! The problem appears to be sedentary *sitting*. After tracking the health of more than one hundred thousand Americans for fourteen years, an American Cancer Society study found that men who sit for six hours or more per day have a 20 percent higher overall death rate compared to men who sit for three hours or less, while women who sit for more than six hours have a 40 percent higher death rate.[3078] A meta-analysis of forty-three such studies found that excess sitting was associated with a shorter lifespan,[3079] and this may be "regardless of physical activity level." In other words, people who religiously hit the gym after work may still have shortened lifespans if they are otherwise sitting throughout the day. Sitting for six or more hours a day appears to increase mortality rates even among people who run or swim for an hour a day, every day, seven days a week.[3080]

I'm not saying we should all quit our desk jobs, but there are other options. For instance, try switching to a standing desk, which elevates the heart rate and may burn as many as fifty extra calories per hour. This may not seem like a lot, but simply standing for three hours a day at work equates to about thirty thousand extra calories burned per year—the equivalent of running ten marathons.[3081] Whether you're at the office, reading the newspaper at home, or, yes, even watching TV, why not find a way to stand while doing it? In fact, most of this book was written while I was walking fifteen miles a day on a treadmill underneath my standing desk. Prebuilt treadmill desks are expensive, but thrift stores are often awash with old exercise equipment. Before upgrading, my treadmill "desk" was just a treadmill slid under some cheap plastic shelving.

If you have been sedentary for a long time, start out slowly. I'm sure you've heard the familiar refrain: "Before starting this or any other exercise program, be sure to check with your doctor." This is definitely true for vigorous exercise, but most people can safely start to take up walking ten or fifteen minutes a few times a day. If, however, you are a man over the age of forty-five or a woman over fifty-five, have diabetes, or experience symptoms such as chest pain, dizziness, or shortness of breath, I would recommend checking with your health professional before starting a new exercise regimen.[3082]

What If You Really Have to Sit All Day?

Why is sitting around so bad for us? One reason may be endothelial dysfunction, the inability of the inner lining of our blood vessels to signal our arteries to relax normally in response to blood flow. Just as our muscles atrophy if we don't use them, "use it or lose it" may apply to arterial function as well. Increased blood flow promotes a healthy endothelium.[3083] Blood flow is what maintains the stability and integrity of the inner lining of our arteries. Without that constant tugging flow with each heartbeat of exertion, we can end up a sitting duck for arterial dysfunction diseases.

What if sitting all day is part of your job? Research suggests treadmill desks may improve the health of office workers without detracting from work performance,[3084] but your office might not accommodate a standing desk. Preliminary evidence from observational[3085] as well as interventional[3086] studies suggests that regular interruptions in sitting time can be beneficial. And they don't have to be long. Breaks could be as short as one minute and not necessarily entail strenuous exercise—just walking up and down stairs may be enough. Another option at a sedentary workplace is to opt for "walking meetings" rather than traditional sit-downs.

What if you have a sitting job in which you can't take frequent breaks, like truck driving? Is there any way to improve your endothelial function sitting on your butt? First you need to get rid of any butts—cigarette butts, that is. Smoking a single cigarette can significantly impair endothelial function.[3087] Diet-wise, drinking green tea every two hours can help keep your endothelium functional,[3088] as can eating meals with greens and other nitrate-rich vegetables. (See chapter 5.)

Turmeric may also help. One head-to-head study found that daily ingestion of the turmeric component curcumin can improve endothelial function just as well as up to an hour a day of aerobic exercise.[3089] Does that mean we can just be a couch potato as long as we eat curried potatoes? No, we still need to move around as much as possible—the combination of curcumin *and* exercise appears to work even better than either option alone.[3090]

Treating Sore Muscles with Plants

Optimizing recovery from exercise is considered the holy grail of exercise science.[3091] Anyone who works out regularly knows about sore muscles. There's the burning sensation during strenuous exercise, which may be related to the buildup of lactic acid in your muscles, and then there's delayed-onset muscle soreness, the kind you get in the days following extreme physical activity. Delayed soreness is likely the result of inflammation caused by microtears in your muscles and can adversely affect athletic performance in the days following a heavy workout. If you're suffering from an inflammatory reaction, might anti-inflammatory phytonutrients help? The bioflavonoids in citrus can help with the lactic acid buildup,[3092] but you may need to ramp up to the anthocyanin flavonoids in berries to deal with the inflammation.

Muscle biopsies of athletes have confirmed that eating blueberries, for example, can significantly reduce exercise-induced inflammation.[3093] Studies using cherries show that this anti-inflammatory effect can translate into faster recovery time, reducing the strength loss from excessive bicep curling from 22 percent down to only 4 percent in male college students over the subsequent four days.[3094] The muscle-soothing effects of berries don't only work for weight lifters; follow-up studies have shown that cherries can also help reduce muscle pain in long-distance runners[3095] and aid in recovery from marathons.[3096]

Eating 300 grams of watermelon prior to intense physical activity was also found to significantly reduce muscle soreness. The researchers concluded that functional compounds in fruits and vegetables can "play a key role in the design of new natural and functional products" like beverages, juices, and energy bars.[3097] But why design *new* products when nature has already designed everything you need?

Preventing Exercise-Induced Oxidative Stress

As discussed in Part 1, when we use oxygen to burn fuel in our body, free radicals can be produced, just as cars burning fuel produce combustion by-products out the exhaust. This happens even if we're just idling, living our day-to-day life. What if we rev things up, start exercising, and really start burning fuel? Might we create more oxidative stress and therefore need to eat even more antioxidant-rich foods?

Studies have demonstrated that ultramarathoners show evidence of DNA damage in about 10 percent of their cells tested during[3098] and up to two weeks following[3099] a race. But most of us aren't ultramarathoners. Might short bouts of exercise still damage our DNA?

Yes. After just five minutes of moderate or intense cycling, we can get an uptick in DNA damage.[3100] Never ones to miss an opportunity, pharmaceutical and supplement companies have investigated ways to block exercise-induced oxidative damage with antioxidant pills, but, ironically, this may lead to a state of *pro*-oxidation. For example, guys doing arm curls taking about 1,000 mg of vitamin C ended up with *more* muscle damage and oxidative stress.[3101]

Instead of using supplements, what about using antioxidant-rich foods to douse the free radicals? Researchers led participants onto treadmills and cranked up the intensity until they nearly collapsed. While a spike in free-radical levels was witnessed in the control group, those who loaded up on watercress two hours before exercising actually ended up with fewer free radicals after the treadmill test than when they started. After two months of eating a daily serving of watercress, no DNA damage resulted, no matter how much it seemed the study participants were punished on the treadmill.[3102] So, with a healthy diet, we can get the best of both worlds—all the benefits of strenuous exercise without excess free-radical damage. As a review in the *Journal of Sports Sciences* put it, those who eat plant-based diets may naturally "have an enhanced antioxidant defence system to counter exercise-induced oxidative stress."[3103] Whether it's about training longer or living longer, the science seems clear. Our quality and quantity of life improves when we choose green-light foods.

How Much Should We Exercise?

In the United States, the current official physical activity guidelines recommend adults get at least 150 minutes a week of moderate aerobic exercise, which comes out to a little more than 20 minutes a day.[3104] That's actually down from previous recommendations from the surgeon general,[3105] the Centers for Disease Control and Prevention, and the American College of Sports Medicine,[3106] which called for a minimum of 30 minutes each day. The exercise authorities seem to have fallen into the same trap as the nutrition authorities, recommending what they think may be achievable, rather than simply informing us what the science says and letting us make up our own mind. They already emphasize that any physical activity is better than none,[3107] so why not stop patronizing the public and just tell everyone the truth?

It is true that walking 150 minutes a week is better than walking 60 minutes a week. Following the current recommendations for 150 minutes appears to reduce our overall mortality rate by 7 percent compared to being sedentary. Walking for only 60 minutes a week only drops our mortality rate about 3 percent, though. But walking 300 minutes a week drops overall mortality by *14 percent*.[3108] So walking twice as long—40 minutes a day compared to the recommended 20—yields twice the benefit. And an hour-long walk each day may reduce mortality by 24 percent.[3109] (I use walking as an example because it's an exercise nearly everyone can do, but the same goes for other moderate-intensity activities, such as gardening or cycling.[3110])

A meta-analysis of physical activity dose and longevity found that the equivalent of about an hour a day of brisk (4 mph or about 6.5 km/h) walking was good, but 90 minutes was even better.[3111] What about more than 90 minutes? Unfortunately, so few people exercise that much every day that there weren't enough studies to compile a higher category.

Mind Your Step

In the Sardinian blue zone, nonagenarians—those in their nineties—average about 12,000 steps a day just living their lives.[3112] Based on a representative sample of thousands of U.S. adults aged forty and older, those getting 12,000 steps a day had a 65 percent lower chance of dying over the subsequent decade compared to those only getting 4,000 daily steps. Even getting just 8,000 steps a day appeared to cut the risk of premature death in half.[3113]

A study of more than 15,000 older U.S. women with an average age of seventy-two found that even 4,400 steps a day also could reduce mortality rates compared to 2,700. This led a group of professors of exercise science to ask, "Is 4,400 steps per day the new 10,000 steps per day?"[3114]

Where did the recommendation for 10,000 steps a day even come from? Surprisingly, it likely originated arbitrarily as the brand name of a Japanese pedometer sold in 1965 called *Manpo-kei*, or "10,000 steps meter."[3115]

In terms of walking, the recommendation for 150 minutes a week of moderate intensity aerobic exercise converts into approximately 7,000 steps a day. The maximal longevity dose of around 90 minutes of exercise a day, which is technically 22.5 to 40 so-called MET-hours a week,[3116] would translate into walking about 30,000 steps a day.

If we know 90 minutes of exercise a day is better than 60 minutes is better than 30 minutes, why is the recommendation only 20 minutes? I understand that only about half of Americans even make the recommended 20 minutes a day,[3117] so the authorities are just hoping to nudge people in the right direction. It's like the dietary guidelines advising us to "eat less candy." If only they'd just give it to us straight.

That's what I've tried to do in this book.

Conclusion

My friend Art was one of those guys you just wanted to be around. Successful, generous, kind, and hilarious, he was more than the public face of the natural foods business empire that he had started. He truly walked the walk, or rather, ran the run. An avid snowboarder and mountain biker, Art ate a whole food, plant-based diet for more than two decades. He was one of the healthiest guys I ever met.

He died while I was writing the first edition of this book.

At just forty-six years old, he was found dead in the shower of a health retreat he owned. My heart couldn't deal with the grief of losing my friend, so my head took over, my mind spinning with possible causes of his death. I thought that if I could figure out what had happened, I could give his family some closure.

I considered all the rare congenital heart disorders that can cause sudden death in young athletes. Maybe it was Brugada syndrome? I remembered there was a case of a marathon runner who had collapsed due to this rare genetic disorder,[3118] which can be triggered by heat.[3119] I looked it up, and indeed, there was a previous case tied to a hot bath,[3120] so it seemed plausible that this was what took Art's life.

The heat of the water was indeed the reason he'd died, but not in the way I had suspected. The sheriff called later that week to inform us that others had collapsed in the very same shower. These victims were medevacked to a nearby hospital and, thankfully, they survived.

It turned out that Art had died of carbon monoxide poisoning. A newly installed hot-water heater must not have been vented properly. It was an unbearable tragedy. I haven't been able to stop thinking about him, and it's been ten years since we lost him.

Art's passing made me realize that no matter how well we eat or how well we live, we can always get hit by a bus—metaphorically or literally. We need to make sure to look both ways in life and before crossing the street. We need to take care of ourselves. We need to wear seat belts and bike helmets and practice safer sex. (After all, practice makes perfect!)

And we need to make each day count by filling it with fresh air, laughter, and love—love for ourselves, for others, and for whatever we are doing with our one precious life. That's what Art taught me.

In Pursuit of Pleasure

The idea of preventive health is that we do something now so that nothing bad happens later. We floss our teeth not because it makes us feel better but because, by doing so, one day we won't feel worse. You could consider the healthy habits described in this book to be preventive—you eat a healthier diet now to avoid disease later.

A healthy diet, however, does more than that.

The food industries bank their billions by manipulating the pleasure centers within our brain, the so-called dopamine reward system. Dopamine is the neurotransmitter the brain evolved to reward us for good behavior, helping to motivate our drive for things like food, water, and sex—all necessary for the perpetuation of our species. This natural response has been and continues to be perverted for profit.

The food industry, like the tobacco companies and other drug lords, has been able to come up with products that tap into the same dopamine reward system that keeps people smoking cigarettes and snorting cocaine. People have chewed coca leaves for at least eight thousand years without any evidence of addiction,[3121] but a problem arises when certain components are isolated and concentrated into cocaine—when the coca leaves are *processed*. The same may be true for sugar. After all, few people binge on bananas. The isolation of sugar from the whole food may be the reason we're more likely to supersize fizzy drinks than sweet potatoes or why we're unlikely to eat too much corn on the cob but can't seem to get enough high-fructose corn syrup.

The overconsumption of sugar-sweetened foods has often been compared to drug addiction. Until recently, this parallel was based more on anecdotal evidence than on solid scientific grounds. But we now have PET scans, imaging technology that allows doctors to measure brain activity in real time. It all started with a study that showed decreased dopamine sensitivity in individuals with obesity. The more the individual being studied weighed, the less responsive to dopamine they appeared to be.[3122] We see the same reduction in sensitivity in cocaine addicts and alcoholics.[3123] The brain gets so overstimulated that it ends up trying to turn down the volume.

It was healthy and adaptive for our primate brains to drive us to eat that banana when there wasn't much food around, but now that fruit is available in Froot Loop form, this evolutionary adaptation has become a liability.[3124] The original Coca-Cola formulation actually included coca leaf, but now, perhaps, its sugar content may be the addictive stand-in.

The brain responds similarly to fat. Within thirty minutes of being fed yogurt packed with butterfat, research subjects exhibited similar brain activity[3125] to those who drank straight sugar water.[3126] People who regularly eat ice cream (sugar *and* fat) have a deadened dopamine response in their brains when drinking a milkshake. It's comparable to the way drug abusers have to use more and more drugs to obtain the same high. A neuroimaging study found that frequent ice cream consumption "is related to a reduction in reward-region [pleasure center] responsivity in humans, paralleling the tolerance observed in drug addiction." Once we've so dulled our dopamine response, we may subsequently overeat in an effort to achieve the degree of gratification experienced previously, contributing to unhealthy weight gain.[3127]

What do fatty and sugary foods have in common? They are both energy dense. It may be less about the number of calories than their concentration. Consumption of green-light foods, which are naturally calorie-dilute, doesn't lead to a deadened dopamine response, but a calorie-dense diet with the same number of calories does.[3128] It's like the difference between cocaine and crack: It's the same stuff chemically, but by smoking crack cocaine, a user can deliver a higher dose more quickly to their brain.

Given our new understanding of the biological basis of food addiction, there have been calls to include obesity as an official mental disorder.[3129] After all, both obesity and addiction share the inability to restrain behavior in spite of an awareness of detrimental health consequences, one of the defining criteria of substance abuse (a phenomenon referred to as the "pleasure trap").[3130] Of course, redefining obesity as an addiction would be a boon to the pharmaceutical companies that are already working on a whole array of drugs to muck with our brain chemistry.[3131]

For example, when researchers tried giving an opiate blocker to binge eaters (similar to how heroin addicts are sometimes treated with opiate blockers to minimize the narcotic's effects), the binge eaters ate significantly fewer fatty and sugary snacks—the snacks just didn't seem to do as much for them when their opiate receptors were blocked.[3132] In addition to new drugs, addiction specialists have urged that the food industry "should be given incentives to develop low calorie foods that are more attractive, palatable and affordable so that people can adhere to diet programs for a long time."[3133] No need—Mother Nature beat them to it. That's what the produce aisle is for.

Rather than taking drugs, we can prevent the numbing of our pleasure center in the first place by sticking to green-light foods. This can help return our dopamine sensitivity to normal levels so that we can again derive the same pleasure from the simplest of foods. When we regularly eat calorie-dense animal products and junk foods like ice cream, it's not just our taste buds that change but our brain chemistry. After eating a bunch of candy bars, not only may a ripe peach no longer taste as sweet on our tongue, but our brain downregulates dopamine receptors to compensate for the repeated jolts of fat and sugar. In fact, an overly rich diet could cause us to experience less enjoyment from other activities as well.

There is a reason cocaine addicts appear to have an impaired neurological capacity for sexual stimulation[3134] and why smokers have an impaired ability to respond to positive stimuli.[3135] Related brain circuits wire all these sensations. Since they all involve overlapping dopamine pathways, what we put into our body—what we eat and what we drink—can affect how we experience all of life's pleasures. Try it and see. Try it and *feel*.

Do you see where I'm going with this?

Eating a diet rich in whole plant foods and returning your brain's dopamine sensitivity to its healthy, normal levels can help you live life to the fullest and allow you to experience greater joy, satisfaction, and pleasure from all the things you do—not just what you eat.

Let Me Help

I hope I've been able to persuade you that nutrition is not the stale, lifeless subject your middle school health class may have led you to believe. It's vibrant and overflowing with opportunity for the betterment of your life. This abundance can create a problem, though. Over the last year alone, more than sixty-five thousand articles on nutrition were published in the medical literature. Who has time to sift through them all?

Every year, my team and I read through every issue of every English-language nutrition journal in the world, so you don't have to. Then I compile all the most interesting, groundbreaking, and practical findings we can uncover to create new videos and articles every day for my nonprofit site, NutritionFacts.org.

Everything on NutritionFacts.org is provided absolutely free of charge. There's no special member area where you pay a fee to get extra life-saving information. What membership websites seem to be saying, in essence, is that if you don't give them money, they'll withhold information that could make you and your loved ones healthier. That's unacceptable to me. Advances in health sciences should be freely available and accessible to all.

Since we refuse to sell products, advertisements, or endorsements, how do the bills get paid? NutritionFacts.org is a 501(c)(3) nonprofit organization that thrives on the Wikipedia model of simply accepting donations from visitors who appreciate the content. We reach so many millions of people that if even one in a thousand makes a small, tax-deductible contribution, we are able to pay for all the staff and server costs. The hope is to offer a public service so valuable that viewers will feel moved to support it and keep this life-changing, life-*saving* resource free for everyone for all time.

I welcome you to make NutritionFacts.org a part of your life. New videos are launched every week on the latest in evidence-based nutrition. You can sign up for daily, weekly, or monthly emails highlighting all the new, fun information, participate in exciting webinars, and join me in my monthly live Q&A. NutritionFacts.org exists to serve you.

Taking Responsibility

My goal is to give you the information to empower and inspire you to make healthy changes in your life, but in the end, it's all up to you. It's your body, your choice. Know, however, that there is only one way of eating that's ever been proven to reverse the progression of heart disease in the majority of patients, a diet centered around whole plant foods. Anytime anyone tries to sell you on some new diet, ask just one simple question: "Has it been proven to reverse heart disease?" (You know, the most likely cause of death for you and everyone you love?) If it hasn't, why would you even consider it?

If that's all a plant-based diet could do—reverse the number one killer of men and women, then shouldn't that be the default diet until proven otherwise? And the fact that it can also be effective in preventing, arresting, and reversing the progression of other leading killers, like high blood pressure, type 2 diabetes, and now maybe even early-stage Alzheimer's disease, would seem to make the case for plant-based eating simply overwhelming. Please give it a try.

It could save your life.

How Not to Die may seem to you a strange title for a book. After all, everyone is going to die eventually. This book is about how not to die *prematurely*. If there is one takeaway message, it's that you have tremendous power over your health destiny. The vast majority of premature deaths can be prevented with simple changes in what you eat and how you live.

In other words, a long and healthy life is largely a matter of choice. After Kim Williams became president of the American College of Cardiology, he was asked why he chose to eat a strictly plant-based diet. "I don't mind dying," Dr. Williams said. "I just don't want it to be my fault."[3136]

That's what this book is about: taking responsibility for your and your friends' and family's health.

Acknowledgments

For this tenth anniversary edition, I want to express special appreciation to my intrepid editor, Miyun Park, and exhaustive fact-checker, Alissa Finley.

Eternal thanks to the thousands upon thousands of individuals around the world who have donated to NutritionFacts.org to enable my work to reach millions. It's been such a dream to spend my days in service to others.

Though it was my grandmother who made me the doctor I am today, it was my mother who made me the person I am today.

I love you, Mom!

APPENDIX

Supplements

By getting our nutrients from green-light foods, not only will we minimize exposure to harmful food components, such as sodium, saturated fat, and cholesterol, but we will maximize our intake of nearly every required nutrient: vitamin A carotenoids; vitamin C; vitamin E; the B vitamins, including thiamin, riboflavin, and folate; magnesium, iron, and potassium; and, of course, fiber.[3137] Dietary quality rating scales consistently rank the most-plant-based diets as the most healthful.[3138]

That said, because of the way we live in our modern world, there are important shortfalls that need to be corrected.

For example, vitamin B12 is not made by plants; it's made by microbes that blanket the earth. But in this sanitized modern world, we now chlorinate the water supply to kill off any bacteria. While we don't get much B12 in the water anymore, we don't get much cholera, either, which is a very good thing. Similarly, we evolved to make all the vitamin D we need from the sun, but most of us are no longer running around naked in equatorial Africa. You may be covered up, inside, at a high northern latitude and therefore need to supplement your diet with this "sunshine vitamin." Thus, these two vitamins must be addressed.

2,000 mcg (μg) Vitamin B12 (Cyanocobalamin) Once a Week

Given modern sanitary standards, a regular, reliable source of vitamin B12 is *critical* for anyone eating a plant-based diet.[3139] Though deficiency for those starting out with adequate stores may take years to develop,[3140] the results of B12 deficiency can be devastating, with cases reported of paralysis,[3141] psychosis,[3142] blindness,[3143] and even death.[3144] Newborn infants of mothers who eat a plant-based diet and fail to supplement can develop deficiency much more rapidly with disastrous results.[3145]

For adults under age sixty-five, the easiest way to get B12 is to take at least one 2,000 mcg supplement each week. If you take too much, you merely get expensive pee. Well, not all that expensive: A five-year supply of vitamin B12 can cost less than twenty dollars. If you'd rather get into the habit of taking it daily, the once-a-day dosing is 50 mcg. Note that these doses are specific to cyanocobalamin, the preferred supplemental form of vitamin B12, as there is insufficient evidence to support the efficacy of the other forms, like methylcobalamin.[3146]

As we age, our ability to absorb vitamin B12 may decline.[3147] For those over sixty-five who eat plant-based diets, the supplementation should probably be increased from at least 2,000 mcg a week (or 50 mcg a day) up to 1,000 mcg of cyanocobalamin each day.[3148,3149]

Instead of taking B12 supplements, it's possible to get sufficient amounts from B12-fortified foods, but you would have to eat three servings a day of foods providing at least 2 mcg (85 percent of the Daily Value on the U.S. Nutrition Facts label).[3150] There are also green-light fortified sources (more at see.nf/b12), but for most people, it would probably be cheaper and more convenient to just take a supplement.

My other supplement recommendations in this section can be considered conditional, but getting enough vitamin B12 is absolutely nonnegotiable for those centering their diets around green-light foods.

Vitamin D from Sun or Supplements

I recommend that people unable to get sufficient sun take one 2,000 IU vitamin D3 supplement each day,[3151] ideally with the largest meal of the day.[3152]

In the Northern Hemisphere, below approximately 30° latitude (south of Los Angeles, Dallas, or Atlanta), fifteen minutes each day of midday sun on the forearms and face without sunblock should produce sufficient vitamin D for Caucasians under the age of sixty. Those who have darker skin[3153] or who are older[3154] may require thirty minutes or more.

Farther north, at 40° latitude (Portland, Chicago, or New York City), the sun's rays are at such an angle during the months of November through February that vitamin D may not be produced. No matter how long you might sunbathe naked in Times Square on New Year's Day, you may not make any vitamin D.[3155]

Above 50° latitude (around London, Berlin, Moscow, and Edmonton, Canada), this "vitamin D winter" may extend for as long as six months of the year.

Vitamin D supplements are therefore recommended for people at higher latitudes during the winter months and year-round for those not getting enough midday sun, regardless of location. This may also apply to those living in smoggy cities, such as Los Angeles or Beijing.[3156]

I do not recommend tanning beds. They can be both ineffective[3157] and dangerous.[3158] The lamps emit mostly UVA,[3159] which increases melanoma skin cancer risk without producing vitamin D.[3160]

Eat Iodine-Rich Foods

Iodine, a mineral essential for thyroid function, is found predominantly in the ocean and in variable amounts in the soils of the world. To ensure everyone was getting enough, table salt was fortified with the mineral starting in the 1920s. So if you do add salt to your food, use iodized salt (*not* sea salt or "natural" salt, which contains about sixty times less iodine[3161]). Given that sodium is considered the leading dietary killer in the world,[3162] however, iodized salt should be considered a red-light source.

There are two yellow-light sources of iodine: seafood and dairy milk. (Iodine leaches into the milk from iodine-containing antiseptic chemicals used to disinfect the cow's teats to prevent mastitis.[3163]) The most concentrated green-light source is seaweed, which has the iodine of seafood without the fat-soluble pollutants that build up in the aquatic food chain.

Sea vegetables are the underwater dark green leafies. I encourage you to experiment with ways to include them in your diet. The recommended daily intake of iodine is 150 mcg, which is what is in about two sheets of nori,[3164] the seaweed that's used to make sushi. There are all sorts of seaweed snacks on the market, but most, if not all of them, seem to have added red-light ingredients. So I buy plain nori and season the sheets myself by brushing them with jarred pickled ginger juice and lightly sprinkling on wasabi powder before recrisping them at 300°F (150°C) for about five minutes.

Sprinkling just half a teaspoon of the seaweeds arame or dulse onto dishes you're preparing may also get you your iodine for the day. Dulse is sold as pretty purple flakes you can just shake onto your food. I do caution *against* hijiki[3165] (also spelled *hiziki*), because it has been found to be contaminated with arsenic. I also caution against kelp, which may have *too much* iodine; just half a teaspoon of kelp could exceed the daily upper limit. For the same reason, you shouldn't get into a regular habit of eating more than fifteen sheets of nori or more than a tablespoon of arame or dulse a day.[3166] Too much iodine can cause excessive thyroid gland activity.[3167]

For those who don't like seaweed, Eden brand's canned beans have a tiny amount of kelp added such that iodine levels average between 36.3 mcg per 130 gram serving (great northern beans) to 71.2 mcg (haricot beans).[3168] Not only are those levels safe—you'd have to eat about twenty cans a day to get too much—but check-marking my three legume servings a day with Eden's beans would fulfill your daily iodine requirement.

One last note about iodine: Although people who avoid seafood and dairy products do not appear to have impaired thyroid function,[3169,3170] I would not leave it to chance during pregnancy, where iodine is critical for proper brain development.[3171] I agree with the American Thyroid Association's recommendation that all North American pregnant and breast-feeding women receive a prenatal vitamin containing 150 mcg of iodine daily.[3172]

Consider Taking 250 mg of Pollutant-Free (Algae-Derived) Long-Chain Omega-3s Daily

According to two of the most credible nutrition authorities, the World Health Organization and the European Food Safety Authority, we should get at least half a percent of our calories from the short-chain omega-3 ALA.[3173] That's easy—the one Daily Dozen tablespoon of ground flaxseeds takes care of that. Our body can then take the short-chain omega-3 from flaxseeds (or chia seeds or walnuts) and elongate it into the long-chain omega-3s EPA and DHA found in fish fat. The question, however, is whether our body can make enough for optimal brain health.[3174,3175] Until we know more, I recommend taking 250 mg of pollutant-free long-chain omega-3s directly.

I don't recommend fish oil, since even purified ("distilled") fish oil has been found to be contaminated with considerable amounts of PCBs and other pollutants, so much so that, when taken as directed, salmon, herring, and tuna oils would exceed the tolerable daily intake of toxicity.[3176] This may help explain the studies that found adverse effects of fish consumption on cognitive function in both adults and children. But many of those studies either were done downstream of a gold-mining area contaminated with mercury, which is used in the mining process,[3177] or included people who ate whale meat or fish caught next to chemical plants or toxic spills.[3178] What about fish you'd just get at a restaurant or supermarket?

An elite group of Floridians (mostly corporate executives) was studied. They ate so much seafood that at least 43 percent of them exceeded the U.S. Environmental Protection Agency's safety limit for mercury, and it appeared to have an effect. The researchers found that excessive seafood intake, which they defined as more than around three to four servings per month of such fish as tuna or snapper, elevates mercury levels and appeared to cause cognitive dysfunction. The effect wasn't large—only about a 5 percent drop in cognitive performance—but "a decrement [in executive function] that no one, let alone a health-conscious and achievement-oriented person, is likely to welcome."[3179]

Thankfully, we can get the benefits without the risks by getting long-chain omega-3s from algae-based supplements instead,[3180] which is where the fish primarily get it from to begin with.[3181] By cutting out the middle-fish and getting EPA and DHA directly from the source at the bottom of the food chain, we don't have to worry about pollutant contamination. In fact, the algae used for supplements are just grown in tanks and never even come in contact with the ocean.[3182] That's why I recommend a contaminant-free source to get the best of both worlds, omega-3 levels associated with brain preservation[3183] and minimized exposure to industrial pollutants.

What About . . . ?

All the other vitamins, minerals, and nutrients should be taken care of by the mountains of nutrition you'll be getting by centering your diet around whole plant foods. And many of those nutrients are ones people normally don't get in sufficient quantity—namely, vitamins A, C, and E and the minerals magnesium and potassium, along with fiber.[3184] At the same time, most people are getting too much saturated fat, sugar, and sodium.[3185] You, my friend, are going to be the one in a thousand who does it right.

If you have a specific question about some obscure nutrient—like, "What about my molybdenum or menaquinones?"—rather than have me bore everyone else with minutiae, allow me to refer you to NutritionFacts.org and an excellent reference book on plant-based nutrition by the preeminent dietitians Brenda Davis and Vesanto Melina.[3186] The authors go into great detail and even have chapters on pregnancy, breast-feeding, and raising bouncing boys and girls.

Vitamin B12-fortified plant-based diets can offer health benefits for all stages of the life cycle.[3187] Dr. Benjamin Spock, the most esteemed pediatrician of all time, wrote perhaps the bestselling American book of the twentieth century: *The Common Sense Book of Baby and Child Care*. In the seventh edition, the final one before Dr. Spock died at ninety-four, he advocated children be raised on a plant-based diet with no exposure to meat or dairy products. Dr. Spock had lived long enough to see the beginnings of the childhood obesity epidemic. "Children who grow up getting their nutrition from plant foods," he wrote, "have a tremendous health advantage and are much less likely to develop health problems as the years go by."[3188]

APPENDIX

Cooking Legumes

Excerpted from The How Not to Age Cookbook

Cooking legumes is fairly formulaic. It's a simple process that results in amazingly delicious—and healthful—food.

Generally, 1 cup (200g) of dried legumes yields about 3 cups (600g) cooked.

COOKING LEGUMES ON THE STOVETOP

When cooking on a stovetop, dried legumes—with the exception of lentils—benefit from soaking prior to cooking. Soaking rehydrates the legumes and shortens their cooking time. It also dissolves some of the complex sugars that cause digestive gas. Before soaking legumes, rinse them, then pick through to remove any small stones or other debris.

To soak the legumes, place them in a bowl with enough water to cover them by about 3 inches (10cm). Soak them overnight and drain before cooking. To quick-soak legumes, put them in a pot with enough water to cover by about 3 inches (10cm) and boil for 2 minutes. Remove the pot from the heat, cover, and let stand for 2 hours before draining. The quick-soaked legumes are then ready for cooking.

Cooking time may vary, depending on the type, quality, and age of the legumes, as well as the altitude at which you are cooking. Cooked legumes should be firm but tender. Once cooked, drain in a colander and rinse with cold water before using.

Cooked legumes will keep well in an airtight container in the refrigerator for up to 5 days or in the freezer for 3 months or longer.

STOVETOP COOKING TIMES FOR SOAKED LEGUMES

LEGUME	QUANTITY	WATER	COOKING TIME (IN MINUTES)
Black beans	1 cup (200g)	4 cups (1L)	50 to 60
Cannellini beans (white)	1 cup (180g)	4 cups (1L)	60
Chickpeas (garbanzo beans)	1 cup (200g)	4 cups (1L)	60 to 70
Great northern beans (white)	1 cup (180g)	3½ cups (875ml)	50
Kidney beans	1 cup (185g)	3½ cups (875ml)	50 to 60
Lentils (brown)*	1 cup (200g)	3 cups (700ml)	25 to 30
Lentils (black or green)*	1 cup (200g)	3 cups (700ml)	30
Lentils (red)*	1 cup (200g)	3 cups (700ml)	10 to 15
Pinto beans	1 cup (200g)	3½ cups (875ml)	50

* Note: Lentils do not require soaking.

COOKING LEGUMES IN A MULTICOOKER OR PRESSURE COOKER

If you have a large (6- to 8-quart/5.5- to 7.5-L) multicooker, such as an Instant Pot, or another pressure cooker, you can cook 1 pound (500g) of legumes at a time. (If you don't have one yet, give one a try. I'll bet you won't go back.)

Cooking time may vary, depending on the type, quality, and age of the legumes.

Rinse the dried legumes, then pick through to remove any small stones or other debris. Add the legumes to your cooker along with the water quantity specified in the following chart. There is no need to presoak any legumes when cooking in an Instant Pot.

Close and lock the lid. Set the valve on the lid to Sealing. Select the Pressure Cook function with High Pressure. Cook on high pressure for the directed time. Let the pressure release naturally for at least 20 minutes.

Remove the lid. The legumes should be firm but tender. Once cooked, drain in a colander and rinse with cold water before using.

Cooked legumes will keep well in an airtight container in the refrigerator for up to 5 days or in the freezer for 3 months or longer.

MULTICOOKER COOKING TIMES FOR UNSOAKED LEGUMES ON HIGH PRESSURE

LEGUME	QUANTITY	WATER	COOKING TIME (IN MINUTES)
Black beans	1 cup (200g)	3 cups (700ml)	25
Cannellini beans (white)	1 cup (180g)	4 cups (1L)	40
Chickpeas (garbanzo beans)	1 cup (200g)	4 cups (1L)	45
Great northern beans (white)	1 cup (180g)	3 cups (700ml)	35
Kidney beans	1 cup (185g)	3 cups (700ml)	30
Lentils (brown)	1 cup (200g)	2 cups (475ml)	8
Lentils (black or green)	1 cup (200g)	2 cups (475ml)	8
Lentils (red)	1 cup (200g)	1¾ cups (415ml)	5
Pinto beans	1 cup (200g)	3 cups (700ml)	25

APPENDIX

Cooking Whole Grains

Adapted from The How Not to Diet Cookbook

As with cooking legumes, cooking whole grains is nothing to fear. Whether on the stovetop or in a multicooker or pressure cooker, it's a snap to prepare perfectly cooked, wholesome whole grains.

Generally, 1 cup (180g) of uncooked whole grains yields about 3 cups (540g) cooked.

COOKING WHOLE GRAINS ON THE STOVETOP

Before cooking any grains, rinse them to remove loose hulls, dust, and other impurities. Longer-cooking grains, such as rye berries and oat groats, are best soaked overnight in a bowl with enough water to cover them by about 3 inches (10cm). The next day, drain before cooking.

To cook grains, add them to a pot and cover with 2 to 3 times as much water. (Adding extra water for longer-cooking grains will help keep them from scorching, and any excess water can be drained off.) Bring the water to a boil, then lower the heat to low, cover, and simmer until tender, for the average time specified in the following chart.

If the grains are not tender before the water is absorbed, add a little more water and continue to cook until the grains are to your liking. After cooking, remove the pot from the heat and let it stand, covered, for 5 to 10 minutes before serving. If any water remains in the pot, drain it off before serving. When ready to serve, fluff the grains with a fork.

Cooked grains will keep well in an airtight container in the refrigerator for up to 5 days or in the freezer for 3 months or longer.

STOVETOP COOKING TIMES FOR DRIED WHOLE GRAINS

GRAIN	QUANTITY	WATER	COOKING TIME (IN MINUTES)
Barley groats	1 cup (190g)	3 to 4 cups (700ml to 1L)	50 to 60
Millet	1 cup (200g)	2½ cups (600ml)	30
Oat groats	1 cup (180g)	3 to 4 cups (700ml to 1L)	50 to 60
Quinoa	1 cup (170g)	2 cups (500 ml)	15 to 20
Rye berries	1 cup (170g)	3 to 4 cups (700ml to 1L)	60
Sorghum	1 cup (190g)	3 to 4 cups (700ml to 1L)	50 to 60
Teff	1 cup (190g)	2 cups (500ml)	15 to 20

COOKING WHOLE GRAINS IN A MULTICOOKER OR PRESSURE COOKER

If you have a large (6- to 8-quart/5.5- to 7.5-L) multicooker, such as an Instant Pot, or another pressure cooker, you can cook 2 cups (360g) of grains at a time.

Before cooking any grains, rinse them to remove loose hulls, dust, and other impurities. There is no need to presoak any grains when cooking in an Instant Pot.

Add the grains and the water quantity specified in the following chart to your multicooker or pressure cooker. Close and lock the lid. Set the valve on the lid to Sealing. Select the Pressure Cook function with High Pressure.

APPENDIX: COOKING WHOLE GRAINS

Cook on high pressure for the directed time. Let the pressure release naturally for at least 20 minutes.

Remove the lid. The grains should be firm but tender.

If any water remains, drain the grains in a colander. When ready to serve, fluff the grains with a fork.

Cooked grains will keep well in an airtight container in the refrigerator for up to 5 days or in the freezer for 3 months or longer.

MULTICOOKER COOKING TIMES FOR DRIED WHOLE GRAINS ON HIGH PRESSURE

GRAIN	QUANTITY	WATER	COOKING TIME (IN MINUTES)
Barley groats	1 cup (190g)	3 cups (700ml)	20 to 30
Millet	1 cup (200g)	2 cups (500ml)	8 to 10
Oat groats	1 cup (180g)	3 cups (700ml)	20 to 30
Quinoa	1 cup (170g)	2 cups (500ml)	1
Rye berries	1 cup (170g)	3 cups (700ml)	20 to 30
Sorghum	1 cup (190g)	3 cups (700ml)	20 to 30
Teff	1 cup (190g)	2 cups (500ml)	2 to 3

Notes

1. How much does it cost to save a life? GiveWell. https://www.givewell.org/how-much-does-it-cost-to-save-a-life. April 2024. Accessed January 26, 2025.
2. Fallows ES. Lifestyle medicine: a cultural shift in medicine that can drive integration of care. *Future Healthc J*. 2023;10(3):226–31.
3. Katz DL, Frates EP, Bonnet JP, Gupta SK, Vartiainen E, Carmona RH. Lifestyle as medicine: the case for a True Health Initiative. *Am J Health Promot*. 2018;32(6):1452–8.
4. Lippman D, Stump M, Veazey E, et al. Foundations of lifestyle medicine and its evolution. *Mayo Clin Proc Innov Qual Outcomes*. 2024;8(1):97–111.
5. Benigas S. A milestone: 2024 marks the 20th anniversary of the founding of the American College of Lifestyle Medicine. *Am J Lifestyle Med*. 2024;18(4):449–55.
6. Sister organizations. Lifestyle Medicine Global Alliance. https://lifestylemedicineglobal.org/sister-organizations/. Accessed January 26, 2025.
7. Morgenstern S, Redwood M, Herby A. An innovative program for hospital nutrition. *Am J Lifestyle Med*. Published online September 12, 2024:15598276241283158.
8. Mayor Adams, NYC Health + Hospitals expand access to lifestyle medicine services city-wide. City of New York. https://www.nyc.gov/office-of-the-mayor/news/063–22/mayor-adams-nyc-health-hospitals-expand-access-lifestyle-medicine-services-city-wide#/0. February 7, 2022. Accessed January 26, 2025.
9. New York City's public school system goes meat-free on Fridays. Reuters. https://www.reuters.com/world/us/new-york-citys-public-school-system-goes-meat-free-fridays-2022-02-04/. February 4, 2022. Accessed January 26, 2025.
10. Mayor Adams announces NYC will serve up healthier meals with enhanced food standards. City of New York. https://www.nyc.gov/office-of-the-mayor/news/176-22/mayor-adams-nyc-will-serve-up-healthier-meals-enhanced-food-standards. April 1, 2022. Accessed January 26, 2025.
11. New York City Food Standards. Meals and snacks purchased and served. NYC Food Policy. https://www.nyc.gov/assets/foodpolicy/downloads/pdf/nycfoodstandards.pdf. Accessed January 26, 2025.
12. Gardner MN, Brandt AM. "The doctors' choice is America's choice": the physician in US cigarette advertisements, 1930–1953. *Am J Public Health*. 2006;96(2):222–32.
13. Proctor RN. The history of the discovery of the cigarette–lung cancer link: evidentiary traditions, corporate denial, global toll. *Tob Control*. 2012;21(2):87–91.
14. The advertising of cigarettes. *JAMA*. 1948;138(9):652–3.
15. Centers for Disease Control and Prevention (CDC). Tobacco use—United States, 1900–1999. *MMWR Morb Mortal Wkly Rep*. 1999;48(43):986–93.
16. The advertising of cigarettes. *JAMA*. 1948;138(9):652–3.
17. Berger VW, Knoll D. Levels of evidence: further insight on Gugiu and Gugiu. *Eval Health Prof*. 2011;34(1):124–6; discussion 127–30.

18. Institute for Health Metrics and Evaluation (IHME). GBD results. University of Washington. https://vizhub.healthdata.org/gbd-results/. 2024. Accessed January 25, 2025.
19. Barnard ND. The physician's role in nutrition-related disorders: from bystander to leader. *Virtual Mentor*. 2013;15(4):367–72.
20. Monte T, Pritikin I. *Pritikin: The Man Who Healed America's Heart*. Emmaus, PA: Rodale Press; 1988.
21. Gould KL, Ornish D, Scherwitz L, et al. Changes in myocardial perfusion abnormalities by positron emission tomography after long-term, intense risk factor modification. *JAMA*. 1995;274:894–901.
22. Ornish D, Scherwitz L, Billings J, et al. Intensive lifestyle changes for reversal of coronary heart disease. Five-year follow-up of the Lifestyle Heart Trial. *JAMA*. 1998;280:2001–7.
23. Ornish DM, Scherwitz LW, Doody RS, et al. Effects of stress management training and dietary changes in treating ischemic heart disease. *JAMA*. 1983;249:54–9.
24. Ornish D. Intensive lifestyle changes and health reform. *Lancet Oncol*. 2009;10(7):638–9.
25. Adams KM, Kohlmeier M, Zeisel SH. Nutrition education in U.S. medical schools: latest update of a national survey. *Acad Med*. 2010;85(9):1537–42.
26. Jamal A, Dube SR, Malarcher AM, Shaw L, Engstrom MC. Tobacco use screening and counseling during physician office visits among adults. National Ambulatory Medical Care Survey and National Health Interview Survey, United States, 2005–2009. *MMWR Morb Mortal Wkly Rep*. 2012;61 Suppl:38–45.
27. Berzlanovich AM, Keil W, Waldhoer T, Sim E, Fasching P, Fazeny-Dörner B. Do centenarians die healthy? An autopsy study. *J Gerontol A Biol Sci Med Sci*. 2005;60(7):862–5.
28. Kohn RR. Cause of death in very old people. *JAMA*. 1982;247(20):2793–7.
29. Berzlanovich AM, Keil W, Waldhoer T, Sim E, Fasching P, Fazeny-Dörner B. Do centenarians die healthy? An autopsy study. *J Gerontol A Biol Sci Med Sci*. 2005;60(7):862–5.
30. Lenders C, Gorman K, Milch H, et al. A novel nutrition medicine education model: the Boston University experience. *Adv Nutr*. 2013;4(1):1–7.
31. Institute for Health Metrics and Evaluation (IHME). GBD 2021 results. University of Washington. https://vizhub.healthdata.org/gbd-results/. Accessed January 16, 2025.
32. Kris-Etherton PM, Akabas SR, Bales CW, et al. The need to advance nutrition education in the training of health care professionals and recommended research to evaluate implementation and effectiveness. *Am J Clin Nutr*. 2014;99(5 Suppl):1153S–66S.
33. Swift CS. Nutrition trends: implications for diabetes health care professionals. *Diabetes Spectr*. 2009;29(1):23–5.
34. Vetter ML, Herring SJ, Sood M, Shah NR, Kalet AL. What do resident physicians know about nutrition? An evaluation of attitudes, self-perceived proficiency and knowledge. *J Am Coll Nutr*. 2008;27(2):287–98.
35. Lazarus K, Weinsier RL, Boker JR. Nutrition knowledge and practices of physicians in a family-practice residency program: the effect of an education program provided by a physician nutrition specialist. *Am J Clin Nutr*. 1993;58(3):319–25.
36. Senate Committee on Business, Professions and Economic Development. Bill Analysis on SB 380. http://www.leginfo.ca.gov/pub/11-12/bill/sen/sb_0351-0400/sb_380_cfa_20110421_125358_sen_comm.html. Hearing held April 25, 2011. Accessed January 10, 2025.
37. Continuing Medical Education. The Medical Board of California. https://www.mbc.ca.gov/Licensing/Physicians-and-Surgeons/Renew/Current-Status/Continuing-Medical-Education.aspx. Accessed January 13, 2025.
38. Wizard Edison says doctors of future will give no medicine. *Newark Advocate*. January 2, 1903.
39. Stange KC, Zyzanski SJ, Jaén CR, et al. Illuminating the "black box." A description of 4454 patient visits to 138 family physicians. *J Fam Pract*. 1998;46(5):377–89.
40. Aitken M, Kleinrock M, Nass D. Outlook for global medicines through 2021. QuintilesIMS Institute. https://www.iqvia.com/-/media/iqvia/pdfs/institute-reports/global-outlook-for-medicines-through-2021.pdf. December 2016. Accessed January 13, 2025.

41. Willett WC. Balancing life-style and genomics research for disease prevention. *Science.* 2002;296(5568):695–8.
42. Willett WC. Balancing life-style and genomics research for disease prevention. *Science.* 2002;296(5568):695–8.
43. Robertson TL, Kato H, Rhoads GG, et al. Epidemiologic studies of coronary heart disease and stroke in Japanese men living in Japan, Hawaii and California. Incidence of myocardial infarction and death from coronary heart disease. *Am J Cardiol.* 1977;39(2):239–43.
44. Nearly 7 in 10 Americans take prescription drugs, Mayo Clinic, Olmsted Medical Center find. Mayo Clinic News Network. http://newsnetwork.mayoclinic.org/discussion/nearly-7-in-10-americans-take-prescription-drugs-mayo-clinic-olmsted-medical-center-find/. June 19, 2013. Accessed January 13, 2025.
45. Murray CJ, Atkinson C, Bhalla K, et al. The state of US health, 1990–2010: burden of diseases, injuries, and risk factors. *JAMA.* 2013;310(6):591–608.
46. Villines TC. Risks of the American lifestyle: insights from a trans-Pacific comparison of coronary artery calcium progression. *Circ Cardiovasc Imaging.* 2019;12(2):e008810.
47. Papanicolas I, Woskie LR, Jha AK. Health care spending in the United States and other high-income countries. *JAMA.* 2018;319(10):1024–39.
48. Institute for Health Metrics and Evaluation (IHME). GBD 2021 results. University of Washington. https://vizhub.healthdata.org/gbd-results/. Accessed January 16, 2025.
49. Olshansky SJ, Passaro DJ, Hershow RC, et al. A potential decline in life expectancy in the United States in the 21st century. *N Engl J Med.* 2005;352(11):1138–45.
50. Xu J, Murphy SL, Kochanek KD, Arias E. Mortality in the United States, 2015. NCHS Data Brief. 2016;(267):1–8.
51. Masters RK, Aron LY, Woolf SH. Changes in life expectancy between 2019 and 2021 in the United States and 21 peer countries. *Public and Global Health*; 2022.
52. Crimmins EM, Beltrán-Sánchez H. Mortality and morbidity trends: is there compression of morbidity? *J Gerontol B Psychol Sci Soc Sci.* 2011; 66(1):75–86.
53. Offord DR. Selection of levels of prevention. *Addict Behav.* 2000;25(6):833–42.
54. Gofrit ON, Shemer J, Leibovici D, Modan B, Shapira SC. Quaternary prevention: a new look at an old challenge. *Isr Med Assoc J.* 2000;2(7):498–500.
55. Strasser T. Reflections on cardiovascular diseases. *Interdiscip Sci Rev.* 1978;3(3):225–30.
56. Lloyd-Jones DM, Hong Y, Labarthe D, et al. Defining and setting national goals for cardiovascular health promotion and disease reduction: the American Heart Association's strategic Impact Goal through 2020 and beyond. *Circulation.* 2010;121(4):586–613.
57. Yancy CW. Is ideal cardiovascular health attainable? *Circulation.* 2011;123(8):835–7.
58. Lloyd-Jones DM, Hong Y, Labarthe D, et al. Defining and setting national goals for cardiovascular health promotion and disease reduction: the American Heart Association's strategic Impact Goal through 2020 and beyond. *Circulation.* 2010;121(4):586–613.
59. Yusuf S, Hawken S, Ounpuu S, et al. Effect of potentially modifiable risk factors associated with myocardial infarction in 52 countries (the INTERHEART study): case-control study. *Lancet.* 2004;364(9438):937–52.
60. Lloyd-Jones DM, Hong Y, Labarthe D, et al. Defining and setting national goals for cardiovascular health promotion and disease reduction: the American Heart Association's strategic Impact Goal through 2020 and beyond. *Circulation.* 2010;121(4):586–613.
61. Shay CM, Ning H, Allen NB, et al. Status of cardiovascular health in US adults: prevalence estimates from the National Health and Nutrition Examination Surveys (NHANES) 2003–2008. *Circulation.* 2012;125(1):45–56.
62. Shay CM, Ning H, Allen NB, et al. Status of cardiovascular health in US adults: prevalence estimates from the National Health and Nutrition Examination Surveys (NHANES) 2003–2008. *Circulation.* 2012;125(1):45–56.
63. Omran AR. The epidemiologic transition. A theory of the epidemiology of population change. *Milbank Mem Fund Q.* 1971;49(4):509–38.

64. US Centers for Disease Control and Prevention. Leading causes of death, 1900–1998. http://www.cdc.gov/nchs/data/dvs/lead1900_98.pdf. Accessed January 13, 2025.
65. US Centers for Disease Control and Prevention. Provisional Mortality Statistics, 2018 through last week results. https://wonder.cdc.gov/controller/datarequest/D176;jsessionid=61B2048DD441F90EFD4A0B3C8360. Accessed January 13, 2025.
66. Lim SS, Vos T, Flaxman AD, et al. A comparative risk assessment of burden of disease and injury attributable to 67 risk factors and risk factor clusters in 21 regions, 1990–2010: a systematic analysis for the Global Burden of Disease Study 2010. *Lancet.* 2012;380(9859):2224–60.
67. Popkin BM. Global nutrition dynamics: the world is shifting rapidly toward a diet linked with noncommunicable diseases. *Am J Clin Nutr.* 2006;84(2):289–98.
68. Zhai F, Wang H, Du S, et al. Prospective study on nutrition transition in China. *Nutr Rev.* 2009;67 Suppl 1:S56–61.
69. Singh PN, Arthur KN, Orlich MJ, et al. Global epidemiology of obesity, vegetarian dietary patterns, and noncommunicable disease in Asian Indians. *Am J Clin Nutr.* 2014;100 Suppl 1:359S–64S.
70. Singh PN, Arthur KN, Orlich MJ, et al. Global epidemiology of obesity, vegetarian dietary patterns, and noncommunicable disease in Asian Indians. *Am J Clin Nutr.* 2014;100 Suppl 1:359S–64S.
71. McCarty MF. Proposal for a dietary "phytochemical index." *Med Hypotheses.* 2004;63(5):813–7.
72. Mirmiran P, Bahadoran Z, Golzarand M, Shiva N, Azizi F. Association between dietary phytochemical index and 3-year changes in weight, waist circumference and body adiposity index in adults: Tehran Lipid and Glucose study. *Nutr Metab (Lond).* 2012;9(1):108.
73. Mirmiran P, Bahadoran Z, Golzarand M, Shiva N, Azizi F. Association between dietary phytochemical index and 3-year changes in weight, waist circumference and body adiposity index in adults: Tehran Lipid and Glucose study. *Nutr Metab (Lond).* 2012;9(1):108.
74. Golzarand M, Bahadoran Z, Mirmiran P, Sadeghian-Sharif S, Azizi F. Dietary phytochemical index is inversely associated with the occurrence of hypertension in adults: a 3-year follow-up (the Tehran Lipid and Glucose Study). *Eur J Clin Nutr.* 2015;69(3):392–8.
75. Golzarand M, Mirmiran P, Bahadoran Z, Alamdari S, Azizi F. Dietary phytochemical index and subsequent changes of lipid profile: a 3-year follow-up in Tehran Lipid and Glucose Study in Iran. *ARYA Atheroscler.* 2014;10(4):203–10.
76. Bahadoran Z, Karimi Z, Houshiar-Rad A, Mirzayi HR, Rashidkhani B. Dietary phytochemical index and the risk of breast cancer: a case control study in a population of Iranian women. *Asian Pac J Cancer Prev.* 2013;14(5):2747–51.
77. U.S. Department of Agriculture Economic Research Service. Loss-adjusted food availability. https://www.ers.usda.gov/data-products/food-availability-per-capita-data-system. September 30, 2014. Accessed February 27, 2025.
78. Wansink B, Kniffin KM, Shimizu M. Death row nutrition. Curious conclusions of last meals. *Appetite.* 2012;59(3):837–43.
79. Bambs C, Kip KE, Dinga A, Mulukutla SR, Aiyer AN, Reis SE. Low prevalence of "ideal cardiovascular health" in a community-based population: the Heart Strategies Concentrating on Risk Evaluation (Heart SCORE) study. *Circulation.* 2011;123(8):850–7.
80. Yancy CW. Is ideal cardiovascular health attainable? *Circulation.* 2011;123(8):835–7.
81. Ford ES, Bergmann MM, Krord J, Schienkiewitz A, Weikert C, Boeing H. Healthy living is the best revenge: findings from the European Prospective Investigation into Cancer and Nutrition-Potsdam study. *Arch Intern Med.* 2009;169(15):1355–62.
82. Platz EA, Willett WC, Colditz GA, Rimm EB, Spiegelman D, Giovannucci E. Proportion of colon cancer risk that might be preventable in a cohort of middle-aged US men. *Cancer Causes Control.* 2000;11(7):579–88.
83. Wahls TL. The seventy percent solution. *J Gen Intern Med.* 2011;26(10):1215–6.
84. Ford ES, Bergmann MM, Boeing H, Li C, Capewell S. Healthy lifestyle behaviors and all-cause mortality among adults in the United States. *Prev Med.* 2012;55(1):23–7.

85. Khaw KT, Wareham N, Bingham S, Welch A, Luben R, Day N. Combined impact of health behaviours and mortality in men and women: the EPIC-Norfolk prospective population study. *PLoS Med.* 2008;5(1):e12.
86. Jiang H, Ju Z, Rudolph KL. Telomere shortening and ageing. *Z Gerontol Geriatr.* 2007;40(5):314–24.
87. Mather KA, Jorm AF, Parslow RA, Christensen H. Is telomere length a biomarker of aging? A review. *J Gerontol A Biol Sci Med Sci.* 2011;66(2):202–13.
88. Tsuji A, Ishiko A, Takasaki T, Ikeda N. Estimating age of humans based on telomere shortening. *Forensic Sci Int.* 2002;126(3):197–9.
89. Shammas MA. Telomeres, lifestyle, cancer, and aging. *Curr Opin Clin Nutr Metab Care.* 2011;14(1):28–34.
90. Huzen J, Wong LS, van Veldhuisen DJ, et al. Telomere length loss due to smoking and metabolic traits. *J Intern Med.* 2014;275(2):155–63.
91. Hou L, Savage SA, Blaser MJ, et al. Telomere length in peripheral leukocyte DNA and gastric cancer risk. *Cancer Epidemiol Biomarkers Prev.* 2009;18(11):3103–9.
92. Gu Y, Honig LS, Schupf N, et al. Mediterranean diet and leukocyte telomere length in a multi-ethnic elderly population. *Age* (Dordr). 2015;37(2):9758.
93. García-Calzón S, Moleres A, Martínez-González MA, et al. Dietary total antioxidant capacity is associated with leukocyte telomere length in a children and adolescent population. *Clin Nutr.* 2014;S0261–5614(14):00191–5.
94. García-Calzón S, Moleres A, Martínez-González MA, et al. Dietary total antioxidant capacity is associated with leukocyte telomere length in a children and adolescent population. *Clin Nutr.* 2014;S0261–5614(14):00191–5.
95. Leung CW, Laraia BA, Needham BL, et al. Soda and cell aging: associations between sugar-sweetened beverage consumption and leukocyte telomere length in healthy adults from the National Health and Nutrition Examination Surveys. *Am J Public Health.* 2014;104(12):2425–31.
96. Nettleton JA, Diez-Roux A, Jenny NS, Fitzpatrick AL, Jacobs DR. Dietary patterns, food groups, and telomere length in the Multi-Ethnic Study of Atherosclerosis (MESA). *Am J Clin Nutr.* 2008;88(5):1405–12.
97. Gu Y, Honig LS, Schupf N, et al. Mediterranean diet and leukocyte telomere length in a multi-ethnic elderly population. *Age* (Dordr). 2015;37(2):9758.
98. Flanary BE, Kletetschka G. Analysis of telomere length and telomerase activity in tree species of various life-spans, and with age in the bristlecone pine Pinus longaeva. *Biogerontology.* 2005;6(2):101–11.
99. Ornish D, Lin J, Daubenmier J, et al. Increased telomerase activity and comprehensive lifestyle changes: a pilot study. *Lancet Oncol.* 2008;9(11):1048–57.
100. Skordalakes E. Telomerase and the benefits of healthy living. *Lancet Oncol.* 2008;9(11):1023–4.
101. Ornish D, Lin J, Chan JM, et al. Effect of comprehensive lifestyle changes on telomerase activity and telomere length in men with biopsy-proven low-risk prostate cancer: 5-year follow-up of a descriptive pilot study. *Lancet Oncol.* 2013;14(11):1112–20.
102. Mason C, Risques RA, Xiao L, et al. Independent and combined effects of dietary weight loss and exercise on leukocyte telomere length in postmenopausal women. *Obesity* (Silver Spring). 2013;21(12):E549–54.
103. Ornish D, Lin J, Daubenmier J, et al. Increased telomerase activity and comprehensive lifestyle changes: a pilot study. *Lancet Oncol.* 2008;9(11):1048–57.
104. Ornish D, Lin J, Chan JM, et al. Effect of comprehensive lifestyle changes on telomerase activity and telomere length in men with biopsy-proven low-risk prostate cancer: 5-year follow-up of a descriptive pilot study. *Lancet Oncol.* 2013;14(11):1112–20.
105. Greger M. *How Not to Age.* New York: Macmillan; 2023.
106. Fiorito G, Caini S, Palli D, et al. DNA methylation-based biomarkers of aging were slowed down in a two-year diet and physical activity intervention trial: the DAMA study. *Aging Cell.* 2021;20(10):e13439.

107. Dwaraka VB, Aronica L, Carreras-Gallo N, et al. Unveiling the epigenetic impact of vegan vs. omnivorous diets on aging: insights from the Twins Nutrition Study (TwiNS). *BMC Med.* 2024;22(1):301.
108. Artandi SE, Depinho RA. Telomeres and telomerase in cancer. *Carcinogenesis.* 2010;31(1):9–18.
109. Tsao CW, Aday AW, Almarzooq ZI, et al. Heart disease and stroke statistics—2023 update: a report from the American Heart Association. *Circulation.* 2023;147(8):e93–e621.
110. U.S. Cancer Statistics Working Group. U.S. Cancer Statistics Data Visualizations Tool. U.S. Department of Health and Human Services, Centers for Disease Control and Prevention and National Cancer Institute. https://www.cdc.gov/cancer/dataviz. June 2024. Accessed January 18, 2025.
111. Centers for Disease Control and Prevention, National Center for Health Statistics. National Vital Statistics System, Mortality 2018–2023 on CDC WONDER Online Database. http://wonder.cdc.gov/ucd-icd10-expanded.html. Accessed January 16, 2025.
112. Tsao CW, Aday AW, Almarzooq ZI, Anderson CAM, Arora P, Avery CL, et al. Heart disease and stroke statistics—2023 update: a report from the American Heart Association. *Circulation.* 2023;147(8):e93–e621.
113. Centers for Disease Control and Prevention, National Center for Health Statistics. National Vital Statistics System, Mortality 2018–2023 on CDC WONDER Online Database. http://wonder.cdc.gov/ucd-icd10-expanded.html. Accessed January 16, 2025.
114. Centers for Disease Control and Prevention, National Center for Health Statistics. National Vital Statistics System, Mortality 2018–2023 on CDC WONDER Online Database. http://wonder.cdc.gov/ucd-icd10-expanded.html. Accessed January 16, 2025.
115. Centers for Disease Control and Prevention. COVID data tracker. U.S. Department of Health and Human Services. https://covid.cdc.gov/covid-data-tracker. Accessed January 19, 2025.
116. Tsao CW, Aday AW, Almarzooq ZI, Anderson CAM, Arora P, Avery CL, et al. Heart disease and stroke statistics—2023 update: a report from the American Heart Association. *Circulation.* 2023;147(8):e93–e621.
117. U.S. Cancer Statistics Working Group. U.S. Cancer Statistics Data Visualizations Tool. U.S. Department of Health and Human Services, Centers for Disease Control and Prevention and National Cancer Institute. https://www.cdc.gov/cancer/dataviz. June 2024. Accessed January 18, 2025.
118. Centers for Disease Control and Prevention, National Center for Health Statistics. National Vital Statistics System, Mortality 2018–2023 on CDC WONDER Online Database. http://wonder.cdc.gov/ucd-icd10-expanded.html. Accessed January 16, 2025.
119. Centers for Disease Control and Prevention, National Center for Health Statistics. National Vital Statistics System, Mortality 2018–2023 on CDC WONDER Online Database. http://wonder.cdc.gov/ucd-icd10-expanded.html. Accessed January 16, 2025.
120. U.S. Cancer Statistics Working Group. U.S. Cancer Statistics Data Visualizations Tool. U.S. Department of Health and Human Services, Centers for Disease Control and Prevention and National Cancer Institute. https://www.cdc.gov/cancer/dataviz. June 2024. Accessed January 18, 2025.
121. U.S. Cancer Statistics Working Group. U.S. Cancer Statistics Data Visualizations Tool. U.S. Department of Health and Human Services, Centers for Disease Control and Prevention and National Cancer Institute. https://www.cdc.gov/cancer/dataviz. June 2024. Accessed January 18, 2025.
122. Centers for Disease Control and Prevention, National Center for Health Statistics. National Vital Statistics System, Mortality 2018–2023 on CDC WONDER Online Database. http://wonder.cdc.gov/ucd-icd10-expanded.html. Accessed January 16, 2025.
123. Centers for Disease Control and Prevention, National Center for Health Statistics. National Vital Statistics System, Mortality 2018–2023 on CDC WONDER Online Database. http://wonder.cdc.gov/ucd-icd10-expanded.html. Accessed January 16, 2025.

124. U.S. Cancer Statistics Working Group. U.S. Cancer Statistics Data Visualizations Tool. U.S. Department of Health and Human Services, Centers for Disease Control and Prevention and National Cancer Institute. https://www.cdc.gov/cancer/dataviz. June 2024. Accessed January 18, 2025.
125. Siegel RL, Kratzer TB, Giaquinto AN, Sung H, Jemal A. Cancer statistics, 2025. *CA Cancer J Clin*. Published online January 16, 2025:caac.21871.
126. Centers for Disease Control and Prevention, National Center for Health Statistics. National Vital Statistics System, Mortality 2018–2023 on CDC WONDER Online Database. http://wonder.cdc.gov/ucd-icd10-expanded.html. Accessed January 16, 2025.
127. U.S. Cancer Statistics Working Group. U.S. Cancer Statistics Data Visualizations Tool. U.S. Department of Health and Human Services, Centers for Disease Control and Prevention and National Cancer Institute. https://www.cdc.gov/cancer/dataviz. June 2024. Accessed January 18, 2025.
128. Tuso PJ, Ismail MH, Ha BP, Bartolotto C. Nutritional update for physicians: plant-based diets. *Perm J*. 2013;17(2):61–6.
129. Egger GJ, Binns AF, Rossner SR. The emergence of "lifestyle medicine" as a structured approach for management of chronic disease. *Med J Aust*. 2009;190(3):143–5.
130. Hyman MA, Ornish D, Roizen M. Lifestyle medicine: treating the causes of disease. *Altern Ther Health Med*. 2009;15(6):12–4.
131. Willett WC. Balancing life-style and genomics research for disease prevention. *Science*. 2002;296(5568):695–8.
132. Hyman MA, Ornish D, Roizen M. Lifestyle medicine: treating the causes of disease. *Altern Ther Health Med*. 2009;15(6):12–4.
133. Allen J, Anderson DR, Baun B, et al. Reflections on developments in health promotion in the past quarter century from founding members of the American Journal of Health Promotion Editorial Board. *Am J Health Promot*. 2011;25(4):ei–eviii.
134. Tuso PJ, Ismail MH, Ha BP, Bartolotto C. Nutritional update for physicians: plant-based diets. *Perm J*. 2013;17(2):61–6.
135. Tuso PJ, Ismail MH, Ha BP, Bartolotto C. Nutritional update for physicians: plant-based diets. *Perm J*. 2013;17(2):61–6.
136. Tuso PJ, Ismail MH, Ha BP, Bartolotto C. Nutritional update for physicians: plant-based diets. *Perm J*. 2013;17(2):61–6.
137. Kono S. Secular trend of colon cancer incidence and mortality in relation to fat and meat intake in Japan. *Eur J Cancer Prev*. 2004;13(2):127–32.
138. Willett WC. Balancing life-style and genomics research for disease prevention. *Science*. 2002;296(5568):695–8.
139. Kono S. Secular trend of colon cancer incidence and mortality in relation to fat and meat intake in Japan. *Eur J Cancer Prev*. 2004;13(2):127–32.
140. Kulshreshtha A, Goyal A, Veledar E, et al. Association between ideal cardiovascular health and carotid intima-media thickness: a twin study. *J Am Heart Assoc*. 2014;3(1):e000282.
141. Corona M, Velarde RA, Remolina S, et al. Vitellogenin, juvenile hormone, insulin signaling, and queen honey bee longevity. *Proc Natl Acad Sci USA*. 2007;104(17):7128–33.
142. Bacalini MG, Friso S, Olivieri F, et al. Present and future of anti-ageing epigenetic diets. *Mech Ageing Dev*. 2014;136–7:101–15.
143. Kucharski R, Maleszka J, Foret S, Maleszka R. Nutritional control of reproductive status in honeybees via DNA methylation. *Science*. 2008;319(5871):1827–30.
144. Gnyszka A, Jastrzebski Z, Flis S. DNA methyltransferase inhibitors and their emerging role in epigenetic therapy of cancer. *Anticancer Res*. 2013;33(8):2989–96.
145. Joven J, Micol V, Segura-Carretero A, Alonso-Villaverde C, Menéndez JA. Polyphenols and the modulation of gene expression pathways: can we eat our way out of the danger of chronic disease? *Crit Rev Food Sci Nutr*. 2014;54(8):985–1001.
146. Fang MZ, Wang Y, Ai N, et al. Tea polyphenol (-)-epigallocatechin-3-gallate inhibits DNA

methyltransferase and reactivates methylation-silenced genes in cancer cell lines. *Cancer Res.* 2003;63(22):7563–70.
147. Myzak MC, Tong P, Dashwood WM, Dashwood RH, Ho E. Sulforaphane retards the growth of human PC-3 xenografts and inhibits HDAC activity in human subjects. *Exp Biol Med* (Maywood). 2007;232(2):227–34.
148. Dashwood RH, Ho E. Dietary histone deacetylase inhibitors: from cells to mice to man. *Semin Cancer Biol.* 2007;17(5):363–9.
149. Gryder BE, Sodji QH, Oyelere AK. Targeted cancer therapy: giving histone deacetylase inhibitors all they need to succeed. *Future Med Chem.* 2012;4(4):505–24.
150. Ornish D, Magbanua MJ, Weidner G, et al. Changes in prostate gene expression in men undergoing an intensive nutrition and lifestyle intervention. *Proc Natl Acad Sci USA.* 2008;105(24):8369–74.
151. Green A. Li Wenliang. *Lancet.* 2020;395(10225):682.
152. World Health Organization. Novel coronavirus (2019-nCoV). Situation report—18. https://www.who.int/docs/default-source/coronaviruse/situation-reports/20200207-sitrep-18-ncov.pdf?sfvrsn=fa644293_2. February 7, 2020. Accessed January 18, 2025.
153. Page J, Fan W, Khan N. How it all started: China's early coronavirus missteps. *Wall Street Journal.* https://www.wsj.com/articles/how-it-all-started-chinas-early-coronavirus-missteps-11583508932. March 6, 2020. Accessed January 18, 2025.
154. McNeil DG. Disease's pioneer is mourned as a victim. *New York Times.* https://www.nytimes.com/2003/04/08/science/disease-s-pioneer-is-mourned-as-a-victim.html. April 8, 2003. Accessed January 18, 2025.
155. Ashour HM, Elkhatib WF, Rahman MM, Elshabrawy HA. Insights into the recent 2019 novel coronavirus (SARS-CoV-2) in light of past human coronavirus outbreaks. *Pathogens.* 2020;9(3):186.
156. World Health Organization. Global excess deaths associated with COVID-19, January 2020–December 2021. https://www.who.int/data/stories/global-excess-deaths-associated-with-covid-19-january-2020-december-2021. Accessed January 18, 2025.
157. World Heart Federation. *World Heart Report 2023: Confronting the World's Number One Killer.* Geneva, Switzerland; 2023.
158. Department of Veterans Affairs. America's Wars. Office of Public Affairs. https://www.va.gov/opa/publications/factsheets/fs_americas_wars.pdf. November 2023. Accessed January 19, 2025.
159. Voller RD, Strong WB. Pediatric aspects of atherosclerosis. *Am Heart J.* 1981;101(6):815–36.
160. Myerburg RJ, Junttila MJ. 2012. Sudden cardiac death caused by coronary heart disease. *Circulation.* 28;125(8):1043–52.
161. Campbell TC, Parpia B, Chen J. Diet, lifestyle, and the etiology of coronary artery disease: the Cornell China study. *Am J Cardiol.* 1998;82(10B):18T–21T.
162. Shaper AG, Jones KW. Serum-cholesterol, diet, and coronary heart-disease in Africans and Asians in Uganda: 1959. *Int J Epidemiol.* 2012;41(5):1221–5.
163. Thomas WA, Davies JN, O'Neal RM, Dimakulangan AA. Incidence of myocardial infarction correlated with venous and pulmonary thrombosis and embolism. A geographic study based on autopsies in Uganda, East Africa and St. Louis, U.S.A. *Am J Cardiol.* 1960;5:41–7.
164. Benfante R. Studies of cardiovascular disease and cause-specific mortality trends in Japanese-American men living in Hawaii and risk factor comparisons with other Japanese populations in the Pacific region: a review. *Hum Biol.* 1992;64(6):791–805.
165. Chen J, Campbell TC, Li J, Peto R. Diet, *Life-style and Mortality in China: A Study of the Characteristics of 65 Chinese Counties.* New York: Oxford University Press; 1990.
166. Shaper AG, Jones KW. Serum-cholesterol, diet, and coronary heart-disease in Africans and Asians in Uganda: 1959. *Int J Epidemiol.* 2012;41(5):1221–5.

167. De Biase SG, Fernandes SF, Gianini RJ, Duarte JL. Vegetarian diet and cholesterol and triglycerides levels. *Arq Bras Cardiol.* 2007;88(1):35–9.
168. Stoy PJ. Dental disease and civilization. *Ulster Med J.* 1951;20(2):144–58.
169. Kris-Etherton PM, Harris WS, Appel LJ, Nutrition Committee. Fish consumption, fish oil, omega-3 fatty acids, and cardiovascular disease. *Arterioscler Thromb Vasc Biol.* 2003;23(2): e20–30.
170. Shepherd CJ, Jackson AJ. Global fishmeal and fish-oil supply: inputs, outputs and markets. *J Fish Biol.* 2013;83(4):1046–66.
171. Rizos EC, Ntzani EE, Bika E, Kostapanos MS, Elisaf MS. Association between omega-3 fatty acid supplementation and risk of major cardiovascular disease events: a systematic review and meta-analysis. *JAMA.* 2012;308(10):1024–33.
172. Kwak SM, Myung SK, Lee YJ, Seo HG. Efficacy of omega-3 fatty acid supplements (eicosapentaenoic acid and docosahexaenoic acid) in the secondary prevention of cardiovascular disease: a meta-analysis of randomized, double-blind, placebo-controlled trials. *Arch Intern Med.* 2012;172(9):686–94.
173. Fodor JG, Helis E, Yazdekhasti N, Vohnout B. "Fishing" for the origins of the "Eskimos and heart disease" story: facts or wishful thinking? *Can J Cardiol.* 2014;30(8):864–8.
174. Burr ML, Fehily AM, Gilbert JF, et al. Effects of changes in fat, fish, and fibre intakes on death and myocardial reinfarction: Diet and Reinfarction Trial (DART). *Lancet.* 1989;2(8666): 757–61.
175. Burr ML. Secondary prevention of CHD in UK men: the Diet and Reinfarction Trial and its sequel. *Proc Nutr Soc.* 2007;66(1):9–15.
176. Burr ML, Ashfield-Watt PAL, Dunstan FDJ, et al. Lack of benefit of dietary advice to men with angina: results of a controlled trial. *Eur J Clin Nutr.* 2003;57(2):193–200.
177. Rizos EC, Ntzani EE, Bika E, Kostapanos MS, Elisaf MS. Association between omega-3 fatty acid supplementation and risk of major cardiovascular disease events: a systematic review and meta-analysis. *JAMA.* 2012;308(10):1024–33.
178. Abdelhamid AS, Brown TJ, Brainard JS, et al. Omega-3 fatty acids for the primary and secondary prevention of cardiovascular disease. *Cochrane Database Syst Rev.* 2020;3(3):CD003177.
179. Smith DA. ACP Journal Club. Review: omega-3 polyunsaturated fatty acid supplements do not reduce major cardiovascular events in adults. *Ann Intern Med.* 2012;157(12):JC6–5.
180. Enos WF, Holmes RH, Beyer J. Coronary disease among United States soldiers killed in action in Korea; preliminary report. *JAMA.* 1953;152(12):1090–3.
181. Strong JP. Landmark perspective: coronary atherosclerosis in soldiers. A clue to the natural history of atherosclerosis in the young. *JAMA.* 1986;256(20):2863–6.
182. Voller RD, Strong WB. Pediatric aspects of atherosclerosis. *Am Heart J.* 1981;101(6):815–36.
183. Napoli C, D'Armiento FP, Mancini FP, et al. Fatty streak formation occurs in human fetal aortas and is greatly enhanced by maternal hypercholesterolemia. Intimal accumulation of low density lipoprotein and its oxidation precede monocyte recruitment into early atherosclerotic lesions. *J Clin Invest.* 1997;100(11):2680–90.
184. Benjamin MM, Roberts WC. Facts and principles learned at the 39th Annual Williamsburg Conference on Heart Disease. *Proc (Bayl Univ Med Cent).* 2013;26(2):124–36.
185. McMahan CA, Gidding SS, Malcom GT, et al. Pathobiological determinants of atherosclerosis in youth risk scores are associated with early and advanced atherosclerosis. *Pediatrics.* 2006;118(4):1447–55.
186. Trumbo PR, Shimakawa T. Tolerable upper intake levels for trans fat, saturated fat, and cholesterol. *Nutr Rev.* 2011;69(5):270–8.
187. Roberts WC. It's the cholesterol, stupid! *Am J Cardiol.* 2010;106(9):1364–6.
188. O'Keefe JH, Cordain L, Harris WH, Moe RM, Vogel R. Optimal low-density lipoprotein is 50 to 70 mg/dl: lower is better and physiologically normal. *J Am Coll Cardiol.* 2004;43(11): 2142–6.

189. Esselstyn CB. In cholesterol lowering, moderation kills. *Cleve Clin J Med.* 2000;67(8):560–4.
190. Roberts WC. The cause of atherosclerosis. *Nutr Clin Pract.* 2008;23(5):464–7.
191. Roberts WC. The cause of atherosclerosis. *Nutr Clin Pract.* 2008;23(5):464–7.
192. King S. The best selling drugs since 1996—why AbbVie's Humira is set to eclipse Pfizer's Lipitor. http://www.forbes.com/sites/simonking/2013/07/15/the-best-selling-drugs-since-1996-why-abbvies-humira-is-set-to-eclipse-pfizers-lipitor/. July 15, 2013. Accessed January 15, 2025.
193. Ginter E, Kajaba I, Sauša M. Addition of statins into the public water supply? Risks of side effects and low cholesterol levels. *Cas Lek Cesk.* 2012;151(5):243–7.
194. Ferenczi EA, Asaria P, Hughes AD, Chaturvedi N, Francis DP. Can a statin neutralize the cardiovascular risk of unhealthy dietary choices? *Am J Cardiol.* 2010;106(4):587–92.
195. Draeger A, Monastyrskaya K, Mohaupt M, et al. Statin therapy induces ultrastructural damage in skeletal muscle in patients without myalgia. *J Pathol.* 2006;210(1):94–102.
196. Scott D, Blizzard L, Fell J, Jones G. Statin therapy, muscle function and falls risk in community-dwelling older adults. *QJM.* 2009;102(9):625–33.
197. U.S. Food and Drug Administration. FDA announces safety changes in labeling for some cholesterol-lowering drugs. https://www.fda.gov/drugs/drug-safety-and-availability/fda-drug-safety-communication-important-safety-label-changes-cholesterol-lowering-statin-drugs#hcp. February 28, 2012. Updated January 19, 2016. Accessed January 2025.
198. Jenkins DJ, Kendall CW, Marchie A, et al. The Garden of Eden—plant based diets, the genetic drive to conserve cholesterol and its implications for heart disease in the 21st century. *Comp Biochem Physiol, Part A Mol Integr Physiol.* 2003;136(1):141–51.
199. Grundy SM, Stone NJ, Bailey AL, et al. 2018 AHA/ACC/AACVPR/AAPA/ABC/ACPM/ADA/AGS/APhA/ASPC/NLA/PCNA guideline on the management of blood cholesterol: a report of the American College of Cardiology/American Heart Association Task Force on Clinical Practice Guidelines. *Circulation.* 2019;139:e1082–143.
200. Jaspers NEM, Ridker PM, Dorresteijn JAN, Visseren FLJ. The prediction of therapy-benefit for individual cardiovascular disease prevention: rationale, implications, and implementation. *Curr Opin Lipidol.* 2018;29(6):436–44.
201. Lloyd-Jones DM, Braun LT, Ndumele CE, et al. Use of risk assessment tools to guide decision-making in the primary prevention of atherosclerotic cardiovascular disease: a special report from the American Heart Association and American College of Cardiology. *J Am Coll Cardiol.* 2019;73(24):3153–67.
202. Lloyd-Jones DM, Braun LT, Ndumele CE, et al. Use of risk assessment tools to guide decision-making in the primary prevention of atherosclerotic cardiovascular disease: a special report from the American Heart Association and American College of Cardiology. *J Am Coll Cardiol.* 2019;73(24):3153–67.
203. Curry SJ, Krist AH, Owens DK, et al. Risk assessment for cardiovascular disease with nontraditional risk factors: US Preventive Services Task Force recommendation statement. *JAMA.* 2018;320(3):272–80.
204. Esselstyn CB. Is the present therapy for coronary artery disease the radical mastectomy of the twenty-first century? *Am J Cardiol.* 2010;106(6):902–4.
205. Kadoch MA. The power of nutrition as medicine. *Prev Med.* 2012;55(1):80.
206. Wakai K, Marugame T, Kuriyama S, et al. Decrease in risk of lung cancer death in Japanese men after smoking cessation by age at quitting: pooled analysis of three large-scale cohort studies. *Cancer Sci.* 2007;98(4):584–9.
207. Vogel RA, Corretti MC, Plotnick GD. Effect of a single high-fat meal on endothelial function in healthy subjects. *Am J Cardiol.* 1997;79(3):350–4.
208. Erridge C. The capacity of foodstuffs to induce innate immune activation of human monocytes in vitro is dependent on food content of stimulants of Toll-like receptors 2 and 4. *Br J Nutr.* 2011;105(1):15–23.

209. Ornish D, Scherwitz LW, Doody RS, et al. Effects of stress management training and dietary changes in treating ischemic heart disease. *JAMA*. 1983;249(1):54–9.
210. Ornish D, Scherwitz LW, Billings JH, et al. Intensive lifestyle changes for reversal of coronary heart disease. *JAMA*. 1998;280(23):2001–7.
211. Ellis FR, Sanders TA. Angina and vegan diet. *Am Heart J*. 1977;93(6):803–5.
212. Sweeney M. Effects of very low-fat diets on anginal symptoms. *Med Hypotheses*. 2004;63(3):553.
213. Savarese G, Rosano G, D'amore C, et al. Effects of ranolazine in symptomatic patients with stable coronary artery disease. A systematic review and meta-analysis. *Int J Cardiol*. 2013;169(4):262–70.
214. Colpo E, Vilanova CD, Brenner Reetz LG, et al. A single consumption of high amounts of the Brazil nuts improves lipid profile of healthy volunteers. *J Nutr Metab*. 2013;2013:1–7.
215. Stern RH, Yang BB, Hounslow NJ, et al. Pharmacodynamics and pharmacokinetic-pharmacodynamic relationships of atorvastatin, an HMG-CoA reductase Inhibitor. *J Clin Pharmacol*. 2000;40(6):616–3.
216. Hegsted M. Washington—dietary guidelines. Food Politics. www.foodpolitics.com/wp-content/uploads/Hegsted.pdf. Accessed January 14, 2025.
217. Campbell TC. *The Low-Carb Fraud*. Dallas, TX: BenBella Books, Inc.; 2014.
218. Herman J. Saving U.S. dietary advice from conflicts of interest. *Food and Drug Law Journal* 2010; 65(20):285–316.
219. Herman J. Saving U.S. dietary advice from conflicts of interest. *Food and Drug Law Journal* 2010; 65(20):285–316.
220. Goodwin JS, Goodwin JM. The tomato effect. Rejection of highly efficacious therapies. *JAMA*. 1984;251(18):2387–90.
221. Adams KM, Kohlmeier M, Zeisel SH. Nutrition education in U.S. medical schools: latest update of a national survey. *Acad Med*. 2010;85(9):1537–42.
222. Hearing of California Senate Bill 380. http://www.leginfo.ca.gov/pub/11–12/bill/sen/sb_0351–0400/sb_380_cfa_20110421_125358_sen_comm.html. April 25, 2011. Accessed January 15, 2025.
223. Murray JL. Coke and the AAFP—the real thing or a dangerous liaison? *Fam Med*. 2010;42(1):57–8.
224. Blum A. AAFP-Coke editorial was music to [our] ears. *J Fam Pract*. 2010;59(2):74.
225. Brownell KD, Warner KE. The perils of ignoring history: Big Tobacco played dirty and millions died. How similar is Big Food? *Milbank Q*. 2009;87(1):259–94.
226. Brownell KD, Warner KE. The perils of ignoring history: Big Tobacco played dirty and millions died. How similar is Big Food? *Milbank Q*. 2009;87(1):259–94.
227. Simon M. And now a word from our sponsors. Eat Drink Politics. http://www.eatdrinkpolitics.com/wp-content/uploads/AND_Corporate_Sponsorship_Report.pdf. January 22, 2013. Accessed January 15, 2025.
228. Bruckert E, Pouchain D, Auboiron S, Mulet C. Cross-analysis of dietary prescriptions and adherence in 356 hypercholesterolaemic patients. *Arch Cardiovasc Dis*. 2012;105(11):557–65.
229. Barnard ND. The physician's role in nutrition-related disorders: from bystander to leader. *Virtual Mentor*. 2013;15(4):367–72.
230. U.S. Cancer Statistics Working Group. U.S. Cancer Statistics Data Visualizations Tool. U.S. Department of Health and Human Services, Centers for Disease Control and Prevention and National Cancer Institute. https://www.cdc.gov/cancer/dataviz. June 2024. Accessed January 18, 2025.
231. Centers for Disease Control and Prevention, National Center for Health Statistics. National Vital Statistics System, Mortality 2018–2023 on CDC WONDER Online Database. http://wonder.cdc.gov/ucd-icd10-expanded.html. Accessed January 16, 2025.
232. Centers for Disease Control and Prevention, National Center for Health Statistics. National

Vital Statistics System, Mortality 2018–2023 on CDC WONDER Online Database. http://wonder.cdc.gov/ucd-icd10-expanded.html. Accessed January 16, 2025.

233. U.S. Cancer Statistics Working Group. U.S. Cancer Statistics Data Visualizations Tool. U.S. Department of Health and Human Services, Centers for Disease Control and Prevention and National Cancer Institute. https://www.cdc.gov/cancer/dataviz. June 2024. Accessed January 18, 2025.

234. U.S. Cancer Statistics Working Group. U.S. Cancer Statistics Data Visualizations Tool. U.S. Department of Health and Human Services, Centers for Disease Control and Prevention and National Cancer Institute. https://www.cdc.gov/cancer/dataviz. June 2024. Accessed January 21, 2025.

235. SEER (Surveillance, Epidemiology, and End Results Program). Cancer Stat Facts: lung and bronchus cancer. https://seer.cancer.gov/statfacts/html/lungb.html. National Cancer Institute. 2024. Accessed January 21, 2025.

236. Lung cancer fact sheet. American Lung Association. http://www.lung.org/lung-disease/lung-cancer/resources/facts-figures/lung-cancer-fact-sheet.html. 2015. Accessed February 14, 2025.

237. Moodie R, Stuckler D, Monteiro C, et al. Profits and pandemics: prevention of harmful effects of tobacco, alcohol, and ultra-processed food and drink industries. *Lancet*. 2013;381(9867):670–9.

238. Health benefits of quitting smoking over time. American Cancer Society. https://www.cancer.org/cancer/risk-prevention/tobacco/guide-quitting-smoking/benefits-of-quitting-smoking-over-time.html. Accessed January 18, 2025.

239. Schwartz R. Legalize marijuana without the smoke. *CMAJ*. 2017;189(4):E137–8.

240. Wei B, Alwis KU, Li Z, et al. Urinary concentrations of PAH and VOC metabolites in marijuana users. *Environ Int*. 2016;88:1–8.

241. Cheng T, Chaousis S, Kodagoda Gamage H, Lam AK, Gopalan V. Polycyclic aromatic hydrocarbons detected in processed meats cause genetic changes in colorectal cancers. *Int J Mol Sci*. 2021;22(20):10959.

242. Institute of Medicine (US) and National Research Council (US) National Cancer Policy Board. *State Programs Can Reduce Tobacco Use*. Washington (DC): National Academies Press (US); 2000.

243. Tashkin DP. Effects of marijuana smoking on the lung. *Ann Am Thorac Soc*. 2013;10(3):239–47.

244. Wu TC, Tashkin DP, Djahed B, Rose JE. Pulmonary hazards of smoking marijuana as compared with tobacco. *N Engl J Med*. 1988;318(6):347–51.

245. Gieringer DH. Cannabis "vaporization": a promising strategy for smoke harm reduction. *J Cannabis Ther*. 2001;1(3–4):153–70.

246. Hoffmann D, Brunnemann KD, Gori GB, Wynder EL. On the carcinogenicity of marijuana smoke. In: Runeckles VC, ed. *Recent Advances in Phytochemistry*. Boston: Springer; 1975:63–81.

247. Hashibe M, Morgenstern H, Cui Y, et al. Marijuana use and the risk of lung and upper aerodigestive tract cancers: results of a population-based case-control study. *Cancer Epidemiol Biomarkers Prev*. 2006;15(10):1829–34.

248. Huang YHJ, Zhang ZF, Tashkin DP, Feng B, Straif K, Hashibe M. An epidemiologic review of marijuana and cancer: an update. *Cancer Epidemiol Biomarkers Prev*. 2015;24(1):15–31.

249. Tashkin DP. Effects of marijuana smoking on the lung. *Ann Am Thorac Soc*. 2013;10(3):239–47.

250. Huang YHJ, Zhang ZF, Tashkin DP, Feng B, Straif K, Hashibe M. An epidemiologic review of marijuana and cancer: an update. *Cancer Epidemiol Biomarkers Prev*. 2015;24(1):15–31.

251. Ghasemiesfe M, Barrow B, Leonard S, Keyhani S, Korenstein D. Association between marijuana use and risk of cancer: a systematic review and meta-analysis. *JAMA Netw Open*. 2019;2(11):e1916318.

252. US Department of Health and Human Services. *A Report of the Surgeon General. How Tobacco Smoke Causes Disease: What It Means to You*. Atlanta: US Department of Health and Human

Services, Centers for Disease Control and Prevention, National Center for Chronic Disease Prevention and Health Promotion, Office on Smoking and Health; 2010.

253. Riso P, Martini D, Møller P, et al. DNA damage and repair activity after broccoli intake in young healthy smokers. *Mutagenesis*. 2010;25(6):595–602.

254. Gupta GP, Massagué J. Cancer metastasis: building a framework. *Cell*. 2006;127(4): 679–95.

255. Wu X, Zhu Y, Yan H, et al. Isothiocyanates induce oxidative stress and suppress the metastasis potential of human non-small cell lung cancer cells. *BMC Cancer*. 2010;10:269.

256. Wang Q, Cui Q, Gao JP, Zhao YH. Plant-based dietary patterns and lung cancer mortality: a perspective cohort study. *Food Funct*. 2023;14(14):6470–81.

257. Kim SY, Yoon S, Kwon SM, Park KS, Lee-Kim YC. Kale juice improves coronary artery disease risk factors in hypercholesterolemic men. *Biomed Environ Sci*. 2008;21(2):91–7.

258. Park W, Amin AR, Chen ZG, Shin DM. New perspectives of curcumin in cancer prevention. *Cancer Prev Res* (Phila). 2013;6(5):387–400.

259. Park W, Amin AR, Chen ZG, Shin DM. New perspectives of curcumin in cancer prevention. *Cancer Prev Res* (Phila). 2013;6(5):387–400.

260. Nagabhushan M, Amonkar AJ, Bhide SV. In vitro antimutagenicity of curcumin against environmental mutagens. *Food Chem Toxicol*. 1987;25(7):545–7.

261. Polasa K, Raghuram TC, Krishna TP, Krishnaswamy K. Effect of turmeric on urinary mutagens in smokers. *Mutagenesis*. 1992;7(2):107–9.

262. Ravindran J, Prasad S, Aggarwal BB. Curcumin and cancer cells: how many ways can curry kill tumor cells selectively? *AAPS J*. 2009;11(3):495–510.

263. Wu SH, Hang LW, Yang JS, et al. Curcumin induces apoptosis in human non-small cell lung cancer NCI-H460 cells through ER stress and caspase cascade-and mitochondria-dependent pathways. *Anticancer Res*. 2010;30(6):2125–33.

264. Su CC, Lin JG, Li TM, et al. Curcumin-induced apoptosis of human colon cancer colo 205 cells through the production of ROS, Ca2+ and the activation of caspase-3. *Anticancer Res*. 2006;26(6B):4379–89.

265. Ravindran J, Prasad S, Aggarwal BB. Curcumin and cancer cells: how many ways can curry kill tumor cells selectively? *AAPS J*. 2009;11(3):495–510.

266. Ravindran J, Prasad S, Aggarwal BB. Curcumin and cancer cells: how many ways can curry kill tumor cells selectively? *AAPS J*. 2009;11(3):495–510.

267. Pallis AG, Syrigos KN. Lung cancer in never smokers: disease characteristics and risk factors. *Crit Rev Oncol Hematol*. 2013;88(3):494–503.

268. Chiang TA, Wu PF, Wang LF, Lee H, Lee CH, Ko YC. Mutagenicity and polycyclic aromatic hydrocarbon content of fumes from heated cooking oils produced in Taiwan. *Mutat Res*. 1997;381(2):157–61.

269. Katragadda HR, Fullana A, Sidhu S, Carbonell-Barrachina AA. Emissions of volatile aldehydes from heated cooking oils. *Food Chem*. 2010;120(1):59–65.

270. Jin ZY, Wu M, Han RQ, et al. Household ventilation may reduce effects of indoor air pollutants for prevention of lung cancer: a case-control study in a Chinese population. *PLoS ONE*. 2014;9(7):e102685.

271. Seow A, Poh WT, Teh M, et al. Fumes from meat cooking and lung cancer risk in Chinese women. *Cancer Epidemiol Biomarkers Prev*. 2000;9(11):1215–21.

272. Jedrychowski W, Perera FP, Tang D, et al. Impact of barbecued meat consumed in pregnancy on birth outcomes accounting for personal prenatal exposure to airborne polycyclic aromatic hydrocarbons: birth cohort study in Poland. *Nutrition*. 2012;28(4):372–7.

273. Perera FP, Li Z, Whyatt R, et al. Prenatal airborne polycyclic aromatic hydrocarbon exposure and child IQ at age 5 years. *Pediatrics*. 2009;124(2):e195–202.

274. Chen JW, Wang SL, Hsieh DP, Yang HH, Lee HL. Carcinogenic potencies of polycyclic aromatic hydrocarbons for back-door neighbors of restaurants with cooking emissions. *Sci Total Environ*. 2012;417–418:68–75.

275. Yang SC, Jenq SN, Kang ZC, Lee H. Identification of benzo[a]pyrene 7,8-diol 9,10-epoxide N2-deoxyguanosine in human lung adenocarcinoma cells exposed to cooking oil fumes from frying fish under domestic conditions. *Chem Res Toxicol.* 2000;13(10):1046–50.

276. Chen JW, Wang SL, Hsieh DP, Yang HH, Lee HL. Carcinogenic potencies of polycyclic aromatic hydrocarbons for back-door neighbors of restaurants with cooking emissions. *Sci Total Environ.* 2012 Feb 15;417–418:68–75.

277. Lijinsky W. N-Nitroso compounds in the diet. *Mutat Res.* 1999;443(1–2):129–38.

278. Thiébaud HP, Knize MG, Kuzmicky PA, Hsieh DP, Felton JS. Airborne mutagens produced by frying beef, pork and a soy-based food. *Food Chem Toxicol.* 1995;33(10):821–8.

279. Thiébaud HP, Knize MG, Kuzmicky PA, Hsieh DP, Felton JS. Airborne mutagens produced by frying beef, pork and a soy-based food. *Food Chem Toxicol.* 1995;33(10):821–8.

280. Mitsakou C, Housiadas C, Eleftheriadis K, Vratolis S, Helmis C, Asimakopoulos D. Lung deposition of fine and ultrafine particles outdoors and indoors during a cooking event and a no activity period. *Indoor Air.* 2007;17(2):143–52.

281. Liu Y, Carlson SA, Watson KB, Xu F, Greenlund KJ. Trends in the prevalence of chronic obstructive pulmonary disease among adults aged ≥18 years—United States, 2011–2021. *MMWR Morb Mortal Wkly Rep.* 2023;72:1250–6.

282. Tabak C, Smit HA, Räsänen L, et al. Dietary factors and pulmonary function: a cross sectional study in middle aged men from three European countries. *Thorax.* 1999;54(11):1021–6.

283. Walda IC, Tabak C, Smit HA, et al. Diet and 20-year chronic obstructive pulmonary disease mortality in middle-aged men from three European countries. *Eur J Clin Nutr.* 2002;56(7):638–43.

284. Varraso R, Jiang R, Barr RG, Willett WC, Camargo CA Jr. Prospective study of cured meats consumption and risk of chronic obstructive pulmonary disease in men. *Am J Epidemiol.* 2007 Dec 15;166(12):1438–45.

285. Jiang R, Paik DC, Hankinson JL, Barr RG. Cured meat consumption, lung function, and chronic obstructive pulmonary disease among United States adults. *Am J Respir Crit Care Med.* 2007 Apr 15;175(8):798–804.

286. Jiang R, Camargo CA, Varraso R, Paik DC, Willett WC, Barr RG. Consumption of cured meats and prospective risk of chronic obstructive pulmonary disease in women. *Am J Clin Nutr.* 2008;87(4):1002–8.

287. Keranis E, Makris D, Rodopoulou P, et al. Impact of dietary shift to higher-antioxidant foods in COPD: a randomised trial. *Eur Respir J.* 2010;36(4):774–80.

288. Varraso R, Dumas O, Tabung FK, et al. Healthful and unhealthful plant-based diets and chronic obstructive pulmonary disease in U.S. adults: prospective study. *Nutrients.* 2023;15(3):765.

289. Lim SS, Vos T, Flaxman AD, et al. A comparative risk assessment of burden of disease and injury attributable to 67 risk factors and risk factor clusters in 21 regions, 1990–2010: a systematic analysis for the Global Burden of Disease Study 2010. *Lancet.* 2012;380(9859):2224–60. Erratum in: *Lancet.* 2013;381(9874):1276 and 2013;381(9867):628.

290. Lee BJ, Kim B, Lee K. Air pollution exposure and cardiovascular disease. *Toxicol Res.* 2014;30(2):71–5.

291. Laden F, Schwartz J, Speizer FE, Dockery DW. Reduction in fine particulate air pollution and mortality: extended follow-up of the Harvard Six Cities study. *Am J Respir Crit Care Med.* 2006;173(6):667–72.

292. Olmo NRS, Saldiva PH do N, Braga ALF, Lin CA, Santos U de P, Pereira LAA. A review of low-level air pollution and adverse effects on human health: implications for epidemiological studies and public policy. *Clinics* (Sao Paulo). 2011;66(4):681–90.

293. Guarnieri M, Balmes JR. Outdoor air pollution and asthma. *Lancet.* 2014;383(9928):1581–92.

294. Kim JW, Park S, Lim CW, Lee K, Kim B. The role of air pollutants in initiating liver disease. *Toxicol Res.* 2014;30(2):65–70.
295. Janghorbani M, Momeni F, Mansourian M. Systematic review and metaanalysis of air pollution exposure and risk of diabetes. *Eur J Epidemiol.* 2014;29(4):231–42.
296. Olmo NRS, do Nascimento Saldiva PH, Braga ALF, Lin CA, de Paula Santos U, Pereira LAA. A review of low-level air pollution and adverse effects on human health: implications for epidemiological studies and public policy. *Clinics* (Sao Paulo). 2011;66(4):681–90.
297. Olmo NRS, do Nascimento Saldiva PH, Braga ALF, Lin CA, de Paula Santos U, Pereira LAA. A review of low-level air pollution and adverse effects on human health: implications for epidemiological studies and public policy. *Clinics* (Sao Paulo). 2011;66(4):681–90.
298. Gilliland FD, Li YF, Saxon A, Diaz-Sanchez D. Effect of glutathione-S-transferase M1 and P1 genotypes on xenobiotic enhancement of allergic responses: randomised, placebo-controlled crossover study. *Lancet.* 2004;363(9403):119–25.
299. Tracy RP, Psaty BM, Macy E, et al. Lifetime smoking exposure affects the association of C-reactive protein with cardiovascular disease risk factors and subclinical disease in healthy elderly subjects. *Arterioscler Thromb Vasc Biol.* 1997;17(10):2167–76.
300. O'Loughlin J, Lambert M, Karp I, et al. Association between cigarette smoking and C-reactive protein in a representative, population-based sample of adolescents. *Nicotine Tob Res.* 2008;10(3):525–32.
301. Jiang Y, Wu SH, Shu XO, et al. Cruciferous vegetable intake is inversely correlated with circulating levels of proinflammatory markers in women. *J Acad Nutr Diet.* 2014;114(5):700–8.e2.
302. Liu X, Chang Y, Li Y, et al. Prospective cohort study of broccoli consumption frequency and all-cause and cause-specific mortality risks. *Front Nutr.* 2024;10:1286658.
303. Ritz SA, Wan J, Diaz-Sanchez D. Sulforaphane-stimulated phase II enzyme induction inhibits cytokine production by airway epithelial cells stimulated with diesel extract. *Am J Physiol Lung Cell Mol Physiol.* 2007;292(1):L33–9.
304. Riedl MA, Saxon A, Diaz-Sanchez D. Oral sulforaphane increases Phase II antioxidant enzymes in the human upper airway. *Clin Immunol.* 2009;130(3):244–51.
305. Heber D, Li Z, Garcia-Lloret M, et al. Sulforaphane-rich broccoli sprout extract attenuates nasal allergic response to diesel exhaust particles. *Food Funct.* 2014;5(1):35–41.
306. Egner PA, Chen JG, Zarth AT, et al. Rapid and sustainable detoxication of airborne pollutants by broccoli sprout beverage: results of a randomized clinical trial in China. *Cancer Prev Res* (Phila). 2014;7(8):813–23.
307. Warner JO. Worldwide variations in the prevalence of atopic symptoms: what does it all mean? *Thorax.* 1999;54 Suppl 2:S46–51.
308. 2021 National Health Interview Survey (NHIS). Most recent national asthma data. U.S. Centers for Disease Control and Prevention. https://www.cdc.gov/asthma/most_recent_national_asthma_data.htm. May 10, 2023. Accessed January 22, 2025.
309. Warner JO. Worldwide variations in the prevalence of atopic symptoms: what does it all mean? *Thorax.* 1999;54 Suppl 2:S46–51.
310. Aït-Khaled N, Pearce N, Anderson HR, et al. Global map of the prevalence of symptoms of rhinoconjunctivitis in children: the International Study of Asthma and Allergies in Childhood (ISAAC) Phase Three. *Allergy.* 2009;64(1):123–48.
311. Asher MI, Stewart AW, Mallol J, et al. Which population level environmental factors are associated with asthma, rhinoconjunctivitis and eczema? Review of the ecological analyses of ISAAC Phase One. *Respir Res.* 2010;11:8.
312. Ellwood P, Asher MI, Björkstén B, Burr M, Pearce N, Robertson CF. Diet and asthma, allergic rhinoconjunctivitis and atopic eczema symptom prevalence: an ecological analysis of the International Study of Asthma and Allergies in Childhood (ISAAC) data. ISAAC Phase One Study Group. *Eur Respir J.* 2001;17(3):436–43.

313. Protudjer JL, Sevenhuysen GP, Ramsey CD, Kozyrskyj AL, Becker AB. Low vegetable intake is associated with allergic asthma and moderate-to-severe airway hyperresponsiveness. *Pediatr Pulmonol.* 2012;47(12):1159–69.
314. Bime C, Wei CY, Holbrook J, Smith LJ, Wise RA. Association of dietary soy genistein intake with lung function and asthma control: a post-hoc analysis of patients enrolled in a prospective multicentre clinical trial. *Prim Care Respir J.* 2012;21(4):398–404.
315. Agrawal S, Pearce N, Ebrahim S. Prevalence and risk factors for self-reported asthma in an adult Indian population: a cross-sectional survey. *Int J Tuberc Lung Dis.* 2013;17(2):275–82.
316. Tsai HJ, Tsai AC. The association of diet with respiratory symptoms and asthma in schoolchildren in Taipei, Taiwan. *J Asthma.* 2007;44(8):599–603.
317. Yusoff NA, Hampton SM, Dickerson JW, Morgan JB. The effects of exclusion of dietary egg and milk in the management of asthmatic children: a pilot study. *J R Soc Promot Health.* 2004;124(2):74–80.
318. Wood LG, Garg ML, Blake RJ, Garcia-Caraballo S, Gibson PG. Airway and circulating levels of carotenoids in asthma and healthy controls. *J Am Coll Nutr.* 2005;24(6):448–55.
319. Miller ER, Appel LJ, Risby TH. Effect of dietary patterns on measures of lipid peroxidation: results from a randomized clinical trial. *Circulation.* 1998;98(22):2390–5.
320. Wood LG, Garg ML, Smart JM, Scott HA, Barker D, Gibson PG. Manipulating antioxidant intake in asthma: a randomized controlled trial. *Am J Clin Nutr.* 2012;96(3):534–43.
321. Ljaljević Grbić M, Unković N, Dimkić I, et al. Frankincense and myrrh essential oils and burn incense fume against micro-inhabitants of sacral ambients. Wisdom of the ancients? *J Ethnopharmacol.* 2018;219:1–14.
322. Mannix RC, Nguyen KP, Tan EW, Ho EE, Phalen RF. Physical characterization of incense aerosols. *Sci Total Environ.* 1996;193(2):149–58.
323. Roberts D, Pontin D. The health risks of incense use in the home: an underestimated source of indoor air pollution? *Community Pract.* 2016;89(3):36–41.
324. Višić B, Kranjc E, Pirker L, et al. Incense powder and particle emission characteristics during and after burning incense in an unventilated room setting. *Air Qual Atmos Health.* 2018;11:649–63.
325. Ho SSH, Yu JZ. Concentrations of formaldehyde and other carbonyls in environments affected by incense burning. *J Environ Monit.* 2002;4(5):728–33.
326. Zhang Z, Tan L, Huss A, et al. Household incense burning and children's respiratory health: a cohort study in Hong Kong. *Pediatr Pulmonol.* 2019;54(4):399–404.
327. Chen YC, Ho WC, Yu YH. Adolescent lung function associated with incense burning and other environmental exposures at home. *Indoor Air.* 2017;27(4):746–52.
328. Pan A, Clark ML, Ang LW, Yu MC, Yuan JM, Koh WP. Incense use and cardiovascular mortality among Chinese in Singapore: the Singapore Chinese Health Study. *Environ Health Perspect.* 2014;122(12):1279–84.
329. Navasumrit P, Arayasiri M, Hiang OMT, et al. Potential health effects of exposure to carcinogenic compounds in incense smoke in temple workers. *Chem Biol Interact.* 2008;173(1):19–31.
330. Seow WJ, Lan Q. Domestic incense use and lung cancer in Asia: a review. *Rev Environ Health.* 2016;31(1):155–8.
331. Friborg JT, Yuan JM, Wang R, Koh WP, Lee HP, Yu MC. Incense use and respiratory tract carcinomas: a prospective cohort study. *Cancer.* 2008;113(7):1676–84.
332. Preston-Martin S, Yu MC, Benton B, Henderson BE. N-Nitroso compounds and childhood brain tumors: a case-control study. *Cancer Res.* 1982;42(12):5240–5.
333. Wei CF, Chen MH, Lin CC, et al. Household incense burning and infant gross motor development: results from the Taiwan Birth Cohort Study. *Environ Int.* 2018;115:110–6.
334. Wong A, Lou W, Ho KF, et al. Indoor incense burning impacts cognitive functions and brain functional connectivity in community older adults. *Sci Rep.* 2020;10(1):7090.

335. Višić B, Kranjc E, Pirker L, et al. Incense powder and particle emission characteristics during and after burning incense in an unventilated room setting. *Air Qual Atmos Health*. 2018;11:649–63.
336. Roberts D, Pontin D. The health risks of incense use in the home: an underestimated source of indoor air pollution? *Community Pract*. 2016;89(3):36–41.
337. Wood LG, Garg ML, Smart JM, Scott HA, Barker D, Gibson PG. Manipulating antioxidant intake in asthma: a randomized controlled trial. *Am J Clin Nutr*. 2012;96(3):534–43.
338. Patel S, Murray CS, Woodcock A, Simpson A, Custovic A. Dietary antioxidant intake, allergic sensitization and allergic diseases in young children. *Allergy*. 2009;64(12):1766–72.
339. Troisi RJ, Willett WC, Weiss ST, Trichopoulos D, Rosner B, Speizer FE. A prospective study of diet and adult-onset asthma. *Am J Respir Crit Care Med*. 1995;151(5):1401–8.
340. Wood LG, Garg ML, Smart JM, Scott HA, Barker D, Gibson PG. Manipulating antioxidant intake in asthma: a randomized controlled trial. *Am J Clin Nutr*. 2012;96(3):534–43.
341. Lindahl O, Lindwall L, Spångberg A, Stenram A, Ockerman PA. Vegan regimen with reduced medication in the treatment of bronchial asthma. *J Asthma*. 1985;22(1):45–55.
342. Lindahl O, Lindwall L, Spångberg A, Stenram A, Ockerman PA. Vegan regimen with reduced medication in the treatment of bronchial asthma. *J Asthma*. 1985;22(1):45–55.
343. Lindahl O, Lindwall L, Spångberg A, Stenram A, Ockerman PA. Vegan regimen with reduced medication in the treatment of bronchial asthma. *J Asthma*. 1985;22(1):45–55.
344. Maștaleru A, Popescu G, Abdulan IM, et al. Association between serum lipids and asthma in adults—a systematic review. *Nutrients*. 2024;16(13):2070.
345. Tsao CW, Aday AW, Almarzooq ZI, Anderson CAM, Arora P, Avery CL, et al. Heart disease and stroke statistics—2023 update: a report from the American Heart Association. *Circulation*. 2023;147(8):e93–e621.
346. Centers for Disease Control and Prevention, National Center for Health Statistics. National Vital Statistics System, Mortality 2018–2023 on CDC WONDER Online Database. http://wonder.cdc.gov/ucd-icd10-expanded.html. Accessed January 16, 2025.
347. Mozaffarian D, Benjamin EJ, Go AS, et al. Heart disease and stroke statistics—2015 update: a report from the American Heart Association. *Circulation*. 2015;131(4):e29–322.
348. Grau-Olivares M, Arboix A. Mild cognitive impairment in stroke patients with ischemic cerebral small-vessel disease: a forerunner of vascular dementia? *Expert Rev Neurother*. 2009;9(8):1201–17.
349. Aune D, Chan DS, Lau R, et al. Dietary fibre, whole grains, and risk of colorectal cancer: systematic review and dose-response meta-analysis of prospective studies. *BMJ*. 2011;343:d6617.
350. Aune D, Chan DS, Greenwood DC, et al. Dietary fiber and breast cancer risk: a systematic review and meta-analysis of prospective studies. *Ann Oncol*. 2012;23(6):1394–402.
351. Yao B, Fang H, Xu W, et al. Dietary fiber intake and risk of type 2 diabetes: a dose-response analysis of prospective studies. *Eur J Epidemiol*. 2014;29(2):79–88.
352. Threapleton DE, Greenwood DC, Evans CE, et al. Dietary fibre intake and risk of cardiovascular disease: systematic review and meta-analysis. *BMJ*. 2013;347:f6879.
353. Maskarinec G, Takata Y, Pagano I, et al. Trends and dietary determinants of overweight and obesity in a multiethnic population. *Obesity* (Silver Spring). 2006;14(4):717–26.
354. Kim Y, Je Y. Dietary fiber intake and total mortality: a meta-analysis of prospective cohort studies. *Am J Epidemiol*. 2014;180(6):565–73.
355. Threapleton DE, Greenwood DC, Evans CE, et al. Dietary fiber intake and risk of first stroke: a systematic review and meta-analysis. *Stroke*. 2013;44(5):1360–8.
356. United States Department of Agriculture, Agricultural Research Service. Usual nutrient intake from food and beverages, by gender and age, What We Eat in America, NHANES 2017–March 2020 prepandemic. www.ars.usda.gov/nea/bhnrc/fsrg. 2023. Accessed January 19, 2025.
357. Threapleton DE, Greenwood DC, Evans CE, et al. Dietary fiber intake and risk of first stroke: a systematic review and meta-analysis. *Stroke*. 2013;44(5):1360–8.

358. Whitehead A, Beck EJ, Tosh S, Wolever TM. Cholesterol-lowering effects of oat β-glucan: a meta-analysis of randomized controlled trials. *Am J Clin Nutr.* 2014;100(6):1413–21.
359. Silva FM, Kramer CK, De Almeida JC, Steemburgo T, Gross JL, Azevedo MJ. Fiber intake and glycemic control in patients with type 2 diabetes mellitus: a systematic review with meta-analysis of randomized controlled trials. *Nutr Rev.* 2013;71(12):790–801.
360. Streppel MT, Arends LR, van 't Veer P, Grobbee DE, Geleijnse JM. Dietary fiber and blood pressure: a meta-analysis of randomized placebo-controlled trials. *Arch Intern Med.* 2005;165(2):150–6.
361. Centers for Disease Control and Prevention. Deaths: final data for 2013 table 10. Number of deaths from 113 selected causes. National Vital Statistics Report. 2016;64(2).
362. van de Laar RJ, Stehouwer CDA, van Bussel BCT, et al. Lower lifetime dietary fiber intake is associated with carotid artery stiffness: the Amsterdam Growth and Health Longitudinal Study. *Am J Clin Nutr.* 2012;96(1):14–23.
363. van de Laar RJ, Stehouwer CDA, van Bussel BCT, et al. Lower lifetime dietary fiber intake is associated with carotid artery stiffness: the Amsterdam Growth and Health Longitudinal Study. *Am J Clin Nutr.* 2012;96(1):14–23.
364. Casiglia E, Tikhonoff V, Caffi S, et al. High dietary fiber intake prevents stroke at a population level. *Clin Nutr.* 2013;32(5):811–8.
365. Tikhonoff V, Palatini P, Casiglia E. Letter by Tikhonoff et al regarding article, "Dietary fiber intake and risk of first stroke: a systematic review and meta-analysis." *Stroke.* 2013;44(9):e109.
366. Threapleton DE, Greenwood DC, Burley VJ. Response to letter regarding article, "Dietary fiber intake and risk of first stroke: a systematic review and meta-analysis." *Stroke.* 2013;44(9):e110.
367. Eaton SB, Konner M. Paleolithic nutrition. A consideration of its nature and current implications. *N Engl J Med.* 1985;312(5):283–9.
368. Cogswell ME, Zhang Z, Carriquiry AL, et al. Sodium and potassium intakes among US adults: NHANES 2003–2008. *Am J Clin Nutr.* 2012;96(3):647–57.
369. Cogswell ME, Zhang Z, Carriquiry AL, et al. Sodium and potassium intakes among US adults: NHANES 2003–2008. *Am J Clin Nutr.* 2012;96(3):647–57.
370. D'Elia L, Barba G, Cappuccio FP, et al. Potassium intake, stroke, and cardiovascular disease a meta-analysis of prospective studies. *J Am Coll Cardiol.* 2011;57(10):1210–9.
371. U.S. Department of Agriculture. USDA National Nutrient Database for Standard Reference. https://web.archive.org/web/20151012070814/http://ndb.nal.usda.gov/ndb/nutrients/report/nutrientsfrm?max=25&offset=0&totCount=0&nutrient1=306&nutrient2=&nutrient3=&subset=0&fg=&sort=c&measureby=m. Accessed January 22, 2025.
372. U.S. Department of Agriculture, Agricultural Research Service. Food sources of potassium. Dietary Guidelines for Americans. https://www.dietaryguidelines.gov/food-sources-potassium. Accessed January 19, 2025.
373. Hu D, Huang J, Wang Y, Zhang D, Qu Y. Fruits and vegetables consumption and risk of stroke: a meta-analysis of prospective cohort studies. *Stroke.* 2014;45(6):1613–9.
374. Morand C, Dubray C, Milenkovic D, et al. Hesperidin contributes to the vascular protective effects of orange juice: a randomized crossover study in healthy volunteers. *Am J Clin Nutr.* 2011;93(1):73–80.
375. Takumi H, Nakamura H, Simizu T, et al. Bioavailability of orally administered water-dispersible hesperetin and its effect on peripheral vasodilatation in human subjects: implication of endothelial functions of plasma conjugated metabolites. *Food Funct.* 2012;3(4):389–98.
376. Patyar S, Patyar RR. Correlation between sleep duration and risk of stroke. *J Stroke Cerebrovasc Dis.* 2015;24(5):905–11.
377. Ikehara S, Iso H, Date C, et al; JACC Study Group. Association of sleep duration with mortality from cardiovascular disease and other causes for Japanese men and women: the JACC study. *Sleep.* 2009;32(3):295–301.

378. Fang J, Wheaton AG, Ayala C. Sleep duration and history of stroke among adults from the USA. *J Sleep Res.* 2014;23(5):531–7.
379. von Ruesten A, Weikert C, Fietze I, et al. Association of sleep duration with chronic diseases in the European Prospective Investigation into Cancer and Nutrition (EPIC)—Potsdam study. *PLoS ONE.* 2012;7(1):e30972.
380. Pan A, De Silva DA, Yuan JM, et al. Sleep duration and risk of stroke mortality among Chinese adults: Singapore Chinese health study. *Stroke.* 2014;45(6):1620–5.
381. Leng Y, Cappuccio FP, Wainwright NW, et al. Sleep duration and risk of fatal and nonfatal stroke: a prospective study and meta-analysis. *Neurology.* 2015;84(11):1072–9.
382. Sansevero TB. *The Profit Machine.* Madrid: Cultiva Libros;2009:59.
383. Harman D. The biologic clock: the mitochondria? *J Am Geriatr Soc.* 1972;20(4):145–7.
384. Graham J, Poole ND, Traylor J. Cyanide toxicity. In: *StatPearls.* Treasure Island (FL): StatPearls Publishing; 2025.
385. Chance B, Sies H, Boveris A. Hydroperoxide metabolism in mammalian organs. *Physiol Rev.* 1979;59(3):527–605.
386. Emerit I. Reactive oxygen species, chromosome mutation, and cancer: possible role of clastogenic factors in carcinogenesis. *Free Radic Biol Med.* 1994;16(1):99–109.
387. Rinnerthaler M, Bischof J, Streubel MK, Trost A, Richter K. Oxidative stress in aging human skin. *Biomolecules.* 2015;5(2):545–89.
388. Logan S, Royce GH, Owen D, et al. Accelerated decline in cognition in a mouse model of increased oxidative stress. *Geroscience.* 2019;41(5):591–607.
389. Hensley K, Floyd RA. Reactive oxygen species and protein oxidation in aging: a look back, a look ahead. *Arch Biochem Biophys.* 2002;397(2):377–83.
390. Rautiainen S, Larsson S, Virtamo J, et al. Total antioxidant capacity of diet and risk of stroke: a population-based prospective cohort of women. *Stroke.* 2012;43(2):335–40.
391. Del Rio D, Agnoli C, Pellegrini N, et al. Total antioxidant capacity of the diet is associated with lower risk of ischemic stroke in a large Italian cohort. *J Nutr.* 2011;141(1):118–23.
392. Satia JA, Littman A, Slatore CG, Galanko JA, White E. Long-term use of beta-carotene, retinol, lycopene, and lutein supplements and lung cancer risk: results from the VITamins And Lifestyle (VITAL) study. *Am J Epidemiol.* 2009;169(7):815–28.
393. Hankey GJ. Vitamin supplementation and stroke prevention. *Stroke.* 2012;43(10):2814–8.
394. Carlsen MH, Halvorsen BL, Holte K, et al. The total antioxidant content of more than 3100 foods, beverages, spices, herbs and supplements used worldwide. *Nutr J.* 2010;9:3.
395. Yang M, Chung SJ, Chung CE, et al. Estimation of total antioxidant capacity from diet and supplements in US adults. *Br J Nutr.* 2011;106(2):254–63.
396. Carlsen MH, Halvorsen BL, Holte K, et al. The total antioxidant content of more than 3100 foods, beverages, spices, herbs and supplements used worldwide. *Nutr J.* 2010;9:3.
397. Bastin S, Henken K. Water content of fruits and vegetables. University of Kentucky College of Agriculture Cooperative Extension Service. https://www.academia.edu/5729963/Water_Content_of_Fruits_and_Vegetables. December 1997. Accessed January 19, 2025.
398. Carlsen MH, Halvorsen BL, Holte K, et al. The total antioxidant content of more than 3100 foods, beverages, spices, herbs and supplements used worldwide. *Nutr J.* 2010;9:3.
399. Liu Y, Zhu L, Li D, Wang L, Tang H, Zhang C. Stroke risk with vegetarian, low-animal and high-animal diets: a systematic review and meta-analysis. *Asia Pac J Clin Nutr.* 2022;31(3):422–32.
400. Carlsen MH, Halvorsen BL, Holte K, et al. The total antioxidant content of more than 3100 foods, beverages, spices, herbs and supplements used worldwide. *Nutr J.* 2010;9:3.
401. Kelly PJ, Morrow JD, Ning M, et al. Oxidative stress and matrix metalloproteinase-9 in acute ischemic stroke: the Biomarker Evaluation for Antioxidant Therapies in Stroke (BEAT-Stroke) study. *Stroke.* 2008;39(1):100–4.
402. Lilamand M, Kelaiditi E, Guyonnet S, et al. Flavonoids and arterial stiffness: promising perspectives. *Nutr Metab Cardiovasc Dis.* 2014;24(7):698–704.

403. Santhakumar AB, Bulmer AC, Singh I. A review of the mechanisms and effectiveness of dietary polyphenols in reducing oxidative stress and thrombotic risk. *J Hum Nutr Diet.* 2014;27(1):1–21.
404. Stoclet JC, Chataigneau T, Ndiaye M, et al. Vascular protection by dietary polyphenols. *Eur J Pharmacol.* 2004;500(1–3):299–313.
405. Moylan S, Berk M, Dean OM, et al. Oxidative & nitrosative stress in depression: why so much stress? *Neurosci Biobehav Rev.* 2014;45:46–62.
406. Watzl B. Anti-inflammatory effects of plant-based foods and of their constituents. *Int J Vitam Nutr Res.* 2008;78(6):293–8.
407. Franzini L, Ardigi D, Valtueña S, et al. Food selection based on high total antioxidant capacity improves endothelial function in a low cardiovascular risk population. *Nutr Metab Cardiovasc Dis.* 2012;22(1):50–7.
408. Alzheimer's Association. 2024 Alzheimer's disease facts and figures. *Alzheimers Dement.* 2024;20(5):3708–21.
409. de la Torre JC. A turning point for Alzheimer's disease? *Biofactors.* 2012;38(2):78–83.
410. de la Torre JC. Alzheimer's disease is incurable but preventable. *J Alzheimers Dis.* 2010;20(3):861–70.
411. Barnes DE, Yaffe K. The projected effect of risk factor reduction on Alzheimer's disease prevalence. *Lancet Neurol.* 2011;10(9):819–28.
412. Singh-Manoux A, Kivimaki M, Glymour MM, et al. Timing of onset of cognitive decline: results from Whitehall II prospective cohort study. *BMJ.* 2012;344:d7622.
413. Roher AE, Tyas SL, Maarouf CL, et al. Intracranial atherosclerosis as a contributing factor to Alzheimer's disease dementia. *Alzheimers Dement.* 2011;7(4):436–44.
414. Ramirez-Bermudez J. Alzheimer's disease: critical notes on the history of a medical concept. *Arch Med Res.* 2012;43(8):595–9.
415. Alzheimer A, Stelzmann RA, Schnitzlein HN, Murtagh FR. An English translation of Alzheimer's 1907 paper, "Uber eine eigenartige Erkankung der Hirnrinde." *Clin Anat.* 1995;8(6):429–31.
416. Kovacic JC, Fuster V. Atherosclerotic risk factors, vascular cognitive impairment, and Alzheimer disease. *Mt Sinai J Med.* 2012;79:664–73.
417. Cardiogenic dementia. *Lancet.* 1977;1(8001):27–8.
418. Roher AE, Tyas SL, Maarouf CL, et al. Intracranial atherosclerosis as a contributing factor to Alzheimer's disease dementia. *Alzheimers Dement.* 2011;7(4):436–44.
419. Roher AE, Tyas SL, Maarouf CL, et al. Intracranial atherosclerosis as a contributing factor to Alzheimer's disease dementia. *Alzheimers Dement.* 2011;7(4):436–44.
420. Yarchoan M, Xie SX, Kling MA, et al. Cerebrovascular atherosclerosis correlates with Alzheimer pathology in neurodegenerative dementias. *Brain.* 2012;135(Pt 12):3749–56.
421. Honig LS, Kukull W, Mayeux R. Atherosclerosis and AD: analysis of data from the US National Alzheimer's Coordinating Center. *Neurology.* 2005;64(3):494–500.
422. de la Torre JC. Vascular risk factors: a ticking time bomb to Alzheimer's disease. *Am J Alzheimers Dis Other Demen.* 2013;28(6):551–9.
423. Roher AE, Tyas SL, Maarouf CL, et al. Intracranial atherosclerosis as a contributing factor to Alzheimer's disease dementia. *Alzheimers Dement.* 2011;7(4):436–44.
424. de la Torre JC. Vascular basis of Alzheimer's pathogenesis. *Ann N Y Acad Sci.* 2002;977:196–215.
425. Zhu J, Wang Y, Li J, et al. Intracranial artery stenosis and progression from mild cognitive impairment to Alzheimer disease. *Neurology.* 2014;82(10):842–9.
426. Deschaintre Y, Richard F, Leys D, Pasquier F. Treatment of vascular risk factors is associated with slower decline in Alzheimer disease. *Neurology.* 2009;73(9):674–80.
427. Mizuno T, Nakata M, Naiki H, et al. Cholesterol-dependent generation of a seeding amyloid beta-protein in cell culture. *J Biol Chem.* 1999;274(21):15110–4.
428. National Academies of Sciences, Engineering, and Medicine. Dietary Reference Intakes

for Energy, Carbohydrate, Fiber, Fat, Fatty Acids, Cholesterol, Protein, and Amino Acids. Washington, DC: The National Academies Press; 2005.
429. Trumbo PR, Shimakawa T. Tolerable upper intake levels for trans fat, saturated fat, and cholesterol. *Nutr Rev.* 2011;69(5):270–8.
430. Benjamin MM, Roberts WC. Facts and principles learned at the 39th Annual Williamsburg Conference on Heart Disease. *Proc (Bayl Univ Med Cent).* 2013;26(2):124–36.
431. Corsinovi L, Biasi F, Poli G, et al. Dietary lipids and their oxidized products in Alzheimer's disease. *Mol Nutr Food Res.* 2011;55 Suppl 2:S161–72.
432. Matsuzaki T, Sasaki K, Hata J, et al. Association of Alzheimer disease pathology with abnormal lipid metabolism: the Hisayama Study. *Neurology.* 2011;77(11):1068–75.
433. Harris JR, Milton NGN. Cholesterol in Alzheimer's disease and other amyloidogenic disorders. *Subcell Biochem.* 2010;51:47–75.
434. Puglielli L, Tanzi RE, Kovacs DM. Alzheimer's disease: the cholesterol connection. *Nat Neurosci.* 2003;6(4):345–51.
435. Harris JR, Milton NGN. Cholesterol in Alzheimer's disease and other amyloidogenic disorders. *Subcell Biochem.* 2010;51:47–75.
436. Reed B, Villeneuve S, Mack W, et al. Associations between serum cholesterol levels and cerebral amyloidosis. *JAMA Neurol.* 2014;71(2):195–200.
437. U.S. Food and Drug Administration. Important safety label changes to cholesterol-lowering statin drugs. U.S. Department of Health and Human Services. http://www.fda.gov/Drugs/DrugSafety/ucm293101.htm. July 7, 2012. Accessed January 19, 2025.
438. Rojas-Fernandez CH, Cameron JC. Is statin-associated cognitive impairment clinically relevant? A narrative review and clinical recommendations. *Ann Pharmacother.* 2012;46(4):549–57.
439. Grant WB. Dietary links to Alzheimer's disease. *Alzheimer Dis Rev.* 1997;2:42–55.
440. Chandra V, Pandav R, Dodge HH, et al. Incidence of Alzheimer's disease in a rural community in India: the Indo-US study. *Neurology.* 2001;57(6):985–9.
441. White L, Petrovitch H, Ross GW, et al. Prevalence of dementia in older Japanese-American men in Hawaii: the Honolulu-Asia Aging Study. *JAMA.* 1996;276(12):955–60.
442. Grant WB. Dietary links to Alzheimer's disease. *Alzheimer Dis Rev.* 1997;2:42–55.
443. Grant WB. Trends in diet and Alzheimer's disease during the nutrition transition in Japan and developing countries. *J Alzheimers Dis.* 2014;38(3):611–20.
444. Chan KY, Wang W, Wu JJ, et al. Epidemiology of Alzheimer's disease and other forms of dementia in China, 1990–2010: a systematic review and analysis. *Lancet.* 2013;381(9882):2016–23.
445. Grant WB. Trends in diet and Alzheimer's disease during the nutrition transition in Japan and developing countries. *J Alzheimers Dis.* 2014;38(3):611–20.
446. Chandra V, Ganguli M, Pandav R, et al. Prevalence of Alzheimer's disease and other dementias in rural India: the Indo-US study. *Neurology.* 1998;51(4):1000–8.
447. Shetty PS. Nutrition transition in India. *Public Health Nutr.* 2002;5(1A):175–82.
448. Giem P, Beeson WL, Fraser GE. The incidence of dementia and intake of animal products: preliminary findings from the Adventist Health Study. *Neuroepidemiology.* 1993;12(1):28–36.
449. Roses AD, Saunders AM. APOE is a major susceptibility gene for Alzheimer's disease. *Curr Opin Biotechnol.* 1994;5(6):663–7.
450. Puglielli L, Tanzi RE, Kovacs DM. Alzheimer's disease: the cholesterol connection. *Nat Neurosci.* 2003;6(4):345–51.
451. Chen X, Hui L, Soliman ML, Geiger JD. Altered cholesterol intracellular trafficking and the development of pathological hallmarks of sporadic AD. *J Parkinsons Dis Alzheimers Dis.* 2014;1(1).
452. Sepehrnia B, Kamboh MI, Adams-Campbell LL, et al. Genetic studies of human apolipoproteins. X. The effect of the apolipoprotein E polymorphism on quantitative levels of lipoproteins in Nigerian blacks. *Am J Hum Genet.* 1989;45(4):586–91.

453. Grant WB. Dietary links to Alzheimer's disease. *Alzheimer Dis Rev.* 1997;2:42–55.
454. Sepehrnia B, Kamboh MI, Adams-Campbell LL, et al. Genetic studies of human apolipoproteins. X. The effect of the apolipoprotein E polymorphism on quantitative levels of lipoproteins in Nigerian blacks. *Am J Hum Genet.* 1989;45(4):586–91.
455. Hendrie HC, Murrell J, Gao S, Unverzagt FW, Ogunniyi A, Hall KS. International studies in dementia with particular emphasis on populations of African origin. *Alzheimer Dis Assoc Disord.* 2006;20(3 Suppl 2):S42–6.
456. Kivipelto M, Helkala EL, Laakso MP, et al. Apolipoprotein E epsilon4 allele, elevated midlife total cholesterol level, and high midlife systolic blood pressure are independent risk factors for late-life Alzheimer disease. *Ann Intern Med.* 2002;137(3):149–55.
457. Kivipelto M, Helkala EL, Laakso MP, et al. Apolipoprotein E epsilon4 allele, elevated midlife total cholesterol level, and high midlife systolic blood pressure are independent risk factors for late-life Alzheimer disease. *Ann Intern Med.* 2002;137(3):149–55.
458. Jost BC, Grossberg GT. The natural history of Alzheimer's disease: a brain bank study. *J Am Geriatr Soc.* 1995;43(11):1248–55.
459. Del Tredici K, Braak H. Neurofibrillary changes of the Alzheimer type in very elderly individuals: neither inevitable nor benign: Commentary on 'No disease in the brain of a 115-year-old woman.' *Neurobiol Aging.* 2008;29(8):1133–6.
460. Barnard ND, Bush AI, Ceccarelli A, et al. Dietary and lifestyle guidelines for the prevention of Alzheimer's disease. *Neurobiol Aging.* 2014;35 Suppl 2:S74–8.
461. Lourida I, Soni M, Thompson-Coon J, et al. Mediterranean diet, cognitive function, and dementia: a systematic review. *Epidemiology.* 2013;24(4):479–89.
462. Roberts RO, Geda YE, Cerhan JR, et al. Vegetables, unsaturated fats, moderate alcohol intake, and mild cognitive impairment. *Dementia and Geriatric Cognitive Disorders.* 2010;29(5):413–23.
463. Okereke OI, Rosner BA, Kim DH, et al. Dietary fat types and 4-year cognitive change in community-dwelling older women. *Ann Neurol.* 2012;72(1):124–34.
464. Parletta N, Milte CM, Meyer BJ. Nutritional modulation of cognitive function and mental health. *J Nutr Biochem.* 2013;24(5):725–43.
465. Essa MM, Vijayan RK, Castellano-Gonzalez G, Memon MA, Braidy N, Guillemin GJ. Neuroprotective effect of natural products against Alzheimer's disease. *Neurochem Res.* 2012;37(9):1829–42.
466. Shukitt-Hale B. Blueberries and neuronal aging. *Gerontology.* 2012;58(6):518–23.
467. Cherniack EP. A berry thought-provoking idea: the potential role of plant polyphenols in the treatment of age-related cognitive disorders. *Br J Nutr.* 2012;108(5):794–800.
468. Johnson EJ. A possible role for lutein and zeaxanthin in cognitive function in the elderly. *Am J Clin Nutr.* 2012;96(5):1161S–5S.
469. Krikorian R, Shidler MD, Nash TA, et al. Blueberry supplementation improves memory in older adults. *J Agric Food Chem.* 2010;58(7):3996–4000.
470. Devore EE, Kang JH, Breteler MMB, et al. Dietary intakes of berries and flavonoids in relation to cognitive decline. *Ann Neurol.* 2012;72(1):135–43.
471. Dai Q, Borenstein AR, Wu Y, et al. Fruit and vegetable juices and Alzheimer's disease: the Kame Project. *Am J Med.* 2006;119(9):751–9.
472. Krikorian R, Nash TA, Shidler MD, Shukitt-Hale B, Joseph JA. Concord grape juice supplementation improves memory function in older adults with mild cognitive impairment. *Br J Nutr.* 2010;103(5):730–4.
473. Nurk E, Refsum H, Drevon CA, et al. Cognitive performance among the elderly in relation to the intake of plant foods. The Hordaland Health Study. *Br J Nutr.* 2010;104(8):1190–201.
474. Mullen W, Marks SC, Crozier A. Evaluation of phenolic compounds in commercial fruit juices and fruit drinks. *J Agric Food Chem.* 2007;55(8):3148–57.
475. Tarozzi A, Morroni F, Merlicco A, et al. Neuroprotective effects of cyanidin 3-O-glucopyranoside on amyloid beta (25–35) oligomer-induced toxicity. *Neurosci Lett.* 2010;473(2):72–6.

476. Hattori M, Sugino E, Minoura K, et al. Different inhibitory response of cyanidin and methylene blue for filament formation of tau microtubule-binding domain. *Biochem Biophys Res Commun.* 2008;374(1):158–63.
477. Mandel SA, Weinreb O, Amit T, Youdim MB. Molecular mechanisms of the neuroprotective/neurorescue action of multi-target green tea polyphenols. *Front Biosci* (Schol Ed). 2012;4:581–98.
478. Ward RJ, Zucca FA, Duyn JH, Crichton RR, Zecca L. The role of iron in brain ageing and neurodegenerative disorders. *Lancet Neurol.* 2014;13(10):1045–60.
479. Hishikawa N, Takahashi Y, Amakusa Y, et al. Effects of turmeric on Alzheimer's disease with behavioral and psychological symptoms of dementia. *Ayu.* 2012;33(4):499–504.
480. Akhondzadeh S, Sabet MS, Harirchian MH, et al. Saffron in the treatment of patients with mild to moderate Alzheimer's disease: a 16-week, randomized and placebo-controlled trial. *J Clin Pharm Ther.* 2010;35(5):581–8.
481. Akhondzadeh S, Shafiee Sabet M, Harirchian MH, et al. A 22-week, multicenter, randomized, double-blind controlled trial of Crocus sativus in the treatment of mild-to-moderate Alzheimer's disease. *Psychopharmacology* (Berl). 2010;207(4):637–43.
482. Hyde C, Peters J, Bond M, et al. Evolution of the evidence on the effectiveness and cost-effectiveness of acetylcholinesterase inhibitors and memantine for Alzheimer's disease: systematic review and economic model. *Age Ageing.* 2013;42(1):14–20.
483. Eisai Inc. ARICEPT® (donepezil hydrochloride tablets) package insert. U.S. Food and Drug Administration. https://www.accessdata.fda.gov/drugsatfda_docs/label/2012/020690s035,021720s008,022568s005lbl.pdf. February 2012. Accessed January 19, 2025.
484. Crowly R. Genetics by the numbers. National Institute of General Medical Sciences. https://biobeat.nigms.nih.gov/2024/04/genetics-by-the-numbers/. April 24, 2024. Accessed January 19, 2025.
485. Mostoslavsky R, Esteller M, Vaquero A. At the crossroad of lifespan, calorie restriction, chromatin and disease: meeting on sirtuins. *Cell Cycle.* 2010;9(10):1907–12.
486. Julien C, Tremblay C, Emond V, et al. Sirtuin 1 reduction parallels the accumulation of tau in Alzheimer disease. *J Neuropathol Exp Neurol.* 2009;68(1):48–58.
487. Cai W, Uribarri J, Zhu L, et al. Oral glycotoxins are a modifiable cause of dementia and the metabolic syndrome in mice and humans. *Proc Natl Acad Sci USA.* 2014;111(13):4940–5.
488. Cai W, Uribarri J, Zhu L, et al. Oral glycotoxins are a modifiable cause of dementia and the metabolic syndrome in mice and humans. *Proc Natl Acad Sci USA.* 2014;111(13):4940–5.
489. Rahmadi A, Steiner N, Münch G. Advanced glycation endproducts as gerontotoxins and biomarkers for carbonyl-based degenerative processes in Alzheimer's disease. *Clin Chem Lab Med.* 2011;49(3):385–91.
490. Semba RD, Nicklett EJ, Ferrucci L. Does accumulation of advanced glycation end products contribute to the aging phenotype? *J Gerontol A Biol Sci Med Sci.* 2010;65(9):963–75.
491. Srikanth V, Westcott B, Forbes J, et al. Methylglyoxal, cognitive function and cerebral atrophy in older people. *J Gerontol A Biol Sci Med Sci.* 2013;68(1):68–73.
492. Cai W, Uribarri J, Zhu L, et al. Oral glycotoxins are a modifiable cause of dementia and the metabolic syndrome in mice and humans. *Proc Natl Acad Sci USA.* 2014;111(13):4940–5.
493. Beeri MS, Moshier E, Schmeidler J, et al. Serum concentration of an inflammatory glycotoxin, methylglyoxal, is associated with increased cognitive decline in elderly individuals. *Mech Ageing Dev.* 2011;132(11–12):583–7.
494. Yaffe K, Lindquist K, Schwartz AV, et al. Advanced glycation end product level, diabetes, and accelerated cognitive aging. *Neurology.* 2011;77(14):1351–6.
495. Angeloni C, Zambonin L, Hrelia S. Role of methylglyoxal in Alzheimer's disease. *Biomed Res Int.* 2014;2014:238485.
496. Vlassara H, Cai W, Goodman S, et al. Protection against loss of innate defenses in adulthood by low advanced glycation end products (AGE) intake: role of the antiinflammatory AGE receptor-1. *J Clin Endocrinol Metab.* 2009;94(11):4483–91.

497. Cerami C, Founds H, Nicholl I, et al. Tobacco smoke is a source of toxic reactive glycation products. *Proc Natl Acad Sci USA.* 1997;94(25):13915–20.
498. Uribarri J, Cai W, Sandu O, Peppa M, Goldberg T, Vlassara H. Diet-derived advanced glycation end products are major contributors to the body's AGE pool and induce inflammation in healthy subjects. *Ann N Y Acad Sci.* 2005;1043:461–6.
499. Uribarri J, Cai W, Sandu O, Peppa M, Goldberg T, Vlassara H. Diet-derived advanced glycation end products are major contributors to the body's AGE pool and induce inflammation in healthy subjects. *Ann N Y Acad Sci.* 2005;1043:461–6.
500. Uribarri J, Woodruff S, Goodman S, et al. Advanced glycation end products in foods and a practical guide to their reduction in the diet. *J Am Diet Assoc.* 2010;110(6):911–6.e12.
501. Uribarri J, Woodruff S, Goodman S, et al. Advanced glycation end products in foods and a practical guide to their reduction in the diet. *J Am Diet Assoc.* 2010;110(6):911–6.e12.
502. Uribarri J, Woodruff S, Goodman S, et al. Advanced glycation end products in foods and a practical guide to their reduction in the diet. *J Am Diet Assoc.* 2010;110(6):911–6.e12.
503. Cai W, Uribarri J, Zhu L, et al. Oral glycotoxins are a modifiable cause of dementia and the metabolic syndrome in mice and humans. *Proc Natl Acad Sci USA.* 2014;111(13):4940–5.
504. Baker LD, Frank LL, Foster-Schubert K, et al. Effects of aerobic exercise on mild cognitive impairment: a controlled trial. *Arch Neurol.* 2010;67(1):71–9.
505. Baker LD, Frank LL, Foster-Schubert K, et al. Effects of aerobic exercise on mild cognitive impairment: a controlled trial. *Arch Neurol.* 2010;67(1):71–9.
506. Erickson KI, Voss MW, Prakash RS, et al. Exercise training increases size of hippocampus and improves memory. *Proc Natl Acad Sci USA.* 2011;108(7):3017–22.
507. ten Brinke LF, Bolandzadeh N, Nagamatsu LS, et al. Aerobic exercise increases hippocampal volume in older women with probable mild cognitive impairment: a 6-month randomised controlled trial. *Br J Sports Med.* 2015;49(4):248–54.
508. Yu Y, Wang J, Xu J. Optimal dose and type of exercise to improve cognitive function in patients with mild cognitive impairment: a systematic review and network meta-analysis of RCTs. *Front Psychiatry.* 2024;15:1436499.
509. Ornish D, Scherwitz LW, Billings JH, et al. Intensive lifestyle changes for reversal of coronary heart disease. *JAMA.* 1998;280(23):2001–7.
510. Silberman A, Banthia R, Estay IS, et al. The effectiveness and efficacy of an intensive cardiac rehabilitation program in 24 sites. *Am J Health Promot.* 2010;24(4):260–6.
511. Ornish D, Weidner G, Fair WR, et al. Intensive lifestyle changes may affect the progression of prostate cancer. *J Urol.* 2005;174(3):1065–9; discussion 1069–70.
512. Ornish D, Lin J, Daubenmier J, et al. Increased telomerase activity and comprehensive lifestyle changes: a pilot study. *Lancet Oncol.* 2008;9(11):1048–57.
513. Barnard ND, Bush AI, Ceccarelli A, et al. Dietary and lifestyle guidelines for the prevention of Alzheimer's disease. *Neurobiol Aging.* 2014;35 Suppl 2:S74–8.
514. Jaqua E, Biddy E, Moore C, Browne G. The impact of the six pillars of lifestyle medicine on brain health. *Cureus.* 2023;15(2):e34605.
515. Giem P, Beeson WL, Fraser GE. The incidence of dementia and intake of animal products: preliminary findings from the Adventist Health Study. *Neuroepidemiology.* 1993;12(1):28–36.
516. Sun Y, Liu B, Snetselaar LG, et al. Association of major dietary protein sources with all-cause and cause-specific mortality: prospective cohort study. *J Am Heart Assoc.* 2021;10(5):e015553.
517. Ornish D, Madison C, Kivipelto M, Kemp C, McCulloch CE, Galasko D, et al. Effects of intensive lifestyle changes on the progression of mild cognitive impairment or early dementia due to Alzheimer's disease: a randomized, controlled clinical trial. *Alzheimers Res Ther.* 2024;16(1):122.
518. Branch A. Ornish study shows lifestyle changes improved cognition in early Alzheimer's patients. American College of Lifestyle Medicine. https://lifestylemedicine.org/articles/ornish-research/. Accessed January 19, 2025.

519. Angelo M, Ward L. Aducanumab fails to produce efficacy results yet obtains US Food and Drug Administration approval. *Popul Health Manag.* 2021;24(6):638–9.
520. Mullard A. Controversial Alzheimer's drug approval could affect other diseases. *Nature.* 2021;595(7866):162–3.
521. Rubin R. Recently approved Alzheimer drug raises questions that might never be answered. *JAMA.* 2021;326(6):469–72.
522. Lundebjerg NE. My head just exploded, now what? Aducanumab. *J Am Geriatr Soc.* 2021;69(9):2689–91.
523. Branch A. Ornish study shows lifestyle changes improved cognition in early Alzheimer's patients. American College of Lifestyle Medicine. https://lifestylemedicine.org/articles/ornish-research/. Accessed January 19, 2025.
524. Civil Practice And Remedies Code. Title 4. Liability in Tort. Chapter 96. False disparagement of perishable food products. Texas Constitution and Statutes. http://www.statutes.legis.state.tx.us/Docs/CP/htm/CP.96.htm. Accessed January 24, 2025.
525. Civil Practice and Remedies Code. Title 4. Liability in Tort. Chapter 96. False disparagement of perishable food products. Texas Constitution and Statutes. http://www.statutes.legis.state.tx.us/Docs/CP/htm/CP.96.htm. Accessed January 24, 2025.
526. Oppel Jr RA. Taping of farm cruelty is becoming the crime. *New York Times.* http://www.nytimes.com/2013/04/07/us/taping-of-farm-cruelty-is-becoming-the-crime.html. April 6, 2013. Accessed January 24, 2025.
527. Shrestha SS, Swerdlow DL, Borse RH, et al. Estimating the burden of 2009 pandemic influenza A (H1N1) in the United States (April 2009–April 2010). *Clin Infect Dis.* 2011;52 Suppl 1:S75–82.
528. Li KSM, Lau SKP, Woo PCY. Bats—the magnificent virus player: SARS, MERS, COVID-19 and beyond. *Viruses.* 2023;15(12):2342.
529. Centers for Disease Control and Prevention. COVID Data Tracker. U.S. Department of Health and Human Services. https://covid.cdc.gov/covid-data-tracker. Accessed January 20, 2025.
530. Woolhouse MEJ, Gowtage-Sequeria S. Host range and emerging and reemerging pathogens. *Emerg Infect Dis.* 2005;11(12):1842–7.
531. Epstein PR, Chivian E, Frith K. Emerging diseases threaten conservation. *Environ Health Perspect.* 2003;111(10):A506–7.
532. Espinosa de los Monteros LE, Galán JC, Gutiérrez M, et al. Allele-specific PCR method based on pncA and oxyR sequences for distinguishing Mycobacterium bovis from Mycobacterium tuberculosis: intraspecific M. bovis pncA sequence polymorphism. *J Clin Microbiol.* 1998;36(1):239–42.
533. Esmail H, Barry CE, Young DB, Wilkinson RJ. The ongoing challenge of latent tuberculosis. *Philos Trans R Soc Lond, B, Biol Sci.* 2014;369(1645):20130437.
534. Daszak P, Cunningham AA. Emerging infectious diseases: a key role for conservation medicine. In: Aguirre AA, Ostfeld RS, Tabor GM, et al. *Conservation Medicine: Ecological Health in Practice.* Oxford: Oxford University Press; 2002:40–61.
535. McMichael AJ. *Human Frontiers, Environments and Disease, Past Patterns, Uncertain Futures.* Cambridge: Cambridge University Press; 2001.
536. Torrey EF, Yolken RH. *Beasts of the Earth, Animals, Humans, and Disease.* New Brunswick, NJ: Rutgers University Press; 2005.
537. McMichael AJ. *Human Frontiers, Environments and Disease, Past Patterns, Uncertain Futures.* Cambridge: Cambridge University Press; 2001.
538. Van Heuverswyn F, Peeters M. The origins of HIV and implications for the global epidemic. *Curr Infect Dis Rep.* 2007;9(4):338–46.
539. Whon TW, Kim MS, Roh SW, Shin NR, Lee HW, Bae JW. Metagenomic characterization of airborne viral DNA diversity in the near-surface atmosphere. *J Virol.* 2012;86(15):8221–31.
540. Agricultural Marketing Service. Microbiological testing of AMS purchased meat, poultry

and egg commodities. United States Department of Agriculture. https://www.ams.usda.gov/resources/microbiological-testing. Accessed January 24, 2025.

541. Centers for Disease Control and Prevention, National Center for Health Statistics. National Vital Statistics System, Mortality 2018–2023 on CDC WONDER Online Database. http://wonder.cdc.gov/ucd-icd10-expanded.html. Accessed January 16, 2025.

542. Centers for Disease Control and Prevention. COVID Data Tracker. U.S. Department of Health and Human Services. https://covid.cdc.gov/covid-data-tracker. Accessed January 19, 2025.

543. Barker J, Stevens D, and Bloomfield SF. Spread and prevention of some common viral infections in community facilities and domestic homes. *J Appl Microbiol.* 2001;91(1):7–21.

544. Boone SA, Gerba CP. The occurrence of influenza A virus on household and day care center fomites. *J Infect.* 2005;51(2):103–9.

545. World Health Organization. *WHO Guidelines on Hand Hygiene in Health Care.* Geneva: World Health Organization; 2009. http://www.ncbi.nlm.nih.gov/books/n/whohand/pdf/. Accessed January 24, 2025.

546. Park GW, Collins N, Barclay L, et al. Strain-specific virolysis patterns of human noroviruses in response to alcohols. *PLoS One.* 2016;11(6):e0157787.

547. InformedHealth.org. How does the immune system work? National Library of Medicine. https://www.ncbi.nlm.nih.gov/books/NBK279364/. Accessed January 24, 2025.

548. Pneumococcal vaccine recommendations. U.S. Centers for Disease Control and Prevention. https://www.cdc.gov/pneumococcal/hcp/vaccine-recommendations/index.html. October 26, 2024. Accessed January 24, 2025.

549. Gibson A, Edgar J, Neville C, et al. Effect of fruit and vegetable consumption on immune function in older people: a randomized controlled trial. *Am J Clin Nutr.* 2012;96(6):1429–36.

550. Nishi K, Kondo A, Okamoto T, et al. Immunostimulatory in vitro and in vivo effects of a water-soluble extract from kale. *Biosci Biotechnol Biochem.* 2011;75(1):40–6.

551. Nishi K, Kondo A, Okamoto T, et al. Immunostimulatory in vitro and in vivo effects of a water-soluble extract from kale. *Biosci Biotechnol Biochem.* 2011;75(1):40–6.

552. Schlotz N, Odongo GA, Herz C, et al. Are raw *brassica* vegetables healthier than cooked ones? A randomized, controlled crossover intervention trial on the health-promoting potential of Ethiopian kale. *Nutrients.* 2018;10(11):1622.

553. Jeppesen PB, Dorner A, Yue Y, et al. Beneficial effects of a freeze-dried kale bar on type 2 diabetes patients: a randomized, double-blinded, placebo-controlled clinical trial. *Nutrients.* 2024;16(21):3641.

554. Chatupos V, Neelawatanasook S, Sangutai T, et al. Comparison of analgesic and anti-inflammatory effects of kale extract versus ibuprofen after impacted mandibular third molar surgery: a randomized, double-blind split-mouth clinical trial. *Nutrients.* 2024;16(22):3821.

555. Nishimoto Y, Salim F, Yamauchi Y, et al. Kale improves bowel movements in constipated women and affects some intestinal microbes and metabolites: a pilot study. *Front Nutr.* 2023;10:1247683.

556. Kondo S, Suzuki A, Kurokawa M, Hasumi K. Intake of kale suppresses postprandial increases in plasma glucose: a randomized, double-blind, placebo-controlled, crossover study. *Biomed Rep.* 2016;5(5):553–8.

557. Jeppesen PB, Dorner A, Yue Y, et al. Beneficial effects of a freeze-dried kale bar on type 2 diabetes patients: a randomized, double-blinded, placebo-controlled clinical trial. *Nutrients.* 2024;16(21):3641.

558. Helander HF, Fändriks L. Surface area of the digestive tract—revisited. *Scand J Gastroenterol.* 2014;49(6):681–9.

559. Sheridan BS, Lefrançois L. Intraepithelial lymphocytes: To serve and protect. *Curr Gastroenterol Rep.* 2010;12(6):513–21.

560. Hooper LV. You AhR what you eat: linking diet and immunity. *Cell*. 2011;147(3):489–91.
561. Esser C. Biology and function of the aryl hydrocarbon receptor: report of an international and interdisciplinary conference. *Arch Toxicol*. 2012;86(8):1323–9.
562. Veldhoen M. Direct interactions between intestinal immune cells and the diet. *Cell Cycle*. 2012;11(3):426–7.
563. Hooper LV. You AhR what you eat: linking diet and immunity. *Cell*. 2011;147(3):489–91.
564. Savouret JF, Berdeaux A, Casper RF. The aryl hydrocarbon receptor and its xenobiotic ligands: a fundamental trigger for cardiovascular diseases. *Nutr Metab Cardiovasc Dis*. 2003;13(2):104–13.
565. Ashida H, Fukuda I, Yamashita T, Kanazawa K. Flavones and flavonols at dietary levels inhibit a transformation of aryl hydrocarbon receptor induced by dioxin. *FEBS Lett*. 2000;476(3):213–7.
566. Ashida H, Fukuda I, Yamashita T, Kanazawa K. Flavones and flavonols at dietary levels inhibit a transformation of aryl hydrocarbon receptor induced by dioxin. *FEBS Lett*. 2000;476(3):213–7.
567. Alhaider AA, El Gendy MAM, Korashy HM, El-Kadi AOS. Camel urine inhibits the cytochrome P450 1a1 gene expression through an AhR-dependent mechanism in Hepa 1c1c7 cell line. *J Ethnopharmacol*. 2011;133(1):184–90.
568. Watts AR, Lennard MS, Mason SL, Tucker GT, Woods HF. Beeturia and the biological fate of beetroot pigments. *Pharmacogenetics*. 1993;3(6):302–11.
569. Yalindag-Ozturk N, Ozdamar M, Cengiz P. Trial of garlic as an adjunct therapy for multidrug resistant Pseudomonas aeruginosa pneumonia in a critically ill infant. *J Altern Complement Med*. 2011;17(4):379–80.
570. Seeram NP. Recent trends and advances in berry health benefits research. *J Agric Food Chem*. 2010;58(7):3869–70.
571. Seeram NP. Berry fruits for cancer prevention: Current status and future prospects. *J Agric Food Chem*. 2008;56(3):630–5.
572. Caligiuri MA. Human natural killer cells. *Blood*. 2008;112(3):461–9.
573. McAnulty LS, Nieman DC, Dumke CL, et al. Effect of blueberry ingestion on natural killer cell counts, oxidative stress, and inflammation prior to and after 2.5 H of running. *Appl Physiol Nutr Metab*. 2011;36(6):976–84.
574. Majdalawieh AF, Carr RI. In vitro investigation of the potential immunomodulatory and anti-cancer activities of black pepper (Piper nigrum) and cardamom (Elettaria cardamomum). *J Med Food*. 2010;13(2):371–81.
575. Lahart I, Darcy P, Gidlow C, Calogiuri G. The effects of green exercise on physical and mental wellbeing: a systematic review. *Int J Environ Res Public Health*. 2019;16(8):1352.
576. Antonelli M, Barbieri G, Donelli D. Effects of forest bathing (shinrin-yoku) on levels of cortisol as a stress biomarker: a systematic review and meta-analysis. *Int J Biometeorol*. 2019;63(8):1117–34.
577. Li Q, Morimoto K, Kobayashi M, et al. Visiting a forest, but not a city, increases human natural killer activity and expression of anti-cancer proteins. *Int J Immunopathol Pharmacol*. 2008;21(1):117–27.
578. Li Q. Effect of forest bathing trips on human immune function. *Environ Health Prev Med*. 2010;15(1):9–17.
579. Li Q, Kobayashi M, Inagaki H, et al. A day trip to a forest park increases human natural killer activity and the expression of anti-cancer proteins in male subjects. *J Biol Regul Homeost Agents*. 2010;24(2):157–65.
580. Rook GA. Regulation of the immune system by biodiversity from the natural environment: an ecosystem service essential to health. *Proc Natl Acad Sci U S A*. 2013;110(46):18360–7.
581. Li Q, Kawada T. Effect of forest environments on human natural killer (NK) activity. *Int J Immunopathol Pharmacol*. 2011;24(1 Suppl):39S–44S.
582. Li Q, Morimoto K, Kobayashi M, et al. Visiting a forest, but not a city, increases human

natural killer activity and expression of anti-cancer proteins. *Int J Immunopathol Pharmacol.* 2008;21(1):117–27.
583. Sumitomo K, Akutsu H, Fukuyama S, et al. Conifer-derived monoterpenes and forest walking. *Mass Spectrom* (Tokyo). 2015;4(1):A0042.
584. Li Q, Nakadai A, Matsushima H, et al. Phytoncides (wood essential oils) induce human natural killer cell activity. *Immunopharmacol Immunotoxicol.* 2006;28(2):319–33.
585. Shibata H, Fujiwara R, Iwamoto M, Matsuoka H, Yokoyama MM. Immunological and behavioral effects of fragrance in mice. *Int J Neurosci.* 1991;57(1–2):151–9.
586. Li Q, Kobayashi M, Wakayama Y, et al. Effect of phytoncide from trees on human natural killer cell function. *Int J Immunopathol Pharmacol.* 2009;22(4):951–9.
587. Li Q. Effect of forest bathing trips on human immune function. *Environ Health Prev Med.* 2010;15(1):9–17.
588. Fujimori H, Hisama M, Shibayama H, Iwaki M. Protecting effect of phytoncide solution, on normal human dermal fibroblasts against reactive oxygen species. *J Oleo Sci.* 2009;58(8):429–36.
589. Li Q, Kobayashi M, Kawada T. Relationships between percentage of forest coverage and standardized mortality ratios (SMR) of cancers in all prefectures in Japan. *Open Public Health J.* 2008;1(1):1–7.
590. Ahmadi F, Ahmadi N. Nature as the most important coping strategy among cancer patients: a Swedish survey. *J Relig Health.* 2015;54(4):1177–90.
591. Liu X, Zhou J, Chen J, et al. Risk of asthma and allergies in children delivered by cesarean section: a comprehensive systematic review. *J Allergy Clin Immunol Pract.* 2024;12(10):2764–73.
592. Benn CS, Thorsen P, Jensen JS, et al. Maternal vaginal microflora during pregnancy and the risk of asthma hospitalization and use of antiasthma medication in early childhood. *J Allergy Clin Immunol.* 2002;110(1):72–7.
593. Sheih YH, Chiang BL, Wang LH, Liao CK, Gill HS. Systemic immunity-enhancing effects in healthy subjects following dietary consumption of the lactic acid bacterium Lactobacillus rhamnosus HN001. *J Am Coll Nutr.* 2001;20(Suppl 2):149–56.
594. Berggren A, Lazou Ahrhiang BL, Wang LH, Liao G. Randomised, double-blind and placebo-controlled study using new probiotic lactobacilli for strengthening the body immune defence against viral infections. *Eur J Nutr.* 2011;50(3):203–10.
595. Hao Q, Lu Z, Dong BR, Huang CQ, Wu T. Probiotics for preventing acute upper respiratory tract infections. *Cochrane Database Syst Rev.* 2011;9:1–42
596. Homayoni Rad A, Akbarzadeh F, Mehrabany EV. Which are more important: prebiotics or probiotics? *Nutrition.* 2012;28(11–12):1196–7.
597. Vitali B, Minervini G, Rizzello CG, et al. Novel probiotic candidates for humans isolated from raw fruits and vegetables. *Food Microbiol.* 2012;31(1):116–25.
598. Kim H, Rebholz CM, Hegde S, et al. Plant-based diets, pescatarian diets and COVID-19 severity: a population-based case-control study in six countries. *BMJ Nutrition, Prevention & Health.* 2021;bmjnph-2021-000272.
599. Dessie ZG, Zewotir T. Mortality-related risk factors of COVID-19: a systematic review and meta-analysis of 42 studies and 423,117 patients. *BMC Infect Dis.* 2021;21(1):855.
600. Greger M. *How Not to Die.* New York: Flatiron Books; 2015.
601. Kim H, Rebholz CM, Hegde S, et al. Plant-based diets, pescatarian diets and COVID-19 severity: a population-based case-control study in six countries. *BMJ Nutrition, Prevention & Health.* 2021;bmjnph-2021-000272.
602. Salazar-Robles E, Kalantar-Zadeh K, Badillo H, et al. Association between severity of COVID-19 symptoms and habitual food intake in adult outpatients. *BMJ Nutr Prev Health.* 2021;4(2):469–78.
603. Merino J, Joshi AD, Nguyen LH, et al. Diet quality and risk and severity of COVID-19: a prospective cohort study. *Gut.* 2021;70(11):2096–104.
604. Storz MA. Lifestyle adjustments in long-COVID management: potential benefits of plant-based diets. *Curr Nutr Rep.* 2021;10(4):352–63.

605. Nieman DC. Moderate exercise improves immunity and decreases illness rates. *Am J Lifestyle Med.* 2011;5(4):338–45.
606. Schwindt CD, Zaldivar F, Wilson L, et al. Do circulating leucocytes and lymphocyte subtypes increase in response to brief exercise in children with and without asthma? *Br J Sports Med.* 2007;41(1):34–40.
607. Nieman DC, Henson DA, Gusewitch G, et al. Physical activity and immune function in elderly women. *Med Sci Sports Exerc.* 1993;25(7):823–31.
608. Neville V, Gleeson M, Folland JP. Salivary IgA as a risk factor for upper respiratory infections in elite professional athletes. *Med Sci Sports Exerc.* 2008;40(7):1228–36.
609. Otsuki T, Shimizu K, Iemitsu M, Kono I. Salivary secretory immunoglobulin A secretion increases after 4-weeks ingestion of chlorella-derived multicomponent supplement in humans: a randomized cross over study. *Nutr J.* 2011 Sep 9;10:91.
610. Klentrou P, Cieslak T, MacNeil M, Vintinner A, Plyley M. Effect of moderate exercise on salivary immunoglobulin A and infection risk in humans. *Eur J Appl Physiol.* 2002;87(2):153–8.
611. There is no note 611.
612. There is no note 612.
613. There is no note 613.
614. There is no note 614.
615. There is no note 615.
616. There is no note 616.
617. Nieman DC. Moderate exercise improves immunity and decreases illness rates. *Am J Lifestyle Med.* 2011;5(4):338–46.
618. Walsh NP, Gleeson M, Shephard RJ, et al. Position statement. Part one: immune function and exercise. *Exerc Immunol Rev.* 2011;17:6–63.
619. Akimoto T, Nakahori C, Aizawa K, Kimura F, Fukubayashi T, Kono I. Acupuncture and responses of immunologic and endocrine markers during competition. *Med Sci Sports Exerc.* 2003;35(8):1296–302.
620. Neville V, Gleeson M, Folland JP. Salivary IgA as a risk factor for upper respiratory infections in elite professional athletes. *Med Sci Sports Exerc.* 2008;40(7):1228–36.
621. Nieman DC. Exercise effects on systemic immunity. *Immunol Cell Biol.* 2000;78(5):496–501.
622. Carpenter KC, Breslin WL, Davidson T, Adams A, McFarlin BK. Baker's yeast β-glucan supplementation increases monocytes and cytokines post-exercise: implications for infection risk? *Br J Nutr.* 2013;109(3):478–86.
623. Carpenter KC, Breslin WL, Davidson T, Adams A, McCarlin BK. Baker's yeast β-glucan supplementation increases monocytes and cytokines post-exercise: implications for infection risk? *Br J Nutr.* 2013;109(3):478–86.
624. Talbott S, Talbott J. Effect of BETA 1, 3/1, 6 GLUCAN on upper respiratory tract infection symptoms and mood state in marathon athletes. *J Sports Sci Med.* 2009;8(4):509–15.
625. Merrill RM, Isakson RT, Beck RE. The association between allergies and cancer: what is currently known? *Ann Allergy Asthma Immunol.* 2007;99(2):102–16.
626. Wakchaure GC. Production and marketing of mushrooms: global and national scenario. In: Singh M, ed. *Mushrooms: Cultivation, Marketing and Consumption.* Indian Council of Agricultural Research Directorate of Mushroom Research; 2011.
627. Jeong SC, Koyyalamudi SR, Pang G. Dietary intake of Agaricus bisporus white button mushroom accelerates salivary immunoglobulin A secretion in healthy volunteers. *Nutrition.* 2012;28(5):527–31.
628. Jeong SC, Koyyalamudi SR, Pang G. Dietary intake of Agaricusbisporus white button mushroom accelerates salivary immunoglobulin A secretion in healthy volunteers. *Nutrition.* 2012;28(5):527–31.
629. Moro C, Palacios I, Lozano M, et al. Anti-inflammatory activity of methanolic extracts from edible mushrooms in LPS activated RAW 264. 7 macrophages. *Food Chemistry.* 2012;130:350–5.
630. Jesenak M, Hrubisko M, Majtan J, Rennerova Z, Banovcin P. Anti-allergic effect of Pleuran

(β-glucan from Pleurotus ostreatus) in children with recurrent respiratory tract infections. *Phytother Res.* 2014;28(3):471–4.
631. Gry J, Andersson C, Krüger L, et al. Mushrooms traded as food: Nordic questionnaire, including guidance list on edible mushrooms suitable and not suitable for marketing. Copenhagen: TemaNord; 2012.
632. Stijve T, Pittet A. Absence of agaritine in *Pleurotus* species and in other cultivated and wild-growing mushrooms not belonging to the genus *Agaricus*. *Dtsch Lebensm-Rundsch.* 2000;96(7):251–4.
633. Heer RS, Patel NB, Mandal AKJ, Lewis F, Missouris CG. Not a fungi to be with: shiitake mushroom flagellate dermatitis. *Am J Emerg Med.* 2020;38(2):412.e1–2.
634. Lagrange E, Vernoux JP. Warning on false or true morels and button mushrooms with potential toxicity linked to hydrazinic toxins: an update. *Toxins* (Basel). 2020;12(8):482.
635. Centers for Disease Control and Prevention. Estimates of foodborne illness in the United States. http://www.cdc.gov/foodborneburden/. Accessed January 24, 2025.
636. Batz MB, Hoffmann S, Morris Jr JG. Ranking the disease burden of 14 pathogens in food sources in the United States using attribution data from outbreak investigations and expert elicitation. *J Food Prot.* 2012;75(7):1278–91.
637. Park S, Navratil S, Gregory A, et al. Multifactorial effects of ambient temperature, precipitation, farm management, and environmental factors determine the level of generic Escherichia coli contamination on preharvested spinach. *Appl Environ Microbiol.* 2015;81(7):2635–50.
638. Hoffmann S, Batz MB, Morris Jr JG. Annual cost of illness and quality-adjusted life year losses in the United States due to 14 foodborne pathogens. *J Food Prot.* 2012;75(7):1292–302.
639. Salmonella infection. Centers for Disease Control and Prevention. https://www.cdc.gov/salmonella/signs-symptoms/index.html. Accessed January 24, 2025.
640. Krouse B. Opposing view on food safety: committed to safety. *USA Today.* http://usatoday30.usatoday.com/news/opinion/editorials/2010-08-30-editorial30_ST1_N.htm. Accessed January 24, 2025.
641. Davis AL, Curtis PA, Conner DE, McKee SR, Kerth LK. Validation of cooking methods using shell eggs inoculated with Salmonella serotypes Enteritidis and Heidelberg. *Poult Sci.* 2008;87(8):1637–42.
642. Stadelman WJ, Muriana PM, Schmieder H. The effectiveness of traditional egg-cooking practices for elimination of Salmonella enteritidis. *Poult Sci.* 1995;74(s1):119.
643. Humphrey TJ, Greenwood M, Gilbert RJ, Rowe B, Chapman PA. The survival of salmonellas in shell eggs cooked under simulated domestic conditions. *Epidemiol Infect.* 1989;103:35–45.
644. Egg Safety Final Rule. U.S. Food and Drug Administration. https://www.fda.gov/food/egg-guidance-regulation-and-other-information/egg-safety-final-rule. August 10, 2022. Accessed January 23, 2025.
645. Batz MB, Hoffmann S, Morris Jr JG. Ranking the disease burden of 14 pathogens in food sources in the United States using attribution data from outbreak investigations and expert elicitation. *J Food Prot.* 2012;75(7):1278–91.
646. Supreme Beef Processors, Inc v United States Dept. of Agriculture, 275 F. 3d 432 (5th Cir 2001). https://casetext.com/case/supreme-beef-processors-v-us-dept-agric. Accessed January 24, 2025.
647. Fravalo P, Laisney MJ, Gillard MO, Salvat G, Chemaly M. Campylobacter transfer from naturally contaminated chicken thighs to cutting boards is inversely related to initial load. *J Food Prot.* 2009;72(9):1836–40.
648. Guyard-Nicodème M, Tresse O, Houard E, et al. Characterization of Campylobacter spp. transferred from naturally contaminated chicken legs to cooked chicken slices via a cutting board. *Int J Food Microbiol.* 2013;164(1):7–14.
649. Foster R. Foster Farms provides food safety update. Close Up Media Inc. http://closeupmedia

.com/food/Foster-Farms-Provides-Food-Safety-Update.html. October 14, 2013. Accessed January 23, 2025.
650. Hoffmann S, Batz MB, Morris Jr JG. Annual cost of illness and quality-adjusted life year losses in the United States due to 14 foodborne pathogens. *J Food Prot.* 2012;75(7):1292–302.
651. Karapetian A. Model EU. *Meatingplace.* March 2010:91.
652. Dangerous contaminated chicken. *Consumer Reports.* http://www.consumerreports.org/cro/magazine/2014/02/the-high-cost-of-cheap-chicken/index.htm. January 2014. Accessed January 24, 2025.
653. Antibiotic resistance threats in the United States, 2019. Centers for Disease Control and Prevention. https://ndc.services.cdc.gov/wp-content/uploads/Antibiotic-Resistance-Threats-in-the-United-States-2019.pdf. December 2019. Accessed January 24, 2025.
654. Balzer D. Signs and symptoms of salmonella infection. The Mayo Clinic. https://newsnetwork.mayoclinic.org/discussion/signs-and-symptoms-of-salmonella-infection/. November 27, 2023. Accessed January 24, 2025.
655. U.S. Food and Drug Administration. NARMS 2011 retail meat annual report. http://www.fda.gov/downloads/AnimalVeterinary/SafetyHealth/AntimicrobialResistance/NationalAntimicrobialResistanceMonitoringSystem/UCM334834.pdf. Accessed April 3, 2015.
656. National Antimicrobial Resistance Monitoring System. 2021 NARMS update: integrated report summary. U.S. Food and Drug Administration. https://www.fda.gov/animal-veterinary/national-antimicrobial-resistance-monitoring-system/2021-narms-update-integrated-report-summary. Updated Aug 20, 2024. Accessed March 1, 2025.
657. Centers for Disease Control and Prevention (CDC). Vital signs: incidence and trends of infection with pathogens transmitted commonly through food—foodborne diseases active surveillance network, 10 U.S. sites, 1996–2010. *MMWR Morb Mortal Wkly Rep.* 2011;60(22):749–55.
658. Chai SJ, White PL, Lathrop SL, et al. Salmonella enterica serotype Enteritidis: increasing incidence of domestically acquired infections. *Clin Infect Dis.* 2012;54-Suppl-5(NA):S488–97.
659. Hoffmann S, Batz MB, Morris Jr JG. Annual cost of illness and quality-adjusted life year losses in the United States due to 14 foodborne pathogens. *J Food Prot.* 2012;75(7):1292–302.
660. American Public Health Association v. Butz, 511 F. 2d 331. http://openjurist.org/511/f2d/331/american-public-health-association-v-butz. Accessed January 24, 2025.
661. Supreme Beef Processors v. U.S. Dept. of Agriculture. United States Court of Appeals, 275 F. 3d 432 (5th Cir 2001). http://www.leagle.com/decision/2001707275F3d432_1672. Accessed January 24, 2025.
662. Stamey TA, Timothy M, Millar M, Mihara G. Recurrent urinary infections in adult women. The role of introital enterobacteria. *Calif Med.* 1971;115(1):1–19.
663. Yamamoto S, Tsukamoto T, Terai A, Kurazono H, Takeda Y, Yoshida O. Genetic evidence supporting the fecal-perineal-urethral hypothesis in cystitis caused by Escherichia coli. *J Urol.* 1997;157(3):1127–9.
664. Bergeron CR, Prussing C, Boerlin P, et al. Chicken as reservoir for extraintestinal pathogenic Escherichia coli in humans, Canada. *Emerg Infect Dis.* 2012;18(3):415–21.
665. Jakobsen L, Garneau P, Bruant G, et al. Is Escherichia coli urinary tract infection a zoonosis? Proof of direct link with production animals and meat. *Eur J Clin Microbiol Infect Dis.* 2012;31(6):1121–9.
666. Foxman B, Barlow R, D'arcy H, Gillespie B, Sobel JD. Urinary tract infection: self-reported incidence and associated costs. *Ann Epidemiol.* 2000;10(8):509–15.
667. Platell JL, Johnson JR, Cobbold RN, Trott DJ. Multidrug-resistant extraintestinal pathogenic Escherichia coli of sequence type ST131 in animals and foods. *Vet Microbiol.* 2011;153(1–2):99–108.
668. Linton AH, Howe K, Bennett PM, Richmond MH, Whiteside EJ. The colonization of the human gut by antibiotic resistant Escherichia coli from chickens. *J Appl Bacteriol.* 1977;43(3):465–9.

669. Linton AH, Howe K, Bennett PM, Richmond MH, Whiteside EJ. The colonization of the human gut by antibiotic resistant Escherichia coli from chickens. *J Appl Bacteriol.* 1977;43(3):465–9.
670. Rusin P, Orosz-Coughlin P, Gerba C. Reduction of faecal coliform, coliform and heterotrophic plate count bacteria in the household kitchen and bathroom by disinfection with hypochlorite cleaners. *J Appl Microbiol.* 1998;85(5):819–28.
671. Cogan TA, Bloomfield SF, Humphrey TJ. The effectiveness of hygiene procedures for prevention of cross-contamination from chicken carcases in the domestic kitchen. *Lett Appl Microbiol.* 1999;29(5):354–8.
672. Cogan TA, Bloomfield SF, Humphrey TJ. The effectiveness of hygiene procedures for prevention of cross-contamination from chicken carcases in the domestic kitchen. *Lett Appl Microbiol.* 1999;29(5):354–8.
673. Cogan TA, Bloomfield SF, Humphrey TJ. The effectiveness of hygiene procedures for prevention of cross-contamination from chicken carcases in the domestic kitchen. *Lett Appl Microbiol.* 1999;29(5):354–8.
674. Linton AH, Howe K, Bennett PM, Richmond MH, Whiteside EJ. The colonization of the human gut by antibiotic resistant Escherichia coli from chickens. *J Appl Bacteriol.* 1977;43(3):465–9.
675. Scallan E, Hoekstra RM, Angulo FJ, et al. Foodborne illness acquired in the United States—major pathogens. *Emerg Infect Dis.* 2011;17:7–15.
676. Batz MB, Hoffmann S, Morris Jr JG. Ranking the disease burden of 14 pathogens in food sources in the United States using attribution data from outbreak investigations and expert elicitation. *J Food Prot.* 2012;75:1278–91.
677. Zheng H, Sun Y, Lin S, Mao Z, Jiang B. Yersinia enterocolitica infection in diarrheal patients. *Eur J Clin Microbiol Infect Dis.* 2008;27:741–52.
678. Bari ML, Hossain MA, Isshiki K, Ukuku D. Behavior of Yersinia enterocolitica in foods. *J Pathog.* 2011;2011:420732.
679. Ternhag A, Törner A, Svensson A, Ekdahl K, Giesecke J. Short-and long-term effects of bacterial gastrointestinal infections. *Emerg Infect Dis.* 2008;14:143–8.
680. Brix TH, Hansen PS, Hegedüs L, Wenzel BE. Too early to dismiss Yersinia enterocolitica infection in the aetiology of Graves' disease: evidence from a twin case-control study. *Clin Endocrinol (Oxf).* 2008;69:491–6.
681. Pork chops and ground pork contaminated with bacteria. *Consumer Reports.* http://www.consumerreports.org/cro/magazine/2013/01/what-s-in-that-pork/index.htm. January 2013. Accessed March 3, 2015.
682. Bari ML, Hossain MA, Isshiki K, Ukuku D. Behavior of Yersinia enterocolitica in foods. *J Pathog.* 2011;2011:420732.
683. Crowding pigs pays—if it's managed properly. *National Hog Farmer.* November 15, 1993;62.
684. Poljak Z, Dewey CE, Martin SW, et al. Prevalence of Yersinia enterocolitica shedding and bioserotype distribution in Ontario finisher pig herds in 2001, 2002, and 2004. *Prev Vet Med.* 2010;93:110–20.
685. Hoffmann S, Batz MB, Morris Jr JG. Annual cost of illness and quality-adjusted life year losses in the United States due to 14 foodborne pathogens. *J Food Prot.* 2012;75:1292–302.
686. Feuerstadt P, Theriault N, Tillotson G. The burden of CDI in the United States: a multifactorial challenge. *BMC Infect Dis.* 2023;23:132.
687. Eyre DW, Cule ML, Wilson DJ, et al. Diverse sources of C. difficile infection identified on whole-genome sequencing. *N Engl J Med.* 2013 Sep 26;369(13):1195–205.
688. Songer JG, Trinh HT, Killgore GE, Thompson AD, McDonald LC, Limbago BM. Clostridium difficile in retail meat products, USA, 2007. *Emerg Infect Dis.* 2009;15(5):819–21.
689. Rupnik M, Songer JG. Clostridium difficile: its potential as a source of foodborne disease. *Adv Food Nutr Res.* 2010;60:53–66.

690. Rodriguez-Palacios A, Borgmann S, Kline TR, LeJeune JT. Clostridium difficile in foods and animals: history and measures to reduce exposure. *Anim Health Res Rev.* 2013;14(1):11–29.
691. Hensgrens MPM, Keessen EC, Squire MM, et al. European Society of Clinical Microbiology and Infectious Diseases Study Group for Clostridium difficile (ESGCD). Clostridium difficile infection in the community: a zoonotic disease? *Clin Microbiol Infect.* 2012;18(7):635–45.
692. Rupnik M, Songer JG. Clostridium difficile: its potential as a source of foodborne disease. *Adv Food Nutr Res.* 2010;60:53–66.
693. Sayedy L, Kothari D, Richards RJ. Toxic megacolon associated Clostridium difficile colitis. *World J Gastrointest Endosc.* 2010;2(8):293–7.
694. Gweon TG, Lee KJ, Kang DH, et al. A case of toxic megacolon caused by Clostridium difficile infection and treated with fecal microbiota transplantation. *Gut Liver.* 2015;9(2):247–50.
695. Weese JS. Clostridium difficile in food—innocent bystander or serious threat? *Clin Microbiol Infect.* 2010;16:3–10.
696. Jabbar U, Leischner J, Kasper D, et al. Effectiveness of alcohol-based hand rubs for removal of Clostridium difficile spores from hands. *Infect Control Hosp Epidemiol.* 2010;31(6):565–70.
697. Bhargava K, Wang X, Donabedian S, Zervos M, de Rocha L, Zhang Y. Methicillin-resistant Staphylococcus aureus in retail meat, Detroit, Michigan, USA. *Emerg Infect Dis.* 2011;17(6):1135–7.
698. Reinberg S. Scientists find MRSA germ in supermarket meats. HealthDay. https://www.healthday.com/health-news/public-health/scientists-find-mrsa-germ-in-supermarket-meats-652855.html. May 11, 2011. Accessed January 24, 2025.
699. Chan M. Antimicrobial resistance in the European Union and the world. World Health Organization. https://www.who.int/director-general/speeches/detail/antimicrobial-resistance-in-the-european-union-and-the-world. March 14, 2012. Accessed January 24, 2025.
700. Wallinga D, Smit LAM, Davis MF, Casey JA, Nachman KE. A review of the effectiveness of current US policies on antimicrobial use in meat and poultry production. *Curr Environ Health Rep.* 2022;9(2):339–54.
701. Ji K, Kho Y, Park C, et al. Influence of water and food consumption on inadvertent antibiotics intake among general population. *Environ Res.* 2010;110(7):641–9.
702. Ji K, Lim Kho YL, Park Y, Choi K. Influence of a five-day vegetarian diet on urinary levels of antibiotics and phthalate metabolites: a pilot study with "Temple Stay" participants. *Environ Res.* 2010;110(4):375–82.
703. Keep Antibiotics Working. Endorsements for "The Preservation of Antibiotics for Medical Treatment Act of 2003." Institute for Agriculture and Trade Policy. https://www.iatp.org/documents/kaws-updated-list-endorsements-preservation-antibiotics-medical-treatment-act-2003. December 20, 2004. Accessed January 26, 2025.
704. Hayes DJ, Jenson HH, Fabiosa J. Technology choice and the economic effects of a ban on the use of antimicrobial feed additives in swine rations. *Food Control.* 2002;13(2):97–101.
705. Rival diet doc leaks Atkins death report. https://www.thesmokinggun.com/file/rival-diet-doc-leaks-atkins-death-report. Accessed January 23, 2025.
706. Greger M. Corporate threat. https://atkinsfacts.org/corporate-threat/. Accessed January 23, 2025.
707. Lozano R, Naghavi M, Foreman K, et al. Global and regional mortality from 235 causes of death for 20 age groups in 1990 and 2010: a systematic analysis for the Global Burden of Disease Study 2010. *Lancet.* 2012;380(9859):2095–128.
708. Murray CJL. The Global Burden of Disease Study at 30 years. *Nat Med.* 2022;28(10):2019–26.
709. Institute for Health Metrics and Evaluation (IHME). GBD 2021 cause and risk summary: diet high in sugar-sweetened beverages—level 3 risk. University of Washington. https://www.healthdata.org/research-analysis/diseases-injuries-risks/factsheets/2021-diet-high-sugar-sweetened-beverages-level. Accessed January 27, 2025.
710. Institute for Health Metrics and Evaluation (IHME). GBD 2021 cause and risk summary: diet high in processed meat—level 3 risk. University of Washington. https://www.healthdata

.org/research-analysis/diseases-injuries-risks/factsheets/2021-diet-high-processed-meat-level-3-risk. Accessed January 27, 2025.
711. Institute for Health Metrics and Evaluation (IHME). GBD 2021 cause and risk summary: diet low in legumes—level 3 risk. University of Washington. https://www.healthdata.org/research-analysis/diseases-injuries-risks/factsheets/2021-diet-low-legumes-level-0-risk. Accessed January 27, 2025.
712. Institute for Health Metrics and Evaluation (IHME). GBD 2021 cause and risk summary: diet low in nuts and seeds—level 3 risk. University of Washington. https://www.healthdata.org/research-analysis/diseases-injuries-risks/factsheets/2021-diet-low-nuts-and-seeds-level-3-risk. Accessed January 27, 2025.
713. Institute for Health Metrics and Evaluation (IHME). GBD 2021 cause and risk summary: diet low in vegetables—level 3 risk. University of Washington. https://www.healthdata.org/research-analysis/diseases-injuries-risks/factsheets/2021-diet-low-vegetables-level-3-risk. Accessed January 27, 2025.
714. Institute for Health Metrics and Evaluation (IHME). GBD 2021 cause and risk summary: diet low in whole grains—level 3 risk. University of Washington. https://www.healthdata.org/research-analysis/diseases-injuries-risks/factsheets/2021-diet-low-whole-grains-level-3-risk. Accessed January 27, 2025.
715. Institute for Health Metrics and Evaluation (IHME). GBD 2021 cause and risk summary: diet low in fruits—level 3 risk. University of Washington. https://www.healthdata.org/research-analysis/diseases-injuries-risks/factsheets/2021-diet-low-fruits-level-3-risk. Accessed January 27, 2025.
716. Chen MM, Zhang X, Liu YM, et al. Heavy disease burden of high systolic blood pressure during 1990–2019: highlighting regional, sex, and age specific strategies in blood pressure control. *Front Cardiovasc Med.* 2021;8:754778.
717. Understanding blood pressure readings. American Heart Association. https://www.heart.org/en/health-topics/high-blood-pressure/understanding-blood-pressure-readings. May 17, 2024. Accessed January 28, 2025.
718. Whelton PK, Carey RM, Aronow WS, et al. 2017 ACC/AHA/AAPA/ABC/ACPM/AGS/APhA/ASH/ASPC/NMA/PCNA guideline for the prevention, detection, evaluation, and management of high blood pressure in adults: executive summary: a report of the American College of Cardiology/American Heart Association Task Force on clinical practice guidelines. *Hypertension.* 2018;71(6):1269–1324.
719. Fryar CD, Kit B, Carroll MD, Afful J. Hypertension prevalence, awareness, treatment, and control among adults age 18 and older: United States, August 2021–August 2023. NCHS Data Brief, no 511. National Center for Health Statistics. https://stacks.cdc.gov/view/cdc/164016. October 2024. Accessed January 28, 2025.
720. Walker AR, Walker BF. High high-density-lipoprotein cholesterol in African children and adults in a population free of coronary heart disease. *Br Med J.* 1978;2(6148):1336–7.
721. Donnison CP. Blood pressure in the African native. *Lancet.* 1929;213(5497):6–7.
722. Macmahon S, Neal B, Rodgers A. Hypertension—time to move on. *Lancet.* 2005;365(9464):1108–9.
723. Law MR, Morris JK, Wald NJ. Use of blood pressure lowering drugs in the prevention of cardiovascular disease: meta-analysis of 147 randomised trials in the context of expectations from prospective epidemiological studies. *BMJ.* 2009;338:b1665.
724. Donnison CP. Blood pressure in the African native. *Lancet.* 1929;213(5497):6–7.
725. West GB, Brown JH, Enquist BJ. A general model for the origin of allometric scaling laws in biology. *Science.* 1997;276(5309):122–6.
726. Levine HJ. Rest heart rate and life expectancy. *J Am Coll Cardiol.* 1997;30(4):1104–6.
727. Levine HJ. Rest heart rate and life expectancy. *J Am Coll Cardiol.* 1997;30(4):1104–6.
728. Levine HJ. Rest heart rate and life expectancy. *J Am Coll Cardiol.* 1997;30(4):1104–6.

729. Cook S, Hess OM. Resting heart rate and cardiovascular events: time for a new crusade? *Eur Heart J.* 2010;31(5):517–9.
730. Jensen MT, Suadicani P, Hein HO, Gyntelberg F. Elevated resting heart rate, physical fitness and all-cause mortality: a 16-year follow-up in the Copenhagen Male Study. *Heart.* 2013;99(12):882–7.
731. Cook S, Hess OM. Resting heart rate and cardiovascular events: time for a new crusade? *Eur Heart J.* 2010;31(5):517–9.
732. Santos RD. Increased resting heart rate and greater progression of subclinical coronary atherosclerosis: another bad fact about fast hearts? Commentary on the study of Rubin et al. *Atherosclerosis.* 2012;220(1):36–7.
733. Woodward M, Webster R, Murakami Y, et al. The association between resting heart rate, cardiovascular disease and mortality: evidence from 112,680 men and women in 12 cohorts. *Eur J Prev Cardiol.* 2014;21(6):719–26.
734. Sloan RP, Shapiro PA, DeMeersman RE, et al. The effect of aerobic training and cardiac autonomic regulation in young adults. *Am J Public Health.* 2009;99(5):921–8.
735. Jenkins DJA, Kendall CWC, Augustin LSA, et al. Effect of legumes as part of a low glycemic index diet on glycemic control and cardiovascular risk factors in type 2 diabetes mellitus: a randomized controlled trial. *Arch Intern Med.* 2012;172(21):1653–60.
736. Sloan RP, Shapiro PA, DeMeersman RE, et al. The effect of aerobic training and cardiac autonomic regulation in young adults. *Am J Public Health.* 2009;99(5):921–8.
737. Schwingshackl L, Schwedhelm C, Hoffmann G, et al. Food groups and risk of all-cause mortality: a systematic review and meta-analysis of prospective studies. *Am J Clin Nutr.* 2017;105(6):1462–73.
738. Institute for Health Metrics and Evaluation (IHME). GBD 2021 cause and risk summary: diet low in fruits—level 3 risk. University of Washington. https://www.healthdata.org/research-analysis/diseases-injuries-risks/factsheets/2021-diet-low-fruits-level-3-risk. Accessed January 27, 2025.
739. Institute for Health Metrics and Evaluation (IHME). GBD 2021 cause and risk summary: diet high in sodium—level 3 risk. University of Washington. https://www.healthdata.org/research-analysis/diseases-injuries-risks/factsheets/2021-diet-high-sodium-level-3-risk. Accessed January 28, 2025.
740. Karppanen H, Mervaala E. Sodium intake and hypertension. *Prog Cardiovasc Dis.* 2006;49(2):59–75.
741. Delahaye F. Should we eat less salt? *Arch Cardiovasc Dis.* 2013;106(5):324–32.
742. Jenkins DJ, Kendall CW. The garden of Eden: plant-based diets, the genetic drive to store fat and conserve cholesterol, and implications for epidemiology in the 21st century. *Epidemiology.* 2006;17(2):128–30.
743. Roberts WC. High salt intake, its origins, its economic impact, and its effect on blood pressure. *Am J Cardiol.* 2001;88(11):1338–46.
744. Roberts WC. High salt intake, its origins, its economic impact, and its effect on blood pressure. *Am J Cardiol.* 2001;88(11):1338–46.
745. Celermajer DS, Neal B. Excessive sodium intake and cardiovascular disease: a-salting our vessels. *J Am Coll Cardiol.* 2013;61(3):344–5.
746. Whelton PK, Appel LJ, Sacco RL, et al. Sodium, blood pressure, and cardiovascular disease: further evidence supporting the American Heart Association sodium reduction recommendations. *Circulation.* 2012;126(24):2880–9.
747. Clarke LS, Overwyk K, Bates M, Park S, Gillespie C, Cogswell ME. Temporal trends in dietary sodium intake among adults aged ≥19 years—United States, 2003–2016. *MMWR Morb Mortal Wkly Rep.* 2021;70:1478–82.
748. Law MR, Frost CD, Wald NJ. By how much does dietary salt reduction lower blood pressure? III—Analysis of data from trials of salt reduction. *BMJ.* 1991;302(6780):819–24.

749. Bibbins-Domingo K, Chertow GM, Coxson PG, et al. Projected effect of dietary salt reductions on future cardiovascular disease. *N Engl J Med*. 2010;362(7):590–9.
750. MacGregor GA, Markandu ND, Best FE, et al. Double-blind randomised crossover trial of moderate sodium restriction in essential hypertension. *Lancet*. 1982;1(8268):351–5.
751. MacGregor GA, Markandu ND, Sagnella GA, Singer DR, Cappuccio FP. Double-blind study of three sodium intakes and long-term effects of sodium restriction in essential hypertension. *Lancet*. 1989;2(8674):1244–7.
752. MacGregor GA, Markandu ND, Sagnella GA, Singer DR, Cappuccio FP. Double-blind study of three sodium intakes and long-term effects of sodium restriction in essential hypertension. *Lancet*. 1989;2(8674):1244–7.
753. Rudelt A, French S, Harnack L. Fourteen-year trends in sodium content of menu offerings at eight leading fast-food restaurants in the USA. *Public Health Nutr*. 2014;17(8):1682–8.
754. Suckling RJ, He FJ, Markandu ND, MacGregor GA. Dietary salt influences postprandial plasma sodium concentration and systolic blood pressure. *Kidney Int*. 2012;81(4):407–11.
755. He FJ, Li J, MacGregor GA. Effect of longer term modest salt reduction on blood pressure: Cochrane systematic review and meta-analysis of randomised trials. *BMJ*. 2013;346:f1325.
756. Celermajer DS, Neal B. Excessive sodium intake and cardiovascular disease: a-salting our vessels. *J Am Coll Cardiol*. 2013;61(3):344–5.
757. Oliver WJ, Cohen EL, Neel JV. Blood pressure, sodium intake, and sodium related hormones in the Yanomamo Indians, a "no-salt" culture. *Circulation*. 1975;52(1):146–51.
758. Mancilha-Carvalho J de J, de Souza e Silva NA. The Yanomami Indians in the INTERSALT Study. *Arq Bras Cardiol*. 2003;80(3):289–300.
759. Celermajer DS, Neal B. Excessive sodium intake and cardiovascular disease: a-salting our vessels. *J Am Coll Cardiol*. 2013;61(3):344–5.
760. Mancilha-Carvalho J de J, de Souza e Silva NA. The Yanomami Indians in the INTERSALT Study. *Arq Bras Cardiol*. 2003;80(3):289–300.
761. Mancilha-Carvalho J de J, Crews DE. Lipid profiles of Yanomamo Indians of Brazil. *Prev Med*. 1990;19(1):66–75.
762. Kempner W. Treatment of heart and kidney disease and of hypertensive and arteriosclerotic vascular disease with the rice diet. *Ann Intern Med*. 1949;31(5):821–56.
763. Klemmer P, Grim CE, Luft FC. Who and what drove Walter Kempner? The rice diet revisited. *Hypertension*. 2014;64(4):684–8.
764. Kempner W. Treatment of heart and kidney disease and of hypertensive and arteriosclerotic vascular disease with the rice diet. *Ann Intern Med*. 1949;31(5):821–56.
765. Roberts WC. High salt intake, its origins, its economic impact, and its effect on blood pressure. *Am J Cardiol*. 2001;88(11):1338–46.
766. Dickinson KM, Clifton PM, Keogh JB. Endothelial function is impaired after a high-salt meal in healthy subjects. *Am J Clin Nutr*. 2011;93(3):500–5.
767. DuPont JJ, Greaney JL, Wenner MM, et al. High dietary sodium intake impairs endothelium-dependent dilation in healthy salt-resistant humans. *J Hypertens*. 2013;31(3):530–6.
768. Dickinson KM, Clifton PM, Keogh JB. Endothelial function is impaired after a high-salt meal in healthy subjects. *Am J Clin Nutr*. 2011;93(3):500–5.
769. Jablonski KL, Racine ML, Geolfos CJ, et al. Dietary sodium restriction reverses vascular endothelial dysfunction in middle-aged/older adults with moderately elevated systolic blood pressure. *J Am Coll Cardiol*. 2013;61(3):335–43.
770. Greaney JL, DuPont JJ, Lennon-Edwards SL, Sanders PW, Edwards DG, Farquhar WB. Dietary sodium loading impairs microvascular function independent of blood pressure in humans: role of oxidative stress. *J Physiol (Lond)*. 2012;590(Pt 21):5519–28.
771. Jablonski KL, Racine ML, Geolfos CJ, et al. Dietary sodium restriction reverses vascular endothelial dysfunction in middle-aged/older adults with moderately elevated systolic blood pressure. *J Am Coll Cardiol*. 2013;61(3):335–43.

772. McCord JM. Analysis of superoxide dismutase activity. *Curr Protoc Toxicol*. 1999;Chapter 7:Unit 7.3.
773. Dickinson KM, Clifton PM, Burrell LM, Barrett PHR, Keogh JB. Postprandial effects of a high salt meal on serum sodium, arterial stiffness, markers of nitric oxide production and markers of endothelial function. *Atherosclerosis*. 2014;232(1):211–6.
774. Huang Ti Nei Ching Su Wua [*The Yellow Emperor's Classic of Internal Medicine*] (Veith I, Trans.) Oakland, CA: University of California Press; 1972:141.
775. Hanneman RL, Satin M. Comments to the Dietary Guidelines Committee on behalf of the Salt Institute. Comment ID: 000447. April 23, 2009.
776. Vital signs: food categories contributing the most to sodium consumption—United States, 2007–2008. *MMWR Morb Mortal Wkly Rep*. 2012;61(5):92–8.
777. Miller GD. Comments to the Dietary Guidelines Committee on behalf of the National Dairy Council. July 27, 2009.
778. Roberts WC. High salt intake, its origins, its economic impact, and its effect on blood pressure. *Am J Cardiol*. 2001;88(11):1338–46.
779. MacGregor G, de Wardener HE. Salt, blood pressure and health. *Int J Epidemiol*. 2002;31(2):320–7.
780. Appel LJ, Anderson CAM. Compelling evidence for public health action to reduce salt intake. *N Engl J Med*. 2010;362(7):650–2.
781. Roberts WC. High salt intake, its origins, its economic impact, and its effect on blood pressure. *Am J Cardiol*. 2001;88(11):1338–46.
782. Buying this chicken? *Consum Rep*. June 2008;7.
783. Drewnowski A, Rehm CD. Sodium intakes of US children and adults from foods and beverages by location of origin and by specific food source. *Nutrients*. 2013;5(6):1840–55.
784. U.S. Department of Agriculture, Agricultural Research Service. Pizza Hut 14" pepperoni pizza, hand-tossed crust. FoodData Central. https://fdc.nal.usda.gov/food-details/172052/nutrients. April 2018. Accessed January 28, 2025.
785. Drewnowski A, Rehm CD. Sodium intakes of US children and adults from foods and beverages by location of origin and by specific food source. *Nutrients*. 2013;5(6):1840–55.
786. Blais CA, Pangborn RM, Borhani NO, Ferrell MF, Prineas RJ, Laing B. Effect of dietary sodium restriction on taste responses to sodium chloride: a longitudinal study. *Am J Clin Nutr*. 1986;44(2):232–43.
787. Tucker RM, Mattes RD. Are free fatty acids effective taste stimuli in humans? Presented at the symposium "The Taste for Fat: New Discoveries on the Role of Fat in Sensory Perception, Metabolism, Sensory Pleasure and Beyond" held at the Institute of Food Technologists 2011 Annual Meeting, New Orleans, LA, June 12, 2011. *J Food Sci*. 2012;77(3):S148–51.
788. Grieve FG, Vander Weg MW. Desire to eat high-and low-fat foods following a low-fat dietary intervention. *J Nutr Educ Behav*. 2003;35(2):98–102.
789. Stewart JE, Newman LP, Keast RS. Oral sensitivity to oleic acid is associated with fat intake and body mass index. *Clin Nutr*. 2011;30(6):838–44.
790. Stewart JE, Keast RS. Recent fat intake modulates fat taste sensitivity in lean and overweight subjects. *Int J Obes* (Lond). 2012;36(6):834–42.
791. Roberts WC. High salt intake, its origins, its economic impact, and its effect on blood pressure. *Am J Cardiol*. 2001;88(11):1338–46.
792. Newson RS, Elmadfa I, Biro G, et al. Barriers for progress in salt reduction in the general population. An international study. *Appetite*. 2013;71:22–31.
793. Neal B, Wu Y, Feng X, et al. Effect of salt substitution on cardiovascular events and death. *N Engl J Med*. 2021;385(12):1067–77.
794. Martin SS, Aday AW, Almarzooq ZI, et al. 2024 heart disease and stroke statistics: a report of US and global data from the American Heart Association. *Circulation*. 2024;149(8):e347–e913.

795. Xu X, Zeng L, Jha V, et al. Potassium-enriched salt substitutes: a review of recommendations in clinical management guidelines. *Hypertension.* 2024;81(3):400–14.
796. Cappuccio FP, Capewell S, Lincoln P, McPherson K. Policy options to reduce population salt intake. *BMJ.* 2011;343:d4995.
797. Toldrá F, Barat JM. Strategies for salt reduction in foods. *Recent Pat Food Nutr Agric.* 2012;4(1):19–25.
798. Lin BH, Guthrie J. Nutritional quality of food prepared at home and away from home, 1977–2008. USDA, Economic Research Service. https://www.ers.usda.gov/publications/pub-details?pubid=43699. December 2012. Accessed January 28, 2025.
799. Newson RS, Elmadfa I, Biro G, et al. Barriers for progress in salt reduction in the general population. An international study. *Appetite.* 2013;71:22–31.
800. Roberts WC. High salt intake, its origins, its economic impact, and its effect on blood pressure. *Am J Cardiol.* 2001;88(11):1338–46.
801. U.S. Department of Agriculture, U.S. Department of Health and Human Services. Dietary Guidelines for Americans, 2020–2025, 9th ed. https://www.dietaryguidelines.gov/sites/default/files/2021-03/Dietary_Guidelines_for_Americans-2020-2025.pdf. December 2020. Accessed January 28, 2025.
802. Karppanen H, Mervaala E. Sodium intake and hypertension. *Prog Cardiovasc Dis.* 2006;49(2):59–75.
803. Law MR, Morris JK, Wald NJ. Use of blood pressure lowering drugs in the prevention of cardiovascular disease: meta-analysis of 147 randomised trials in the context of expectations from prospective epidemiological studies. *BMJ.* 2009;338:b1665.
804. Tighe P, Duthie G, Vaughan N, et al. Effect of increased consumption of whole-grain foods on blood pressure and other cardiovascular risk markers in healthy middle-aged persons: a randomized controlled trial. *Am J Clin Nutr.* 2010;92(4):733–40.
805. Diaconu CC, Balaceanu A, Bartos D. Diuretics, first-line antihypertensive agents: are they always safe in the elderly? *Rom J Intern Med.* 2014;52(2):87–90.
806. Li CI, Daling JR, Tang MT, Haugen KL, Porter PL, Malone KE. Use of antihypertensive medications and breast cancer risk among women aged 55 to 74 years. *JAMA Intern Med.* 2013;173(17):1629–37.
807. Kaiser EA, Lotze U, Schiser HH. Increasing complexity: which drug class to choose for treatment of hypertension in the elderly? *Clin Interv Aging.* 2014;9:459–75.
808. Rasmussen ER, Mey K, Bygum A. Angiotensin-converting enzyme inhibitor-induced angioedema—a dangerous new epidemic. *Acta Derm Venereol.* 2014;94(3):260–4.
809. Tinetti ME, Han L, Lee DS, et al. Antihypertensive medications and serious fall injuries in a nationally representative sample of older adults. *JAMA Intern Med.* 2014;174(4):588–95.
810. Ye EQ, Chacko SA, Chou EL, Kugizaki M, Liu S. Greater whole-grain intake is associated with lower risk of type 2 diabetes, cardiovascular disease, and weight gain. *J Nutr.* 2012;142(7):1304–13.
811. Aune D, Chan DS, Lau R, et al. Dietary fibre, whole grains, and risk of colorectal cancer: systematic review and dose-response meta-analysis of prospective studies. *BMJ.* 2011;343:d6617.
812. Tighe P, Duthie G, Vaughan N, et al. Effect of increased consumption of whole-grain foods on blood pressure and other cardiovascular risk markers in healthy middle-aged persons: a randomized controlled trial. *Am J Clin Nutr.* 2010;92(4):733–40.
813. Sun Q, Spiegelman D, van Dam RM, et al. White rice, brown rice, and risk of type 2 diabetes in US men and women. *Arch Intern Med.* 2010;170(11):961–9.
814. Ye EQ, Chacko SA, Chou EL, Kugizaki M, Liu S. Greater whole-grain intake is associated with lower risk of type 2 diabetes, cardiovascular disease, and weight gain. *J Nutr.* 2012;142(7):1304–13.
815. Mellen PB, Liese AD, Tooze JA, Vitolins MZ, Wagenknecht LE, Herrington DM. Whole-grain intake and carotid artery atherosclerosis in a multiethnic cohort: the Insulin Resistance Atherosclerosis Study. *Am J Clin Nutr.* 2007;85(6):1495–502.

816. Erkkilä AT, Herrington DM, Mozaffarian D, et al. Cereal fiber and whole-grain intake are associated with reduced progression of coronary-artery atherosclerosis in postmenopausal women with coronary artery disease. *Am Heart J*. 2005;150(1):94–101.
817. Centers for Disease Control and Prevention. Hypertension cascade: hypertension prevalence, treatment and control estimates among US adults aged 18 years and older applying the criteria from the American College of Cardiology and American Heart Association's 2017 Hypertension Guideline—NHANES 2017–March 2020. https://millionhearts.hhs.gov/data-reports/hypertension-prevalence.html. May 12, 2023. Accessed January 28, 2025.
818. Go AS, Bauman MA, Coleman King SM, et al. An effective approach to high blood pressure control: a science advisory from the American Heart Association, the American College of Cardiology, and the Centers for Disease Control and Prevention. *J Am Coll Cardiol*. 2014;63(12):1230–8.
819. Mahmud A, Feely J. Low-dose quadruple antihypertensive combination: more efficacious than individual agents—a preliminary report. *Hypertension*. 2007;49(2):272–5.
820. Kronish IM, Woodward M, Sergie Z, Ogedegbe G, Falzon L, Mann DM. Meta-analysis: impact of drug class on adherence to antihypertensives. *Circulation*. 2011;123(15):1611–21.
821. Messerli FH, Bangalore S. Half a century of hydrochlorothiazide: facts, fads, fiction, and follies. *Am J Med*. 2011;124(10):896–9.
822. Law MR, Morris JK, Wald NJ. Use of blood pressure lowering drugs in the prevention of cardiovascular disease: meta-analysis of 147 randomised trials in the context of expectations from prospective epidemiological studies. *BMJ*. 2009;338:b1665.
823. Donnison CP. Blood pressure in the African native. *Lancet*. 1929;213(5497):6–7.
824. Morse WR, McGill MD, Beh YT. Blood pressure amongst aboriginal ethnic groups of Szechwan Province, West China. *Lancet*. 1937;229(5929):966–8.
825. Sacks FM, Kass EH. Low blood pressure in vegetarians: effects of specific foods and nutrients. *Am J Clin Nutr*. 1988;48(3 Suppl):795–800.
826. Go AS, Bauman MA, Coleman King SM, et al. An effective approach to high blood pressure control: a science advisory from the American Heart Association, the American College of Cardiology, and the Centers for Disease Control and Prevention. *J Am Coll Cardiol*. 2014;63(12):1230–8.
827. Sharma AM, Schorr U. Dietary patterns and blood pressure. *N Engl J Med*. 1997;337(9):637.
828. Chen Q, Turban S, Miller ER, Appel LJ. The effects of dietary patterns on plasma renin activity: results from the Dietary Approaches to Stop Hypertension trial. *J Hum Hypertens*. 2012;26(11):664–9.
829. Sacks FM, Rosner B, Kass EH. Blood pressure in vegetarians. *Am J Epidemiol*. 1974;100(5):390–8.
830. Donaldson AN. The relation of protein foods to hypertension. *Cal West Med*. 1926;24(3):328–31.
831. Appel LJ, Brands MW, Daniels SR, et al. Dietary approaches to prevent and treat hypertension: a scientific statement from the American Heart Association. *Hypertension*. 2006;47(2):296–308.
832. Sacks FM, Obarzanek E, Windhauser MM, et al. Rationale and design of the Dietary Approaches to Stop Hypertension trial (DASH). A multicenter controlled-feeding study of dietary patterns to lower blood pressure. *Ann Epidemiol*. 1995;5(2):108–18.
833. Karanja NM, Obarzanek E, Lin PH, et al. Descriptive characteristics of the dietary patterns used in the Dietary Approaches to Stop Hypertension trial. DASH Collaborative Research Group. *J Am Diet Assoc*. 1999;99(8 Suppl):S19–27.
834. Sacks FM, Kass EH. Low blood pressure in vegetarians: effects of specific foods and nutrients. *Am J Clin Nutr*. 1988;48(3 Suppl):795–800.
835. Fuhrman J. *The End of Dieting: How to Live for Life*. HarperOne; 2014.
836. de Paula TP, Steemburgo T, de Almeida JC, Dall'Alba V, Gross JL, de Azevedo MJ. The role of Dietary Approaches to Stop Hypertension (DASH) diet food groups in blood pressure in type 2 diabetes. *Br J Nutr*. 2012;108(1):155–62.

837. Tomé-Carneiro J, Visioli F. Plant-based diets reduce blood pressure: a systematic review of recent evidence. *Curr Hypertens Rep.* 2023;25(7):127–50.
838. Le LT, Sabaté J. Beyond meatless, the health effects of vegan diets: findings from the Adventist cohorts. *Nutrients.* 2014;6(6):2131–47.
839. Erlich MN, Ghidanac D, Blanco Mejia S, et al. A systematic review and meta-analysis of randomized trials of substituting soymilk for cow's milk and intermediate cardiometabolic outcomes: understanding the impact of dairy alternatives in the transition to plant-based diets on cardiometabolic health. *BMC Med.* 2024;22(1):33.
840. Fraser GE. Vegetarian diets: what do we know of their effects on common chronic diseases? *Am J Clin Nutr.* 2009;89(5):1607S–12S.
841. Tonstad S, Stewart K, Oda K, Batech M, Herring RP, Fraser GE. Vegetarian diets and incidence of diabetes in the Adventist Health Study-2. *Nutr Metab Cardiovasc Dis.* 2013;23(4):292–9.
842. Fraser GE. Vegetarian diets: what do we know of their effects on common chronic diseases? *Am J Clin Nutr.* 2009;89(5):1607S–12S.
843. Fontana L, Meyer TE, Klein S, Holloszy JO. Long-term low-calorie low-protein vegan diet and endurance exercise are associated with low cardiometabolic risk. *Rejuvenation Res.* 2007;10(2):225–34.
844. Rodriguez-Leyva D, Weighell W, Edel AL, et al. Potent antihypertensive action of dietary flaxseed in hypertensive patients. *Hypertension.* 2013;62(6):1081–9.
845. Cornelissen VA, Buys R, Smart NA. Endurance exercise beneficially affects ambulatory blood pressure: a systematic review and meta-analysis. *J Hypertens.* 2013;31(4):639–48.
846. Geleijnse JM. Relation of raw and cooked vegetable consumption to blood pressure: the INTERMAP study. *J Hum Hypertens.* 2014;28(6):343–4.
847. Jayalath VH, de Souza RJ, Sievenpiper JL, et al. Effect of dietary pulses on blood pressure: a systematic review and meta-analysis of controlled feeding trials. *Am J Hypertens.* 2014;27(1):56–64.
848. Chiva-Blanch G, Urpi-Sarda M, Ros E, et al. Dealcoholized red wine decreases systolic and diastolic blood pressure and increases plasma nitric oxide: short communication. *Circ Res.* 2012;111(8):1065–8.
849. Figueroa A, Sanchez-Gonzalez MA, Wong A, Arjmandi BH. Watermelon extract supplementation reduces ankle blood pressure and carotid augmentation index in obese adults with prehypertension or hypertension. *Am J Hypertens.* 2012;25(6):640–3.
850. Gammon CS, Kruger R, Brown SJ, Conlon CA, von Hurst PR, Stonehouse W. Daily kiwifruit consumption did not improve blood pressure and markers of cardiovascular function in men with hypercholesterolemia. *Nutr Res.* 2014;34(3):235–40.
851. Anderson JW, Weiter KM, Christian AL, Ritchey MB, Bays HE. Raisins compared with other snack effects on glycemia and blood pressure: a randomized, controlled trial. *Postgrad Med.* 2014;126(1):37–43.
852. Akhtar S, Ismail T, Riaz M. Flaxseed—a miraculous defense against some critical maladies. *Pak J Pharm Sci.* 2013;26(1):199–208.
853. Rodriguez-Leyva D, Weighell W, Edel AL, et al. Potent antihypertensive action of dietary flaxseed in hypertensive patients. *Hypertension.* 2013;62(6):1081–9.
854. Ninomiya T, Perkovic V, Turnbull F, et al. Blood pressure lowering and major cardiovascular events in people with and without chronic kidney disease: meta-analysis of randomised controlled trials. *BMJ.* 2013;347:f5680.
855. Goyal A, Sharma V, Upadhyay N, Gill S, Sihag M. Flax and flaxseed oil: an ancient medicine & modern functional food. *J Food Sci Technol.* 2014;51(9):1633–53.
856. Carlsen MH, Halvorsen BL, Holte K, et al. The total antioxidant content of more than 3100 foods, beverages, spices, herbs and supplements used worldwide. *Nutr J.* 2010;9:3.
857. Frank T, Netzel G, Kammerer DR, et al. Consumption of Hibiscus sabdariffa L. aqueous extract and its impact on systemic antioxidant potential in healthy subjects. *J Sci Food Agric.* 2012;92(10):2207–18.

858. Chang HC, Peng CH, Yeh DM, Kao ES, Wang CJ. Hibiscus sabdariffa extract inhibits obesity and fat accumulation, and improves liver steatosis in humans. *Food Funct.* 2014;5(4):734–9.
859. Mozaffari-Khosravi H, Jalali-Khanabadi BA, Afkhami-Ardekani M, Fatehi F. Effects of sour tea (Hibiscus sabdariffa) on lipid profile and lipoproteins in patients with type II diabetes. *J Altern Complement Med.* 2009;15(8):899–903.
860. Aziz Z, Wong SY, Chong NJ. Effects of Hibiscus sabdariffa L. on serum lipids: a systematic review and meta-analysis. *J Ethnopharmacol.* 2013;150(2):442–50.
861. Lin TL, Lin HH, Chen CC, et al. Hibiscus sabdariffa extract reduces serum cholesterol in men and women. *Nutr Res.* 2007;27:140–5.
862. Hopkins AL, Lamm MG, Funk JL, Ritenbaugh C. Hibiscus sabdariffa L. in the treatment of hypertension and hyperlipidemia: a comprehensive review of animal and human studies. *Fitoterapia.* 2013;85:84–94.
863. McKay DL, Chen CY, Saltzman E, Blumberg JB. Hibiscus sabdariffa L. tea (tisane) lowers blood pressure in prehypertensive and mildly hypertensive adults. *J Nutr.* 2010;140(2):298–303.
864. Chobanian AV, Bakris GL, Black HR, et al. Seventh report of the Joint National Committee on prevention, detection, evaluation, and treatment of high blood pressure. *Hypertension.* 2003;42(6):1206–52.
865. McKay DL, Chen CY, Saltzman E, Blumberg JB. Hibiscus sabdariffa L. tea (tisane) lowers blood pressure in prehypertensive and mildly hypertensive adults. *J Nutr.* 2010;140(2):298–303.
866. Herrera-Arellano A, Flores-Romero S, Chávez-Soto MA, Tortoriello J. Effectiveness and tolerability of a standardized extract from Hibiscus sabdariffa in patients with mild to moderate hypertension: a controlled and randomized clinical trial. *Phytomedicine.* 2004;11(5):375–82.
867. U.S. Food and Drug Administration. CAPOTEN® (Captopril Tablets, USP) http://www.accessdata.fda.gov/drugsatfda_docs/label/2012/018343s084lbl.pdf. Accessed January 28, 2025.
868. Hendricks JL, Marshall TA, Harless JD, Hogan MM, Qian F, Wefel JS. Erosive potentials of brewed teas. *Am J Dent.* 2013;26(5):278–82.
869. Malik J, Frankova A, Drabek O, Szakova J, Ash C, Kokoska L. Aluminium and other elements in selected herbal tea plant species and their infusions. *Food Chem.* 2013;139(1–4):728–34.
870. Förstermann U. Janus-faced role of endothelial NO synthase in vascular disease: uncoupling of oxygen reduction from NO synthesis and its pharmacological reversal. *Biol Chem.* 2006;387(12):1521–33.
871. Franzini L, Ardigò D, Valtueña S, et al. Food selection based on high total antioxidant capacity improves endothelial function in a low cardiovascular risk population. *Nutr Metab Cardiovasc Dis.* 2012;22(1):50–7.
872. Webb AJ, Patel N, Loukogeorgakis S, et al. Acute blood pressure lowering, vasoprotective, and antiplatelet properties of dietary nitrate via bioconversion to nitrite. *Hypertension.* 2008;51(3):784–90.
873. Smith RE, Ashiya M. Antihypertensive therapies. *Nat Rev Drug Discov.* 2007;6(8):597–8.
874. Kapil V, Khambata RS, Robertson A, Caulfield MJ, Ahluwalia A. Dietary nitrate provides sustained blood pressure lowering in hypertensive patients: a randomized, phase 2, double-blind, placebo-controlled study. *Hypertension.* 2015;65(2):320–7.
875. Wylie LJ, Kelly J, Bailey SJ, et al. Beetroot juice and exercise: pharmacodynamic and dose-response relationships. *J Appl Physiol.* 2013;115(3):325–36.
876. European Food Safety Authority. Nitrate in vegetables: scientific opinion of the Panel on Contaminants in the Food Chain. *EFSA J.* 2008;689:1–79.
877. Murphy M, Eliot K, Heuertz RM, Weiss E. Whole beetroot consumption acutely improves running performance. *J Acad Nutr Diet.* 2012;112(4):548–52.
878. Clements WT, Lee SR, Bloomer RJ. Nitrate ingestion: a review of the health and physical performance effects. *Nutrients.* 2014;6(11):5224–64.

879. Hord NG, Tang Y, Bryan NS. Food sources of nitrates and nitrites: the physiologic context for potential health benefits. *Am J Clin Nutr.* 2009;90(1):1–10.
880. Bhupathiraju SN, Wedick NM, Pan A, et al. Quantity and variety in fruit and vegetable intake and risk of coronary heart disease. *Am J Clin Nutr.* 2013;98(6):1514–23.
881. Tamakoshi A, Tamakoshi K, Lin Y, Yagyu K, Kikuchi S. Healthy lifestyle and preventable death: findings from the Japan Collaborative Cohort (JACC) Study. *Prev Med.* 2009;48(5):486–92.
882. Wang F, Dai S, Wang M, Morrison H. Erectile dysfunction and fruit/vegetable consumption among diabetic Canadian men. *Urology.* 2013;82(6):1330–5.
883. Presley TD, Morgan AR, Bechtold E, et al. Acute effect of a high nitrate diet on brain perfusion in older adults. *Nitric Oxide.* 2011;24(1):34–42.
884. Engan HK, Jones AM, Ehrenberg F, Schagatay E. Acute dietary nitrate supplementation improves dry static apnea performance. *Respir Physiol Neurobiol.* 2012;182(2–3):53–9.
885. Bailey SJ, Winyard P, Vanhatalo A, et al. Dietary nitrate supplementation reduces the O2 cost of low-intensity exercise and enhances tolerance to high-intensity exercise in humans. *J Appl Physiol.* 2009;107(4):1144–55.
886. Murphy M, Eliot K, Heuertz RM, Weiss E. Whole beetroot consumption acutely improves running performance. *J Acad Nutr Diet.* 2012;112(4):548–52.
887. Lidder S, Webb AJ. Vascular effects of dietary nitrate (as found in green leafy vegetables and beetroot) via the nitrate-nitrite-nitric oxide pathway. *Br J Clin Pharmacol.* 2013;75(3):677–96.
888. Wylie LJ, Kelly J, Bailey SJ, et al. Beetroot juice and exercise: pharmacodynamic and dose-response relationships. *J Appl Physiol.* 2013;115(3):325–36.
889. Kario K, Okura A, Hoshide S, et al. The WHO Global Report 2023 on hypertension warning the emerging hypertension burden in globe and its treatment strategy. *Hypertens Res.* 2024;47:1099–102.
890. Liu PH, Wang JD, Keating NL. Expected years of life lost for six potentially preventable cancers in the United States. *Prev Med.* 2013;56(5):309–13.
891. Bertram JS, Kolonel LN, Meyskens FL. Rationale and strategies for chemoprevention of cancer in humans. *Cancer Res.* 1987;47(11):3012–31.
892. Combs MP, Dickson RP. Turning the lungs inside out: the intersecting microbiomes of the lungs and the built environment. *Am J Respir Crit Care Med.* 2020;202(12):1618–20.
893. U.S. Cancer Statistics Working Group. U.S. Cancer Statistics Data Visualizations Tool. U.S. Department of Health and Human Services, Centers for Disease Control and Prevention and National Cancer Institute. https://www.cdc.gov/cancer/dataviz. June 2024. Accessed January 18, 2025.
894. U.S. Cancer Statistics Working Group. U.S. Cancer Statistics Data Visualizations Tool. U.S. Department of Health and Human Services, Centers for Disease Control and Prevention and National Cancer Institute. https://www.cdc.gov/cancer/dataviz. June 2024. Accessed January 18, 2025.
895. U.S. Cancer Statistics Working Group. U.S. Cancer Statistics Data Visualizations Tool. U.S. Department of Health and Human Services, Centers for Disease Control and Prevention and National Cancer Institute. https://www.cdc.gov/cancer/dataviz. June 2024. Accessed January 18, 2025.
896. Key statistics for colorectal cancer. American Cancer Society. https://www.cancer.org/cancer/types/colon-rectal-cancer/about/key-statistics.html. January 16, 2025. Accessed January 23, 2025.
897. Cancer prevalence: how many people have cancer? American Cancer Society. https://www.cancer.org/cancer/survivorship/cancer-prevalence.html. January 19, 2023. Accessed January 23, 2025.
898. Survival rates for colorectal cancer. American Cancer Society. https://www.cancer.org

/cancer/types/colon-rectal-cancer/detection-diagnosis-staging/survival-rates.html. January 16, 2025. Accessed January 23, 2025.
899. US Preventive Services Task Force, Davidson KW, Barry MJ, et al. Screening for colorectal cancer: US Preventive Services Task Force recommendation statement. *JAMA.* 2021;325(19):1965–77.
900. Rastogi T, Devesa S, Mangtani P, et al. Cancer incidence rates among South Asians in four geographic regions: India, Singapore, UK and US. *Int J Epidemiol.* 2008;37(1):147–60.
901. Babu GR. Response to "Cancer incidence rates among South Asians in four geographic regions: India, Singapore, UK and US." *Int J Epidemiol.* 2009;38(4):1157–8; author reply 1158–9.
902. Hutchins-Wolfbrandt A, Mistry AM. Dietary turmeric potentially reduces the risk of cancer. *Asian Pac J Cancer Prev.* 2011;12(12):3169–73.
903. Sharma RA, Euden SA, Platton SL, et al. Phase I clinical trial of oral curcumin: biomarkers of systemic activity and compliance. *Clin Cancer Res.* 2004;10(20):6847–54.
904. Carroll RE, Benya RV, Turgeon DK, et al. Phase IIa clinical trial of curcumin for the prevention of colorectal neoplasia. *Cancer Prev Res* (Phila). 2011;4(3):354–64.
905. Cruz-Correa M, Shoskes DA, Sanchez P, et al. Combination treatment with curcumin and quercetin of adenomas in familial adenomatous polyposis. *Clin Gastroenterol Hepatol.* 2006;4(8):1035–8.
906. Sharma RA, McLelland HR, Hill KA, et al. Pharmacodynamic and pharmacokinetic study of oral Curcuma extract in patients with colorectal cancer. *Clin Cancer Res.* 2001;7(7):1894–900.
907. Singh S. From exotic spice to modern drug? *Cell.* 2007;130(5):765–8.
908. International Institute for Population Sciences & Macro International. *National Family Health Survey (NFHS-3), 2005–06: India: Vol. I.* Mumbai: IIPS; 2007.
909. Cummings JH, Bingham SA, Heaton KW, Eastwood MA. Fecal weight, colon cancer risk, and dietary intake of nonstarch polysaccharides (dietary fiber). *Gastroenterology.* 1992;103(6):1783–9.
910. Cummings JH, Bingham SA, Heaton KW, Eastwood MA. Fecal weight, colon cancer risk, and dietary intake of nonstarch polysaccharides (dietary fiber). *Gastroenterology.* 1992;103(6):1783–9.
911. Gear JS, Brodribb AJ, Ware A, Mann JI. Fibre and bowel transit times. *Br J Nutr.* 1981;45(1):77–82.
912. Burkitt DP, Walker AR, Painter NS. Effect of dietary fibre on stools and the transit-times, and its role in the causation of disease. *Lancet.* 1972;2(7792):1408–12.
913. Sonnenberg A, Koch TR. Physician visits in the United States for constipation: 1958 to 1986. *Dig Dis Sci.* 1989;34(4):606–11.
914. Burkitt DP. A deficiency of dietary fiber may be one cause of certain colonic and venous disorders. *Am J Dig Dis.* 1976;21(2):104–8.
915. Fox A, Tietze PH, Ramakrishnan K. Anorectal conditions: anal fissure and anorectal fistula. *FP Essent.* 2014;419:20–7.
916. Burkitt DP. A deficiency of dietary fiber may be one cause of certain colonic and venous disorders. *Am J Dig Dis.* 1976;21(2):104–8.
917. Sanjoaquin MA, Appleby PN, Spencer EA, Key TJ. Nutrition and lifestyle in relation to bowel movement frequency: a cross-sectional study of 20630 men and women in EPIC-Oxford. *Public Health Nutr.* 2004;7(1):77–83.
918. Siegel RL, Wagle NS, Cercek A, Smith RA, Jemal A. Colorectal cancer statistics, 2023. *CA Cancer J Clin.* 2023;73(3):233–54.
919. Doll R. The geographical distribution of cancer. *Br J Cancer.* 1969;23(1):1–8.
920. Lipski E. Traditional non-Western diets. *Nutr Clin Pract.* 2010;25(6):585–93.
921. Burkitt DP. Epidemiology of cancer of the colon and rectum. 1971. *Dis Colon Rectum.* 1993;36(11):1071–82.

922. Shaper AG, Jones KW. Serum-cholesterol, diet, and coronary heart-disease in Africans and Asians in Uganda: 1959. *Int J Epidemiol.* 2012;41(5):1221–5.
923. Malila N, Hakulinen T. Epidemiological trends of colorectal cancer in the Nordic countries. *Scand J Surg.* 2003;92(1):5–9.
924. Englyst HN, Bingham SA, Wiggins HS, et al. Nonstarch polysaccharide consumption in four Scandinavian populations. *Nutr Cancer.* 1982;4(1):50–60.
925. Graf E, Eaton JW. Dietary suppression of colonic cancer. Fiber or phytate? *Cancer.* 1985;56(4):717–8.
926. Fonseca-Nunes A, Jakszyn P, Agudo A. Iron and cancer risk—a systematic review and meta-analysis of the epidemiological evidence. *Cancer Epidemiol Biomarkers Prev.* 2014;23(1):12–31.
927. Mellanby E. The rickets-producing and anti-calcifying action of phytate. *J Physiol.* 1949;109(3–4):488–533.
928. House WA, Welch RM, Van Campen DR. Effect of phytic acid on the absorption, distribution, and endogenous excretion of zinc in rats. *J Nutr.* 1982;112(5):941–53.
929. Urbano G, López-Jurado M, Aranda P, Vidal-Valverde C, Tenorio E, Porres J. The role of phytic acid in legumes: antinutrient or beneficial function? *J Physiol Biochem.* 2000;56(3):283–94.
930. López-González AA, Grases F, Roca P, Mari B, Vicente-Herrero MT, Costa-Bauzá A. Phytate (myo-inositol hexaphosphate) and risk factors for osteoporosis. *J Med Food.* 2008;11(4):747–52.
931. López-González AA, Grases F, Monroy N, et al. Protective effect of myo-inositol hexaphosphate (phytate) on bone mass loss in postmenopausal women. *Eur J Nutr.* 2013;52(2):717–26.
932. Arriero Mdel M, Ramis JM, Perelló J, Monjo M. Inositol hexakisphosphate inhibits osteoclastogenesis on RAW 264.7 cells and human primary osteoclasts. *PLoS ONE.* 2012;7(8):e43187.
933. Khosla S, Burr D, Cauley J, et al. Bisphosphonate-associated osteonecrosis of the jaw: report of a task force of the American Society for Bone and Mineral Research. *J Bone Miner Res.* 2007;22(10):1479–91.
934. Singh PN, Fraser GE. Dietary risk factors for colon cancer in a low-risk population. *Am J Epidemiol.* 1998;148(8):761–74.
935. Manousos O, Day NE, Trichopoulos D, Gerovassilis F, Tzonou A, Polychronopoulou A. Diet and colorectal cancer: a case-control study in Greece. *Int J Cancer.* 1983;32(1):1–5.
936. Lanza E, Hartman TJ, Albert PS, et al. High dry bean intake and reduced risk of advanced colorectal adenoma recurrence among participants in the polyp prevention trial. *J Nutr.* 2006;136(7):1896–903.
937. Vucenik I, Shamsuddin AM. Protection against cancer by dietary IP6 and inositol. *Nutr Cancer.* 2006;55(2):109–25.
938. Vucenik I, Shamsuddin AM. Cancer inhibition by inositol hexaphosphate (IP6) and inositol: from laboratory to clinic. *J Nutr.* 2003;133(11-Suppl-1):3778S–84S.
939. Ogawa S, Kobayashi H, Amada S, et al. Sentinel node detection with (99m)Tc phytate alone is satisfactory for cervical cancer patients undergoing radical hysterectomy and pelvic lymphadenectomy. *Int J Clin Oncol.* 2010;15(1):52–8.
940. Vucenik I, Shamsuddin AM. Protection against cancer by dietary IP6 and inositol. *Nutr Cancer.* 2006;55(2):109–25.
941. Vucenik I, Passaniti A, Vitolo MI, Tantivejkul K, Eggleton P, Shamsuddin AM. Anti-angiogenic activity of inositol hexaphosphate (IP6). *Carcinogenesis.* 2004;25(11):2115–23.
942. Wang H, Khor TO, Shu L, et al. Plants vs. cancer: a review on natural phytochemicals in preventing and treating cancers and their druggability. *Anticancer Agents Med Chem.* 2012;12(10):1281–305.
943. Yang GY, Shamsuddin AM. IP6-induced growth inhibition and differentiation of HT-29 human colon cancer cells: involvement of intracellular inositol phosphates. *Anticancer Res.* 1995;15(6B):2479–87.

944. Shamsuddin AM, Yang GY, Vucenik I. Novel anti-cancer functions of IP6: growth inhibition and differentiation of human mammary cancer cell lines in vitro. *Anticancer Res.* 1996;16(6A):3287–92.
945. Vucenik I, Tantivejkul K, Zhang ZS, Cole KE, Saied I, Shamsuddin AM. IP6 in treatment of liver cancer. I. IP6 inhibits growth and reverses transformed phenotype in HepG2 human liver cancer cell line. *Anticancer Res.* 1998;18(6A):4083–90.
946. Shamsuddin AM, Yang GY. Inositol hexaphosphate inhibits growth and induces differentiation of PC-3 human prostate cancer cells. *Carcinogenesis.* 1995;16(8):1975–9.
947. Shamsuddin AM. Anti-cancer function of phytic acid. *Int J Food Sci Tech.* 2002;37(7):769–82.
948. Sun J, Chu YF, Wu X, Liu RH. Antioxidant and antiproliferative activities of common fruits. *J Agric Food Chem.* 2002;50(25):7449–54.
949. Olsson ME, Andersson CS, Oredsson S, Berglund RH, Gustavsson KE. Antioxidant levels and inhibition of cancer cell proliferation in vitro by extracts from organically and conventionally cultivated strawberries. *J Agric Food Chem.* 2006;54(4):1248–55.
950. Graham DJ, Campen D, Hui R, et al. Risk of acute myocardial infarction and sudden cardiac death in patients treated with cyclo-oxygenase 2 selective and non-selective non-steroidal anti-inflammatory drugs: nested case-control study. *Lancet.* 2005;365(9458):475–81.
951. Wang LS, Burke CA, Hasson H, et al. A phase Ib study of the effects of black raspberries on rectal polyps in patients with familial adenomatous polyposis. *Cancer Prev Res* (Phila). 2014;7(7):666–74.
952. Wang LS, Burke CA, Hasson H, et al. A phase Ib study of the effects of black raspberries on rectal polyps in patients with familial adenomatous polyposis. *Cancer Prev Res* (Phila). 2014;7(7):666–74.
953. Pan A, Sun Q, Bernstein AM, et al. Red meat consumption and mortality: results from 2 prospective cohort studies. *Arch Intern Med.* 2012;172(7):555–63.
954. Sinha R, Cross AJ, Graubard BI, Leitzmann MF, Schatzkin A. Meat intake and mortality: a prospective study of over half a million people. *Arch Intern Med.* 2009;169(6):562–71.
955. Popkin BM. Reducing meat consumption has multiple benefits for the world's health. *Arch Intern Med.* 2009;169(6):543.
956. Dixon SJ, Stockwell BR. The role of iron and reactive oxygen species in cell death. *Nat Chem Biol.* 2014;10(1):9–17.
957. Hurrell R, Egli I. Iron bioavailability and dietary reference values. *Am J Clin Nutr.* 2010;91(5):1461S–7S.
958. Cook JD. Adaptation in iron metabolism. *Am J Clin Nutr.* 1990;51(2):301–8.
959. Fonseca-Nunes A, Jakszyn P, Agudo A. Iron and cancer risk—a systematic review and meta-analysis of the epidemiological evidence. *Cancer Epidemiol Biomarkers Prev.* 2014;23(1):12–31.
960. Yang W, Li B, Dong X, et al. Is heme iron intake associated with risk of coronary heart disease? A meta-analysis of prospective studies. *Eur J Nutr.* 2014;53(2):395–400.
961. Bao W, Rong Y, Rong S, Liu L. Dietary iron intake, body iron stores, and the risk of type 2 diabetes: a systematic review and meta-analysis. *BMC Med.* 2012;10:119.
962. Zacharski LR, Chow BK, Howes PS, et al. Decreased cancer risk after iron reduction in patients with peripheral arterial disease: results from a randomized trial. *J Natl Cancer Inst.* 2008;100(14):996–1002.
963. Edgren G, Nyrén O, Melbye M. Cancer as a ferrotoxic disease: are we getting hard stainless evidence? *J Natl Cancer Inst.* 2008;100(14):976–7.
964. Corpet DE. Red meat and colon cancer: should we become vegetarians, or can we make meat safer? *Meat Sci.* 2011;89(3):310–6.
965. Farmer B, Larson BT, Fulgoni VL 3rd, Rainville AJ, Liepa GU. A vegetarian dietary pattern as a nutrient-dense approach to weight management: an analysis of the National Health and Nutrition Examination Survey 1999–2004. *J Am Diet Assoc.* 2011;111(6):819–27.
966. Iron deficiency—United States, 1999–2000. *MMWR Morb Mortal Wkly Rep.* 2002;51(40):897–9.

967. Munro MG. Heavy menstrual bleeding, iron deficiency, and iron deficiency anemia: framing the issue. *Int J Gynaecol Obstet.* 2023;162 Suppl 2:7–13.
968. Matteson KA, Rahn DD, Wheeler TL 2nd, et al. Nonsurgical management of heavy menstrual bleeding: a systematic review. *Obstet Gynecol.* 2013;121(3):632–43.
969. Stoffel NU, von Siebenthal HK, Moretti D, Zimmermann MB. Oral iron supplementation in iron-deficient women: how much and how often? *Mol Aspects Med.* 2020;75:100865.
970. Auerbach M, Macdougall IC, Rodgers GM, Deloughery T, Richards T. The iron revolution: keeping abreast of the developments in iron therapy. *Am J Hematol.* 2022;97(3):250–2.
971. Auerbach M, Macdougall IC, Rodgers GM, Deloughery T, Richards T. The iron revolution: keeping abreast of the developments in iron therapy. *Am J Hematol.* 2022;97(3):250–2.
972. Malesza IJ, Bartkowiak-Wieczorek J, Winkler-Galicki J, et al. The dark side of iron: the relationship between iron, inflammation and gut microbiota in selected diseases associated with iron deficiency anaemia—a narrative review. *Nutrients.* 2022;14(17):3478.
973. Skolmowska D, Głąbska D, Kołota A, Guzek D. Effectiveness of dietary interventions to treat iron-deficiency anemia in women: a systematic review of randomized controlled trials. *Nutrients.* 2022;14(13):2724.
974. Skolmowska D, Głąbska D, Kołota A, Guzek D. Effectiveness of dietary interventions to treat iron-deficiency anemia in women: a systematic review of randomized controlled trials. *Nutrients.* 2022;14(13):2724.
975. Łuszczki E, Boakye F, Zielińska M, et al. Vegan diet: nutritional components, implementation, and effects on adults' health. *Front Nutr.* 2023;10:1294497. Erratum in: *Front Nutr.* 2024;10:1354336.
976. Armah SM, Carriquiry A, Sullivan D, Cook JD, Reddy MB. A complete diet-based algorithm for predicting nonheme iron absorption in adults. *J Nutr.* 2013;143(7):1136–40.
977. Survival rates for pancreatic cancer. American Cancer Society. https://www.cancer.org/cancer/types/pancreatic-cancer/detection-diagnosis-staging/survival-rates.html. January 16, 2025. Accessed January 23, 2025.
978. U.S. Cancer Statistics Working Group. U.S. Cancer Statistics Data Visualizations Tool. U.S. Department of Health and Human Services, Centers for Disease Control and Prevention and National Cancer Institute. https://www.cdc.gov/cancer/dataviz. June 2024. Accessed January 18, 2025.
979. Iodice S, Gandini S, Maisonneuve P, Lowenfels AB. Tobacco and the risk of pancreatic cancer: a review and meta-analysis. *Langenbecks Arch Surg.* 2008;393(4):535–45.
980. Kolodecik T, Shugrue C, Ashat M, Thrower EC. Risk factors for pancreatic cancer: underlying mechanisms and potential targets. *Front Physiol.* 2013;4:415.
981. Thiébaut AC, Jiao L, Silverman DT, et al. Dietary fatty acids and pancreatic cancer in the NIH-AARP Diet and Health Study. *J Natl Cancer Inst.* 2009;101(14):1001–11.
982. Landrigan PJ. Preface. *Ann N Y Acad Sci.* 1991;643:xv–xvi.
983. Weiner R, Rees D, Lunga FJ, Felix MA. Third wave of asbestos-related disease from secondary use of asbestos. A case report from industry. *S Afr Med J.* 1994;84(3):158–60.
984. Johnson ES, Zhou Y, Lillian Yau C, et al. Mortality from malignant diseases—update of the Baltimore union poultry cohort. *Cancer Causes Control.* 2010;21(2):215–21.
985. Felini M, Johnson E, Preacely N, Sarda V, Ndetan H, Bangara S. A pilot case-cohort study of liver and pancreatic cancers in poultry workers. *Ann Epidemiol.* 2011;21(10):755–66.
986. Lynch SM, Vrieling A, Lubin JH, et al. Cigarette smoking and pancreatic cancer: a pooled analysis from the pancreatic cancer cohort consortium. *Am J Epidemiol.* 2009;170(4):403–13.
987. Rohrmann S, Linseisen J, Nöthlings U, et al. Meat and fish consumption and risk of pancreatic cancer: results from the European Prospective Investigation into Cancer and Nutrition. *Int J Cancer.* 2013;132(3):617–24.
988. Rohrmann S, Linseisen J, Jakobsen MU, et al. Consumption of meat and dairy and lymphoma risk in the European Prospective Investigation into Cancer and Nutrition. *Int J Cancer.* 2011;128(3):623–34.

989. Gao Y, Ma Y, Yu M, et al. Poultry and fish intake and pancreatic cancer risk: a systematic review and meta-analysis. *Nutr Cancer.* 2022;74(1):55–67.
990. Lotti M, Bergamo L, Murer B. Occupational toxicology of asbestos-related malignancies. *Clin Toxicol* (Phila). 2010;48(6):485–96.
991. Marvisi M, Balzarini L, Mancini C, Mouzakiti P. A new type of hypersensitivity pneumonitis: salami brusher's disease. *Monaldi Arch Chest Dis.* 2012;77(1):35–7.
992. Yang ZY, Yuan JQ, Di MY, et al. Gemcitabine plus erlotinib for advanced pancreatic cancer: a systematic review with meta-analysis. *PLoS ONE.* 2013;8(3):e57528.
993. Li L, Aggarwal BB, Shishodia S, Abbruzzese J, Kurzrock R. Nuclear factor-kappaB and IkappaB kinase are constitutively active in human pancreatic cells, and their down-regulation by curcumin (diferuloylmethane) is associated with the suppression of proliferation and the induction of apoptosis. *Cancer.* 2004;101(10):2351–62.
994. Dhillon N, Aggarwal BB, Newman RA, et al. Phase II trial of curcumin in patients with advanced pancreatic cancer. *Clin Cancer Res.* 2008;14(14):4491–9.
995. Dhillon N, Aggarwal BB, Newman RA, et al. Phase II trial of curcumin in patients with advanced pancreatic cancer. *Clin Cancer Res.* 2008;14(14):4491–9.
996. Bosetti C, Bravi F, Turati F, et al. Nutrient-based dietary patterns and pancreatic cancer risk. *Ann Epidemiol.* 2013;23(3):124–8.
997. Mills PK, Beeson WL, Abbey DE, Fraser GE, Phillips RL. Dietary habits and past medical history as related to fatal pancreas cancer risk among Adventists. *Cancer.* 1988;61(12):2578–85.
998. Ren HG, Luu HN, Liu Y, Wang DW, Guo X. High intake of cruciferous vegetables reduces the risk of gastrointestinal cancers: results from observational studies. *Crit Rev Food Sci Nutr.* 2024;64(23):8493–9.
999. U.S. Cancer Statistics Working Group. U.S. Cancer Statistics Data Visualizations Tool. U.S. Department of Health and Human Services, Centers for Disease Control and Prevention and National Cancer Institute. https://www.cdc.gov/cancer/dataviz. June 2024. Accessed January 18, 2025.
1000. Bagnardi V, Rota M, Botteri E, et al. Light alcohol drinking and cancer: a meta-analysis. *Ann Oncol.* 2013;24(2):301–8.
1001. Wang SM, Katki HA, Graubard BI, et al. Population attributable risks of subtypes of esophageal and gastric cancers in the United States. *Am J Gastroenterol.* 2021;116(9):1844–52.
1002. Rubenstein JH, Chen JW. Epidemiology of gastroesophageal reflux disease. *Gastroenterol Clin North Am.* 2014;43(1):1–14.
1003. Lagergren J, Bergström R, Lindgren A, Nyrén O. Symptomatic gastroesophageal reflux as a risk factor for esophageal adenocarcinoma. *N Engl J Med.* 1999;340(11):825–31.
1004. Rodriguez GM, DePuy D, Aljehani M, et al. Trends in epidemiology of esophageal cancer in the US, 1975–2018. *JAMA Netw Open.* 2023;6(8):e2329497.
1005. Parasa S, Sharma P. Complications of gastro-oesophageal reflux disease. *Best Pract Res Clin Gastroenterol.* 2013;27(3):433–42.
1006. El-Serag HB. Time trends of gastroesophageal reflux disease: a systematic review. *Clin Gastroenterol Hepatol.* 2007;5(1):17–26.
1007. De Ceglie A, Fisher DA, Filiberti R, Blanchi S, Conio M. Barrett's esophagus, esophageal and esophagogastric junction adenocarcinomas: the role of diet. *Clin Res Hepatol Gastroenterol.* 2011;35(1):7–16.
1008. Navarro Silvera SA, Mayne ST, Risch H, et al. Food group intake and risk of subtypes of esophageal and gastric cancer. *Int J Cancer.* 2008;123(4):852–60.
1009. Nebel OT, Castell DO. Lower esophageal sphincter pressure changes after food ingestion. *Gastroenterology.* 1972;63(5):778–83.
1010. Becker DJ, Sinclair J, Castell DO, Wu WC. A comparison of high and low fat meals on postprandial esophageal acid exposure. *Am J Gastroenterol.* 1989;84(7):782–6.
1011. Charlton KE, Tapsell LC, Batterham MJ, et al. Pork, beef and chicken have similar effects on acute satiety and hormonal markers of appetite. *Appetite.* 2011;56(1):1–8.

1012. Mitsukawa T, Takemura J, Ohgo S, et al. Gallbladder function and plasma cholecystokinin levels in diabetes mellitus. *Am J Gastroenterol*. 1990;85(8):981–5.
1013. Matsuki N, Fujita T, Watanabe N, et al. Lifestyle factors associated with gastroesophageal reflux disease in the Japanese population. *J Gastroenterol*. 2013;48(3):340–9.
1014. Jung JG, Kang HW, Hahn SJ, et al. Vegetarianism as a protective factor for reflux esophagitis: a retrospective, cross-sectional study between Buddhist priests and general population. *Dig Dis Sci*. 2013;58(8):2244–52.
1015. Fashner J, Gitu AC. Common gastrointestinal symptoms: risks of long-term proton pump inhibitor therapy. *FP Essent*. 2013;413:29–39.
1016. Terry P, Lagergren J, Ye W, Nyrén O, Wolk A. Antioxidants and cancers of the esophagus and gastric cardia. *Int J Cancer*. 2000;87(5):750–4.
1017. Ekström AM, Serafini M, Nyrén O, Hansson LE, Ye W, Wolk A. Dietary antioxidant intake and the risk of cardia cancer and noncardia cancer of the intestinal and diffuse types: a population-based case-control study in Sweden. *Int J Cancer*. 2000;87(1):133–40.
1018. Luo H, Fan Q, Xiao S, Chen K. Changes in proton pump inhibitor prescribing trend over the past decade and pharmacists' effect on prescribing practice at a tertiary hospital. *BMC Health Serv Res*. 2018;18(1):537.
1019. Savarino E, Marabotto E, Zentilin P, et al. A safety review of proton pump inhibitors to treat acid-related digestive diseases. *Expert Opin Drug Saf*. 2018;17(8):785–94.
1020. Ayoub J, White ND. GERD management: the case for lifestyle in an era of PPIs. *Am J Lifestyle Med*. 2017;11(1):24–8.
1021. Poly TN, Islam MM, Yang HC, Wu CC, Li YCJ. Proton pump inhibitors and risk of hip fracture: a meta-analysis of observational studies. *Osteoporos Int*. 2019;30(1):103–14.
1022. Safer DJ. Overprescribed medications for US adults: four major examples. *J Clin Med Res*. 2019;11(9):617–22.
1023. Abrahami D, McDonald EG, Schnitzer M, Azoulay L. Trends in prescribing patterns of proton pump inhibitors surrounding new guidelines. *Ann Epidemiol*. 2021;55:24–6.
1024. Sheikh I, Waghray A, Waghray N, Dong C, Wolfe MM. Consumer use of over-the-counter proton pump inhibitors in patients with gastroesophageal reflux disease. *Am J Gastroenterol*. 2014;109(6):789–94.
1025. Safer DJ. Overprescribed medications for US adults: four major examples. *J Clin Med Res*. 2019;11(9):617–22.
1026. Reimer C, Søndergaard B, Hilsted L, Bytzer P. Proton-pump inhibitor therapy induces acid-related symptoms in healthy volunteers after withdrawal of therapy. *Gastroenterology*. 2009;137(1):80–7,87.e1.
1027. Xun X, Yin Q, Fu Y, He X, Dong Z. Proton pump inhibitors and the risk of community-acquired pneumonia: an updated meta-analysis. *Ann Pharmacother*. 2022;56(5):524–32.
1028. Moayyedi P, Lewis MA. Proton pump inhibitors and dementia: deciphering the data. *Am J Gastroenterol*. 2017;112(12):1809–11.
1029. Vengrus CS, Delfino VD, Bignardi PR. Proton pump inhibitors use and risk of chronic kidney disease and end-stage renal disease. *Minerva Urol Nephrol*. 2021;73(4):462–70.
1030. D'Silva KM, Mehta R, Mitchell M, et al. Proton pump inhibitor use and risk for recurrent *Clostridioides difficile* infection: a systematic review and meta-analysis. *Clin Microbiol Infect*. 2021;27(5):697–703.
1031. Salvo EM, Ferko NC, Cash SB, Gonzalez A, Kahrilas PJ. Umbrella review of 42 systematic reviews with meta-analyses: the safety of proton pump inhibitors. *Aliment Pharmacol Ther*. 2021;54(2):129–43.
1032. Sun S, Cui Z, Zhou M, et al. Proton pump inhibitor monotherapy and the risk of cardiovascular events in patients with gastro-esophageal reflux disease: a meta-analysis. *Neurogastroenterol Motil*. 2017;29(2):e12926.
1033. Perry TW. Abrupt-onset, profound erectile dysfunction in a healthy young man after initiating over-the-counter omeprazole: a case report. *J Med Case Reports*. 2021;15(1):360.

1034. Ben-Eltriki M, Green CJ, Maclure M, Musini V, Bassett KL, Wright JM. Do proton pump inhibitors increase mortality? A systematic review and in-depth analysis of the evidence. *Pharmacol Res Perspect*. 2020;8(5):e00651.
1035. Poly TN, Islam MM, Yang HC, Wu CC, Li YCJ. Proton pump inhibitors and risk of hip fracture: a meta-analysis of observational studies. *Osteoporos Int*. 2019;30(1):103–14.
1036. Ren D, Gurney E, Hornecker JR. Appropriate use and stewardship of proton-pump inhibitors. *US Pharm*. 2019.44(22):25–31.
1037. Nilsson M, Johnsen R, Ye W, Hveem K, Lagergren J. Lifestyle related risk factors in the aetiology of gastro-oesophageal reflux. *Gut*. 2004;53(12):1730–5.
1038. Coleman HG, Murray LJ, Hicks B, et al. Dietary fiber and the risk of precancerous lesions and cancer of the esophagus: a systematic review and meta-analysis. *Nutr Rev*. 2013;71(7):474–82.
1039. Burkitt DP. Hiatus hernia: is it preventable? *Am J Clin Nutr*. 1981;34(3):428–31.
1040. Burkitt DP, James PA. Low-residue diets and hiatus hernia. *Lancet*. 1973;2(7821):128–30.
1041. Burkitt DP, James PA. Low-residue diets and hiatus hernia. *Lancet*. 1973;2(7821):128–30.
1042. Burkitt DP. Two blind spots in medical knowledge. *Nurs Times*. 1976;72(1):24–7.
1043. Burkitt DP. Hiatus hernia: is it preventable? *Am J Clin Nutr*. 1981;34(3):428–31.
1044. Survival rates for esophageal cancer. American Cancer Society. https://www.cancer.org/cancer/types/pancreatic-cancer/detection-diagnosis-staging/survival-rates.html. January 16, 2025. Accessed January 23, 2025.
1045. SEER*Explorer. Surveillance Research Program, National Cancer Institute. https://seer.cancer.gov/statistics-network/explorer/. November 5, 2024. Accessed January 23, 2025.
1046. Chen T, Yan F, Qian J, et al. Randomized phase II trial of lyophilized strawberries in patients with dysplastic precancerous lesions of the esophagus. *Cancer Prev Res* (Phila). 2012;5(1):41–50.
1047. Chen T, Yan F, Qian J, et al. Randomized phase II trial of lyophilized strawberries in patients with dysplastic precancerous lesions of the esophagus. *Cancer Prev Res* (Phila). 2012;5(1):41–50.
1048. Eaton SB, Konner M, Shostak M. Stone agers in the fast lane: chronic degenerative diseases in evolutionary perspective. *Am J Med*. 1988;84(4):739–49.
1049. King DE, Mainous AG, Lambourne CA. Trends in dietary fiber intake in the United States, 1999–2008. *J Acad Nutr Diet*. 2012;112(5):642–8.
1050. Zhang N, Huang C, Ou S. In vitro binding capacities of three dietary fibers and their mixture for four toxic elements, cholesterol, and bile acid. *J Hazard Mater*. 2011;186(1):236–9.
1051. United States Department of Agriculture, Agricultural Research Service. Usual nutrient intake from food and beverages, by gender and age, What We Eat in America, NHANES 2017–March 2020 prepandemic. www.ars.usda.gov/nea/bhnrc/fsrg. 2023. Accessed January 20, 2025.
1052. Matthews DR, Matthews PC. Banting Memorial Lecture 2010. Type 2 diabetes as an 'infectious' disease: is this the Black Death of the 21st century? *Diabet Med*. 2011;28(1):2–9.
1053. Centers for Disease Control and Prevention. A report card: diabetes in the United States. https://www.cdc.gov/diabetes/communication-resources/diabetes-statistics.html. May 15, 2024. Accessed January 26, 2025.
1054. Boyle JP, Thompson TJ, Gregg EW, Barker LE, Williamson DF. Projection of the year 2050 burden of diabetes in the US adult population: dynamic modeling of incidence, mortality, and prediabetes prevalence. *Popul Health Metr*. 2010;8:29.
1055. Centers for Disease Control and Prevention. National diabetes statistics report. https://www.cdc.gov/diabetes/php/data-research/index.html. May 15, 2024. Accessed January 26, 2025.
1056. Centers for Disease Control and Prevention. National diabetes statistics report. https://www.cdc.gov/diabetes/php/data-research/index.html. May 15, 2024. Accessed January 26, 2025.
1057. Lempainen J, Tauriainen S, Vaarala O, et al. Interaction of enterovirus infection and cow's

milk-based formula nutrition in type 1 diabetes-associated autoimmunity. *Diabetes Metab Res Rev.* 2012;28(2):177–85.
1058. U.S. Centers for Disease Control and Prevention. National diabetes statistics report. https://www.cdc.gov/diabetes/php/data-research/index.html. May 15, 2024. Accessed January 26, 2025.
1059. Rachek LI. Free fatty acids and skeletal muscle insulin resistance. *Prog Mol Biol Transl Sci.* 2014;121:267–92.
1060. Sweeney JS. Dietary factors that influence the dextrose tolerance test. *Arch Intern Med.* 1927;40(6):818–30.
1061. Roden M, Price TB, Perseghin G, et al. Mechanism of free fatty acid-induced insulin resistance in humans. *J Clin Invest.* 1996;97(12):2859–65.
1062. Roden M, Krssak M, Stingl H, et al. Rapid impairment of skeletal muscle glucose transport/phosphorylation by free fatty acids in humans. *Diabetes.* 1999;48(2):358–64.
1063. Santomauro AT, Boden G, Silva ME, et al. Overnight lowering of free fatty acids with Acipimox improves insulin resistance and glucose tolerance in obese diabetic and nondiabetic subjects. *Diabetes.* 1999;48(9):1836–41.
1064. Krssak M, Falk Petersen K, Dresner A, et al. Intramyocellular lipid concentrations are correlated with insulin sensitivity in humans: a ^{1}H NMR spectroscopy study. *Diabetologia.* 1999;42(1):113–6.
1065. Lee S, Boesch C, Kuk JL, Arslanian S. Effects of an overnight intravenous lipid infusion on intramyocellular lipid content and insulin sensitivity in African-American versus Caucasian adolescents. *Metab Clin Exp.* 2013;62(3):417–23.
1066. Roden M, Krssak M, Stingl H, et al. Rapid impairment of skeletal muscle glucose transport/phosphorylation by free fatty acids in humans. *Diabetes.* 1999;48(2):358–64.
1067. Himsworth HP. Dietetic factors influencing the glucose tolerance and the activity of insulin. *J Physiol* (Lond). 1934;81(1):29–48.
1068. Tabák AG1, Herder C, Rathmann W, Brunner EJ, Kivimäki M. Prediabetes: a high-risk state for diabetes. *Lancet.* 2012;379(9833):2279–90.
1069. Pratley RE. The early treatment of type 2 diabetes. *Am J Med.* 2013;126(9 Suppl 1):S2–9.
1070. Reinehr T. Type 2 diabetes mellitus in children and adolescents. *World J Diabetes.* 2013;4(6):270–81.
1071. Sawatsky L, Halipchuk J, Wicklow B. Type 2 diabetes in a four-year-old child. *CMAJ.* 2017;189(26):E888–90.
1072. Dean H, Flett B. Natural history of type 2 diabetes diagnosed in childhood: long term follow-up in young adult years. *Diabetes.* 2002;51(s1):A24.
1073. Hannon TS, Rao G, Arslanian SA. Childhood obesity and type 2 diabetes mellitus. *Pediatrics.* 2005;116(2):473–80.
1074. U.S. Centers for Disease Control and Prevention. Childhood obesity facts. https://www.cdc.gov/obesity/childhood-obesity-facts/childhood-obesity-facts.html. April 2, 2024. Accessed January 26, 2025.
1075. Lifshitz F. Obesity in children. *J Clin Res Pediatr Endocrinol.* 2008;1(2):53–60.
1076. Must A, Jacques PF, Dallal GE, Bajema CJ, Dietz WH. Long-term morbidity and mortality of overweight adolescents. A follow-up of the Harvard Growth Study of 1922 to 1935. *N Engl J Med.* 1992;327(19):1350–5.
1077. Sabaté J, Wien M. Vegetarian diets and childhood obesity prevention. *Am J Clin Nutr.* 2010;91(5):1525S–9S.
1078. Tonstad S, Butler T, Yan R, Fraser GE. Type of vegetarian diet, body weight, and prevalence of type 2 diabetes. *Diabetes Care.* 2009;32(5):791–6.
1079. Sabaté J, Lindsted KD, Harris RD, Sanchez A. Attained height of lacto-ovo vegetarian children and adolescents. *Eur J Clin Nutr.* 1991;45(1):51–8.
1080. Sabaté J, Wien M. Vegetarian diets and childhood obesity prevention. *Am J Clin Nutr.* 2010;91(5):1525S–9S.

1081. Cali AM, Caprio S. Prediabetes and type 2 diabetes in youth: an emerging epidemic disease? *Curr Opin Endocrinol Diabetes Obes.* 2008;15(2):123–7.
1082. Puhl R, Brownell KD. Bias, discrimination, and obesity. *Obes Res.* 2001;9(12):788–805.
1083. Seacat JD, Dougal SC, Roy D. A daily diary assessment of female weight stigmatization. *J Health Psychol.* 2016;21(2):228–40.
1084. Puhl RM, Andreyeva T, Brownell KD. Perceptions of weight discrimination: prevalence and comparison to race and gender discrimination in America. *Int J Obes* (Lond). 2008;32(6):992–1000.
1085. Cramer P, Steinwert T. Thin is good, fat is bad: how early does it begin? *J Appl Dev Psychol.* 1998;19(3):429–51.
1086. Richardson S, Goodman N, Hastorf A, Dornbusch S. Cultural uniformity in reaction to physical disabilities. *Am Sociol Rev.* 1961;26(2):241.
1087. Latner JD, Stunkard AJ. Getting worse: the stigmatization of obese children. *Obes Res.* 2003;11(3):452–6.
1088. Andreyeva T, Puhl RM, Brownell KD. Changes in perceived weight discrimination among Americans, 1995–1996 through 2004–2006. *Obesity* (Silver Spring). 2008;16(5):1129–34.
1089. Neumark-Sztainer D, Story M, Harris T. Beliefs and attitudes about obesity among teachers and school health care providers working with adolescents. *J Nutr Educ Behav.* 1999;31(1):3–9.
1090. Crandall C. Do parents discriminate against their heavyweight daughters? *Pers Soc Psychol Bull.* 1995;21(7):724–35.
1091. Puhl R, Brownell KD. Bias, discrimination, and obesity. *Obes Res.* 2001;9(12):788–805.
1092. Foster GD, Wadden TA, Makris AP, et al. Primary care physicians' attitudes about obesity and its treatment. *Obes Res.* 2003;11(10):1168–77.
1093. Bagley CR, Conklin DN, Isherwood RT, Pechiulis DR, Watson LA. Attitudes of nurses toward obesity and obese patients. *Percept Mot Skills.* 1989;68(3 Pt 1):954.
1094. Poorolajal J, Jenabi E. The association between BMI and cervical cancer risk: a meta-analysis. *Eur J Cancer Prev.* 2016;25(3):232–8.
1095. Adams CH, Smith NJ, Wilbur DC, Grady KE. The relationship of obesity to the frequency of pelvic examinations: do physician and patient attitudes make a difference? *Women Health.* 1993;20(2):45–57.
1096. Hernandez-Boussard T, Ahmed SM, Morton JM. Obesity disparities in preventive care: findings from the National Ambulatory Medical Care Survey, 2005–2007. *Obesity* (Silver Spring). 2012;20(8):1639–44.
1097. LaMendola B. Overweight women: some ob-gyns in South Florida turn away overweight women. *Sun Sentinel.* Published May 16, 2011. Available at: http://articles.sun-sentinel.com/2011-05-16/health/fl-hk-no-obesity-doc-20110516_1_gyn-ob-gyn-obese-patients. Accessed April 17, 2019.
1098. Hebl MR, Xu J. Weighing the care: physicians' reactions to the size of a patient. *Int J Obes Relat Metab Disord.* 2001;25(8):1246–52.
1099. Gudzune KA, Beach MC, Roter DL, Cooper LA. Physicians build less rapport with obese patients. *Obesity* (Silver Spring). 2013;21(10):2146–52.
1100. Gudzune KA, Huizinga MM, Beach MC, Cooper LA. Obese patients overestimate physicians' attitudes of respect. *Patient Educ Couns.* 2012;88(1):23–8.
1101. Ginter E, Simko V. Type 2 diabetes mellitus, pandemic in 21st century. *Adv Exp Med Biol.* 2012;771:42–50.
1102. Spalding KL, Arner E, Westermark PO, et al. Dynamics of fat cell turnover in humans. *Nature.* 2008;453(7196):783–7.
1103. Roden M. How free fatty acids inhibit glucose utilization in human skeletal muscle. *News Physiol Sci.* 2004;19:92–6.
1104. Fraser GE. Vegetarian diets: what do we know of their effects on common chronic diseases? *Am J Clin Nutr.* 2009;89(5):1607S–12S.

1105. Tonstad S, Stewart K, Oda K, Batech M, Herring RP, Fraser GE. Vegetarian diets and incidence of diabetes in the Adventist Health Study-2. *Nutr Metab Cardiovasc Dis.* 2013;23(4): 292–9.
1106. Nolan CJ, Larter CZ. Lipotoxicity: why do saturated fatty acids cause and monounsaturates protect against it? *J Gastroenterol Hepatol.* 2009;24(5):703–6.
1107. Evans WJ. Oxygen-carrying proteins in meat and risk of diabetes mellitus. *JAMA Intern Med.* 2013;173(14):1335–6.
1108. Egnatchik RA, Leamy AK, Jacobson DA, Shiota M, Young JD. ER calcium release promotes mitochondrial dysfunction and hepatic cell lipotoxicity in response to palmitate overload. *Mol Metab.* 2014;3(5):544–53.
1109. Estadella D, da Penha Oller do Nascimento CM, Oyama LM, Ribeiro EB, Dâmaso AR, de Piano A. Lipotoxicity: effects of dietary saturated and transfatty acids. *Mediators Inflamm.* 2013;2013:137579.
1110. Perseghin G, Scifo P, De Cobelli F, et al. Intramyocellular triglyceride content is a determinant of in vivo insulin resistance in humans: a 1H-13C nuclear magnetic resonance spectroscopy assessment in offspring of type 2 diabetic parents. *Diabetes.* 1999;48(8):1600–6.
1111. Nolan CJ, Larter CZ. Lipotoxicity: why do saturated fatty acids cause and monounsaturates protect against it? *J Gastroenterol Hepatol.* 2009;24(5):703–6.
1112. Goff LM, Bell JD, So PW, Dornhorst A, Frost GS. Veganism and its relationship with insulin resistance and intramyocellular lipid. *Eur J Clin Nutr.* 2005;59(2):291–8.
1113. Gojda J, Patková J, Jaček M, et al. Higher insulin sensitivity in vegans is not associated with higher mitochondrial density. *Eur J Clin Nutr.* 2013;67(12):1310–5.
1114. Goff LM, Bell JD, So PW, Dornhorst A, Frost GS. Veganism and its relationship with insulin resistance and intramyocellular lipid. *Eur J Clin Nutr.* 2005;59(2):291–8.
1115. Papanikolaou Y, Fulgoni VL. Bean consumption is associated with greater nutrient intake, reduced systolic blood pressure, lower body weight, and a smaller waist circumference in adults: results from the National Health and Nutrition Examination Survey 1999–2002. *J Am Coll Nutr.* 2008;27(5):569–76.
1116. Mollard RC, Luhovyy BL, Panahi S, Nunez M, Hanley A, Anderson GH. Regular consumption of pulses for 8 weeks reduces metabolic syndrome risk factors in overweight and obese adults. *Br J Nutr.* 2012;108 Suppl 1:S111–22.
1117. Cnop M, Hughes SJ, Igoillo-Esteve M, et al. The long lifespan and low turnover of human islet beta cells estimated by mathematical modelling of lipofuscin accumulation. *Diabetologia.* 2010;53(2):321–30.
1118. Taylor R. Banting Memorial lecture 2012: reversing the twin cycles of type 2 diabetes. *Diabet Med.* 2013;30(3):267–75.
1119. Cunha DA, Igoillo-Esteve M, Gurzov EN, et al. Death protein 5 and p53-upregulated modulator of apoptosis mediate the endoplasmic reticulum stress-mitochondrial dialog triggering lipotoxic rodent and human β-cell apoptosis. *Diabetes.* 2012;61(11):2763–75.
1120. Cnop M, Hannaert JC, Grupping AY, Pipeleers DG. Low density lipoprotein can cause death of islet beta-cells by its cellular uptake and oxidative modification. *Endocrinology.* 2002;143(9):3449–53.
1121. Maedler K, Oberholzer J, Bucher P, Spinas GA, Donath MY. Monounsaturated fatty acids prevent the deleterious effects of palmitate and high glucose on human pancreatic beta-cell turnover and function. *Diabetes.* 2003;52(3):726–33.
1122. Xiao C, Giacca A, Carpentier A, Lewis GF. Differential effects of monounsaturated, polyunsaturated and saturated fat ingestion on glucose-stimulated insulin secretion, sensitivity and clearance in overweight and obese, non-diabetic humans. *Diabetologia.* 2006;49(6):1371–9.
1123. Wang L, Folsom AR, Zheng ZJ, Pankow JS, Eckfeldt JH. Plasma fatty acid composition and incidence of diabetes in middle-aged adults: the Atherosclerosis Risk in Communities (ARIC) Study. *Am J Clin Nutr.* 2003;78(1):91–8.
1124. Cunha DA, Igoillo-Esteve M, Gurzov EN, et al. Death protein 5 and p53-upregulated modu-

lator of apoptosis mediate the endoplasmic reticulum stress-mitochondrial dialog triggering lipotoxic rodent and human β-cell apoptosis. *Diabetes.* 2012;61(11):2763–75.
1125. Welch RW. Satiety: have we neglected dietary non-nutrients? *Proc Nutr Soc.* 2011;70(2):145–54.
1126. Wright N, Wilson L, Smith M, Duncan B, McHugh P. The BROAD study: a randomised controlled trial using a whole food plant-based diet in the community for obesity, ischaemic heart disease or diabetes. *Nutr Diabetes.* 2017;7(3):e256.
1127. Trapp CB, Barnard ND. Usefulness of vegetarian and vegan diets for treating type 2 diabetes. *Curr Diab Rep.* 2010;10(2):152–8.
1128. Pratley RE. The early treatment of type 2 diabetes. *Am J Med.* 2013;126(9 Suppl 1):S2–9.
1129. Juutilainen A, Lehto S, Rönnemaa T, Pyörälä K, Laakso M. Type 2 diabetes as a "coronary heart disease equivalent": an 18-year prospective population-based study in Finnish subjects. *Diabetes Care.* 2005;28(12):2901–7.
1130. Kahleova H, Matoulek M, Malinska H, et al. Vegetarian diet improves insulin resistance and oxidative stress markers more than conventional diet in subjects with type 2 diabetes. *Diabet Med.* 2011;28(5):549–59.
1131. Ornish D. Statins and the soul of medicine. *Am J Cardiol.* 2002;89(11):1286–90.
1132. Kahleova H, Hrachovinova T, Hill M, et al. Vegetarian diet in type 2 diabetes—improvement in quality of life, mood and eating behaviour. *Diabet Med.* 2013;30(1):127–9.
1133. Chiu THT, Huang HY, Chiu YF, et al. Taiwanese vegetarians and omnivores: dietary composition, prevalence of diabetes and IFG. *PLoS One.* 2014;9(2):e88547.
1134. Chiu THT, Huang HY, Chiu YF, et al. Taiwanese vegetarians and omnivores: dietary composition, prevalence of diabetes and IFG. *PLoS One.* 2014;9(2):e88547.
1135. Magliano DJ, Loh VHY, Harding JL, et al. Persistent organic pollutants and diabetes: a review of the epidemiological evidence. *Diabetes Metab.* 2014;40(1):1–14.
1136. Lee DH, Lee IK, Song K, et al. A strong dose-response relation between serum concentrations of persistent organic pollutants and diabetes: results from the National Health and Examination Survey 1999–2002. *Diabetes Care.* 2006;29(7):1638–44.
1137. Wu H, Bertrand KA, Choi AL, et al. Persistent organic pollutants and type 2 diabetes: a prospective analysis in the Nurses' Health Study and meta-analysis. *Environ Health Perspect.* 2013;121(2):153–61.
1138. Schecter A, Colacino J, Haffner D, et al. Perfluorinated compounds, polychlorinated biphenyls, and organochlorine pesticide contamination in composite food samples from Dallas, Texas, USA. *Environ Health Perspect.* 2010;118(6):796–802.
1139. Crinnion WJ. The role of persistent organic pollutants in the worldwide epidemic of type 2 diabetes mellitus and the possible connection to farmed Atlantic salmon (Salmo salar). *Altern Med Rev.* 2011;16(4):301–13.
1140. Lee DH, Lee IK, Song K, et al. A strong dose-response relation between serum concentrations of persistent organic pollutants and diabetes: results from the National Health and Examination Survey 1999–2002. *Diabetes Care.* 2006;29(7):1638–44.
1141. Crinnion WJ. The role of persistent organic pollutants in the worldwide epidemic of type 2 diabetes mellitus and the possible connection to farmed Atlantic salmon (Salmo salar). *Altern Med Rev.* 2011;16(4):301–13.
1142. Farmer B, Larson BT, Fulgoni VL III, et al. A vegetarian dietary pattern as a nutrient-dense approach to weight management: an analysis of the National Health and Nutrition Examination Survey 1999–2004. *J Am Diet Assoc.* 2011;111(6):819–27.
1143. Farmer B, Larson BT, Fulgoni VL III, et al. A vegetarian dietary pattern as a nutrient-dense approach to weight management: an analysis of the National Health and Nutrition Examination Survey 1999–2004. *J Am Diet Assoc.* 2011;111(6):819–27.
1144. Toth MJ, Poehlman ET. Sympathetic nervous system activity and resting metabolic rate in vegetarians. *Metabolism.* 1994;43(5):621–5.
1145. Karlic H, Schuster D, Varga F, et al. Vegetarian diet affects genes of oxidative metabolism and collagen synthesis. *Ann Nutr Metab.* 2008;53(1):29–32.

1146. Vergnaud AC, Norat T, Romaguera D, et al. Meat consumption and prospective weight change in participants of the EPIC-PANACEA study. *Am J Clin Nutr.* 2010;92(2):398–407.
1147. The Action to Control Cardiovascular Risk in Diabetes Study Group, Gerstein HC, Miller ME, et al. Effects of intensive glucose lowering in type 2 diabetes. *N Engl J Med.* 2008;358(24):2545–59.
1148. The Action to Control Cardiovascular Risk in Diabetes Study Group, Gerstein HC, Miller ME, et al. Effects of intensive glucose lowering in type 2 diabetes. *N Engl J Med.* 2008;358(24):2545–59.
1149. Luan FL, Nguyen K. Intensive glucose control in type 2 diabetes. *N Engl J Med.* 2008;359(14):1519–20.
1150. Blagosklonny MV. Prospective treatment of age-related diseases by slowing down aging. *Am J Pathol.* 2012;181(4):1142–6.
1151. Madonna R, Pandolfi A, Massaro M, et al. Insulin enhances vascular cell adhesion molecule-1 expression in human cultured endothelial cells through a pro-atherogenic pathway mediated by p38 mitogen-activated protein-kinase. *Diabetologia.* 2004;47(3):532–6.
1152. Lingvay I, Guth E, Islam A, et al. Rapid improvement in diabetes after gastric bypass surgery: is it the diet or surgery? *Diabetes Care.* 2013;36(9):2741–7.
1153. Lingvay I, Guth E, Islam A, et al. Rapid improvement in diabetes after gastric bypass surgery: is it the diet or surgery? *Diabetes Care.* 2013;36(9):2741–7.
1154. Taylor R. Type 2 diabetes: etiology and reversibility. *Diabetes Care.* 2013;36(4):1047–55.
1155. Lim EL, Hollingsworth KG, Aribisala BS, Chen MJ, Mathers JC, Taylor R. Reversal of type 2 diabetes: normalisation of beta cell function in association with decreased pancreas and liver triacylglycerol. *Diabetologia.* 2011;54(10):2506–14.
1156. Taheri S, Tahrani A, Barnett A. Bariatric surgery: a cure for diabetes? *Pract Diabetes Int.* 2009;26:356–8.
1157. Vergnaud AC, Norat T, Romaguera D, et al. Meat consumption and prospective weight change in participants of the EPIC-PANACEA study. *Am J Clin Nutr.* 2010;92(2):398–407.
1158. Gilsing AM, Weijenberg MP, Hughes LA, et al. Longitudinal changes in BMI in older adults are associated with meat consumption differentially, by type of meat consumed. *J Nutr.* 2012;142(2):340–9.
1159. Wang Y, Lehane C, Ghebremeskel K, et al. Modern organic and broiler chickens sold for human consumption provide more energy from fat than protein. *Public Health Nutr.* 2010;13(3):400–8.
1160. National Cattlemen's Beef Association, Young MK, Redson BA. New USDA data show 29 beef cuts now meet government guidelines for lean. https://web.archive.org/web/20140617162653/http://www.beef.org/udocs/29leancuts.pdf. 2005. Accessed January 26, 2025.
1161. Steven S, Lim EL, Taylor R. Dietary reversal of type 2 diabetes motivated by research knowledge. *Diabet Med.* 2010;27(6):724–5.
1162. Taylor R. Pathogenesis of type 2 diabetes: tracing the reverse route from cure to cause. *Diabetologia.* 2008;51(10):1781–9.
1163. American Diabetes Association. Standards of medical care in diabetes—2015. *Diabetes Care.* 2015;38(suppl 1):S1–S93.
1164. Dunaief DM, Fuhrman J, Dunaief JL, et al. Glycemic and cardiovascular parameters improved in type 2 diabetes with the high nutrient density (HND) diet. *Open Journal of Preventive Medicine.* 2012;2(3):364–71.
1165. Lim EL, Hollingsworth KG, Aribisala BS, Chen MJ, Mathers JC, Taylor R. Reversal of type 2 diabetes: normalisation of beta cell function in association with decreased pancreas and liver triacylglycerol. *Diabetologia.* 2011;54(10):2506–14.
1166. Steven S, Lim EL, Taylor R. Population response to information on reversibility of type 2 diabetes. *Diabet Med.* 2013;30(4):e135–8.
1167. Dunaief DM, Fuhrman J, Dunaief JL, et al. Glycemic and cardiovascular parameters improved in type 2 diabetes with the high nutrient density (HND) diet. *Open J Prev Med.* 2012;2(3):364–71.

1168. Anderson JW, Ward K. High-carbohydrate, high-fiber diets for insulin-treated men with diabetes mellitus. *Am J Clin Nutr.* 1979;32(11):2312–21.
1169. Anderson JW, Ward K. High-carbohydrate, high-fiber diets for insulin-treated men with diabetes mellitus. *Am J Clin Nutr.* 1979;32(11):2312–21.
1170. Rosenfeld RM, Kelly JH, Agarwal M, et al. Dietary interventions to treat type 2 diabetes in adults with a goal of remission: an expert consensus statement from the American College of Lifestyle Medicine. *Am J Lifestyle Med.* 2022;16(3):342–62.
1171. Callaghan BC, Cheng H, Stables CL, et al. Diabetic neuropathy: clinical manifestations and current treatments. *Lancet Neurol.* 2012;11(6):521–34.
1172. Said G. Diabetic neuropathy—a review. *Nat Clin Pract Neurol.* 2007;3(6):331–40.
1173. Crane MG, Sample C. Regression of diabetic neuropathy with total vegetarian (vegan) diet. *J Nutr Med.* 1994;4(4):431–9.
1174. Crane MG, Sample C. Regression of diabetic neuropathy with total vegetarian (vegan) diet. *J Nutr Med.* 1994;4(4):431–9.
1175. Rabinowitch IM. Effects of the high carbohydrate-low calorie diet upon carbohydrate tolerance in diabetes mellitus. *Can Med Assoc J.* 1935;33(2):136–44.
1176. Newborg B, Kempner W. Analysis of 177 cases of hypertensive vascular disease with papilledema; one hundred twenty-six patients treated with rice diet. *Am J Med.* 1955;19(1):33–47.
1177. Crane MG, Sample C. Regression of diabetic neuropathy with total vegetarian (vegan) diet. *J Nutr Med.* 1994;4(4):431–9.
1178. Crane MG, Sample C. Regression of diabetic neuropathy with total vegetarian (vegan) diet. *J Nutr Med.* 1994;4(4):431–9.
1179. Crane MG, Sample C. Regression of diabetic neuropathy with total vegetarian (vegan) diet. *J Nutr Med.* 1994;4(4):431–9.
1180. Crane MG, Zielinski R, Aloia R. Cis and trans fats in omnivores, lacto-ovo vegetarians and vegans. *Am J Clin Nutr.* 1988;48:920.
1181. Tesfaye S, Chaturvedi N, Eaton SEM, et al. Vascular risk factors and diabetic neuropathy. *N Engl J Med.* 2005;352(4):341–50.
1182. Newrick PG, Wilson AJ, Jakubowski J, et al. Sural nerve oxygen tension in diabetes. *Br Med J (Clin Res Ed).* 1986;293(6554):1053–4.
1183. McCarty MF. Favorable impact of a vegan diet with exercise on hemorheology: implications for control of diabetic neuropathy. *Med Hypotheses.* 2002;58(6):476–86.
1184. Kempner W, Peschel RL, Schlayer C. Effect of rice diet on diabetes mellitus associated with vascular disease. *Postgrad Med.* 1958;24(4):359–71.
1185. McCarty MF. Favorable impact of a vegan diet with exercise on hemorheology: implications for control of diabetic neuropathy. *Med Hypotheses.* 2002;58(6):476–86.
1186. Browning LM, Hsieh SD, Ashwell M. A systematic review of waist-to-height ratio as a screening tool for the prediction of cardiovascular disease and diabetes: 0·5 could be a suitable global boundary value. *Nutr Res Rev.* 2010;23(2):247–69.
1187. Bigaard J, Tjønneland A, Thomsen BL, Overvad K, Heitmann BL, Sørensen TIA. Waist circumference, BMI, smoking, and mortality in middle-aged men and women. *Obes Res.* 2003;11(7):895–903.
1188. Bigaard J, Tjønneland A, Thomsen BL, Overvad K, Heitmann BL, Sørensen TIA. Waist circumference, BMI, smoking, and mortality in middle-aged men and women. *Obes Res.* 2003;11(7):895–903.
1189. Leitzmann MF, Moore SC, Koster A, et al. Waist circumference as compared with body-mass index in predicting mortality from specific causes. *PLoS One.* 2011;6(4):e18582.
1190. Browning LM, Hsieh SD, Ashwell M. A systematic review of waist-to-height ratio as a screening tool for the prediction of cardiovascular disease and diabetes: 0·5 could be a suitable global boundary value. *Nutr Res Rev.* 2010;23(2):247–69.
1191. U.S. Centers for Disease Control and Prevention. National diabetes statistics report. https:

//www.cdc.gov/diabetes/php/data-research/index.html. May 15, 2024. Accessed January 26, 2025.
1192. Nathan DM, Davidson MB, Defronzo RA, et al. Impaired fasting glucose and impaired glucose tolerance: implications for care. *Diabetes Care.* 2007;30(3):753–9.
1193. Karve A, Hayward RA. Prevalence, diagnosis, and treatment of impaired fasting glucose and impaired glucose tolerance in nondiabetic U.S. adults. *Diabetes Care.* 2010;33(11):2355–9.
1194. Cardona-Morrell M, Rychetnik L, Morrell SL, Espinel PT, Bauman A. Reduction of diabetes risk in routine clinical practice: are physical activity and nutrition interventions feasible and are the outcomes from reference trials replicable? A systematic review and meta-analysis. *BMC Public Health.* 2010;10:653.
1195. Holman H. Chronic disease—the need for a new clinical education. *JAMA.* 2004;292(9):1057–9.
1196. Institute of Medicine. *Crossing the Quality Chasm: A New Health System for the 21st Century.* Washington, D.C.: The National Academies Press; 2001:213.
1197. Chiras, DD. *Human Biology.* Burlington, MA: Jones & Bartlett Learning; 2015.
1198. U.S. Centers for Disease Control and Prevention, National Center for Health Statistics. National Vital Statistics System, Mortality 2018–2023 on CDC WONDER Online Database. http://wonder.cdc.gov/ucd-icd10-expanded.html. Accessed January 16, 2025.
1199. U.S. Cancer Statistics Working Group. U.S. Cancer Statistics Data Visualizations Tool. U.S. Department of Health and Human Services, Centers for Disease Control and Prevention and National Cancer Institute. https://www.cdc.gov/cancer/dataviz. June 2024. Accessed January 18, 2025.
1200. Abboud Y, Mathew AG, Meybodi MA, et al. Chronic liver disease and cirrhosis mortality rates are disproportionately increasing in younger women in the United States between 2000–2020. *Clin Gastroenterol Hepatol.* 2024;22(4):798–809.e28.
1201. Holubek WJ, Kalman S, Hoffman RS. Acetaminophen-induced acute liver failure: results of a United States multicenter, prospective study. *Hepatology.* 2006;43(4):880.
1202. Institute for Health Metrics and Evaluation (IHME). GBD 2021 cause and risk summary: high alcohol use—level 2 risk. University of Washington. https://www.healthdata.org/research-analysis/diseases-injuries-risks/factsheets/2021-high-alcohol-use-level-2-risk. Accessed December 7, 2024.
1203. Global status report on alcohol and health and treatment of substance use disorders. World Health Organization. https://iris.who.int/handle/10665/377960. 2024. Accessed December 23, 2024.
1204. Institute for Health Metrics and Evaluation (IHME). GBD 2021 cause and risk summary: drug use—level 2 risk. University of Washington. https://www.healthdata.org/research-analysis/diseases-injuries-risks/factsheets/2021-drug-use-level-2-risk. Accessed December 7, 2024.
1205. U.S. Centers for Disease Control and Prevention (CDC). Alcohol-attributable deaths and years of potential life lost—United States, 2001. *MMWR Morb Mortal Wkly Rep.* 2004;53(37):866–70.
1206. Martinez P, Kerr WC, Subbaraman MS, Roberts SCM. New estimates of the mean ethanol content of beer, wine, and spirits sold in the United States show a greater increase in per capita alcohol consumption than previous estimates. *Alcohol Clin Exp Res.* 2019;43(3):509–21.
1207. Editorial. Alcohol and health: time for an overdue conversation. *Lancet Gastroenterol Hepatol.* 2020;5(3):229.
1208. Esser MB, Sherk A, Subbaraman MS, et al. Improving estimates of alcohol-attributable deaths in the United States: impact of adjusting for the underreporting of alcohol consumption. *J Stud Alcohol Drugs.* 2022;83(1):134–44.
1209. Alcohol use and your health. Centers for Disease Control and Prevention. https://www.cdc.gov/alcohol/about-alcohol-use/index.html. January 14, 2025. Accessed January 29, 2025.
1210. Schwartz JM, Reinus JF. Prevalence and natural history of alcoholic liver disease. *Clin Liver Dis.* 2012;16(4):659–66.

1211. Lane BP, Lieber CS. Ultrastructural alterations in human hepatocytes following ingestion of ethanol with adequate diets. *Am J Pathol.* 1966;49(4):593–603.
1212. Mendenhall CL. Anabolic steroid therapy as an adjunct to diet in alcoholic hepatic steatosis. *Am J Dig Dis.* 1968;13(9):783–91.
1213. O'Shea RS, Dasarathy S, McCullough AJ. Alcoholic liver disease. *Hepatology.* 2010;51(1):307–28.
1214. Mandayam S, Jamal MM, Morgan TR. Epidemiology of alcoholic liver disease. *Semin Liver Dis.* 2004;24(3):217–32.
1215. Galambos JT. Natural history of alcoholic hepatitis. 3. Histological changes. *Gastroenterology.* 1972;63(6):1026–35.
1216. Woerle S, Roeber J, Landen MG. Prevalence of alcohol dependence among excessive drinkers in New Mexico. *Alcohol Clin Exp Res.* 2007;31(2):293–8.
1217. Kaskutas LA. Alcoholics Anonymous effectiveness: faith meets science. *J Addict Dis.* 2009;28(2):145–57.
1218. Xi B, Veeranki SP, Zhao M, Ma C, Yan Y, Mi J. Relationship of alcohol consumption to all-cause, cardiovascular, and cancer-related mortality in U.S. adults. *J Am Coll Cardiol.* 2017;70(8):913–22.
1219. Stockwell T, Zhao J. Alcohol's contribution to cancer is underestimated for exactly the same reason that its contribution to cardioprotection is overestimated. *Addiction.* 2017;112(2):230–2.
1220. Doll R, Peto R, Boreham J, Sutherland I. Mortality from cancer in relation to smoking: 50 years observations on British doctors. *Br J Cancer.* 2005;92(3):426–9.
1221. Stockwell T, Zhao J, Panwar S, Roemer A, Naimi T, Chikritzhs T. Do "moderate" drinkers have reduced mortality risk? A systematic review and meta-analysis of alcohol consumption and all-cause mortality. *J Stud Alcohol Drugs.* 2016;77(2):185–98.
1222. Burton R, Sheron N. No level of alcohol consumption improves health. *Lancet.* 2018;392(10152):987–8.
1223. Manolis TA, Manolis AA, Manolis AS. Cardiovascular effects of alcohol: a double-edged sword / how to remain at the nadir point of the J-curve? *Alcohol.* 2019;76:117–29.
1224. Arora M, ElSayed A, Beger B, et al. The impact of alcohol consumption on cardiovascular health: myths and measures. *Glob Heart.* 2022;17(1):45.
1225. Mukamal KJ. A safe level of alcohol consumption: the right answer demands the right question. *J Intern Med.* 2020;288(5):550–9.
1226. Griswold MG, Fullman N, Hawley C, et al. Alcohol use and burden for 195 countries and territories, 1990–2016: a systematic analysis for the Global Burden of Disease Study 2016. *Lancet.* 2018;392(10152):1015–35.
1227. Rinella ME, Sookoian S. From NAFLD to MASLD: updated naming and diagnosis criteria for fatty liver disease. *J Lipid Res.* 2024;65(1):100485.
1228. Kechagias S, Ernersson Å, Dahlqvist O, et al. Fast-food-based hyper-alimentation can induce rapid and profound elevation of serum alanine aminotransferase in healthy subjects. *Gut.* 2008;57(5):649–54.
1229. Le P, Tatar M, Dasarathy S, et al. Estimated burden of metabolic dysfunction–associated steatotic liver disease in US adults, 2020 to 2050. *JAMA Netw Open.* 2025;8(1):e2454707.
1230. Silverman JF, Pories WJ, Caro JF. Liver pathology in diabetes mellitus and morbid obesity: clinical, pathological and biochemical considerations. *Pathol Annu.* 1989;24:275–302.
1231. Singh S, Allen AM, Wang Z, Prokop LJ, Murad MH, Loomba R. Fibrosis progression in nonalcoholic fatty liver vs nonalcoholic steatohepatitis: a systematic review and meta-analysis of paired-biopsy studies. *Clin Gastroenterol Hepatol.* 2014;S1542–3565(14):00602–8.
1232. Zelber-Sagi S, Nitzan-Kaluski D, Goldsmith R, et al. Long term nutritional intake and the risk for non-alcoholic fatty liver disease (NAFLD): a population based study. *J Hepatol.* 2007;47(5):711–7.

1233. Zelber-Sagi S, Nitzan-Kaluski D, Goldsmith R, et al. Long term nutritional intake and the risk for non-alcoholic fatty liver disease (NAFLD): a population based study. *J Hepatol.* 2007;47(5):711–7.
1234. Longato L. Non-alcoholic fatty liver disease (NAFLD): a tale of fat and sugar? *Fibrogenesis Tissue Repair.* 2013;6(1):14.
1235. Musso G, Gambino R, De Michieli F, et al. Dietary habits and their relations to insulin resistance and postprandial lipemia in nonalcoholic steatohepatitis. *Hepatology.* 2003;37(4):909–16.
1236. Kontogianni MD, Tileli N, Margariti A, et al. Adherence to the Mediterranean diet is associated with the severity of non-alcoholic fatty liver disease. *Clin Nutr.* 2014;33(4):678–83.
1237. Kim EJ, Kim BH, Seo HS, et al. Cholesterol-induced non-alcoholic fatty liver disease and atherosclerosis aggravated by systemic inflammation. *PLoS ONE.* 2014;9(6):e97841.
1238. Yasutake K, Nakamuta M, Shima Y, et al. Nutritional investigation of non-obese patients with non-alcoholic fatty liver disease: the significance of dietary cholesterol. *Scand J Gastroenterol.* 2009;44(4):471–7.
1239. Duewell P, Kono H, Rayner KJ, et al. NLRP3 inflammasomes are required for atherogenesis and activated by cholesterol crystals that form early in disease. *Nature.* 2010;464(7293):1357–61.
1240. Ioannou GN, Haigh WG, Thorning D, Savard C. Hepatic cholesterol crystals and crown-like structures distinguish NASH from simple steatosis. *J Lipid Res.* 2013;54(5):1326–34.
1241. U.S. Department of Agriculture, Agricultural Research Service. McDonald's, sausage McMuffin with egg. FoodData Central. https://fdc.nal.usda.gov/food-details/172068/nutrients. April 1, 2019. Accessed February 1, 2025.
1242. Ioannou GN, Morrow OB, Connole ML, Lee SP. Association between dietary nutrient composition and the incidence of cirrhosis or liver cancer in the United States population. *Hepatology.* 2009;50(1):175–84.
1243. Treatment of hepatitis C. U.S. Centers for Disease Control and Prevention. https://www.cdc.gov/hepatitis-c/treatment/index.html. December 20, 2023. Accessed February 5, 2025.
1244. Lock G, Dirscherl M, Obermeier F, et al. Hepatitis C—contamination of toothbrushes: myth or reality? *J Viral Hepat.* 2006;13(9):571–3.
1245. Bocket L, Chevaliez S, Talbodec N, Sobaszek A, Pawlotsky JM, Yazdanpanah Y. Occupational transmission of hepatitis C virus resulting from use of the same supermarket meat slicer. *Clin Microbiol Infect.* 2011;17(2):238–41.
1246. Teo CG. Much meat, much malady: changing perceptions of the epidemiology of hepatitis E. *Clin Microbiol Infect.* 2010;16(1):24–32.
1247. Yazaki Y, Mizuo H, Takahashi M, et al. Sporadic acute or fulminant hepatitis E in Hokkaido, Japan, may be food-borne, as suggested by the presence of hepatitis E virus in pig liver as food. *J Gen Virol.* 2003;84(Pt 9):2351–7.
1248. Feagins AR, Opriessnig T, Guenette DK, Halbur PG, Meng XJ. Detection and characterization of infectious Hepatitis E virus from commercial pig livers sold in local grocery stores in the USA. *J Gen Virol.* 2007;88(Pt 3):912–7.
1249. Feagins AR, Opriessnig T, Guenette DK, Halbur PG, Meng XJ. Detection and characterization of infectious Hepatitis E virus from commercial pig livers sold in local grocery stores in the USA. *J Gen Virol.* 2007;88(Pt 3):912–7.
1250. Dalton HR, Bendall RP, Pritchard C, Henley W, Melzer D. National mortality rates from chronic liver disease and consumption of alcohol and pig meat. *Epidemiol Infect.* 2010;138(2):174–82.
1251. Emerson SU, Arankalle VA, Purcell RH. Thermal stability of hepatitis E virus. *J Infect Dis.* 2005;192(5):930–3.
1252. About four steps to food safety. U. S. Centers for Disease Control and Prevention. https://www.cdc.gov/food-safety/prevention/index.html. April 29, 2024. Accessed February 2, 2025.

1253. Shinde NR, Patil TB, Deshpande AS, Gulhane RV, Patil MB, Bansod YV. Clinical profile, maternal and fetal outcomes of acute hepatitis E in pregnancy. *Ann Med Health Sci Res.* 2014;4(Suppl 2):S133–9.
1254. Navarro VJ, Barnhart H, Bonkovsky HL, et al. Liver injury from herbals and dietary supplements in the U.S. Drug-Induced Liver Injury Network. *Hepatology.* 2014;60(4):1399–408.
1255. Yu EL, Sivagnanam M, Ellis L, Huang JS. Acute hepatotoxicity after ingestion of Morinda citrifolia (noni berry) juice in a 14-year-old boy. *J Pediatr Gastroenterol Nutr.* 2011;52(2):222–4.
1256. Licata A, Craxt A. Considerations regarding the alleged association between Herbalife products and cases of hepatotoxicity: a rebuttal. *Intern Emerg Med.* 2014;9(5):601–2.
1257. Lobb AL. Science in liquid dietary supplement promotion: the misleading case of mangosteen juice. *Hawaii J Med Public Health.* 2012;71(2):46–8.
1258. Lobb AL. Science in liquid dietary supplement promotion: the misleading case of mangosteen juice. *Hawaii J Med Public Health.* 2012;71(2):46–8.
1259. Boozer CN, Nasser JA, Heymsfield SB, Wang V, Chen G, Solomon JL. An herbal supplement containing Ma Huang-Guarana for weight loss: a randomized, double-blind trial. *Int J Obes Relat Metab Disord.* 2001;25(3):316–24.
1260. Dietary supplements containing ephedra: health risks and FDA's oversight. US Government Accountability Office. http://www.gao.gov/assets/120/110228.pdf. July 23, 2003. Accessed February 3, 2025.
1261. Preuss HG, Bagchi D, Bagchi M, Rao CV, Dey DK, Satyanarayana S. Effects of a natural extract of (-)-hydroxycitric acid (HCA-SX) and a combination of HCA-SX plus niacin-bound chromium and Gymnema sylvestre extract on weight loss. *Diabetes Obes Metab.* 2004;6(3):171–80.
1262. Fong TL, Klontz KC, Canas-Coto A, et al. Hepatotoxicity due to Hydroxycut: a case series. *Am J Gastroenterol.* 2010;105(7):1561–6.
1263. Ye EQ, Chacko SA, Chou EL, Kugizaki M, Liu S. Greater whole-grain intake is associated with lower risk of type 2 diabetes, cardiovascular disease, and weight gain. *J Nutr.* 2012;142(7):1304–13.
1264. Karl JP, Saltzman E. The role of whole grains in body weight regulation. *Adv Nutr.* 2012;3(5):697–707.
1265. Ye EQ, Chacko SA, Chou EL, Kugizaki M, Liu S. Greater whole-grain intake is associated with lower risk of type 2 diabetes, cardiovascular disease, and weight gain. *J Nutr.* 2012;142(7):1304–13.
1266. Chang HC, Huang CN, Yeh DM, Wang SJ, Peng CH, Wang CJ. Oat prevents obesity and abdominal fat distribution, and improves liver function in humans. *Plant Foods Hum Nutr.* 2013;68(1):18–23.
1267. Chang HC, Huang CN, Yeh DM, Wang SJ, Peng CH, Wang CJ. Oat prevents obesity and abdominal fat distribution, and improves liver function in humans. *Plant Foods Hum Nutr.* 2013;68(1):18–23.
1268. Georgoulis M, Kontogianni MD, Tileli N, et al. The impact of cereal grain consumption on the development and severity of non-alcoholic fatty liver disease. *Eur J Nutr.* 2014;53(8):1727–35.
1269. Valenti L, Riso P, Mazzocchi A, Porrini M, Fargion S, Agostoni C. Dietary anthocyanins as nutritional therapy for nonalcoholic fatty liver disease. *Oxid Med Cell Longev.* 2013;2013:145421.
1270. Suda I, Ishikawa F, Hatakeyama M, et al. Intake of purple sweet potato beverage affects on serum hepatic biomarker levels of healthy adult men with borderline hepatitis. *Eur J Clin Nutr.* 2008;62(1):60–7.
1271. Sun J, Chu YF, Wu X, Liu RH. Antioxidant and antiproliferative activities of common fruits. *J Agric Food Chem.* 2002;50(25):7449–54.
1272. Ferguson PJ, Kurowska EM, Freeman DJ, Chambers AF, Koropatnick J. In vivo inhibition of growth of human tumor lines by flavonoid fractions from cranberry extract. *Nutr Cancer.* 2006;56(1):86–94.

1273. Sun J, Hai Liu R. Cranberry phytochemical extracts induce cell cycle arrest and apoptosis in human MCF-7 breast cancer cells. *Cancer Lett*. 2006;241(1):124–34.
1274. Ferguson PJ, Kurowska EM, Freeman DJ, Chambers AF, Koropatnick J. In vivo inhibition of growth of human tumor lines by flavonoid fractions from cranberry extract. *Nutr Cancer*. 2006;56(1):86–94.
1275. Kresty LA, Howell AB, Baird M. Cranberry proanthocyanidins mediate growth arrest of lung cancer cells through modulation of gene expression and rapid induction of apoptosis. *Molecules*. 2011;16(3):2375–90.
1276. Seeram NP, Adams LS, Zhang Y, et al. Blackberry, black raspberry, blueberry, cranberry, red raspberry, and strawberry extracts inhibit growth and stimulate apoptosis of human cancer cells in vitro. *J Agric Food Chem*. 2006;54(25):9329–39.
1277. Kim KK, Singh AP, Singh RK, et al. Anti-angiogenic activity of cranberry proanthocyanidins and cytotoxic properties in ovarian cancer cells. *Int J Oncol*. 2012;40(1):227–35.
1278. Déziel B, MacPhee J, Patel K, et al. American cranberry (Vaccinium macrocarpon) extract affects human prostate cancer cell growth via cell cycle arrest by modulating expression of cell cycle regulators. *Food Funct*. 2012;3(5):556–64.
1279. Liu M, Lin LQ, Song BB, et al. Cranberry phytochemical extract inhibits SGC-7901 cell growth and human tumor xenografts in Balb/c nu/nu mice. *J Agric Food Chem*. 2009;57(2):762–8.
1280. Seeram NP, Adams LS, Hardy ML, Heber D. Total cranberry extract versus its phytochemical constituents: antiproliferative and synergistic effects against human tumor cell lines. *J Agric Food Chem*. 2004;52(9):2512–7.
1281. Grace MH, Massey AR, Mbeunkui F, Yousef GG, Lila MA. Comparison of health-relevant flavonoids in commonly consumed cranberry products. *J Food Sci*. 2012;77(8):H176–83.
1282. Grace MH, Massey AR, Mbeunkui F, Yousef GG, Lila MA. Comparison of health-relevant flavonoids in commonly consumed cranberry products. *J Food Sci*. 2012;77(8):H176–83.
1283. Vinson JA, Bose P, Proch J, Al kharrat H, Samman N. Cranberries and cranberry products: powerful in vitro, ex vivo, and in vivo sources of antioxidants. *J Agric Food Chem*. 2008;56(14):5884–91.
1284. White BL, Howard LR, Prior RL. Impact of different stages of juice processing on the anthocyanin, flavonol, and procyanidin contents of cranberries. *J Agric Food Chem*. 2011;59(9):4692–8.
1285. Arnesen E, Huseby NE, Brenn T, Try K. The Tromsø Heart Study: distribution of, and determinants for, gamma-glutamyltransferase in a free-living population. *Scand J Clin Lab Invest*. 1986;46(1):63–70.
1286. Ruhl CE, Everhart JE. Coffee and tea consumption are associated with a lower incidence of chronic liver disease in the United States. *Gastroenterology*. 2005;129(6):1928–36.
1287. SEER*Explorer. Surveillance Research Program, National Cancer Institute. https://seer.cancer.gov/statistics-network/explorer/. November 5, 2024. Accessed February 5, 2025.
1288. Qiu S, Cai J, Yang Z, et al. Trends in hepatocellular carcinoma mortality rates in the US and projections through 2040. *JAMA Netw Open*. 2024;7(11):e2445525.
1289. Yu J, Liang D, Li J, et al. Coffee, green tea intake, and the risk of hepatocellular carcinoma: a systematic review and meta-analysis of observational studies. *Nutr Cancer*. 2023;75(5):1295–308.
1290. Lai GY, Weinstein SJ, Albanes D, et al. The association of coffee intake with liver cancer incidence and chronic liver disease mortality in male smokers. *Br J Cancer*. 2013;109(5):1344–51.
1291. Fujita Y, Shibata A, Ogimoto I, et al. The effect of interaction between hepatitis C virus and cigarette smoking on the risk of hepatocellular carcinoma. *Br J Cancer*. 2006;94(5):737–9.
1292. Danielsson J, Kangastupa P, Laatikainen T, Aalto M, Niemelä O. Dose- and gender-dependent interactions between coffee consumption and serum GGT activity in alcohol consumers. *Alcohol Alcohol*. 2013;48(3):303–7.

1293. Bravi F, Bosetti C, Tavani A, Gallus S, La Vecchia C. Coffee reduces risk for hepatocellular carcinoma: an meta-analysis. *Clin Gastroenterol Hepatol.* 2013;11(11):1413–21.e1.
1294. Pipitone RM, Ciccioli C, Infantino G, et al. MAFLD: a multisystem disease. *Ther Adv Endocrinol Metab.* 2023;14:20420188221145549.
1295. Cardin R, Piciocchi M, Martines D, Scribano L, Petracco M, Farinati F. Effects of coffee consumption in chronic hepatitis C: a randomized controlled trial. *Dig Liver Dis.* 2013;45(6):499–504.
1296. Torres DM, Harrison SA. Is it time to write a prescription for coffee? Coffee and liver disease. *Gastroenterology.* 2013;144(4):670–2.
1297. Ng V, Saab S. Can daily coffee consumption reduce liver disease-related mortality? *Clin Gastroenterol Hepatol.* 2013;11(11):1422–3.
1298. Torres DM, Harrison SA. Is it time to write a prescription for coffee? Coffee and liver disease. *Gastroenterology.* 2013;144(4):670–2.
1299. Hunger SP, Lu X, Devidas M, et al. Improved survival for children and adolescents with acute lymphoblastic leukemia between 1990 and 2005: a report from the Children's Oncology Group. *J Clin Oncol.* 2012;30(14):1663–9.
1300. SEER*Explorer. SEER Incidence Data, November 2023 submission. Surveillance Research Program, National Cancer Institute. https://seer.cancer.gov/statistics-network/explorer/. November 5, 2024. Accessed February 4, 2025.
1301. U.S. Cancer Statistics Working Group. U.S. Cancer Statistics Data Visualizations Tool. U.S. Department of Health and Human Services, Centers for Disease Control and Prevention and National Cancer Institute. https://www.cdc.gov/cancer/dataviz. Accessed February 3, 2025.
1302. U.S. Cancer Statistics Working Group. U.S. Cancer Statistics Data Visualizations Tool. U.S. Department of Health and Human Services, Centers for Disease Control and Prevention and National Cancer Institute. https://www.cdc.gov/cancer/dataviz. Accessed February 3, 2025.
1303. U.S. Cancer Statistics Working Group. U.S. Cancer Statistics Data Visualizations Tool. U.S. Department of Health and Human Services, Centers for Disease Control and Prevention and National Cancer Institute. https://www.cdc.gov/cancer/dataviz. Accessed February 3, 2025.
1304. Key TJ, Appleby PN, Spencer EA, et al. Cancer incidence in British vegetarians. *Br J Cancer.* 2009;101(1):192–7.
1305. Vegetarians less likely to develop cancer than meat eaters. *Cancer Research UK.* https://news.cancerresearchuk.org/2009/07/01/vegetarians-less-likely-to-develop-cancer-than-meat-eaters/. July 1, 2009. Accessed February 3, 2025.
1306. Suppipat K, Park CS, Shen Y, Zhu X, Lacorazza HD. Sulforaphane induces cell cycle arrest and apoptosis in acute lymphoblastic leukemia cells. *PLoS One.* 2012;7(12):e51251.
1307. Han X, Zheng T, Foss F, et al. Vegetable and fruit intake and non-Hodgkin lymphoma survival in Connecticut women. *Leuk Lymphoma.* 2010;51(6):1047–54.
1308. Thompson CA, Cerhan JR. Fruit and vegetable intake and survival from non-Hodgkin lymphoma: does an apple a day keep the doctor away? *Leuk Lymphoma.* 2010;51(6):963–4.
1309. Thompson CA, Habermann TM, Wang AH, et al. Antioxidant intake from fruits, vegetables and other sources and risk of non-Hodgkin's lymphoma: the Iowa Women's Health Study. *Int J Cancer.* 2010;126(4):992–1003.
1310. Holtan SG, O'Connor HM, Fredericksen ZS, et al. Food-frequency questionnaire-based estimates of total antioxidant capacity and risk of non-Hodgkin lymphoma. *Int J Cancer.* 2012;131(5):1158–68.
1311. Holtan SG, O'Connor HM, Fredericksen ZS, et al. Food-frequency questionnaire-based estimates of total antioxidant capacity and risk of non-Hodgkin lymphoma. *Int J Cancer.* 2012;131(5):1158–68.
1312. Thompson CA, Habermann TM, Wang AH, et al. Antioxidant intake from fruits, vegetables

and other sources and risk of non-Hodgkin's lymphoma: the Iowa Women's Health Study. *Int J Cancer.* 2010;126(4):992–1003.
1313. Bjelakovic G, Nikolova D, Simonetti RG, Gluud C. Antioxidant supplements for prevention of gastrointestinal cancers: a systematic review and meta-analysis. *Lancet.* 2004;364(9441): 1219–28.
1314. Jacobs DR, Tapsell LC. Food synergy: the key to a healthy diet. *Proc Nutr Soc.* 2013;72(2):200–6.
1315. Elsayed RK, Glisson JK, Minor DS. Rhabdomyolysis associated with the use of a mislabeled "acai berry" dietary supplement. *Am J Med Sci.* 2011;342(6):535–8.
1316. Zhang Y, Wang D, Lee RP, Henning SM, Heber D. Absence of pomegranate ellagitannins in the majority of commercial pomegranate extracts: implications for standardization and quality control. *J Agric Food Chem.* 2009;57(16):7395–400.
1317. Zhang Y, Krueger D, Durst R, et al. International multidimensional authenticity specification (IMAS) algorithm for detection of commercial pomegranate juice adulteration. *J Agric Food Chem.* 2009;57(6):2550–7.
1318. Del Pozo-Insfran D, Percival SS, Talcott ST. Açai (Euterpe oleracea Mart.) polyphenolics in their glycoside and aglycone forms induce apoptosis of HL-60 leukemia cells. *J Agric Food Chem.* 2006;54(4):1222–9.
1319. Schauss AG, Wu X, Prior RL, et al. Antioxidant capacity and other bioactivities of the freeze-dried Amazonian palm berry, Euterpe oleraceae mart. (aSch). *J Agric Food Chem.* 2006;54(22):8604–10.
1320. Haytowitz DB, Bhagwat SA. *USDA database for the oxygen radical capacity (ORAC) of selected foods, release 2.* Washington, D.C.: United States Department of Agriculture; 2010.
1321. Landgren O, Kyle RA, Pfeiffer RM, et al. Monoclonal gammopathy of undetermined significance (MGUS) consistently precedes multiple myeloma: a prospective study. *Blood.* 2009;113(22):5412–7.
1322. Landgren O, Kyle RA, Pfeiffer RM, et al. Monoclonal gammopathy of undetermined significance (MGUS) consistently precedes multiple myeloma: a prospective study. *Blood.* 2009;113(22):5412–7.
1323. Mouhieddine TH, Weeks LD, Ghobrial IM. Monoclonal gammopathy of undetermined significance. *Blood.* 2019;133(23):2484–94.
1324. Kyle RA, Therneau TM, Rajkumar SV, et al. A long-term study of prognosis in monoclonal gammopathy of undetermined significance. *N Engl J Med.* 2002;346(8):564–9.
1325. Bharti AC, Donato N, Singh S, Aggarwal BB. Curcumin (diferuloylmethane) down-regulates the constitutive activation of nuclear factor-kappa B and IkappaBalpha kinase in human multiple myeloma cells, leading to suppression of proliferation and induction of apoptosis. *Blood.* 2003;101(3):1053–62.
1326. Golombick T, Diamond TH, Badmaev V, Manoharan A, Ramakrishna R. The potential role of curcumin in patients with monoclonal gammopathy of undefined significance—its effect on paraproteinemia and the urinary N-telopeptide of type I collagen bone turnover marker. *Clin Cancer Res.* 2009;15(18):5917–22.
1327. Golombick T, Diamond TH, Manoharan A, Ramakrishna R. Monoclonal gammopathy of undetermined significance, smoldering multiple myeloma, and curcumin: a randomized, double-blind placebo-controlled cross-over 4g study and an open-label 8g extension study. *Am J Hematol.* 2012;87(5):455–60.
1328. Santosa D, Suharti C, Riwanto I, et al. Curcumin as adjuvant therapy to improve remission in myeloma patients: a pilot randomized clinical trial. *Caspian J Intern Med.* 2022;13(2): 375–84.
1329. Key TJ, Appleby PN, Spencer EA, et al. Cancer incidence in British vegetarians. *Br J Cancer.* 2009;101(1):192–7.
1330. Rohrmann S, Linseisen J, Jakobsen MU, et al. Consumption of meat and dairy and lymphoma risk in the European Prospective Investigation into Cancer and Nutrition. *Int J Cancer.* 2011;128(3):623–34.

1331. U.S. Department of Agriculture, Agricultural Research Service. Chicken, broiler, rotisserie, BBQ, breast meat and skin. FoodData Central. https://fdc.nal.usda.gov/food-details/171125/nutrients. April 1, 2019. Accessed February 4, 2025.
1332. Rohrmann S, Linseisen J, Jakobsen MU, et al. Consumption of meat and dairy and lymphoma risk in the European Prospective Investigation into Cancer and Nutrition. Int J Cancer. 2011;128(3):623–34.
1333. Chiu BC, Cerhan JR, Folsom AR, et al. Diet and risk of non-Hodgkin lymphoma in older women. JAMA. 1996;275(17):1315–21.
1334. Daniel CR, Sinha R, Park Y, et al. Meat intake is not associated with risk of non-Hodgkin lymphoma in a large prospective cohort of U.S. men and women. J Nutr. 2012;142(6):1074–80.
1335. Puangsombat K, Gadgil P, Houser TA, Hunt MC, Smith JS. Occurrence of heterocyclic amines in cooked meat products. Meat Sci. 2012;90(3):739–46.
1336. 't Mannetje A, Eng A, Pearce N. Farming, growing up on a farm, and haematological cancer mortality. Occup Environ Med. 2012;69(2):126–32.
1337. Johnson ES, Zhou Y, Yau LC, et al. Mortality from malignant diseases–update of the Baltimore union poultry cohort. Cancer Causes Control. 2010;21(2):215–21.
1338. Neasham D, Sifi A, Nielsen KR, et al. Occupation and risk of lymphoma: a multicentre prospective cohort study (EPIC). Occup Environ Med. 2011;68(1):77–81.
1339. Kalland KH, Ke XS, Øyan AM. Tumour virology—history, status and future challenges. APMIS. 2009;117(5–6):382–99.
1340. Centers for Disease Control and Prevention. Human Orf virus infection from household exposures—United States, 2009–2011. MMWR Morb Mortal Wkly Rep. 2012;61(14):245–8.
1341. Benton EC. Warts in butchers—a cause for concern? Lancet. 1994;343(8906):1114.
1342. Gubéran E, Usel M, Raymond L, Fioretta G. Mortality and incidence of cancer among a cohort of self employed butchers from Geneva and their wives. Br J Ind Med. 1993;50(11):1008–16.
1343. Johnson ES, Zhou Y, Yau LC, et al. Mortality from malignant diseases—update of the Baltimore union poultry cohort. Cancer Causes Control. 2010;21(2):215–21.
1344. Johnson ES, Ndetan H, Lo KM. Cancer mortality in poultry slaughtering/processing plant workers belonging to a union pension fund. Environ Res. 2010;110(6):588–94.
1345. Gandhi S, Felini MJ, Ndetan H, et al. A pilot case-cohort study of brain cancer in poultry and control workers. Nutr Cancer. 2014;66(3):343–50.
1346. Choi KM, Johnson ES. Occupational exposure assessment using antibody levels: exposure to avian leukosis/sarcoma viruses in the poultry industry. Int J Environ Health Res. 2011;21(4):306–16.
1347. Choi KM, Johnson ES. Industrial hygiene assessment of reticuloendotheliosis viruses exposure in the poultry industry. Int Arch Occup Environ Health. 2011;84(4):375–82.
1348. Choi KM, Johnson ES. Industrial hygiene assessment of reticuloendotheliosis viruses exposure in the poultry industry. Int Arch Occup Environ Health. 2011;84(4):375–82.
1349. Johnson ES, Ndetan H, Lo KM. Cancer mortality in poultry slaughtering/processing plant workers belonging to a union pension fund. Environ Res. 2010;110(6):588–94.
1350. 't Mannetje A, Eng A, Pearce N. Farming, growing up on a farm, and haematological cancer mortality. Occup Environ Med. 2012;69(2):126–32.
1351. Tranah GJ, Bracci PM, Holly EA. Domestic and farm-animal exposures and risk of non-Hodgkin's lymphoma in a population-based study in the San Francisco Bay Area. Cancer Epidemiol Biomarkers Prev. 2008;17(9):2382–7.
1352. Buehring GC, Philpott SM, Choi KY. Humans have antibodies reactive with Bovine leukemia virus. AIDS Res Hum Retroviruses. 2003;19(12):1105–13.
1353. Veterinary Services, Centers for Epidemiology and Animal Health. Bovine Leukosis Virus (BLV) on U.S. dairy operations, 2007. U.S. Department of Agriculture, Animal and Plant Health Inspection Service. http://www.aphis.usda.gov/animal_health/nahms/dairy/downloads/dairy07/Dairy07_is_BLV.pdf. October 2008. Accessed February 4, 2025.

1354. Buehring GC, Shen HM, Jensen HM, Choi KY, Sun D, Nuovo G. Bovine leukemia virus DNA in human breast tissue. *Emerg Infect Dis.* 2014;20(5):772–82.
1355. de Quadros DL, Ribeiro VA, Rezende MA, et al. Oncogenic viral DNA related to human breast cancer found on cattle milk and meat. *Comp Immunol Microbiol Infect Dis.* 2023;101: 102053.
1356. Buehring GC, Sans HM. Breast cancer gone viral? Review of possible role of bovine leukemia virus in breast cancer, and related opportunities for cancer prevention. *Int J Environ Res Public Health.* 2019;17(1):209.
1357. Tranah GJ, Bracci PM, Holly EA. Domestic and farm-animal exposures and risk of non-Hodgkin's lymphoma in a population-based study in the San Francisco Bay Area. *Cancer Epidemiol Biomarkers Prev.* 2008;17(9):2382–7.
1358. Kramer CK, Mehmood S, Suen RS. Dog ownership and survival: a systematic review and meta-analysis. *Circ Cardiovasc Qual Outcomes.* 2019;12(10):e005554.
1359. Nagasawa M, Mitsui S, En S, et al. Oxytocin-gaze positive loop and the coevolution of human-dog bonds. *Science.* 2015;348(6232):333–6.
1360. Friedmann E, Katcher AH, Lynch JJ, Thomas SA. Animal companions and one-year survival of patients after discharge from a coronary care unit. *Public Health Rep.* 1980;95(4):307–12.
1361. Herzog H. The impact of pets on human health and psychological well-being: fact, fiction, or hypothesis? *Curr Dir Psychol Sci.* 2011;20(4):236–9.
1362. Kramer CK, Mehmood S, Suen RS. Dog ownership and survival: a systematic review and meta-analysis. *Circ Cardiovasc Qual Outcomes.* 2019;12(10):e005554.
1363. Kojima G, Aoyama R, Taniguchi Y. Associations between pet ownership and frailty: a systematic review. *Geriatrics (Basel).* 2020;5(4):89.
1364. Kazi DS. Who is rescuing whom? Dog ownership and cardiovascular health. *Circ Cardiovasc Qual Outcomes.* 2019;12(10):e005887.
1365. Kazi DS. Who is rescuing whom? Dog ownership and cardiovascular health. *Circ Cardiovasc Qual Outcomes.* 2019;12(10):e005887.
1366. Bauman A, Owen KB, Torske MO, Ding D, Krokstad S, Stamatakis E. Does dog ownership really prolong survival? A revised meta-analysis and reappraisal of the evidence. *Circ Cardiovasc Qual Outcomes.* 2020;13(10):e006907.
1367. Friedmann E, Thomas SA, Son H. Pets, depression and long-term survival in community living patients following myocardial infarction. *Anthrozoös.* 2011;24(3):273–85.
1368. Friedmann E, Thomas SA. Pet ownership, social support, and one-year survival after acute myocardial infarction in the Cardiac Arrhythmia Suppression Trial (CAST). *Am J Cardiol.* 1995;76(17):1213–7.
1369. Serpell J. Beneficial effects of pet ownership on some aspects of human health and behaviour. *J R Soc Med.* 1991;84(12):717–20.
1370. Ko HJ, Youn CH, Kim SH, Kim SY. Effect of pet insects on the psychological health of community-dwelling elderly people: a single-blinded, randomized, controlled trial. *Gerontology.* 2016;62(2):200–9.
1371. Friedmann E, Gee NR. Critical review of research methods used to consider the impact of human-animal interaction on older adults' health. *Gerontologist.* 2019;59(5):964–72.
1372. Thorpe RJ Jr, Simonsick EM, Brach JS, et al. Dog ownership, walking behavior, and maintained mobility in late life. *J Am Geriatr Soc.* 2006;54(9):1419–24.
1373. Puterbaugh JS. The emperor's tailors: the failure of the medical weight loss paradigm and its causal role in the obesity of America. *Diabetes Obes Metab.* 2009;11(6):557–70.
1374. Schernhammer ES, Bertrand KA, Birmann BM, Sampson L, Willett WC, Feskanich D. Consumption of artificial sweetener-and sugar-containing soda and risk of lymphoma and leukemia in men and women. *Am J Clin Nutr.* 2012;96(6):1419–28.
1375. Lim U, Subar AF, Mouw T, et al. Consumption of aspartame-containing beverages and incidence of hematopoietic and brain malignancies. *Cancer Epidemiol Biomarkers Prev.* 2006;15(9):1654–9.

1376. McCullough ML, Teras LR, Shah R, Diver WR, Gaudet MM, Gapstur SM. Artificially and sugar-sweetened carbonated beverage consumption is not associated with risk of lymphoid neoplasms in older men and women. *J Nutr*. 2014;144(12):2041–9.
1377. Beigrezaei S, Raeisi-Dehkordi H, Hernández Vargas JA, et al. Non-sugar-sweetened beverages and risk of chronic diseases: an umbrella review of meta-analyses of prospective cohort studies. *Nutr Rev*. Published online September 26, 2024:nuae135.
1378. United States Renal Data System. 2020 USRDS Annual Data Report: epidemiology of kidney disease in the United States. National Institutes of Health, National Institute of Diabetes and Digestive and Kidney Diseases. https://usrds-adr.niddk.nih.gov/2020. Accessed February 5, 2025.
1379. Chronic kidney disease in the United States, 2023. US Department of Health and Human Services, Centers for Disease Control and Prevention. https://www.cdc.gov/kidney-disease/php/data-research/index.html. May 15, 2024. Accessed February 5, 2025.
1380. Hoerger TJ, Simpson SA, Yarnoff BO, et al. The future burden of CKD in the United States: a simulation model for the CDC CKD Initiative. *Am J Kidney Dis*. 2015;65(3):403–11.
1381. Dalrymple LS, Katz R, Kestenbaum B, et al. Chronic kidney disease and the risk of end-stage renal disease versus death. *J Gen Intern Med*. 2011;26(4):379–85.
1382. Kumar S, Bogle R, Banerjee D. Why do young people with chronic kidney disease die early? *World J Nephrol*. 2014;3(4):143–55.
1383. Lin J, Hu FB, Curhan GC. Associations of diet with albuminuria and kidney function decline. *Clin J Am Soc Nephrol*. 2010;5(5):836–43.
1384. Lin J, Hu FB, Curhan GC. Associations of diet with albuminuria and kidney function decline. *Clin J Am Soc Nephrol*. 2010;5(5):836–43.
1385. Virchow, R. *Cellular Pathology as Based upon Physiological and Pathological Histology. Twenty Lectures Delivered in the Pathological Institute of Berlin During the Months of February, March and April, 1858*. Philadelpia, PA: J. B. Lippincott and Co.; 1863.
1386. Moorhead JF, Chan MK, El-Nahas M, Varghese Z. Lipid nephrotoxicity in chronic progressive glomerular and tubulo-interstitial disease. *Lancet*. 1982;2(8311):1309–11.
1387. Hartroft WS. Fat emboli in glomerular capillaries of choline-deficient rats and of patients with diabetic glomerulosclerosis. *Am J Pathol*. 1955;31(3):381–97.
1388. Gyebi L, Soltani Z, Reisin E. Lipid nephrotoxicity: new concept for an old disease. *Curr Hypertens Rep*. 2012;14(2):177–81.
1389. US Burden of Disease Collaborators. The state of US health, 1990–2010: burden of diseases, injuries, and risk factors. *JAMA*. 2013;310(6):591–608.
1390. Odermatt A. The Western-style diet: a major risk factor for impaired kidney function and chronic kidney disease. *Am J Physiol Renal Physiol*. 2011;301(5):F919–31.
1391. van den Berg E, Hospers FA, Navis G, et al. Dietary acid load and rapid progression to end-stage renal disease of diabetic nephropathy in Westernized South Asian people. *J Nephrol*. 2011;24(1):11–7.
1392. Piccoli GB, Vigotti FN, Leone F, et al. Low-protein diets in CKD: how can we achieve them? A narrative, pragmatic review. *Clin Kidney J*. 2015;8(1):61–70.
1393. Brenner BM, Meyer TW, Hostetter TH. Dietary protein intake and the progressive nature of kidney disease: the role of hemodynamically mediated glomerular injury in the pathogenesis of progressive glomerular sclerosis in aging, renal ablation, and intrinsic renal disease. *N Engl J Med*. 1982;307(11):652–9.
1394. Wiseman MJ, Hunt R, Goodwin A, Gross JL, Keen H, Viberti GC. Dietary composition and renal function in healthy subjects. *Nephron*. 1987;46(1):37–42.
1395. Nakamura H, Takasawa M, Kashara S, et al. Effects of acute protein loads of different sources on renal function of patients with diabetic nephropathy. *Tohoku J Exp Med*. 1989;159(2):153–62.
1396. Simon AH, Lima PR, Almerinda M, Alves VF, Bottini PV, de Faria JB. Renal haemodynamic responses to a chicken or beef meal in normal individuals. *Nephrol Dial Transplant*. 1998;13(9):2261–4.

1397. Kontessis P, Jones S, Dodds R, et al. Renal, metabolic and hormonal responses to ingestion of animal and vegetable proteins. *Kidney Int.* 1990;38(1):136–44.
1398. Nakamura H, Takasawa M, Kashara S, et al. Effects of acute protein loads of different sources on renal function of patients with diabetic nephropathy. *Tohoku J Exp Med.* 1989;159(2):153–62.
1399. Azadbakht L, Shakerhosseini R, Atabak S, Jamshidian M, Mehrabi Y, Esmaill-Zadeh A. Beneficiary effect of dietary soy protein on lowering plasma levels of lipid and improving kidney function in type II diabetes with nephropathy. *Eur J Clin Nutr.* 2003;57(10):1292–4.
1400. Kontessis PA, Bossinakou I, Sarika L, et al. Renal, metabolic, and hormonal responses to proteins of different origin in normotensive, nonproteinuric type I diabetic patients. *Diabetes Care.* 1995;18(9):1233–40.
1401. Teixeira SR, Tappenden KA, Carson L, et al. Isolated soy protein consumption reduces urinary albumin excretion and improves the serum lipid profile in men with type 2 diabetes mellitus and nephropathy. *J Nutr.* 2004;134(8):1874–80.
1402. Stephenson TJ, Setchell KD, Kendall CW, Jenkins DJ, Anderson JW, Fanti P. Effect of soy protein-rich diet on renal function in young adults with insulin-dependent diabetes mellitus. *Clin Nephrol.* 2005;64(1):1–11.
1403. Jibani MM, Bloodworth LL, Foden E, Griffiths KD, Galpin OP. Predominantly vegetarian diet in patients with incipient and early clinical diabetic nephropathy: effects on albumin excretion rate and nutritional status. *Diabet Med.* 1991;8(10):949–53.
1404. Bosch JP, Saccaggi A, Lauer A, Ronco C, Belledonne M, Glabman S. Renal functional reserve in humans. Effect of protein intake on glomerular filtration rate. *Am J Med.* 1983;75(6):943–50.
1405. Liu ZM, Ho SC, Chen YM, Tang N, Woo J. Effect of whole soy and purified isoflavone daidzein on renal function—a 6-month randomized controlled trial in equol-producing postmenopausal women with prehypertension. *Clin Biochem.* 2014;47(13–14):1250–6.
1406. Fioretto P, Trevisan R, Valerio A, et al. Impaired renal response to a meat meal in insulin-dependent diabetes: role of glucagon and prostaglandins. *Am J Physiol.* 1990;258(3 Pt 2):F675–83.
1407. Frassetto L, Morris RC, Sellmeyer DE, Todd K, Sebastian A. Diet, evolution and aging—the pathophysiologic effects of the post-agricultural inversion of the potassium-to-sodium and base-to-chloride ratios in the human diet. *Eur J Nutr.* 2001;40(5):200–13.
1408. Mofrad MD, Daneshzad E, Azadbakht L. Dietary acid load, kidney function and risk of chronic kidney disease: a systematic review and meta-analysis of observational studies. *Int J Vitam Nutr Res.* 2021;91(3–4):343–55.
1409. Poyourow CN, Leonberg K, Ghajar M, Chung M, Byham-Gray L. The role of dietary acid load on progression of estimated glomerular filtration rate among individuals diagnosed with chronic kidney disease. *J Ren Nutr.* 2024;34(4):273–82.
1410. Sebastian A, Frassetto LA, Sellmeyer DE, Merriam RL, Morris RC. Estimation of the net acid load of the diet of ancestral preagricultural Homo sapiens and their hominid ancestors. *Am J Clin Nutr.* 2002;76(6):1308–16.
1411. van den Berg E, Hospers FA, Navis G, et al. Dietary acid load and rapid progression to end-stage renal disease of diabetic nephropathy in Westernized South Asian people. *J Nephrol.* 2011;24(1):11–7.
1412. Uribarri J, Oh MS. The key to halting progression of CKD might be in the produce market, not in the pharmacy. *Kidney Int.* 2012;81(1):7–9.
1413. Cohen E, Nardi Y, Krause I, et al. A longitudinal assessment of the natural rate of decline in renal function with age. *J Nephrol.* 2014;27(6):635–41.
1414. Brenner BM, Meyer TW, Hostetter TH. Dietary protein intake and the progressive nature of kidney disease: the role of hemodynamically mediated glomerular injury in the pathogenesis of progressive glomerular sclerosis in aging, renal ablation, and intrinsic renal disease. *N Engl J Med.* 1982;307(11):652–9.
1415. Frassetto LA, Todd KM, Morris RC, Sebastian A. Estimation of net endogenous noncar-

bonic acid production in humans from diet potassium and protein contents. *Am J Clin Nutr.* 1998;68(3):576–83.

1416. Wiseman MJ, Hunt R, Goodwin A, Gross JL, Keen H, Viberti GC. Dietary composition and renal function in healthy subjects. *Nephron.* 1987;46(1):37–42.

1417. Kempner W. Treatment of heart and kidney disease and of hypertensive and arteriosclerotic vascular disease with the rice diet. *Ann Intern Med.* 1949;31(5):821–56.

1418. Barsotti G, Morelli E, Cupisti A, Meola M, Dani L, Giovannetti S. A low-nitrogen low-phosphorus vegan diet for patients with chronic renal failure. *Nephron.* 1996;74(2):390–4.

1419. Deriemaeker P, Aerenhouts D, Hebbelinck M, Clarys P. Nutrient based estimation of acid-base balance in vegetarians and non-vegetarians. *Plant Foods Hum Nutr.* 2010;65(1):77–82.

1420. Cotter T, Kotov A, Wang S, Murukutla N. 'Warning: ultra-processed'—a call for warnings on foods that aren't really foods. *BMJ Glob Health.* 2021;6(12):e007240.

1421. Monteiro CA, Cannon G, Moubarac JC, Levy RB, Louzada MLC, Jaime PC. The UN Decade of Nutrition, the NOVA food classification and the trouble with ultra-processing. *Public Health Nutr.* 2018;21(1):5–17.

1422. Taneri PE, Wehrli F, Roa-Díaz ZM, et al. Association between ultra-processed food intake and all-cause mortality: a systematic review and meta-analysis. *Am J Epidemiol.* 2022;191(7):1323–35.

1423. Orlich MJ, Sabaté J, Mashchak A, et al. Ultra-processed food intake and animal-based food intake and mortality in the Adventist Health Study-2. *Am J Clin Nutr.* 2022;115(6):1589–601.

1424. Rauber F, Laura da Costa Louzada M, Chang K, et al. Implications of food ultra-processing on cardiovascular risk considering plant origin foods: an analysis of the UK Biobank cohort. *Lancet Reg Health Eur.* 2024;43:100948.

1425. Cordova R, Viallon V, Fontvieille E, et al. Consumption of ultra-processed foods and risk of multimorbidity of cancer and cardiometabolic diseases: a multinational cohort study. *Lancet Reg Health Eur.* 2023;35:100771.

1426. Crimarco A, Springfield S, Petlura C, et al. A randomized crossover trial on the effect of plant-based compared with animal-based meat on trimethylamine-N-oxide and cardiovascular disease risk factors in generally healthy adults: Study With Appetizing Plantfood-Meat Eating Alternative Trial (SWAP-MEAT). *Am J Clin Nutr.* 2020;112(5):1188–99.

1427. Azadbakht L, Atabak S, Esmaillzadeh A. Soy protein intake, cardiorenal indices, and C-reactive protein in type 2 diabetes with nephropathy: a longitudinal randomized clinical trial. *Diabetes Care.* 2008;31(4):648–54.

1428. Institute for Health Metrics and Evaluation (IHME). GBD 2021 results. University of Washington. https://vizhub.healthdata.org/gbd-results/. Accessed December 13, 2024.

1429. Institute for Health Metrics and Evaluation (IHME). GBD 2021 cause and risk summary: diet high in processed meat—level 3 risk. University of Washington. https://www.healthdata.org/research-analysis/diseases-injuries-risks/factsheets/2021-diet-high-processed-meat-level-3-risk. Accessed January 27, 2025.

1430. Institute for Health Metrics and Evaluation (IHME). GBD 2021 cause and risk summary: diet high in processed meat—level 3 risk. University of Washington. https://www.healthdata.org/research-analysis/diseases-injuries-risks/factsheets/2021-diet-high-red-meat-level-3-risk. Accessed January 27, 2025.

1431. Grosso G, La Vignera S, Condorelli RA, et al. Total, red and processed meat consumption and human health: an umbrella review of observational studies. *Int J Food Sci Nutr.* 2022;73(6):726–37.

1432. Springmann M, Godfray HC, Rayner M, Scarborough P. Analysis and valuation of the health and climate change cobenefits of dietary change. *Proc Natl Acad Sci U S A.* 2016;113(15):4146–51.

1433. Goraya N, Simoni J, Jo C, Wesson DE. Dietary acid reduction with fruits and vegetables or bicarbonate attenuates kidney injury in patients with a moderately reduced glomerular filtration rate due to hypertensive nephropathy. *Kidney Int.* 2012;81(1):86–93.

1434. Yaqoob MM. Treatment of acidosis in CKD. *Clin J Am Soc Nephrol.* 2013;8(3):342–3.
1435. Goraya N, Simoni J, Jo C, Wesson DE. Dietary acid reduction with fruits and vegetables or bicarbonate attenuates kidney injury in patients with a moderately reduced glomerular filtration rate due to hypertensive nephropathy. *Kidney Int.* 2012;81(1):86–93.
1436. Wright JA, Cavanaugh KL. Dietary sodium in chronic kidney disease: a comprehensive approach. *Semin Dial.* 2010;23(4):415–21.
1437. Uribarri J, Oh MS. The key to halting progression of CKD might be in the produce market, not in the pharmacy. *Kidney Int.* 2012;81(1):7–9.
1438. Goldfarb S. Dietary factors in the pathogenesis and prophylaxis of calcium nephrolithiasis. *Kidney Int.* 1988;34(4):544–55.
1439. Hill AJ, Basourakos SP, Lewicki P, Wu X, Arenas-Gallo C, Chuang D, et al. Incidence of kidney stones in the United States: the continuous National Health and Nutrition Examination Survey. *J Urol.* 2022;207(4):851–6.
1440. Scales CD Jr, Smith AC, Hanley JM, Saigal CS; Urologic Diseases in America Project. Prevalence of kidney stones in the United States. *Eur Urol.* 2012;62(1):160–5.
1441. Robertson WG, Peacock M, Hodgkinson A. Dietary changes and the incidence of urinary calculi in the U.K. between 1958 and 1976. *J Chronic Dis.* 1979;32(6):469–76.
1442. Robertson WG, Heyburn PJ, Peacock M, Hanes FA, Swaminathan R. The effect of high animal protein intake on the risk of calcium stone-formation in the urinary tract. *Clin Sci* (Lond). 1979;57(3):285–8.
1443. Robertson WG, Heyburn PJ, Peacock M, Hanes FA, Swaminathan R. The effect of high animal protein intake on the risk of calcium stone-formation in the urinary tract. *Clin Sci* (Lond). 1979;57(3):285–8.
1444. Robertson WG, Peacock M, Heyburn PJ, et al. Should recurrent calcium oxalate stone formers become vegetarians? *Br J Urol.* 1979;51(6):427–31.
1445. Turney BW, Appleby PN, Reynard JM, Noble JG, Key TJ, Allen NE. Diet and risk of kidney stones in the Oxford cohort of the European Prospective Investigation into Cancer and Nutrition (EPIC). *Eur J Epidemiol.* 2014;29(5):363–9.
1446. Tracy CR, Best S, Bagrodia A, et al. Animal protein and the risk of kidney stones: a comparative metabolic study of animal protein sources. *J Urol.* 2014;192:137–41.
1447. Bushinsky DA. Recurrent hypercalciuric nephrolithiasis—does diet help? *N Engl J Med.* 2002;346(2):124–5.
1448. Borghi L, Schianchi T, Meschi T, et al. Comparison of two diets for the prevention of recurrent stones in idiopathic hypercalciuria. *N Engl J Med.* 2002;346(2):77–84.
1449. Sorensen MD, Hsi RS, Chi T, et al. Dietary intake of fiber, fruit and vegetables decreases the risk of incident kidney stones in women: a Women's Health Initiative report. *J Urol.* 2014;192(6):1694–9.
1450. Albersmeyer M, Hilge R, Schröttle A, Weiss M, Sitter T, Vielhauer V. Acute kidney injury after ingestion of rhubarb: secondary oxalate nephropathy in a patient with type 1 diabetes. *BMC Nephrol.* 2012;13:141.
1451. Barman AK, Goel R, Sharma M, Mahanta PJ. Acute kidney injury associated with ingestion of star fruit: acute oxalate nephropathy. *Indian J Nephrol.* 2016;26(6):446–8.
1452. Kikuchi Y, Seta K, Ogawa Y, et al. Chaga mushroom-induced oxalate nephropathy. *Clin Nephrol.* 2014;81(6):440–4.
1453. Gandhi A, Nasser S, Kassis Akl N, Kotadia S. Quiz page June 2016: rapidly progressive kidney failure. *Am J Kidney Dis.* 2016;67(6):A15–7.
1454. Syed F, Mena-Gutierrez A, Ghaffar U. A case of iced-tea nephropathy. *N Engl J Med.* 2015;372(14):1377–8.
1455. Bernardino M, Parmar MS. Oxalate nephropathy from cashew nut intake. *CMAJ.* 2017;189(10):E405–8.
1456. Haaskjold YL, Drotningsvik A, Leh S, Marti HP, Svarstad E. Renal failure due to excessive intake of almonds in the absence of Oxalobacter formigenes. *Am J Med.* 2015;128(12):e29–30.

1457. Mehta TH, Goldfarb DS. Uric acid stones and hyperuricosuria. *Adv Chronic Kidney Dis.* 2012;19(6):413–8.
1458. de Vries A, Frank M, Liberman UA, Sperling O. Allopurinol in the prophylaxis of uric acid stones. *Ann Rheum Dis.* 1966;25(6 Suppl):691–3.
1459. Siener R, Hesse A. The effect of a vegetarian and different omnivorous diets on urinary risk factors for uric acid stone formation. *Eur J Nutr.* 2003;42(6):332–7.
1460. Siener R, Hesse A. The effect of a vegetarian and different omnivorous diets on urinary risk factors for uric acid stone formation. *Eur J Nutr.* 2003;42(6):332–7.
1461. Trinchieri A. Development of a rapid food screener to assess the potential renal acid load of diet in renal stone formers (LAKE score). *Arch Ital Urol Androl.* 2012;84(1):36–8.
1462. Chae JY, Kim JW, Kim JW, et al. Increased fluid intake and adequate dietary modification may be enough for the successful treatment of uric acid stone. *Urolithiasis.* 2013;41(2):179–82.
1463. Deriemaeker P, Aerenhouts D, Hebbelinck M, Clarys P. Nutrient based estimation of acid-base balance in vegetarians and non-vegetarians. *Plant Foods Hum Nutr.* 2010;65(1):77–82.
1464. Adeva MM, Souto G. Diet-induced metabolic acidosis. *Clin Nutr.* 2011;30(4):416–21.
1465. Dawson-Hughes B, Harris SS, Ceglia L. Alkaline diets favor lean tissue mass in older adults. *Am J Clin Nutr.* 2008;87(3):662–5.
1466. Ritz E, Hahn K, Ketteler M, Kuhlmann MK, Mann J. Phosphate additives in food—a health risk. *Dtsch Arztebl Int.* 2012;109(4):49–55.
1467. Ritz E, Hahn K, Ketteler M, Kuhlmann MK, Mann J. Phosphate additives in food—a health risk. *Dtsch Arztebl Int.* 2012;109(4):49–55.
1468. Calvo MS, Uribarri J. Public health impact of dietary phosphorus excess on bone and cardiovascular health in the general population. *Am J Clin Nutr.* 2013;98(1):6–15.
1469. Moe SM, Zidehsarai MP, Chambers MA, et al. Vegetarian compared with meat dietary protein source and phosphorus homeostasis in chronic kidney disease. *Clin J Am Soc Nephrol.* 2011;6(2):257–64.
1470. Fukagawa M, Komaba H, Miyamoto K. Source matters: from phosphorus load to bioavailability. *Clin J Am Soc Nephrol.* 2011;6(2):239–40.
1471. Murphy-Gutekunst L, Uribarri J. Hidden phosphorus-enhanced meats: part 3. *J Ren Nutr.* 2005;15(4):E1–4.
1472. Ritz E, Hahn K, Ketteler M, Kuhlmann MK, Mann J. Phosphate additives in food—a health risk. *Dtsch Arztebl Int.* 2012;109(4):49–55.
1473. Karp H, Ekholm P, Kemi V, et al. Differences among total and in vitro digestible phosphorus content of plant foods and beverages. *J Ren Nutr.* 2012;22(4):416–22.
1474. Karp H, Ekholm P, Kemi V, Hirvonen T, Lamberg-Allardt C. Differences among total and in vitro digestible phosphorus content of meat and milk products. *J Ren Nutr.* 2012;22(3):344–9.
1475. Karp H, Ekholm P, Kemi V, et al. Differences among total and in vitro digestible phosphorus content of plant foods and beverages. *J Ren Nutr.* 2012;22(4):416–22.
1476. Murphy-Gutekunst L, Uribarri J. Hidden phosphorus-enhanced meats: part 3. *J Ren Nutr.* 2005;15(4):E1–4.
1477. Sherman RA, Mehta O. Phosphorus and potassium content of enhanced meat and poultry products: implications for patients who receive dialysis. *Clin J Am Soc Nephrol.* 2009;4(8):1370–3.
1478. Benini O, D'Alessandro C, Gianfaldoni D, Cupisti A. Extra-phosphate load from food additives in commonly eaten foods: a real and insidious danger for renal patients. *J Ren Nutr.* 2011;21(4):303–8.
1479. Sherman RA, Mehta O. Phosphorus and potassium content of enhanced meat and poultry products: implications for patients who receive dialysis. *Clin J Am Soc Nephrol.* 2009;4(8):1370–3.
1480. Benini O, D'Alessandro C, Gianfaldoni D, Cupisti A. Extra-phosphate load from food additives in commonly eaten foods: a real and insidious danger for renal patients. *J Ren Nutr.* 2011;21(4):303–8.

1481. Shroff R. Phosphate is a vascular toxin. *Pediatr Nephrol.* 2013;28(4):583–93.
1482. Shuto E, Taketani Y, Tanaka R, et al. Dietary phosphorus acutely impairs endothelial function. *J Am Soc Nephrol.* 2009;20(7):1504–12.
1483. Gunther NW, He Y, Fratamico P. Effects of polyphosphate additives on the pH of processed chicken exudates and the survival of Campylobacter. *J Food Prot.* 2011;74(10):1735–40.
1484. Sherman RA, Mehta O. Dietary phosphorus restriction in dialysis patients: potential impact of processed meat, poultry, and fish products as protein sources. *Am J Kidney Dis.* 2009;54(1):18–23.
1485. Sherman RA, Mehta O. Dietary phosphorus restriction in dialysis patients: potential impact of processed meat, poultry, and fish products as protein sources. *Am J Kidney Dis.* 2009;54(1):18–23.
1486. Sullivan CM, Leon JB, Sehgal AR. Phosphorus-containing food additives and the accuracy of nutrient databases: implications for renal patients. *J Ren Nutr.* 2007;17(5):350–4.
1487. Trans fat. Food and Drug Administration, Department of Health and Human Services. https://www.fda.gov/food/food-additives-petitions/trans-fat. April 30, 2024. Accessed February 5, 2025.
1488. Food and Drug Administration, Department of Health and Human Services. Tentative determination regarding partially hydrogenated oils; request for comments and for scientific data and information. Federal Register Docket No. D78 FR 67169–75. https://www.federalregister.gov/articles/2013/11/08/2013-26854/tentative-determination-regarding-partially-hydrogenated-oils-request-for-comments-and-for. November 8, 2013. Accessed February 5, 2025.
1489. Food and Drug Administration, Department of Health and Human Services. Tentative determination regarding partially hydrogenated oils; request for comments and for scientific data and information. Federal Register Docket No. D78 FR 67169–75. https://www.federalregister.gov/articles/2013/11/08/2013-26854/tentative-determination-regarding-partially-hydrogenated-oils-request-for-comments-and-for. November 8, 2013. Accessed February 5, 2025.
1490. Neltner TG, Kulkami NR, Alger HM, et al. Navigating the U.S. food additive regulatory program. *Compr Rev Food Sci Food Saf.* 2011;10(6):342–68.
1491. Neltner TG, Alger HM, O'Reilly JT, Krimsky S, Bero LA, Maffini MV. Conflicts of interest in approvals of additives to food determined to be generally recognized as safe: out of balance. *JAMA Intern Med.* 2013;173(22):2032–6.
1492. Stuckler D, Basu S, McKee M. Commentary: UN high level meeting on non-communicable diseases: an opportunity for whom? *BMJ.* 2011;343:d5336.
1493. Moodie R, Stuckler D, Monteiro C, et al. Profits and pandemics: prevention of harmful effects of tobacco, alcohol, and ultra-processed food and drink industries. *Lancet.* 2013;381(9867):670–9.
1494. U.S. Cancer Statistics Working Group. U.S. Cancer Statistics Data Visualizations Tool. U.S. Department of Health and Human Services, Centers for Disease Control and Prevention and National Cancer Institute. https://www.cdc.gov/cancer/dataviz. June 2024. Accessed February 5, 2025.
1495. Kirkali Z, Cal C. Renal Cell Carcinoma: Overview. In Nargund VH, Raghavan D, Sandler HM, eds. *Urological Oncology.* London, UK: Springer; 2008:263–80.
1496. Kirkali Z, Cal C. Renal Cell Carcinoma: Overview. In Nargund VH, Raghavan D, Sandler HM, eds. *Urological Oncology.* London, UK: Springer; 2008:263–80.
1497. Ramírez N, Özel MZ, Lewis AC, Marcé RM, Borrull F, Hamilton JF. Exposure to nitrosamines in thirdhand tobacco smoke increases cancer risk in non-smokers. *Environ Int.* 2014;71:139–47.
1498. Schick SF, Farraro KF, Perrino C, et al. Thirdhand cigarette smoke in an experimental chamber: evidence of surface deposition of nicotine, nitrosamines and polycyclic aromatic hydrocarbons and de novo formation of NNK. *Tob Control.* 2014;23(2):152–9.

1499. Hecht SS. It is time to regulate carcinogenic tobacco-specific nitrosamines in cigarette tobacco. *Cancer Prev Res* (Phila). 2014;7(7):639–47.
1500. Rodgman A, Perfetti TA. *The Chemical Components of Tobacco and Tobacco Smoke.* Boca Raton, FL: CRC Press, Taylor & Francis Group; 2009.
1501. Haorah J, Zhou L, Wang X, Xu G, Mirvish SS. Determination of total N-nitroso compounds and their precursors in frankfurters, fresh meat, dried salted fish, sauces, tobacco, and tobacco smoke particulates. *J Agric Food Chem.* 2001;49(12):6068–78.
1502. Rohrmann S, Overvad K, Bueno-de-Mesquita HB, et al. Meat consumption and mortality—results from the European Prospective Investigation into Cancer and Nutrition. *BMC Med.* 2013;11:63.
1503. Sinha R, Cross AJ, Graubard BI, Leitzmann MF, Schatzkin A. Meat intake and mortality: a prospective study of over half a million people. *Arch Intern Med.* 2009;169(6):562–71.
1504. IARC Working Group on the Evaluation of Carcinogenic Risks to Humans. *IARC Monographs on the Evaluation of Carcinogenic Risks to Humans: Red Meat and Processed Meat.* Vol 11. Lyon (France): WHO; 2018.
1505. Office on Smoking and Health (US). The health consequences of involuntary exposure to tobacco smoke: a report of the Surgeon General. U.S. Centers for Disease Control and Prevention. https://www.ncbi.nlm.nih.gov/books/NBK44324/. 2006. Accessed February 6, 2025.
1506. De Smet S, Van Hecke T. Meat products in human nutrition and health—about hazards and risks. *Meat Sci.* 2024;218:109628.
1507. Additives in meat and poultry products. Food Safety and Inspection Service, United States Department of Agriculture. https://www.fsis.usda.gov/food-safety/safe-food-handling-and-preparation/food-safety-basics/additives-meat-and-poultry. September 27, 2024. Accessed February 5, 2025.
1508. Sebranek JG, Jackson-Davis AL, Myers KL, Lavieri NA. Beyond celery and starter culture: advances in natural/organic curing processes in the United States. *Meat Sci.* 2012;92(3):267–73.
1509. Dellavalle CT, Daniel CR, Aschebrook-Kilfoy B, et al. Dietary intake of nitrate and nitrite and risk of renal cell carcinoma in the NIH-AARP Diet and Health Study. *Br J Cancer.* 2013;108(1):205–12.
1510. Bartsch H, Ohshima H, Pignatelli B. Inhibitors of endogenous nitrosation. Mechanisms and implications in human cancer prevention. *Mutat Res.* 1988;202(2):307–24.
1511. Dellavalle CT, Daniel CR, Aschebrook-Kilfoy B, et al. Dietary intake of nitrate and nitrite and risk of renal cell carcinoma in the NIH-AARP Diet and Health Study. *Br J Cancer.* 2013;108(1):205–12.
1512. Liu B, Mao Q, Wang X, et al. Cruciferous vegetables consumption and risk of renal cell carcinoma: a meta-analysis. *Nutr Cancer.* 2013;65(5):668–76.
1513. U. S. Centers for Disease Control and Prevention, National Center for Health Statistics. National Vital Statistics System, Mortality 2018–2023 on CDC WONDER Online Database. http://wonder.cdc.gov/ucd-icd10-expanded.html. Accessed January 16, 2025.
1514. Sartorius N. The economic and social burden of depression. *J Clin Psychiatry.* 2001;62 Suppl 15:8–11.
1515. Preamble to the Constitution of the World Health Organization as adopted by the International Health Conference, New York, 19–22 June 1946; signed on 22 July 1946 by the representatives of 61 States (Official Records of the World Health Organization, no. 2, p. 100) and entered into force on 7 April 1948.
1516. Kessler RC, Chiu WT, Demler O, Merikangas KR, Walters EE. Prevalence, severity, and comorbidity of 12-month DSM-IV disorders in the National Comorbidity Survey Replication. *Arch Gen Psychiatry.* 2005;62(6):617–27.
1517. Chida Y, Steptoe A. Positive psychological well-being and mortality: a quantitative review of prospective observational studies. *Psychosom Med.* 2008;70(7):741–56.
1518. Chida Y, Steptoe A. Positive psychological well-being and mortality: a quantitative review of prospective observational studies. *Psychosom Med.* 2008;70(7):741–56.

1519. Grant N, Wardle J, Steptoe A. The relationship between life satisfaction and health behavior: a cross-cultural analysis of young adults. *Int J Behav Med.* 2009;16(3):259–68.
1520. Cohen S, Doyle WJ, Turner RB, Alper CM, Skoner DP. Emotional style and susceptibility to the common cold. *Psychosom Med.* 2003;65(4):652–7.
1521. Cohen S, Alper CM, Doyle WJ, Treanor JJ, Turner RB. Positive emotional style predicts resistance to illness after experimental exposure to rhinovirus or influenza A virus. *Psychosom Med.* 2006;68(6):809–15.
1522. Beezhold BL, Johnston CS, Daigle DR. Vegetarian diets are associated with healthy mood states: a cross-sectional study in Seventh Day Adventist adults. *Nutr J.* 2010;9:26.
1523. Beezhold BL, Johnston CS, Daigle DR. Vegetarian diets are associated with healthy mood states: a cross-sectional study in Seventh Day Adventist adults. *Nutr J.* 2010;9:26.
1524. Knutsen SF. Lifestyle and the use of health services. *Am J Clin Nutr.* 1994;59(5 Suppl):1171S–1175S.
1525. Beezhold BL, Johnston CS, Daigle DR. Vegetarian diets are associated with healthy mood states: a cross-sectional study in Seventh Day Adventist adults. *Nutr J.* 2010;9:26.
1526. Fisher M, Levine PH, Weiner B, et al. The effect of vegetarian diets on plasma lipid and platelet levels. *Arch Intern Med.* 1986;146(6):1193–7.
1527. Institute of Medicine. *Dietary Reference Intakes: The Essential Guide to Nutrient Requirements.* Washington, D.C.: National Academies Press; 2006.
1528. Vaz JS, Kac G, Nardi AE, Hibbeln JR. Omega-6 fatty acids and greater likelihood of suicide risk and major depression in early pregnancy. *J Affect Disord.* 2014;152–154:76–82.
1529. National Cancer Institute. Identification of top food sources of various dietary components. Epidemiology and Genomics Research Program. https://epi.grants.cancer.gov/diet/foodsources. November 30, 2019. Accessed February 12, 2025.
1530. Hirota S, Adachi N, Gomyo T, Kawashima H, Kiso Y, Kawabata T. Low-dose arachidonic acid intake increases erythrocytes and plasma arachidonic acid in young women. *Prostaglandins Leukot Essent Fatty Acids.* 2010;83(2):83–8.
1531. Beezhold BL, Johnston CS, Daigle DR. Vegetarian diets are associated with healthy mood states: a cross-sectional study in Seventh Day Adventist adults. *Nutr J.* 2010;9:26.
1532. Beezhold BL, Johnston CS. Restriction of meat, fish, and poultry in omnivores improves mood: a pilot randomized controlled trial. *Nutr J.* 2012;11:9.
1533. Beezhold BL, Johnston CS, Daigle DR. Restriction of flesh foods in omnivores improves mood: a pilot randomized controlled trial. American Public Health Association Annual Conference, November 7–11, 2009. Philadelphia, PA.
1534. Katcher HI, Ferdowsian HR, Hoover VJ, Cohen JL, Barnard ND. A worksite vegan nutrition program is well-accepted and improves health-related quality of life and work productivity. *Ann Nutr Metab.* 2010;56(4):245–52.
1535. Katcher HI, Ferdowsian HR, Hoover VJ, Cohen JL, Barnard ND. A worksite vegan nutrition program is well-accepted and improves health-related quality of life and work productivity. *Ann Nutr Metab.* 2010;56(4):245–52.
1536. Mishra S, Xu J, Agarwal U, Gonzales J, Levin S, Barnard ND. A multicenter randomized controlled trial of a plant-based nutrition program to reduce body weight and cardiovascular risk in the corporate setting: the GEICO study. *Eur J Clin Nutr.* 2013;67(7):718–24.
1537. Agarwal U, Mishra S, Xu J, Levin S, Gonzales J, Barnard ND. A multicenter randomized controlled trial of a nutrition intervention program in a multiethnic adult population in the corporate setting reduces depression and anxiety and improves quality of life: the GEICO Study. *Am J Health Promot.* 2015;29(4):245–54.
1538. Sarris J, Logan AC, Akbaraly TN, et al. Nutritional medicine as mainstream in psychiatry. *Lancet Psych.* 2015;2(3):271–4.
1539. Firth J, Marx W, Dash S, et al. The effects of dietary improvement on symptoms of depression and anxiety: a meta-analysis of randomized controlled trials. *Psychosom Med.* 2019;81(3):265–80.

1540. Jacka FN, O'Neil A, Opie R, et al. A randomised controlled trial of dietary improvement for adults with major depression (the 'SMILES' trial). *BMC Med.* 2017;15(1):23.
1541. Jacka FN, O'Neil A, Opie R, et al. A randomised controlled trial of dietary improvement for adults with major depression (the 'SMILES' trial). *BMC Med.* 2017;15(1):23.
1542. Parletta N, Zarnowiecki D, Cho J, et al. A Mediterranean-style dietary intervention supplemented with fish oil improves diet quality and mental health in people with depression: a randomized controlled trial (HELFIMED). *Nutr Neurosci.* 2019;22(7):474–87.
1543. Appleton KM, Voyias PD, Sallis HM, et al. Omega-3 fatty acids for depression in adults. *Cochrane Database Syst Rev.* 2021;11(11):CD004692.
1544. Parletta N, Zarnowiecki D, Cho J, et al. A Mediterranean-style dietary intervention supplemented with fish oil improves diet quality and mental health in people with depression: a randomized controlled trial (HELFIMED). *Nutr Neurosci.* 2019;22(7):474–87.
1545. Tsai AC, Chang TL, Chi SH. Frequent consumption of vegetables predicts lower risk of depression in older Taiwanese—results of a prospective population-based study. *Public Health Nutr.* 2012;15(6):1087–92.
1546. Gomez-Pinilla F, Nguyen TTJ. Natural mood foods: the actions of polyphenols against psychiatric and cognitive disorders. *Nutr Neurosci.* 2012;15(3):127–33.
1547. Meyer JH, Ginovart N, Boovariwala A, et al. Elevated monoamine oxidase A levels in the brain: an explanation for the monoamine imbalance of major depression. *Arch Gen Psychiatry.* 2006;63(11):1209–16.
1548. de Villiers JC. Intracranial haemorrhage in patients treated with monoamineoxidase inhibitors. *Br J Psychiatry.* 1966;112(483):109–18.
1549. Dixon Clarke SE, Ramsay RR. Dietary inhibitors of monoamine oxidase A. *J Neural Transm.* 2011;118(7):1031–41.
1550. Lai JS, Hiles S, Bisquera A, Hure AJ, McEvoy M, Attia J. A systematic review and meta-analysis of dietary patterns and depression in community-dwelling adults. *Am J Clin Nutr.* 2014;99(1):181–97.
1551. White BA, Horwath CC, Conner TS. Many apples a day keep the blues away—daily experiences of negative and positive affect and food consumption in young adults. *Br J Health Psychol.* 2013;18(4):782–98.
1552. Odjakova M, Hadjiivanova C. Animal neurotransmitter substances in plants. *Bulg J Plant Physiol.* 1997;23:94–102.
1553. Ghirri A, Cannella C, Bignetti E. The psychoactive effects of aromatic amino acids. *Curr Nutr Food Science.* 2011;7(1):21–32.
1554. Allen JA, Peterson A, Sufit R, et al. Post-epidemic eosinophilia-myalgia syndrome associated with L-tryptophan. *Arthritis Rheum.* 2011;63(11):3633–9.
1555. Fernstrom JD, Faller DV. Neutral amino acids in the brain: changes in response to food ingestion. *J Neurochem.* 1978;30(6):1531–8.
1556. Wurtman RJ, Wurtman JJ, Regan MM, McDermott JM, Tsay RH, Breu JJ. Effects of normal meals rich in carbohydrates or proteins on plasma tryptophan and tyrosine ratios. *Am J Clin Nutr.* 2003;77(1):128–32.
1557. Wurtman JJ, Brzezinski A, Wurtman RJ, Laferrere B. Effect of nutrient intake on premenstrual depression. *Am J Obstet Gynecol.* 1989;161(5):1228–34.
1558. Brinkworth GD, Buckley JD, Noakes M, Clifton PM, Wilson CJ. Long-term effects of a very low-carbohydrate diet and a low-fat diet on mood and cognitive function. *Arch Intern Med.* 2009;169(20):1873–80.
1559. Fernstrom JD, Wurtman RJ. Brain serotonin content: physiological regulation by plasma neutral amino acids. *Science.* 1972;178(4059):414–6.
1560. Hudson C, Hudson S, MacKenzie J. Protein-source tryptophan as an efficacious treatment for social anxiety disorder: a pilot study. *Can J Physiol Pharmacol.* 2007;85(9):928–32.
1561. Schweiger U, Laessle R, Kittl S, Dickhaut B, Schweiger M, Pirke KM. Macronutrient intake,

plasma large neutral amino acids and mood during weight-reducing diets. *J Neural Transm.* 1986;67(1–2):77–86.
1562. Ferrence SC, Bendersky G. Therapy with saffron and the goddess at Thera. *Perspect Biol Med.* 2004;47(2):199–226.
1563. Noorbala AA, Akhondzadeh S, Tahmacebi-Pour N, Jamshidi AH. Hydro-alcoholic extract of Crocus sativus L. versus fluoxetine in the treatment of mild to moderate depression: a double-blind, randomized pilot trial. *J Ethnopharmacol.* 2005;97(2):281–4.
1564. Gohari AR, Saeidnia S, Mahmoodabadi MK. An overview on saffron, phytochemicals, and medicinal properties. *Pharmacogn Rev.* 2013;7(13):61–6.
1565. Fukui H, Toyoshima K, Komaki R. Psychological and neuroendocrinological effects of odor of saffron (Crocus sativus). *Phytomedicine.* 2011;18(8–9):726–30.
1566. Araj-Khodaei M, Noorbala AA, Yarani R, et al. A double-blind, randomized pilot study for comparison of Melissa officinalis L. and Lavandula angustifolia Mill. with fluoxetine for the treatment of depression. *BMC Complement Med Ther.* 2020;20(1):207.
1567. Ghazizadeh J, Sadigh-Eteghad S, Marx W, et al. The effects of lemon balm (Melissa officinalis L.) on depression and anxiety in clinical trials: a systematic review and meta-analysis. *Phytother Res.* 2021;35(12):6690–705.
1568. Bazrafshan MR, Jokar M, Shokrpour N, Delam H. The effect of lavender herbal tea on the anxiety and depression of the elderly: a randomized clinical trial. *Complement Ther Med.* 2020;50:102393.
1569. Lucas M, O'Reilly EJ, Pan A, et al. Coffee, caffeine, and risk of completed suicide: results from three prospective cohorts of American adults. *World J Biol Psychiatry.* 2014;15(5):377–86.
1570. Klatsky AL, Armstrong MA, Friedman GD. Coffee, tea, and mortality. *Ann Epidemiol.* 1993;3(4):375–81.
1571. Tanskanen A, Tuomilehto J, Viinamnen H, Vartiainen E, Lehtonen J, Puska P. Heavy coffee drinking and the risk of suicide. *Eur J Epidemiol.* 2000;16(9):789–91.
1572. Guo X, Park Y, Freedman ND, et al. Sweetened beverages, coffee, and tea and depression risk among older US adults. *PLoS One.* 2014;9(4):e94715.
1573. Maher TJ, Wurtman RJ. Possible neurologic effects of aspartame, a widely used food additive. *Environ Health Perspect.* 1987;75:53–7.
1574. Walton RG, Hudak R, Green-Waite RJ. Adverse reactions to aspartame: double-blind challenge in patients from a vulnerable population. *Biol Psychiatry.* 1993;34(1–2):13–7.
1575. Lindseth GN, Coolahan SE, Petros TV, Lindseth PD. Neurobehavioral effects of aspartame consumption. *Res Nurs Health.* 2014;37(3):185–93.
1576. U.S. Food and Drug Administration. Aspartame: Commissioner's final decision. *Fed Reg.* 1981;46:38285–308.
1577. Lindseth GN, Coolahan SE, Petros TV, Lindseth PD. Neurobehavioral effects of aspartame consumption. *Res Nurs Health.* 2014;37(3):185–93.
1578. Riboli E, Beland FA, Lachenmeier DW, et al. Carcinogenicity of aspartame, methyleugenol, and isoeugenol. *Lancet Oncol.* 2023;24(8):848–50.
1579. Whitehouse CR, Boullata J, McCauley LA. The potential toxicity of artificial sweeteners. *AAOHN J.* 2008;56(6):251–9.
1580. Aspartame products. Calorie Control Council. https://aspartame.org/aspartame-products/#.VF_cyr74tSU. 2019. Accessed February 11, 2025.
1581. Whitehouse CR, Boullata J, McCauley LA. The potential toxicity of artificial sweeteners. *AAOHN J.* 2008;56(6):251–9.
1582. Yeung RR. The acute effects of exercise on mood state. *J Psychosom Res.* 1996;40(2):123–41.
1583. Goodwin RD. Association between physical activity and mental disorders among adults in the United States. *Prev Med.* 2003;36(6):698–703.
1584. Blumenthal JA, Babyak MA, Moore KA, et al. Effects of exercise training on older patients with major depression. *Arch Intern Med.* 1999;159(19):2349–56.

1585. Blumenthal JA, Babyak MA, Doraiswamy PM, et al. Exercise and pharmacotherapy in the treatment of major depressive disorder. *Psychosom Med.* 2007;69(7):587–96.
1586. Pandya CD, Howell KR, Pillai A. Antioxidants as potential therapeutics for neuropsychiatric disorders. *Prog Neuropsychopharmacol Biol Psychiatry.* 2013;46:214–23.
1587. Michel TM, Pülschen D, Thome J. The role of oxidative stress in depressive disorders. *Curr Pharm Des.* 2012;18(36):5890–9.
1588. McMartin SE, Jacka FN, Colman I. The association between fruit and vegetable consumption and mental health disorders: evidence from five waves of a national survey of Canadians. *Prev Med.* 2013;56(3–4):225–30.
1589. Beydoun MA, Beydoun HA, Boueiz A, Shroff MR, Zonderman AB. Antioxidant status and its association with elevated depressive symptoms among US adults: National Health and Nutrition Examination Surveys 2005–6. *Br J Nutr.* 2013;109(9):1714–29.
1590. Niu K, Guo H, Kakizaki M, et al. A tomato-rich diet is related to depressive symptoms among an elderly population aged 70 years and over: a population-based, cross-sectional analysis. *J Affect Disord.* 2013;144(1–2):165–70.
1591. Fisk J, Khalid S, Reynolds SA, Williams CM. Effect of 4 weeks daily wild blueberry supplementation on symptoms of depression in adolescents. *Br J Nutr.* 2020;124(2):181–8.
1592. Payne ME, Steck SE, George RR, Steffens DC. Fruit, vegetable, and antioxidant intakes are lower in older adults with depression. *J Acad Nutr Diet.* 2012;112(12):2022–7.
1593. Gilbody S, Lightfoot T, Sheldon T. Is low folate a risk factor for depression? A meta-analysis and exploration of heterogeneity. *J Epidemiol Community Health.* 2007;61(7):631–7.
1594. Tolmunen T, Hintikka J, Ruusunen A, et al. Dietary folate and the risk of depression in Finnish middle-aged men. A prospective follow-up study. *Psychother Psychosom.* 2004;73(6):334–9.
1595. Sharpley AL, Hockney R, McPeake L, Geddes JR, Cowen PJ. Folic acid supplementation for prevention of mood disorders in young people at familial risk: a randomised, double blind, placebo controlled trial. *J Affect Disord.* 2014;167:306–11.
1596. Penn E, Tracy DK. The drugs don't work? Antidepressants and the current and future pharmacological management of depression. *Ther Adv Psychopharmacol.* 2012;2(5):179–88.
1597. Turner EH, Matthews AM, Linardatos E, Tell RA, Rosenthal R. Selective publication of antidepressant trials and its influence on apparent efficacy. *N Engl J Med.* 2008;358(3):252–60.
1598. Kirsch I. Antidepressants and the placebo effect. *Z Psychol.* 2014;222(3):128–34.
1599. Kirsch I. Antidepressants and the placebo response. *Epidemiol Psichiatr Soc.* 2009;18(4):318–22.
1600. Spence D. Are antidepressants overprescribed? Yes. *BMJ.* 2013;346:f191.
1601. Brody DJ, Gu Q. Antidepressant use among adults: United States, 2015–2018. *NCHS Data Brief.* 2020;(377):1–8.
1602. Kirsch I. Antidepressants and the placebo effect. *Z Psychol.* 2014;222(3):128–34.
1603. Blease C. Deception as treatment: the case of depression. *J Med Ethics.* 2011;37(1):13–6.
1604. Kirsch I. Antidepressants and the placebo effect. *Z Psychol.* 2014;222(3):128–34.
1605. Kirsch I. Antidepressants and the placebo effect. *Z Psychol.* 2014;222(3):128–34.
1606. Lariscy JT, Hummer RA, Rogers RG. Lung cancer mortality among never-smokers in the United States: estimating smoking-attributable mortality with nationally representative data. *Ann Epidemiol.* 2020;45:5–11.
1607. Giaquinto AN, Sung H, Newman LA, et al. Breast cancer statistics 2024. *CA Cancer J Clin.* 2024; 74(6):477–95.
1608. Sanders ME, Schuyler PA, Dupont WD, Page DL. The natural history of low-grade ductal carcinoma in situ of the breast in women treated by biopsy only revealed over 30 years of long-term follow-up. *Cancer.* 2005;103(12):2481–4.
1609. Nielsen M, Thomsen JL, Primdahl S, Dyreborg U, Andersen JA. Breast cancer and atypia among young and middle-aged women: a study of 110 medicolegal autopsies. *Br J Cancer.* 1987;56(6):814–9.

1610. Soto AM, Brisken C, Schaeberle C, Sonnenschein C. Does cancer start in the womb? Altered mammary gland development and predisposition to breast cancer due to in utero exposure to endocrine disruptors. *J Mammary Gland Biol Neoplasia*. 2013;18(2):199–208.
1611. Del Monte U. Does the cell number 10^9 still really fit one gram of tumor tissue? *Cell Cycle*. 2009;8(3):505–6.
1612. Black WC, Welch HG. Advances in diagnostic imaging and overestimations of disease prevalence and the benefits of therapy. *N Engl J Med*. 1993;328(17):1237–43.
1613. Friberg S, Mattson S. On the growth rates of human malignant tumors: implications for medical decision making. *J Surg Oncol*. 1997;65(4):284–97.
1614. Philippe E, Le Gal Y. Growth of seventy-eight recurrent mammary cancers. Quantitative study. *Cancer*. 1968;21(3):461–7.
1615. Kuroishi T, Tominaga S, Morimoto T, et al. Tumor growth rate and prognosis of breast cancer mainly detected by mass screening. *Jpn J Cancer Res*. 1990;81(5):454–62.
1616. American Association for Cancer Research. Studies weigh cost, effectiveness of mammography. *Cancer Discov*. 2014;4(5):OF5.
1617. Nielsen M, Thomsen JL, Primdahl S, Dyreborg U, Andersen JA. Breast cancer and atypia among young and middle-aged women: a study of 110 medicolegal autopsies. *Br J Cancer*. 1987;56(6):814–9.
1618. Brawley OW, O'Regan RM. Breast cancer screening: time for rational discourse. *Cancer*. 2014;120(18):2800–2.
1619. Biller-Andorno N, Jüni P. Abolishing mammography screening programs? A view from the Swiss Medical Board. *N Engl J Med*. 2014;370(21):1965–7.
1620. Nelson AL. Controversies regarding mammography, breast self-examination, and clinical breast examination. *Obstet Gynecol Clin North Am*. 2013;40(3):413–27.
1621. Loh KP, Stefan MS, Friderici J, et al. Healthcare professionals' perceptions and knowledge of the USPSTF guidelines on breast self-examination. *South Med J*. 2015;108(8):459–62.
1622. Welch HG. Screening mammography—a long run for a short slide? *N Engl J Med*. 2010;363(13):1276–8.
1623. Gigerenzer G. Women's perception of the benefit of breast cancer screening. *Maturitas*. 2010;67(1):5–6.
1624. Atkins CD. Potential hazards of mammography. *J Clin Oncol*. 2007;25(5):604.
1625. Barratt A. Overdiagnosis in mammography screening: a 45 year journey from shadowy idea to acknowledged reality. *BMJ*. 2015;350:h867.
1626. Gøtzsche PC, Jørgensen KJ, Zahl PH, Mæhlen J. Why mammography screening has not lived up to expectations from the randomised trials. *Cancer Causes Control*. 2012;23(1):15–21.
1627. Pace LE, Keating NL. A systematic assessment of benefits and risks to guide breast cancer screening decisions. *JAMA*. 2014;311(13):1327–35.
1628. Gøtzsche PC, Jørgensen KJ, Zahl PH, Mæhlen J. Why mammography screening has not lived up to expectations from the randomised trials. *Cancer Causes Control*. 2012;23(1):15–21.
1629. Sohn E. Screening: don't look now. *Nature*. 2015;527(7578):S118–9.
1630. Gotzsche P. Commentary: screening: a seductive paradigm that has generally failed us. *Int J Epidemiol*. 2015;44(1):278–80.
1631. Derbyshire SWG. Second opinion: doctors, diseases and decisions in modern medicine. *BMJ*. 2003;327(7411):399.
1632. Jørgensen KJ, Gøtzsche PC. The background review for the USPSTF recommendation on screening for breast cancer. *Ann Intern Med*. 2010;152(8):538; author reply 538–9.
1633. American Institute for Cancer Research. Healthy 10 Challenge. https://healthy10challenge .org/. Accessed February 7, 2025.
1634. AICR, the China Study, and *Forks Over Knives*. American Institute for Cancer Research. https: //web.archive.org/web/20130725055418/http://www.aicr.org/about/advocacy/the-china -study.html. July 24, 2013. Accessed February 8, 2025.
1635. Hastert TA, Beresford SAA, Patterson RE, Kristal AR, White E. Adherence to WCRF/

AICR cancer prevention recommendations and risk of postmenopausal breast cancer. *Cancer Epidemiol Biomarkers Prev.* 2013;22(9):1498–508.
1636. Barnard RJ, Gonzalez JH, Liva ME, Ngo TH. Effects of a low-fat, high-fiber diet and exercise program on breast cancer risk factors in vivo and tumor cell growth and apoptosis in vitro. *Nutr Cancer.* 2006;55(1):28–34.
1637. Ngo TH, Barnard RJ, Tymchuk CN, Cohen P, Aronson WJ. Effect of diet and exercise on serum insulin, IGF-I, and IGFBP-1 levels and growth of LNCaP cells in vitro (United States). *Cancer Causes Control.* 2002;13(10):929–35.
1638. Allen NE, Appleby PN, Davey GK, Kaaks R, Rinaldi S, Key TJ. The associations of diet with serum insulin-like growth factor I and its main binding proteins in 292 women meat-eaters, vegetarians, and vegans. *Cancer Epidemiol Biomarkers Prev.* 2002;11(11):1441–8.
1639. Office of the U.S. Surgeon General. *Alcohol and Cancer Risk: The U.S. Surgeon General's Advisory, 2025.* https://www.hhs.gov/sites/default/files/oash-alcohol-cancer-risk.pdf. Accessed January 4, 2025.
1640. International Agency for Research on Cancer. Alcohol drinking. *IARC Monogr Eval Carcinog Risks Hum.* 1988;44:1–378.
1641. Bagnardi V, Rota M, Botteri E, et al. Alcohol consumption and site-specific cancer risk: a comprehensive dose-response meta-analysis. *Br J Cancer.* 2015;112(3):580–93.
1642. Choi YJ, Myung SK, Lee JH. Light alcohol drinking and risk of cancer: a meta-analysis of cohort studies. *Cancer Res Treat.* 2018;50(2):474–87.
1643. Jun S, Park H, Kim UJ, et al. Cancer risk based on alcohol consumption levels: a comprehensive systematic review and meta-analysis. *Epidemiol Health.* 2023;45:e2023092.
1644. SEER*Explorer. Surveillance Research Program, National Cancer Institute. https://seer.cancer.gov/statistics-network/explorer/. November 5, 2024. Accessed February 5, 2025.
1645. Bagnardi V, Rota M, Botteri E, et al. Light alcohol drinking and cancer: a meta-analysis. *Ann Oncol.* 2013;24(2):301–8.
1646. Bagnardi V, Blangiardo M, La Vecchia C, Corrao G. Alcohol consumption and the risk of cancer: a meta-analysis. *Alcohol Res Health.* 2001;25(4):263–70.
1647. Rani S, Laupacis A. "Less is better" is the best message when talking to patients about alcohol. *CMAJ.* 2023;195(36):E1232–3.
1648. Testino G, Caputo F, Patussi V, Scafato E. Alcohol and cancer: no threshold exists. *Minerva Med.* 2020;111(6):523–5.
1649. Rock CL, Thomson C, Gansler T, et al. American Cancer Society guideline for diet and physical activity for cancer prevention. *CA Cancer J Clin.* 2020;70(4):245–71.
1650. Linderborg K, Salaspuro M, Väkeväinen S. A single sip of a strong alcoholic beverage causes exposure to carcinogenic concentrations of acetaldehyde in the oral cavity. *Food Chem Toxicol.* 2011;49(9):2103–6.
1651. Lachenmeier DW, Gumbel-Mako S, Sohnius EM, Keck-Wilhelm A, Kratz E, Mildau G. Salivary acetaldehyde increase due to alcohol-containing mouthwash use: a risk factor for oral cancer. *Int J Cancer.* 2009;125(3):730–5.
1652. Chen WY, Rosner B, Hankinson SE, Colditz GA, Willett WC. Moderate alcohol consumption during adult life, drinking patterns, and breast cancer risk. *JAMA.* 2011;306(17):1884–90.
1653. Shufelt C, Merz CN, Yang Y, et al. Red versus white wine as a nutritional aromatase inhibitor in premenopausal women: a pilot study. *J Womens Health* (Larchmt). 2012;21(3):281–4.
1654. Eng ET, Williams D, Mandava U, Kirma N, Tekmal RR, Chen S. Anti-aromatase chemicals in red wine. *Ann N Y Acad Sci.* 2002;963:239–46.
1655. Shufelt C, Merz CN, Yang Y, et al. Red versus white wine as a nutritional aromatase inhibitor in premenopausal women: a pilot study. *J Womens Health* (Larchmt). 2012;21(3):281–4.
1656. Chen S, Sun XZ, Kao YC, Kwon A, Zhou D, Eng E. Suppression of breast cancer cell growth with grape juice. *Pharmaceutical Biology.* 1998;36(Suppl 1):53–61.
1657. Chen S, Sun XZ, Kao YC, Kwon A, Zhou D, Eng E. Suppression of breast cancer cell growth with grape juice. *Pharmaceutical Biology.* 1998;36(Suppl 1):53–61.

1658. Adams LS, Zhang Y, Seeram NP, Heber D, Chen S. Pomegranate ellagitannin-derived compounds exhibit anti-proliferative and anti-aromatase activity in breast cancer cells in vitro. *Cancer Prev Res* (Phila). 2010;3(1):108–13.
1659. Chen S, Oh SR, Phung S, et al. Anti-aromatase activity of phytochemicals in white button mushrooms (Agaricus bisporus). *Cancer Res*. 2006;66(24):12026–34.
1660. Mishal AA. Effects of different dress styles on vitamin D levels in healthy young Jordanian women. *Osteoporos Int*. 2001;12(11):931–5.
1661. Cardinali DP, Pévet P. Basic aspects of melatonin action. *Sleep Med Rev*. 1998;2(3):175–90.
1662. Sehgal A. Physiology flies with time. *Cell*. 2017;171(6):1232–5.
1663. Froy O, Miskin R. Effect of feeding regimens on circadian rhythms: implications for aging and longevity. *Aging* (Albany NY). 2010;2(1):7–27.
1664. Ruddick-Collins LC, Johnston JD, Morgan PJ, Johnstone AM. The big breakfast study: chrono-nutrition influence on energy expenditure and bodyweight. *Nutr Bull*. 2018;43(2):174–83.
1665. Challet E. Circadian clocks, food intake, and metabolism. *Prog Mol Biol Transl Sci*. 2013;119:105–35.
1666. Green CB, Takahashi JS, Bass J. The meter of metabolism. *Cell*. 2008;134(5):728–42.
1667. Van Someren EJ, Riemersma-Van Der Lek RF. Live to the rhythm, slave to the rhythm. *Sleep Med Rev*. 2007;11(6):465–84.
1668. Panda S. Circadian physiology of metabolism. *Science*. 2016;354(6315):1008–15.
1669. Oda H. Chrononutrition. *J Nutr Sci Vitaminol*. 2015;61 Suppl:S92–4.
1670. Carroll R, Metcalfe C, Gunnell D, Mohamed F, Eddleston M. Diurnal variation in probability of death following self-poisoning in Sri Lanka—evidence for chronotoxicity in humans. *Int J Epidemiol*. 2012;41(6):1821–8.
1671. Dallmann R, Okyar A, Lévi F. Dosing-time makes the poison: circadian regulation and pharmacotherapy. *Trends Mol Med*. 2016;22(5):430–45.
1672. Kirley K, Sharma U, Rowland K. PURLs: BP meds: this simple change improves outcomes. *J Fam Pract*. 2012;61(3):153–5.
1673. Hermida RC, Ayala DE, Mojón A, Fernández JR. Influence of circadian time of hypertension treatment on cardiovascular risk: results of the MAPEC study. *Chronobiol Int*. 2010;27(8):1629–51.
1674. Beccuti G, Monagheddu C, Evangelista A, et al. Timing of food intake: sounding the alarm about metabolic impairments? A systematic review. *Pharmacol Res*. 2017;125(Pt B):132–41.
1675. Blask DE, Dauchy RT, Sauer LA. Putting cancer to sleep at night: the neuroendocrine/circadian melatonin signal. *Endocrine*. 2005;27(2):179–88.
1676. Flynn-Evans EE, Stevens RG, Tabandeh H, Schernhammer ES, Lockley SW. Total visual blindness is protective against breast cancer. *Cancer Causes Control*. 2009;20(9):1753–6.
1677. He C, Anand ST, Ebell MH, Vena JE, Robb SW. Circadian disrupting exposures and breast cancer risk: a meta-analysis. *Int Arch Occup Environ Health*. 2015 Jul;88(5):533–47.
1678. Hurley S, Goldberg D, Nelson D, et al. Light at night and breast cancer risk among California teachers. *Epidemiology*. 2014;25(5):697–706.
1679. Bauer SE, Wagner SE, Burch J, Bayakly R, Vena JE. A case-referent study: light at night and breast cancer risk in Georgia. *Int J Health Geogr*. 2013;12:23.
1680. Kloog I, Haim A, Stevens RG, Barchana M, Portnov BA. Light at night co-distributes with incident breast but not lung cancer in the female population of Israel. *Chronobiol Int*. 2008;25(1):65–81.
1681. Li Q, Zheng T, Holford TR, Boyle P, Zhang Y, Dai M. Light at night and breast cancer risk: results from a population-based case-control study in Connecticut, USA. *Cancer Causes Control*. 2010;21(12):2281–5.
1682. Basler M, Jetter A, Fink D, Seifert B, Kullak-Ublick GA, Trojan A. Urinary excretion of melatonin and association with breast cancer: meta-analysis and review of the literature. *Breast Care* (Basel). 2014;9(3):182–7.

1683. Nagata C, Nagao Y, Shibuya C, Kashiki Y, Shimizu H. Association of vegetable intake with urinary 6-sulfatoxymelatonin level. *Cancer Epidemiol Biomarkers Prev.* 2005;14(5):1333–5.
1684. Schernhammer ES, Feskanich D, Niu C, Dopfel R, Holmes MD, Hankinson SE. Dietary correlates of urinary 6-sulfatoxymelatonin concentrations in the Nurses' Health Study cohorts. *Am J Clin Nutr.* 2009;90(4):975–85.
1685. Gonçalves AK, Dantas Florencio GL, Maisonnette de Atayde Silva MJ, Cobucci RN, Giraldo PC, Cote NM. Effects of physical activity on breast cancer prevention: a systematic review. *J Phys Act Health.* 2014;11(2):445–54.
1686. Friedenreich CM, Woolcott CG, McTiernan A, et al. Alberta physical activity and breast cancer prevention trial: sex hormone changes in a year-long exercise intervention among postmenopausal women. *J Clin Oncol.* 2010;28(9):1458–66.
1687. Kossman DA, Williams NI, Domchek SM, Kurzer MS, Stopfer JE, Schmitz KH. Exercise lowers estrogen and progesterone levels in premenopausal women at high risk of breast cancer. *J Appl Physiol.* 2011;111(6):1687–93.
1688. Thune I, Furberg AS. Physical activity and cancer risk: dose-response and cancer, all sites and site-specific. *Med Sci Sports Exerc.* 2001;33(6 Suppl):S530–50.
1689. Carpenter CL, Ross RK, Paganini-Hill A, Bernstein L. Lifetime exercise activity and breast cancer risk among post-menopausal women. *Br J Cancer.* 1999;80(11):1852–8.
1690. Peters TM, Moore SC, Gierach GL, et al. Intensity and timing of physical activity in relation to postmenopausal breast cancer risk: the prospective NIH-AARP diet and health study. *BMC Cancer.* 2009;9:349.
1691. Friedenreich CM, Cust AE. Physical activity and breast cancer risk: impact of timing, type and dose of activity and population subgroup effects. *Br J Sports Med.* 2008;42(8):636–47.
1692. Hildebrand JS, Gapstur SM, Campbell PT, Gaudet MM, Patel AV. Recreational physical activity and leisure-time sitting in relation to postmenopausal breast cancer risk. *Cancer Epidemiol Biomarkers Prev.* 2013;22(10):1906–12.
1693. Widmark EMP. Presence of cancer-producing substances in roasted food. *Nature.* 1939;143:984.
1694. Chemicals in meat cooked at high temperatures and cancer risk. National Cancer Institute. https://www.cancer.gov/about-cancer/causes-prevention/risk/diet/cooked-meats-fact-sheet. July 11, 2017. Accessed February 7, 2025.
1695. Shaughnessy DT, Gangarosa LM, Schliebe B, et al. Inhibition of fried meat-induced colorectal DNA damage and altered systemic genotoxicity in humans by crucifera, chlorophyllin, and yogurt. *PLoS ONE.* 2011;6(4):e18707.
1696. Zaidi R, Kumar S, Rawat PR. Rapid detection and quantification of dietary mutagens in food using mass spectrometry and ultra performance liquid chromatography. *Food Chem.* 2012;135(4):2897–903.
1697. Thiébaud HP, Knize MG, Kuzmicky PA, Hsieh DP, Felton JS. Airborne mutagens produced by frying beef, pork and a soy-based food. *Food Chem Toxicol.* 1995;33(10):821–8.
1698. Zheng W, Lee SA. Well-done meat intake, heterocyclic amine exposure, and cancer risk. *Nutr Cancer.* 2009;61(4):437–46.
1699. Goldfinger SE. By the way, doctor. In your May issue you say that eating medium or well-done beef increases one's risk for stomach cancer. But what about the dangers of eating rare beef? *Harv Health Lett.* 1999;24(5):7.
1700. Frandsen H, Frederiksen H, Alexander J. 2-Amino-1-methyl-6-(5-hydroxy-)phenylimidazo[4,5-b]pyridine (5-OH-PhIP), a biomarker for the genotoxic dose of the heterocyclic amine, 2-amino-1-methyl-6-phenylimidazo[4,5-b]pyridine (PhIP). *Food Chem Toxicol.* 2002;40(8):1125–30.
1701. Frandsen H. Biomonitoring of urinary metabolites of 2-amino-1-methyl-6-phenylimidazo[4,5-b]pyridine (PhIP) following human consumption of cooked chicken. *Food Chem Toxicol.* 2008;46(9):3200–5.
1702. Steck SE, Gaudet MM, Eng SM, et al. Cooked meat and risk of breast cancer—lifetime versus recent dietary intake. *Epidemiology.* 2007;18(3):373–82.

1703. Zheng W, Gustafson DR, Sinha R, et al. Well-done meat intake and the risk of breast cancer. *J Natl Cancer Inst.* 1998;90(22):1724–9.
1704. Rohrmann S, Lukas Jung SU, Linseisen J, Pfau W. Dietary intake of meat and meat-derived heterocyclic aromatic amines and their correlation with DNA adducts in female breast tissue. *Mutagenesis.* 2009;24(2):127–32.
1705. Santella RM, Gammon M, Terry M, et al. DNA adducts, DNA repair genotype/phenotype and cancer risk. *Mutat Res.* 2005;592(1–2):29–35.
1706. Lauber SN, Ali S, Gooderham NJ. The cooked food derived carcinogen 2-amino-1-methyl-6-phenylimidazo[4,5-b] pyridine is a potent oestrogen: a mechanistic basis for its tissue-specific carcinogenicity. *Carcinogenesis.* 2004;25(12):2509–17.
1707. Debruin LS, Martos PA, Josephy PD. Detection of PhIP (2-amino-1-methyl-6-phenylimidazo [4,5-b]pyridine) in the milk of healthy women. *Chem Res Toxicol.* 2001;14(11):1523–8.
1708. Lauber SN, Ali S, Gooderham NJ. The cooked food derived carcinogen 2-amino-1-methyl-6-phenylimidazo[4,5-b] pyridine is a potent oestrogen: a mechanistic basis for its tissue-specific carcinogenicity. *Carcinogenesis.* 2004;25(12):2509–17.
1709. Debruin LS, Martos PA, Josephy PD. Detection of PhIP (2-amino-1-methyl-6-phenylimidazo [4,5-b]pyridine) in the milk of healthy women. *Chem Res Toxicol.* 2001;14(11):1523–8.
1710. Bessette EE, Yasa I, Dunbar D, Wilkens LR, Le Marchand L, Turesky RJ. Biomonitoring of carcinogenic heterocyclic aromatic amines in hair: a validation study. *Chem Res Toxicol.* 2009;22(8):1454–63.
1711. Grose KR, Grant JL, Bjeldanes LF, et al. Isolation of the carcinogen IQ from fried egg patties. *J Agric Food Chem.* 1986;34(2):201–2.
1712. Holland RD, Gehring T, Taylor J, Lake BG, Gooderham NJ, Turesky RJ. Formation of a mutagenic heterocyclic aromatic amine from creatinine in urine of meat eaters and vegetarians. *Chem Res Toxicol.* 2005;18(3):579–90.
1713. Magagnotti C, Orsi F, Bagnati R, et al. Effect of diet on serum albumin and hemoglobin adducts of 2-amino-1-methyl-6-phenylimidazo[4,5-b]pyridine (PhIP) in humans. *Int J Cancer.* 2000;88(1):1–6.
1714. Lauber SN, Gooderham NJ. The cooked meat-derived mammary carcinogen 2-amino-1-methyl-6-phenylimidazo[4,5-b]pyridine promotes invasive behaviour of breast cancer cells. *Toxicology.* 2011;279(1–3):139–45.
1715. Lauber SN, Gooderham NJ. The cooked meat-derived mammary carcinogen 2-amino-1-methyl-6-phenylimidazo[4,5-b]pyridine promotes invasive behaviour of breast cancer cells. *Toxicology.* 2011;279(1–3):139–45.
1716. Maunsell E, Drolet M, Brisson J, Robert J, Deschell L. Dietary change after breast cancer: extent, predictors, and relation with psychological distress. *J Clin Oncol.* 2002;20(4):1017–25.
1717. Pierce JP, Stefanick ML, Flatt SW, et al. Greater survival after breast cancer in physically active women with high vegetable-fruit intake regardless of obesity. *J Clin Oncol.* 2007;25(17):2345–51.
1718. Parise CA, Caggiano V. Breast cancer survival defined by the ER/PR/HER2 subtypes and a surrogate classification according to tumor grade and immunohistochemical biomarkers. *J Cancer Epidemiol.* 2014;2014:469251.
1719. Romanos-Nanclares A, Willett WC, Rosner BA, et al. Healthful and unhealthful plant-based diets and risk of breast cancer in U.S. women: results from the Nurses' Health Studies. *Cancer Epidemiol Biomarkers Prev.* 2021;30(10):1921–31.
1720. Link LB, Canchola AJ, Bernstein L, et al. Dietary patterns and breast cancer risk in the California Teachers Study cohort. *Am J Clin Nutr.* 2013;98(6):1524–32.
1721. Hankinson SE. Circulating levels of sex steroids and prolactin in premenopausal women and risk of breast cancer. In: Li JJ, Li SA, Mohla S, Rochefort H, Maudelonde T, eds. *Hormonal Carcinogenesis V.* Springer; 2008:161–9.
1722. Key T, Appleby P, Barnes I, et al. Endogenous sex hormones and breast cancer in postmenopausal women: reanalysis of nine prospective studies. *J Natl Cancer Inst.* 2002;94(8):606–16.

1723. Hankinson SE. Circulating levels of sex steroids and prolactin in premenopausal women and risk of breast cancer. In: Li JJ, Li SA, Mohla S, Rochefort H, Maudelonde T, eds. *Hormonal Carcinogenesis V.* Springer; 2008:161–9.
1724. Cleary MP, Grossmann ME. Minireview: obesity and breast cancer: the estrogen connection. *Endocrinology.* 2009;150(6):2537–42.
1725. Shultz TD, Leklem JE. Nutrient intake and hormonal status of premenopausal vegetarian Seventh-day Adventists and premenopausal nonvegetarians. *Nutr Cancer.* 1983;4(4):247–59.
1726. Barbosa JC, Shultz TD, Filley SJ, Nieman DC. The relationship among adiposity, diet, and hormone concentrations in vegetarian and nonvegetarian postmenopausal women. *Am J Clin Nutr.* 1990;51(5):798–803.
1727. Shultz TD, Howie BJ. In vitro binding of steroid hormones by natural and purified fibers. *Nutr Cancer.* 1986;8(2):141–7.
1728. Goldin BR, Woods MN, Spiegelman DL, et al. The effect of dietary fat and fiber on serum estrogen concentrations in premenopausal women under controlled dietary conditions. *Cancer.* 1994;74(3 Suppl):1125–31.
1729. Jew S, AbuMweis SS, Jones PJH. Evolution of the human diet: linking our ancestral diet to modern functional foods as a means of chronic disease prevention. *J Med Food.* 2009;12(5):925–34.
1730. Goldin BR, Adlercreutz H, Dwyer JT, Swenson L, Warram JH, Gorbach SL. Effect of diet on excretion of estrogens in pre- and postmenopausal women. *Cancer Res.* 1981;41(9 Pt 2):3771–3.
1731. Goldin BR, Adlercreutz H, Gorbach SL, et al. Estrogen excretion patterns and plasma levels in vegetarian and omnivorous women. *N Engl J Med.* 1982;307(25):1542–7.
1732. Li Q, Holford TR, Zhang Y, et al. Dietary fiber intake and risk of breast cancer by menopausal and estrogen receptor status. *Eur J Nutr.* 2013;52(1):217–23.
1733. Li Q, Holford TR, Zhang Y, et al. Dietary fiber intake and risk of breast cancer by menopausal and estrogen receptor status. *Eur J Nutr.* 2013;52(1):217–23.
1734. Howe GR, Hirohata T, Hislop TG, et al. Dietary factors and risk of breast cancer: combined analysis of 12 case-control studies. *J Natl Cancer Inst.* 1990;82(7):561–9.
1735. Dong JY, He K, Wang P, Qin LQ. Dietary fiber intake and risk of breast cancer: a meta-analysis of prospective cohort studies. *Am J Clin Nutr.* 2011;94(3):900–5.
1736. Aune D, Chan DS, Greenwood DC, et al. Dietary fiber and breast cancer risk: a systematic review and meta-analysis of prospective studies. *Ann Oncol.* 2012;23(6):1394–402.
1737. Clemens R, Kranz S, Mobley AR, et al. Filling America's fiber intake gap: summary of a roundtable to probe realistic solutions with a focus on grain-based foods. *J Nutr.* 2012;142(7):1390S–401S.
1738. Farmer B, Larson BT, Fulgoni VL, Rainville AJ, Liepa GU. A vegetarian dietary pattern as a nutrient-dense approach to weight management: an analysis of the National Health and Nutrition Examination Survey 1999–2004. *J Am Diet Assoc.* 2011;111(6):819–27.
1739. Rizzo NS, Jaceldo-Siegl K, Sabate J, Fraser GE. Nutrient profiles of vegetarian and nonvegetarian dietary patterns. *J Acad Nutr Diet.* 2013;113(12):1610–9.
1740. Dewell A, Weidner G, Sumner MD, Chi CS, Ornish D. A very-low-fat vegan diet increases intake of protective dietary factors and decreases intake of pathogenic dietary factors. *J Am Diet Assoc.* 2008;108(2):347–56.
1741. Gallus S, Talamini R, Giacosa A, et al. Does an apple a day keep the oncologist away? *Ann Oncol.* 2005;16(11):1841–4.
1742. Wolfe K, Wu X, Liu RH. Antioxidant activity of apple peels. *J Agric Food Chem.* 2003;51(3):609–14.
1743. Sun J, Liu RH. Apple phytochemical extracts inhibit proliferation of estrogen-dependent and estrogen-independent human breast cancer cells through cell cycle modulation. *J Agric Food Chem.* 2008;56(24):11661–7.
1744. Wolfe K, Wu X, Liu RH. Antioxidant activity of apple peels. *J Agric Food Chem.* 2003;51(3):609–14.

1745. Reagan-Shaw S, Eggert D, Mukhtar H, Ahmad N. Antiproliferative effects of apple peel extract against cancer cells. *Nutr Cancer*. 2010;62(4):517–24.
1746. Steck SE, Gaudet MM, Eng SM, et al. Cooked meat and risk of breast cancer—lifetime versus recent dietary intake. *Epidemiology*. 2007;18(3):373–82.
1747. Murray S, Lake BG, Gray S, et al. Effect of cruciferous vegetable consumption on heterocyclic aromatic amine metabolism in man. *Carcinogenesis*. 2001;22(9):1413–20.
1748. Murray S, Lake BG, Gray S, et al. Effect of cruciferous vegetable consumption on heterocyclic aromatic amine metabolism in man. *Carcinogenesis*. 2001;22(9):1413–20.
1749. Murray S, Lake BG, Gray S, et al. Effect of cruciferous vegetable consumption on heterocyclic aromatic amine metabolism in man. *Carcinogenesis*. 2001;22(9):1413–20.
1750. Thiébaud HP, Knize MG, Kuzmicky PA, Hsieh DP, Felton JS. Airborne mutagens produced by frying beef, pork and a soy-based food. *Food Chem Toxicol*. 1995;33(10):821–8.
1751. Boggs DA, Palmer JR, Wise LA, et al. Fruit and vegetable intake in relation to risk of breast cancer in the Black Women's Health Study. *Am J Epidemiol*. 2010;172(11):1268–79.
1752. Boggs DA, Palmer JR, Wise LA, et al. Fruit and vegetable intake in relation to risk of breast cancer in the Black Women's Health Study. *Am J Epidemiol*. 2010;172(11):1268–79.
1753. Tiede B, Kang Y. From milk to malignancy: the role of mammary stem cells in development, pregnancy and breast cancer. *Cell Res*. 2011;21(2):245–57.
1754. Clevers H. The cancer stem cell: premises, promises and challenges. *Nat Med*. 2011;17(3):313–9.
1755. Karrison TG, Ferguson DJ, Meier P. Dormancy of mammary carcinoma after mastectomy. *J Natl Cancer Inst*. 1999;91(1):80–5.
1756. Aguirre-Ghiso JA. Models, mechanisms and clinical evidence for cancer dormancy. *Nat Rev Cancer*. 2007;7(11):834–46.
1757. Clevers H. The cancer stem cell: premises, promises and challenges. *Nat Med*. 2011;17(3):313–9.
1758. Li Y, Zhang T, Korkaya H, et al. Sulforaphane, a dietary component of broccoli/broccoli sprouts, inhibits breast cancer stem cells. *Clin Cancer Res*. 2010;16(9):2580–90.
1759. Cornblatt BS, Ye L, Dinkova-Kostova AT, et al. Preclinical and clinical evaluation of sulforaphane for chemoprevention in the breast. *Carcinogenesis*. 2007;28(7):1485–90.
1760. Fahey JW, Zhang Y, Talalay P. Broccoli sprouts: an exceptionally rich source of inducers of enzymes that protect against chemical carcinogens. *Proc Natl Acad Sci USA*. 1997;94(19):10367–72.
1761. Goyal A, Sharma V, Upadhyay N, Gill S, Sihag M. Flax and flaxseed oil: an ancient medicine & modern functional food. *J Food Sci Technol*. 2014;51(9):1633–53.
1762. Smeds AI, Eklund PC, Sjöholm RE, et al. Quantification of a broad spectrum of lignans in cereals, oilseeds, and nuts. *J Agric Food Chem*. 2007;55(4):1337–46.
1763. Rosolowich V, Saettler E, Szuck B, et al. Mastalgia. *J Obstet Gynaecol Can*. 2006;170:49–57.
1764. Phipps WR, Martini MC, Lampe JW, Slavin JL, Kurzer MS. Effect of flax seed ingestion on the menstrual cycle. *J Clin Endocrinol Metab*. 1993;77(5):1215–9.
1765. Kelsey JL, Gammon MD, John EM. Reproductive factors and breast cancer. *Epidemiol Rev*. 1993;15(1):36–47.
1766. Knekt P, Adlercreutz H, Rissanen H, Aromaa A, Teppo L, Heliövaara M. Does antibacterial treatment for urinary tract infection contribute to the risk of breast cancer? *Br J Cancer*. 2000;82(5):1107–10.
1767. Buck K, Zaineddin AK, Vrieling A, Linseisen J, Chang-Claude J. Meta-analyses of lignans and enterolignans in relation to breast cancer risk. *Am J Clin Nutr*. 2010;92(1):141–53.
1768. Abarzua S, Serikawa T, Szewczyk M, Richter DU, Piechulla B, Briese V. Antiproliferative activity of lignans against the breast carcinoma cell lines MCF 7 and BT 20. *Arch Gynecol Obstet*. 2012;285(4):1145–51.
1769. Fabian CJ, Kimler BF, Zalles CM, et al. Reduction in Ki-67 in benign breast tissue of

high-risk women with the lignan secoisolariciresinol diglycoside. *Cancer Prev Res* (Phila). 2010;3(10):1342–50.
1770. Buck K, Vrieling A, Zaineddin AK, et al. Serum enterolactone and prognosis of postmenopausal breast cancer. *J Clin Oncol*. 2011;29(28):3730–8.
1771. Guglielmini P, Rubagotti A, Boccardo F. Serum enterolactone levels and mortality outcome in women with early breast cancer: a retrospective cohort study. *Breast Cancer Res Treat*. 2012;132(2):661–8.
1772. McCann SE, Thompson LU, Nie J, et al. Dietary lignan intakes in relation to survival among women with breast cancer: the Western New York Exposures and Breast Cancer (WEB) Study. *Breast Cancer Res Treat*. 2010;122(1):229–35.
1773. Åberg UW, Saarinen N, Abrahamsson A, Nurmi T, Engblom S, Dabrosin C. Tamoxifen and flaxseed alter angiogenesis regulators in normal human breast tissue in vivo. *PLoS ONE*. 2011;6(9):e25720.
1774. Thompson LU, Chen JM, Li T, Strasser-Weippl K, Goss PE. Dietary flaxseed alters tumor biological markers in postmenopausal breast cancer. *Clin Cancer Res*. 2005;11(10):3828–35.
1775. Mueller SO, Simon S, Chae K, Metzler M, Korach KS. Phytoestrogens and their human metabolites show distinct agonistic and antagonistic properties on estrogen receptor alpha (ERalpha) and ERbeta in human cells. *Toxicol Sci*. 2004;80(1):14–25.
1776. Oseni T, Patel R, Pyle J, Jordan VC. Selective estrogen receptor modulators and phytoestrogens. *Planta Med*. 2008;74(13):1656–65.
1777. Oseni T, Patel R, Pyle J, Jordan VC. Selective estrogen receptor modulators and phytoestrogens. *Planta Med*. 2008;74(13):1656–65.
1778. Nagata C, Mizoue T, Tanaka K, et al. Soy intake and breast cancer risk: an evaluation based on a systematic review of epidemiologic evidence among the Japanese population. *Jpn J Clin Oncol*. 2014;44(3):282–95.
1779. Chen MN, Lin CC, Liu CF. Efficacy of phytoestrogens for menopausal symptoms: a meta-analysis and systematic review. *Climacteric*. 2015;18(2):260–9.
1780. van Die MD, Bone KM, Visvanathan K, et al. Phytonutrients and outcomes following breast cancer: a systematic review and meta-analysis of observational studies. *JNCI Cancer Spectr*. 2024;8(1):pkad104.
1781. Bhagwat S, Haytowitz DB, Holden JM. USDA database for the isoflavone content of selected foods, release 2.0. https://www.ars.usda.gov/ARSUserFiles/80400525/Data/isoflav/Isoflav_R2.pdf. September 2008. Accessed February 7, 2025.
1782. Nechuta SJ, Caan BJ, Chen WY, et al. Soy food intake after diagnosis of breast cancer and survival: an in-depth analysis of combined evidence from cohort studies of US and Chinese women. *Am J Clin Nutr*. 2012;96(1):123–32.
1783. Kang HB, Zhang YF, Yang JD, Lu KL. Study on soy isoflavone consumption and risk of breast cancer and survival. *Asian Pac J Cancer Prev*. 2012;13(3):995–8.
1784. Bosviel R, Dumollard E, Déchelotte P, Bignon YJ, Bernard-Gallon D. Can soy phytoestrogens decrease DNA methylation in BRCA1 and BRCA2 oncosuppressor genes in breast cancer? *OMICS*. 2012;16(5):235–44.
1785. National Breast Cancer Coalition survey reveals that heightened breast cancer awareness has insufficient impact on knowledge. Imaging Technology News. https://www.itnonline.com/content/many-women-misinformed-about-breast-cancer-causes-detection. October 16, 2007. Accessed February 7, 2025.
1786. Colditz GA, Willett WC, Hunter DJ, et al. Family history, age, and risk of breast cancer. Prospective data from the Nurses' Health Study. *JAMA*. 1993;270(3):338–43.
1787. Bal A, Verma S, Joshi K, et al. BRCA1-methylated sporadic breast cancers are BRCA-like in showing a basal phenotype and absence of ER expression. *Virchows Arch*. 2012;461(3):305–12.
1788. Bosviel R, Dumollard E, Déchelotte P, Bignon YJ, Bernard-Gallon D. Can soy phytoestro-

gens decrease DNA methylation in BRCA1 and BRCA2 oncosuppressor genes in breast cancer? *OMICS*. 2012;16(5):235–44.
1789. Magee PJ, Rowland I. Soy products in the management of breast cancer. *Curr Opin Clin Nutr Metab Care*. 2012;15(6):586–91.
1790. Internation Agency for Research on Cancer. Age-standardized rate (world) per 100 000, incidence, females, in 2022, breast. Cancer Today. https://gco.iarc.fr/today/en/dataviz/bars?types=0&mode=population&sort_by=value0&sexes=2&cancers=20&populations=840_995. Accessed February 9, 2025.
1791. Wu AH, Butler LM. Green tea and breast cancer. *Mol Nutr Food Res*. 2011;55(6):921–30.
1792. Korde LA, Wu AH, Fears T, et al. Childhood soy intake and breast cancer risk in Asian American women. *Cancer Epidemiol Biomarkers Prev*. 2009;18(4):1050–9.
1793. Wakchaure GC. Chapter 3: Production and marketing of mushrooms: global and national scenario. In : Mushrooms: Singh N, Cijay B, Kamal S, Wakchaure GC, eds. *Cultivation, Marketing and Consumption*. Himachal Pradesh-173213, India: Directorate of Mushroom Research; 2014:15–22.
1794. Zhang M, Huang J, Xie X, Holman CD. Dietary intakes of mushrooms and green tea combine to reduce the risk of breast cancer in Chinese women. *Int J Cancer*. 2009;124(6):1404–8.
1795. Ganz PA. A teachable moment for oncologists: cancer survivors, 10 million strong and growing! *J Clin Oncol*. 2005;23(24):5458–60.
1796. Ganz PA. A teachable moment for oncologists: cancer survivors, 10 million strong and growing! *J Clin Oncol*. 2005;23(24):5458–60.
1797. Jafari S, Etminan M, Aminzadeh F, Samii A. Head injury and risk of Parkinson disease: a systematic review and meta-analysis. *Mov Disord*. 2013;28(9):1222–9.
1798. The President's Cancer Panel. Reducing environmental cancer risk: what we can do now. National Cancer Institute. http://deainfo.nci.nih.gov/advisory/pcp/annualReports/pcp08–09rpt/PCP_Report_08–09_508.pdf. April 2010. Accessed February 13, 2025.
1799. Zeliger HI. Exposure to lipophilic chemicals as a cause of neurological impairments, neurodevelopmental disorders and neurodegenerative diseases. *Interdiscip Toxicol*. 2013;6(3):103–10.
1800. National Center for Environmental Health. National Report on Human Exposure to Environmental Chemicals. U.S. Department of Health and Human Services, Centers for Disease Control and Prevention. https://dx.doi.org/10.15620/cdc:133100. 2022. Updated March 2024. Accessed February 13, 2025.
1801. Woodruff TJ, Zota AR, Schwartz JM. Environmental chemicals in pregnant women in the United States: NHANES 2003–2004. *Environ Health Perspect*. 2011;119(6):878–85.
1802. Woodruff TJ, Zota AR, Schwartz JM. Environmental chemicals in pregnant women in the United States: NHANES 2003–2004. *Environ Health Perspect*. 2011;119(6):878–85.
1803. Mariscal-Arcas M, Lopez-Martinez C, Granada A, Olea N, Lorenzo-Tovar ML, Olea-Serrano F. Organochlorine pesticides in umbilical cord blood serum of women from Southern Spain and adherence to the Mediterranean diet. *Food Chem Toxicol*. 2010;48(5):1311–5.
1804. Bjermo H, Darnerud PO, Lignell S, et al. Fish intake and breastfeeding time are associated with serum concentrations of organochlorines in a Swedish population. *Environ Int*. 2013;51:88–96.
1805. Glynn A, Larsdotter M, Aune M, Darnerud PO, Bjerselius R, Bergman A. Changes in serum concentrations of polychlorinated biphenyls (PCBs), hydroxylated PCB metabolites and pentachlorophenol during pregnancy. *Chemosphere*. 2011;83(2):144–51.
1806. Soechitram SD, Athanasiadou M, Hovander L, Bergman A, Sauer PJ. Fetal exposure to PCBs and their hydroxylated metabolites in a Dutch cohort. *Environ Health Perspect*. 2004;112(11):1208–12.
1807. Ulaszewska MM, Zuccato E, Davoli E. PCDD/Fs and dioxin-like PCBs in human milk and estimation of infants' daily intake: a review. *Chemosphere*. 2011;83(6):774–82.

1808. Gallo MV, Schell LM, Decaprio AP, Jacobs A. Levels of persistent organic pollutant and their predictors among young adults. *Chemosphere.* 2011;83(10):1374–82.
1809. Ulaszewska MM, Zuccato E, Davoli E. PCDD/Fs and dioxin-like PCBs in human milk and estimation of infants' daily intake: a review. *Chemosphere.* 2011;83(6):774–82.
1810. Aliyu MH, Alio AP, Salihu HM. To breastfeed or not to breastfeed: a review of the impact of lactational exposure to polychlorinated biphenyls (PCBs) on infants. *J Environ Health.* 2010;73(3):8–14.
1811. Vogt R, Bennett D, Cassady D, Frost J, Ritz B, Hertz-Picciotto I. Cancer and non-cancer health effects from food contaminant exposures for children and adults in California: a risk assessment. *Environ Health.* 2012;11:83.
1812. Vogt R, Bennett D, Cassady D, Frost J, Ritz B, Hertz-Picciotto I. Cancer and non-cancer health effects from food contaminant exposures for children and adults in California: a risk assessment. *Environ Health.* 2012;11:83.
1813. Vogt R, Bennett D, Cassady D, Frost J, Ritz B, Hertz-Picciotto I. Cancer and non-cancer health effects from food contaminant exposures for children and adults in California: a risk assessment. *Environ Health.* 2012;11:83.
1814. Dórea JG, Bezerra VL, Fajon V, Horvat M. Speciation of methyl-and ethyl-mercury in hair of breastfed infants acutely exposed to thimerosal-containing vaccines. *Clin Chim Acta.* 2011;412(17–18):1563–6.
1815. Azevedo LF, Karpova N, Rocha BA, Barbosa Junior F, Gobe GC, Hornos Carneiro MF. Evidence on neurotoxicity after intrauterine and childhood exposure to organomercurials. *Int J Environ Res Public Health.* 2023;20(2):1070.
1816. Zeilmaker MJ, Hoekstra J, van Eijkeren JC, et al. Fish consumption during child bearing age: a quantitative risk-benefit analysis on neurodevelopment. *Food Chem Toxicol.* 2013;54:30–4.
1817. Fromberg A, Granby K, Højgård A, Fagt S, Larsen JC. Estimation of dietary intake of PCB and organochlorine pesticides for children and adults. *Food Chem.* 2011;125:1179–87.
1818. Saktrakulkla P, Lan T, Hua J, Marek RF, Thorne PS, Hornbuckle KC. Polychlorinated biphenyls in food. *Environ Sci Technol.* 2020;54(18):11443–52.
1819. European Food Safety Authority. Results of the monitoring of non dioxin-like PCBs in food and feed. *EFSA Journal.* 2010;8(7):1701.
1820. Fromberg A, Granby K, Højgård A, Fagt S, Larsen JC. Estimation of dietary intake of PCB and organochlorine pesticides for children and adults. *Food Chem.* 2011;125:1179–87.
1821. Zhang T, Sun HW, Wu Q, Zhang XZ, Yun SH, Kannan K. Perfluorochemicals in meat, eggs and indoor dust in China: assessment of sources and pathways of human exposure to perfluorochemicals. *Environ Sci Technol.* 2010;44(9):3572–9.
1822. Schecter A, Cramer P, Boggess K, et al. Intake of dioxins and related compounds from food in the U.S. population. *J Toxicol Environ Health Part A.* 2001;63(1):1–18.
1823. Aune D, De Stefani E, Ronco AL, et al. Egg consumption and the risk of cancer: a multisite case-control study in Uruguay. *Asian Pac J Cancer Prev.* 2009;10(5):869–76.
1824. Yaginuma-Sakurai K, Murata K, Iwai-Shimada M, et al. Hair-to-blood ratio and biological half-life of mercury: experimental study of methylmercury exposure through fish consumption in humans. *J Toxicol Sci.* 2012;37(1):123–30.
1825. Wimmerová S, Lancz K, Tihányi J, et al. Half-lives of serum PCB congener concentrations in environmentally exposed early adolescents. *Chemosphere.* 2011;82(5):687–91.
1826. Hageman KJ, Hafner WD, Campbell DH, Jaffe DA, Landers DH, Simonich SL. Variability in pesticide deposition and source contributions to snowpack in Western U.S. national parks. *Environ Sci Technol.* 2010;44(12):4452–8.
1827. Schecter A, Startin J, Wright C, et al. Congener-specific levels of dioxins and dibenzofurans in U.S. food and estimated daily dioxin toxic equivalent intake. *Environ Health Perspect.* 1994;102(11):962–6.
1828. Fiedler H, Cooper KR, Bergek S, Hjelt M, Rappe C. Polychlorinated dibenzo-p-dioxins and

polychlorinated dibenzofurans (PCDD/PCDF) in food samples collected in southern Mississippi, USA. *Chemosphere.* 1997;34(5–7):1411–9.
1829. Rappe C, Bergek S, Fiedler H, Cooper KR. PCDD and PCDF contamination in catfish feed from Arkansas, USA. *Chemosphere.* 1998;36(13):2705–20.
1830. Ferrario JB, Byrne CJ, Cleverly DH. 2,3,7,8-Dibenzo-p-dioxins in mined clay products from the United States: evidence for possible natural origin. *Environ Sci Technol.* 2000;34(21):4524–32.
1831. U.S. Department of Commerce. Broiler, turkey, and egg production: 1980 to 1999, No. 1143, p. 684. In: *Statistical Abstract of the United States, 2000.* Washington, D.C.: Government Printing Office; 2000.
1832. Hayward DG, Nortrup D, Gardner A, Clower M. Elevated TCDD in chicken eggs and farm-raised catfish fed a diet with ball clay from a Southern United States mine. *Environ Res.* 1999;81(3):248–56.
1833. Hayward DG, Nortrup D, Gardner A, Clower M. Elevated TCDD in chicken eggs and farm-raised catfish fed a diet with ball clay from a Southern United States mine. *Environ Res.* 1999;81(3):248–56.
1834. Tollefson L. Letter to producers or users of clay products in animal feeds. U.S. Food and Drug Administration, U.S. Department of Health and Human Services. https://web.archive.org/web/20081107120600/http://www.fda.gov/cvm/Documents/ballclay.pdf. October 7, 1997. Accessed February 13, 2025.
1835. Hanson T, Sites D. 2012 U.S. catfish database. Fisheries and Allied Aquacultures Department Series No 6, Auburn University. http://aurora.auburn.edu/bitstream/handle/11200/44174/2012%20Catfish%20Database.pdf. March 2013. Accessed February 13, 2025.
1836. Huwe JK, Archer JC. Dioxin congener patterns in commercial catfish from the United States and the indication of mineral clays as the potential source. *Food Addit Contam Part A Chem Anal Control Expo Risk Assess.* 2013;30(2):331–8.
1837. Rappe C, Bergek S, Fiedler H, Cooper KR. PCDD and PCDF contamination in catfish feed from Arkansas, USA. *Chemosphere.* 1998;36(13):2705–20.
1838. Bedi M, Sapozhnikova Y, Ng C. Evaluating contamination of seafood purchased from U.S. retail stores by persistent environmental pollutants, pesticides and veterinary drugs. *Food Addit Contam Part A Chem Anal Control Expo Risk Assess.* 2024;41(3):325–38.
1839. Yaktine AL, Harrison GG, Lawrence RS. Reducing exposure to dioxins and related compounds through foods in the next generation. *Nutr Rev.* 2006;64(9):403–9.
1840. Schecter A, Startin J, Wright C, et al. Congener-specific levels of dioxins and dibenzofurans in U.S. food and estimated daily dioxin toxic equivalent intake. *Environ Health Perspect.* 1994;102(11):962–6.
1841. U.S. Department of Health and Human Services. *The Health Consequences of Smoking: 50 Years of Progress. A Report of the Surgeon General.* Atlanta, GA: US Department of Health and Human Services, Centers for Disease Control and Prevention, National Center for Chronic Disease Prevention and Health Promotion, Office on Smoking and Health; 2014.
1842. Lee PN. 1979 surgeon general's report. University of California San Francisco Library. https://www.industrydocuments.ucsf.edu/tobacco/docs/#id=fqgp0034. September 2, 1979. Accessed February 13, 2025.
1843. Lee PN. 1979 surgeon general's report. University of California San Francisco Library. https://www.industrydocuments.ucsf.edu/tobacco/docs/#id=fqgp0034. September 2, 1979. Accessed February 13, 2025.
1844. PM Exhibit, JD 047710. Hearings before the Subcommittee on Public Buildings and Grounds of the Committee on Public Works and Transportation to Prohibit Smoking in Federal Buildings. University of California San Francisco Library. https://www.industrydocuments.ucsf.edu/tobacco/docs/#id=klvl0154. March 11; April 22, 1993. Accessed February 13, 2025.
1845. Noyce AJ, Bestwick JP, Silveira-Moriyama L, et al. Meta-analysis of early nonmotor features and risk factors for Parkinson disease. *Ann Neurol.* 2012;72(6):893–901.
1846. Morens DM, Grandinetti A, Davis JW, Ross GW, White LR, Reed D. Evidence against the

operation of selective mortality in explaining the association between cigarette smoking and reduced occurrence of idiopathic Parkinson disease. *Am J Epidemiol.* 1996;144(4):400–4.
1847. Noyce AJ, Bestwick JP, Silveira-Moriyama L, et al. Meta-analysis of early nonmotor features and risk factors for Parkinson disease. *Ann Neurol.* 2012;72(6):893–901.
1848. Allam MF, Campbell MJ, Del Castillo AS, Fernández-Crehuet Navajas R. Parkinson's disease protects against smoking? *Behav Neurol.* 2004;15(3–4):65–71.
1849. Tanner CM, Goldman SM, Aston DA, et al. Smoking and Parkinson's disease in twins. *Neurology.* 2002;58(4):581–8.
1850. O'Reilly EJ, Chen H, Gardener H, Gao X, Schwarzschild MA, Ascherio A. Smoking and Parkinson's disease: using parental smoking as a proxy to explore causality. *Am J Epidemiol.* 2009;169(6):678–82.
1851. U.S. Department of Health and Human Services. *The Health Consequences of Smoking: 50 Years of Progress. A Report of the Surgeon General.* Atlanta, GA: US Department of Health and Human Services, Centers for Disease Control and Prevention, National Center for Chronic Disease Prevention and Health Promotion, Office on Smoking and Health; 2014.
1852. Wolf PA, D'Agostino RB, Kannel WB, Bonita R, Belanger AJ. Cigarette smoking as a risk factor for stroke. The Framingham Study. *JAMA.* 1988;259(7):1025–9.
1853. Quik M, Perez XA, Bordia T. Nicotine as a potential neuroprotective agent for Parkinson's disease. *Mov Disord.* 2012;27(8):947–57.
1854. Siegmund B, Leitner E, Pfannhauser W. Determination of the nicotine content of various edible nightshades (Solanaceae) and their products and estimation of the associated dietary nicotine intake. *J Agric Food Chem.* 1999;47(8):3113–20.
1855. Brody AL, Mandelkern MA, London ED, et al. Cigarette smoking saturates brain alpha 4 beta 2 nicotinic acetylcholine receptors. *Arch Gen Psychiatry.* 2006;63(8):907–15.
1856. Searles Nielsen S, Gallagher LG, Lundin JI, et al. Environmental tobacco smoke and Parkinson's disease. *Mov Disord.* 2012;27(2):293–6.
1857. Siegmund B, Leitner E, Pfannhauser W. Determination of the nicotine content of various edible nightshades (Solanaceae) and their products and estimation of the associated dietary nicotine intake. *J Agric Food Chem.* 1999;47(8):3113–20.
1858. Nielsen SS, Franklin GM, Longstreth WT, Swanson PD, Checkoway H. Nicotine from edible Solanaceae and risk of Parkinson disease. *Ann Neurol.* 2013;74(3):472–7.
1859. Nielsen SS, Franklin GM, Longstreth WT, Swanson PD, Checkoway H. Nicotine from edible Solanaceae and risk of Parkinson disease. *Ann Neurol.* 2013;74(3):472–7.
1860. Ma C, Molsberry S, Li Y, Schwarzschild M, Ascherio A, Gao X. Dietary nicotine intake and risk of Parkinson disease: a prospective study. *Am J Clin Nutr.* 2020;112(4):1080–7.
1861. Langston JW, Palfreman J. *The Case of the Frozen Addicts: How the Solution of a Medical Mystery Revolutionized the Understanding of Parkinson's Disease.* IOS Press; 2014.
1862. Langston JW, Ballard P, Tetrud JW, Irwin I. Chronic Parkinsonism in humans due to a product of meperidine-analog synthesis. *Science.* 1983;219(4587):979–80.
1863. Kuhn W, Müller T, Grosse H, Rommelspacher H. Elevated levels of harman and norharman in cerebrospinal fluid of Parkinsonian patients. *J Neural Transm (Vienna).* 1996;103(12):1435–40.
1864. Louis ED, Ferreira JJ. How common is the most common adult movement disorder? Update on the worldwide prevalence of essential tremor. *Mov Disord.* 2010;25(5):534–41.
1865. Louis ED. Essential tremor then and now: how views of the most common tremor diathesis have changed over time. *Parkinsonism Relat Disord.* 2018;46(Suppl 1):S70–4.
1866. Haubenberger D, Hallett M. Essential tremor. *N Engl J Med.* 2018;378(19):1802–10.
1867. Beilin LJ. The fifth Sir George Pickering memorial lecture. Epitaph to essential hypertension—a preventable disorder of known aetiology? *J Hypertens.* 1988;6(2):85–94.
1868. Lenka A, Louis ED. Essential tremor: is the word "essential" really essential? *Parkinsonism Relat Disord.* 2020;81:103–5.

1869. Tanner CM, Goldman SM, Lyons KE, et al. Essential tremor in twins: an assessment of genetic vs environmental determinants of etiology. *Neurology*. 2001;57(8):1389–91.
1870. Louis ED, Jurewicz EC, Applegate L, et al. Association between essential tremor and blood lead concentration. *Environ Health Perspect*. 2003;111(14):1707–11.
1871. Dogu O, Louis ED, Tamer L, Unal O, Yilmaz A, Kaleagasi H. Elevated blood lead concentrations in essential tremor: a case-control study in Mersin, Turkey. *Environ Health Perspect*. 2007;115(11):1564–8.
1872. Hopfner F, Helmich RC. The etiology of essential tremor: genes versus environment. *Parkinsonism Relat Disord*. 2018;46 Suppl 1:S92–6.
1873. Pan MK, Ni CL, Wu YC, Li YS, Kuo SH. Animal models of tremor: relevance to human tremor disorders. *Tremor Other Hyperkinet Mov (N Y)*. 2018;8:587.
1874. Martin FC, Thu Le A, Handforth A. Harmaline-induced tremor as a potential preclinical screening method for essential tremor medications. *Mov Disord*. 2005;20(3):298–305.
1875. Battista AF, Nakatani S, Goldstein M, Anagnoste B. Effect of harmaline in monkeys with central nervous system lesions. *Exp Neurol*. 1970;28(3):513–24.
1876. Louis ED, Zheng W. β-carboline alkaloids and essential tremor: exploring the environmental determinants of one of the most prevalent neurological diseases. *Sci World J*. 2010;10:1783–94.
1877. Ong Y, Deng X, Tan E. Etiologic links between environmental and lifestyle factors and essential tremor. *Ann Clin Transl Neurol*. 2019;6(5):979–89.
1878. Pennes HH, Hoch PH. Psychotomimetics, clinical and theoretical considerations: harmine, Win-2299 and nalline. *Am J Psychiatry*. 1957;113(10):887–92.
1879. Louis ED, Factor-Litvak P, Gerbin M, et al. Blood harmane, blood lead, and severity of hand tremor: evidence of additive effects. *Neurotoxicology*. 2011;32(2):227–32.
1880. Louis ED, Zheng W, Jurewicz EC, et al. Elevation of blood β-carboline alkaloids in essential tremor. *Neurology*. 2002;59(12):1940–4.
1881. Louis ED, Benito-León J, Moreno-García S, et al. Blood harmane (1-methyl-9H-pyrido[3,4-b]indole) concentration in essential tremor cases in Spain. *Neurotoxicology*. 2013;34:264–8.
1882. Louis ED, Jiang W, Pellegrino KM, et al. Elevated blood harmane (1-methyl-9h-pyrido[3,4-b]indole) concentrations in essential tremor. *Neurotoxicology*. 2008;29(2):294–300.
1883. Louis ED, Jiang W, Gerbin M, Viner AS, Factor-Litvak P, Zheng W. Blood harmane (1-methyl-9H-pyrido[3,4-b]indole) concentrations in essential tremor: repeat observation in cases and controls in New York. *J Toxicol Environ Health A*. 2012;75(12):673–83.
1884. Louis ED, Factor-Litvak P, Gerbin M, et al. Blood harmane, blood lead, and severity of hand tremor: evidence of additive effects. *Neurotoxicology*. 2011;32(2):227–32.
1885. Louis ED, Pellegrino KM, Factor-Litvak P, et al. Cancer and blood concentrations of the comutagen harmane in essential tremor. *Mov Disord*. 2008;23(12):1747–51.
1886. Louis ED, Factor-Litvak P, Liu X, et al. Elevated brain harmane (1-methyl-9H-pyrido[3,4-b]indole) in essential tremor cases vs. controls. *Neurotoxicology*. 2013;38:131–5.
1887. Louis ED, Zheng W. β-carboline alkaloids and essential tremor: exploring the environmental determinants of one of the most prevalent neurological diseases. *Sci World J*. 2010;10:1783–94.
1888. Louis ED, Zheng W, Mao X, Shungu DC. Blood harmane is correlated with cerebellar metabolism in essential tremor: a pilot study. *Neurology*. 2007;69(6):515–20.
1889. Pfau W, Skog K. Exposure to β-carbolines norharman and harman. *J Chromatogr B Analyt Technol Biomed Life Sci*. 2004;802(1):115–26.
1890. Skog K, Solyakov A, Arvidsson P, Jägerstad M. Analysis of nonpolar heterocyclic amines in cooked foods and meat extracts using gas chromatography-mass spectrometry. *J Chromatogr A*. 1998;803(1–2):227–33.
1891. Pfau W, Skog K. Exposure to β-carbolines norharman and harman. *J Chromatogr B Analyt Technol Biomed Life Sci*. 2004;802(1):115–26.
1892. Totsuka Y, Ushiyama H, Ishihara J, et al. Quantification of the co-mutagenic beta-carbolines,

norharman and harman, in cigarette smoke condensates and cooked foods. *Cancer Lett.* 1999;143(2):139–43.

1893. Pfau W, Skog K. Exposure to β-carbolines norharman and harman. *J Chromatogr B Analyt Technol Biomed Life Sci.* 2004;802(1):115–26.
1894. Pfau W, Skog K. Exposure to β-carbolines norharman and harman. *J Chromatogr B Analyt Technol Biomed Life Sci.* 2004;802(1):115–26.
1895. Louis ED, Jiang W, Gerbin M, Viner AS, Factor-Litvak P, Zheng W. Blood harmane (1-methyl-9H-pyrido[3,4-b]indole) concentrations in essential tremor: repeat observation in cases and controls in New York. *J Toxicol Environ Health A.* 2012;75(12):673–83.
1896. Louis ED, Keating GA, Bogen KT, Rios E, Pellegrino KM, Factor-Litvak P. Dietary epidemiology of essential tremor: meat consumption and meat cooking practices. *Neuroepidemiology.* 2008;30(3):161–6.
1897. Doll R, Hill AB. Smoking and carcinoma of the lung; preliminary report. *Br Med J.* 1950;2(4682):739–48.
1898. Thun MJ. When truth is unwelcome: the first reports on smoking and lung cancer. *Bull World Health Organ.* 2005;83(2):144–5.
1899. Louis ED, Keating GA, Bogen KT, Rios E, Pellegrino KM, Factor-Litvak P. Dietary epidemiology of essential tremor: meat consumption and meat cooking practices. *Neuroepidemiology.* 2008;30(3):161–6.
1900. Ferrer M, Eliasen EH, Petersen MS, Jiang W, Zheng W, Louis ED. Meat consumption and meat cooking practices in essential tremor: a population-based study in the Faroe Islands. *Tremor Other Hyperkinet Mov (N Y).* 2020;10:30.
1901. Laviţă SI, Aro R, Kiss B, Manto M, Duez P. The role of β-carboline alkaloids in the pathogenesis of essential tremor. *Cerebellum.* 2016;15(3):276–84.
1902. Ferrer M, Eliasen EH, Petersen MS, Jiang W, Zheng W, Louis ED. Meat consumption and meat cooking practices in essential tremor: a population-based study in the Faroe Islands. *Tremor Other Hyperkinet Mov (N Y).* 2020;10:30.
1903. Louis ED, Zheng W. β-carboline alkaloids and essential tremor: exploring the environmental determinants of one of the most prevalent neurological diseases. *Sci World J.* 2010;10:1783–94.
1904. Gibis M, Weiss J. Inhibitory effect of marinades with hibiscus extract on formation of heterocyclic aromatic amines and sensory quality of fried beef patties. *Meat Sci.* 2010;85(4):735–42.
1905. Busquets R, Puignou L, Galceran MT, Skog K. Effect of red wine marinades on the formation of heterocyclic amines in fried chicken breast. *J Agric Food Chem.* 2006;54(21):8376–84.
1906. Smith JS, Ameri F, Gadgil P. Effect of marinades on the formation of heterocyclic amines in grilled beef steaks. *J Food Sci.* 2008;73(6):T100–5.
1907. Khan MR, Busquets R, Azam M. Blueberry, raspberry, and strawberry extracts reduce the formation of carcinogenic heterocyclic amines in fried camel, beef and chicken meats. *Food Control.* 2021;123:107852.
1908. Abdulrahman AA, Faisal K, Meshref AAA, Arshaduddin M. Low-dose acute vanillin is beneficial against harmaline-induced tremors in rats. *Neurol Res.* 2017;39(3):264–70.
1909. Richardson JR, Shalat SL, Buckley B, et al. Elevated serum pesticide levels and risk of Parkinson disease. *Arch Neurol.* 2009;66(7):870–5.
1910. Corrigan FM, Wienburg CL, Shore RF, Daniel SE, Mann D. Organochlorine insecticides in substantia nigra in Parkinson's disease. *J Toxicol Environ Health Part A.* 2000;59(4):229–34.
1911. Hatcher-Martin JM, Gearing M, Steenland K, Levey AI, Miller GW, Pennell KD. Association between polychlorinated biphenyls and Parkinson's disease neuropathology. *Neurotoxicology.* 2012;33(5):1298–304.
1912. Kanthasamy AG, Kitazawa M, Kanthasamy A, Anantharam V. Dieldrin-induced neurotoxicity: relevance to Parkinson's disease pathogenesis. *Neurotoxicology.* 2005;26(4):701–19.
1913. Arguin H, Sánchez M, Bray GA, et al. Impact of adopting a vegan diet or an olestra supplementation on plasma organochlorine concentrations: results from two pilot studies. *Br J Nutr.* 2010;103(10):1433–41.

1914. Jiang W, Ju C, Jiang H, Zhang D. Dairy foods intake and risk of Parkinson's disease: a dose-response meta-analysis of prospective cohort studies. *Eur J Epidemiol.* 2014;29(9):613–9.

1915. Park M, Ross GW, Petrovitch H, et al. Consumption of milk and calcium in midlife and the future risk of Parkinson disease. *Neurology.* 2005;64(6):1047–51.

1916. Kotake Y, Yoshida M, Ogawa M, Tasaki Y, Hirobe M, Ohta S. Chronic administration of 1-benzyl-1,2,3,4-tetrahydroisoquinoline, an endogenous amine in the brain, induces parkinsonism in a primate. *Neurosci Lett.* 1996;217(1):69–71.

1917. Niwa T, Yoshizumi H, Takeda N, Tatematsu A, Matsuura S, Nagatsu T. Detection of tetrahydroisoquinoline, a parkinsonism-related compound, in parkinsonian brains and foods by gas chromatography-mass spectrometry. *Advances in Behavioral Biology.* 1990;38A:313–6.

1918. Niwa T, Yoshizumi H, Tatematsu A, Matsuura S, Nagatsu T. Presence of tetrahydroisoquinoline, a parkinsonism-related compound, in foods. *J Chromatogr.* 1989;493(2):347–52.

1919. Niwa T, Takeda N, Kaneda N, Hashizume Y, Nagatsu T. Presence of tetrahydroisoquinoline and 2-methyl-tetrahydroquinoline in parkinsonian and normal human brains. *Biochem Biophys Res Commun.* 1987;144(2):1084–9.

1920. Ułamek-Kozioł M, Bogucka-Kocka A, Kocki J, Pluta R. Good and bad sides of diet in Parkinson's disease. *Nutrition.* 2013;29(2):474–5.

1921. Ułamek-Kozioł M, Bogucka-Kocka A, Kocki J, Pluta R. Good and bad sides of diet in Parkinson's disease. *Nutrition.* 2013;29(2):474–5.

1922. Kistner A, Krack P. Parkinson's disease: no milk today? *Front Neurol.* 2014;5:172.

1923. Chen H, Zhang SM, Hernn MA, Willett WC, Ascherio A. Diet and Parkinson's disease: a potential role of dairy products in men. *Ann Neurol.* 2002;52(6):793–801.

1924. Jiang W, Ju C, Jiang H, Zhang D. Dairy foods intake and risk of Parkinson's disease: a dose-response meta-analysis of prospective cohort studies. *Eur J Epidemiol.* 2014;29(9):613–9.

1925. Michaëlsson K, Wolk A, Langenskiöld S, et al. Milk intake and risk of mortality and fractures in women and men: cohort studies. *BMJ.* 2014;349:g6015.

1926. Ridel KR, Leslie ND, Gilbert DL. An updated review of the long-term neurological effects of galactosemia. *Pediatr Neurol.* 2005;33(3):153–61.

1927. Marder K, Gu Y, Eberly S, et al. Relationship of Mediterranean diet and caloric intake to phenoconversion in Huntington disease. *JAMA Neurol.* 2013;70(11):1382–8.

1928. Ames BN, Cathcart R, Schwiers E, Hochstein P. Uric acid provides an antioxidant defense in humans against oxidant-and radical-caused aging and cancer: a hypothesis. *Proc Natl Acad Sci USA.* 1981;78(11):6858–62.

1929. Duan W, Ladenheim B, Cutler RG, Kruman II, Cadet JL, Mattson MP. Dietary folate deficiency and elevated homocysteine levels endanger dopaminergic neurons in models of Parkinson's disease. *J Neurochem.* 2002;80(1):101–10.

1930. Auinger P, Kieburtz K, McDermott MP. The relationship between uric acid levels and Huntington's disease progression. *Mov Disord.* 2010;25(2):224–8.

1931. Schwarzschild MA, Schwid SR, Marek K, et al. Serum urate as a predictor of clinical and radiographic progression in Parkinson disease. *Arch Neurol.* 2008;65(6):716–23.

1932. Shen C, Guo Y, Luo W, Lin C, Ding M. Serum urate and the risk of Parkinson's disease: results from a meta-analysis. *Can J Neurol Sci.* 2013;40(1):73–9.

1933. Fang P, Li X, Luo JJ, Wang H, Yang X. A double-edged sword: uric acid and neurological disorders. *Brain Disord Ther.* 2013;2(2):109.

1934. Kutzing MK, Firestein BL. Altered uric acid levels and disease states. *J Pharmacol Exp Ther.* 2008;324(1):1–7.

1935. Schmidt JA, Crowe FL, Appleby PN, Key TJ, Travis RC. Serum uric acid concentrations in meat eaters, fish eaters, vegetarians and vegans: a cross-sectional analysis in the EPIC-Oxford cohort. *PLoS ONE.* 2013;8(2):e56339.

1936. Kuo CF, See LC, Yu KH, Chou IJ, Chiou MJ, Luo SF. Significance of serum uric acid levels on the risk of all-cause and cardiovascular mortality. *Rheumatology* (Oxford). 2013;52(1):127–34.

1937. Arguin H, Sánchez M, Bray GA, et al. Impact of adopting a vegan diet or an olestra supplementation on plasma organochlorine concentrations: results from two pilot studies. *Br J Nutr.* 2010;103(10):1433–41.
1938. Siddiqui MK, Saxena MC, Krishna Murti CR. Storage of DDT and BHC in adipose tissue of Indian males. *Int J Environ Anal Chem.* 1981;10(3–4):197–204.
1939. Norén K. Levels of organochlorine contaminants in human milk in relation to the dietary habits of the mothers. *Acta Paediatr Scand.* 1983;72(6):811–6.
1940. Schecter A, Papke O. Comparison of blood dioxin, dibenzofuran and coplanar PCB levels in strict vegetarians (vegans) and the general United States population. *Org Comps.* 1998;38:179–82.
1941. Schecter A, Harris TR, Päpke O, Tunga KC, Musumba A. Polybrominated diphenyl ether (PBDE) levels in the blood of pure vegetarians (vegans). *Tox Env Chem.* 2006;88(1):107–12.
1942. Eskenazi B, Chevrier J, Rauch SA, et al. In utero and childhood polybrominated diphenyl ether (PBDE) exposures and neurodevelopment in the CHAMACOS study. *Environ Health Perspect.* 2013;121(2):257–62.
1943. Schecter A, Päpke O, Harris TR, et al. Polybrominated diphenyl ether (PBDE) levels in an expanded market basket survey of U.S. food and estimated PBDE dietary intake by age and sex. *Environ Health Perspect.* 2006;114(10):1515–20.
1944. Fraser AJ, Webster TF, McClean MD. Diet contributes significantly to the body burden of PBDEs in the general U.S. population. *Environ Health Perspect.* 2009;117(10):1520–5.
1945. Schecter A, Harris TR, Päpke O, Tunga KC, Musumba A. Polybrominated diphenyl ether (PBDE) levels in the blood of pure vegetarians (vegans). *Tox Env Chem.* 2006;88(1):107–12.
1946. Huwe JK, West M. Polybrominated diphenyl ethers in U.S. meat and poultry from two statistically designed surveys showing trends and levels from 2002 to 2008. *J Agric Food Chem.* 2011;59(10):5428–34.
1947. Dickman MD, Leung CK, Leong MK. Hong Kong male subfertility links to mercury in human hair and fish. *Sci Total Environ.* 1998;214:165–74.
1948. Srikumar TS, Johansson GK, Ockerman PA, Gustafsson JA, Akesson B. Trace element status in healthy subjects switching from a mixed to a lactovegetarian diet for 12 mo. *Am J Clin Nutr.* 1992;55(4):885–90.
1949. Wimmerová S, Lancz K, Tihányi J, et al. Half-lives of serum PCB congener concentrations in environmentally exposed early adolescents. *Chemosphere.* 2011;82(5):687–91.
1950. Parkinson J. *An Essay on the Shaking Palsy.* London: Whittingham and Rowland for Sherwood, Neely and Jones;1817:7.
1951. Abbott RD, Petrovitch H, White LR, et al. Frequency of bowel movements and the future risk of Parkinson's disease. *Neurology.* 2001;57(3):456–62.
1952. Ueki A, Otsuka M. Life style risks of Parkinson's disease: association between decreased water intake and constipation. *J Neurol.* 2004;251 Suppl 7:vII18–23.
1953. Gao X, Chen H, Schwarzschild MA, Ascherio A. A prospective study of bowel movement frequency and risk of Parkinson's disease. *Am J Epidemiol.* 2011;174(5):546–51.
1954. Kamel F. Epidemiology. Paths from pesticides to Parkinson's. *Science.* 2013;341(6147):722–3.
1955. Barnhill LM, Bronstein JM. Pesticides and Parkinson's disease: is it in your genes? *Neurodegener Dis Manag.* 2014;4(3):197–200.
1956. Wang A, Cockburn M, Ly TT, Bronstein JM, Ritz B. The association between ambient exposure to organophosphates and Parkinson's disease risk. *Occup Environ Med.* 2014;71(4):275–81.
1957. Narayan S, Liew Z, Paul K, et al. Household organophosphorus pesticide use and Parkinson's disease. *Int J Epidemiol.* 2013;42(5):1476–85.
1958. Liu X, Ma T, Qu B, Ji Y, Liu Z. Pesticide-induced gene mutations and Parkinson disease risk: a meta-analysis. *Genet Test Mol Biomarkers.* 2013;17(11):826–32.
1959. Lee SJ, Lim HS, Masliah E, Lee HJ. Protein aggregate spreading in neurodegenerative diseases: problems and perspectives. *Neurosci Res.* 2011;70(4):339–48.

1960. Dunnett SB, Björklund SBA. Prospects for new restorative and neuroprotective treatments in Parkinson's disease. *Nature*. 1999;399(6738 Suppl):A32–9.
1961. Campdelacreu J. Parkinson disease and Alzheimer disease: environmental risk factors. *Neurologia*. 2014;29(9):541–9.
1962. Meng X, Munishkina LA, Fink AL, Uversky VN. Effects of various flavonoids on the α-synuclein fibrillation process. *Parkinson's Dis*. 2010;2010:650794.
1963. Strathearn KE, Yousef GG, Grace MH, Roy SA, et al. Neuroprotective effects of anthocyanin-and proanthocyanidin-rich extracts in cellular models of Parkinson's disease. *Brain Res*. 2014;1555:60–77.
1964. Golbe LI, Farrell TM, Davis PH. Case-control study of early life dietary factors in Parkinson's disease. *Arch Neurol*. 1988;45(12):1350–3.
1965. Gao X, Cassidy A, Schwarzschild MA, Rimm EB, Ascherio A. Habitual intake of dietary flavonoids and risk of Parkinson disease. *Neurol*. 2012;78(15):1138–45.
1966. Zhang X, Molsberry SA, Yeh TS, et al. Intake of flavonoids and flavonoid-rich foods and mortality risk among individuals with parkinson disease: a prospective cohort study. *Neurology*. 2022;98(10):e1064-e1076.
1967. Kukull WA. An apple a day to prevent Parkinson disease: reduction of risk by flavonoids. *Neurol*. 2012;78(15):1112–3.
1968. Gao X, Cassidy A, Schwarzschild MA, Rimm EB, Ascherio A. Habitual intake of dietary flavonoids and risk of Parkinson disease. *Neurology*. 2012;78(15):1138–45.
1969. Serafini M, Testa MF, Villain D, et al. Antioxidant activity of blueberry fruit is impaired by association with milk. *Free Radic Biol Med*. 2009;46(6):769–74.
1970. Jekanowski M. Survey says: a snapshot of rendering. *Render Magazine*. 2011;April:58–61.
1971. Schepens PJ, Covaci A, Jorens PG, Hens L, Scharpé S, van Larebeke N. Surprising findings following a Belgian food contamination with polychlorobiphenyls and dioxins. *Environ Health Perspect*. 2001;109(2):101–3.
1972. Dórea JG. Vegetarian diets and exposure to organochlorine pollutants, lead, and mercury. *Am J Clin Nutr*. 2004;80(1):237–8.
1973. Dórea JG. Fish meal in animal feed and human exposure to persistent bioaccumulative and toxic substances. *J Food Prot*. 2006;69(11):2777–85.
1974. Moser GA, McLachlan MS. The influence of dietary concentration on the absorption and excretion of persistent lipophilic organic pollutants in the human intestinal tract. *Chemosphere*. 2001;45(2):201–11.
1975. Dórea JG. Vegetarian diets and exposure to organochlorine pollutants, lead, and mercury. *Am J Clin Nutr*. 2004;80(1):237–8.
1976. Grazina R, Massano J. Physical exercise and Parkinson's disease: influence on symptoms, disease course and prevention. *Rev Neurosci*. 2013;24(2):139–52.
1977. Chen J, Guan Z, Wang L, Song G, Ma B, Wang Y. Meta-analysis: overweight, obesity, and Parkinson's disease. *Int J Endocrinol*. 2014;2014:203930.
1978. Nelson WG, De Marzo AM, Isaacs WB. Prostate cancer. *N Engl J Med*. 2003;349(4):366–81.
1979. Draisma G, Etzioni R, Tsodikov A, et al. Lead time and overdiagnosis in prostate-specific antigen screening: importance of methods and context. *J Natl Cancer Inst*. 2009;101(6):374–83.
1980. U.S. Cancer Statistics Working Group. U.S. cancer statistics data visualizations tool. U.S. Department of Health and Human Services, Centers for Disease Control and Prevention, National Cancer Institute. https://www.cdc.gov/cancer/dataviz. June 2024. Accessed February 12, 2025.
1981. Nelson WG, De Marzo AM, Isaacs WB. Prostate cancer. *N Engl J Med*. 2003;349(4):366–81.
1982. Grossman DC, Curry SJ, Owens DK, et al. Screening for prostate cancer: US Preventive Services Task Force recommendation statement. *JAMA*. 2018;319(18):1901–13.
1983. Moyer VA, LeFevre ML, Sui AL, et al. Screening for prostate cancer: U.S. Preventive Services Task Force recommendation statement. *Ann Intern Med*. 2012;157(2):120–34.

1984. Livingston CJ, Freeman RJ, Mohammad A, et al. Choosing Wisely® in preventive medicine. *Am J Prev Med*. 2016;51(1):141–9.
1985. Mulhem E, Fulbright N, Duncan N. Prostate cancer screening. *Am Fam Physician*. 2015;92(8):683–8.
1986. Ivlev I, Jerabkova S, Mishra M, Cook LA, Eden KB. Prostate cancer screening patient decision aids: a systematic review and meta-analysis. *Am J Prev Med*. 2018;55(6):896–907.
1987. Grossman DC, Curry SJ, Owens DK, et al. Screening for prostate cancer: US Preventive Services Task Force recommendation statement. *JAMA*. 2018;319(18):1901–13.
1988. Carter HB. American Urological Association (AUA) guideline on prostate cancer detection: process and rationale. *BJU Int*. 2013;112(5):543–7.
1989. Wilt TJ, Harris RP, Qaseem A, et al. Screening for cancer: advice for high-value care from the American College of Physicians. *Ann Intern Med*. 2015;162(10):718–25.
1990. American Cancer Society recommendations for prostate cancer early detection. American Cancer Society. https://www.cancer.org/cancer/prostate-cancer/detection-diagnosis-staging/acs-recommendations.html. Updated November 22, 2023. Accessed February 12, 2025.
1991. Grossman DC, Curry SJ, Owens DK, et al. Screening for prostate cancer: US Preventive Services Task Force recommendation statement. *JAMA*. 2018;319(18):1901–13.
1992. Tikkinen KAO, Dahm P, Lytvyn L, et al. Prostate cancer screening with prostate-specific antigen (PSA) test: a clinical practice guideline. *BMJ*. 2018;362:k3581.
1993. Gigerenzer G, Mata J, Frank R. Public knowledge of benefits of breast and prostate cancer screening in Europe. *J Natl Cancer Inst*. 2009;101(17):1216–20.
1994. Grossman DC, Curry SJ, Owens DK, et al. Screening for prostate cancer: US Preventive Services Task Force recommendation statement. *JAMA*. 2018;319(18):1901–13.
1995. Tikkinen KAO, Dahm P, Lytvyn L, et al. Prostate cancer screening with prostate-specific antigen (PSA) test: a clinical practice guideline. *BMJ*. 2018;362:k3581.
1996. Grossman DC, Curry SJ, Owens DK, et al. Screening for prostate cancer: US Preventive Services Task Force recommendation statement. *JAMA*. 2018;319(18):1901–13.
1997. Grossman DC, Curry SJ, Owens DK, et al. Screening for prostate cancer: US Preventive Services Task Force recommendation statement. *JAMA*. 2018;319(18):1901–13.
1998. Early detection of prostate cancer. Harding Center for Risk Literacy. https://www.hardingcenter.de/en/transfer-and-impact/fact-boxes/early-detection-of-cancer/early-detection-of-prostate-cancer-with-psa-testing. Updated November 2020. Accessed February 12, 2025.
1999. Early detection of prostate cancer. Harding Center for Risk Literacy. https://www.hardingcenter.de/en/transfer-and-impact/fact-boxes/early-detection-of-cancer/early-detection-of-prostate-cancer-with-psa-testing. Updated November 2020. Accessed February 12, 2025.
2000. Maruyama K, Oshima T, Ohyama K. Exposure to exogenous estrogen through intake of commercial milk produced from pregnant cows. *Pediatr Int*. 2010;52(1):33–8.
2001. Danby FW. Acne and milk, the diet myth, and beyond. *J Am Acad Dermatol*. 2005;52(2):360–2.
2002. Afeiche M, Williams PL, Mendiola J, et al. Dairy food intake in relation to semen quality and reproductive hormone levels among physically active young men. *Hum Reprod*. 2013;28(8):2265–75.
2003. Maruyama K, Oshima T, Ohyama K. Exposure to exogenous estrogen through intake of commercial milk produced from pregnant cows. *Pediatr Int*. 2010;52(1):33–8.
2004. Steinman G. Mechanisms of twinning: VII. Effect of diet and heredity on the human twinning rate. *J Reprod Med*. 2006;51(5):405–10.
2005. Melnik BC, John SM, Schmitz G. Milk is not just food but most likely a genetic transfection system activating mTORC1 signaling for postnatal growth. *Nutr J*. 2013;12:103.

2006. Ludwig DS, Willett WC. Three daily servings of reduced-fat milk: an evidence-based recommendation? *JAMA Pediatr.* 2013;167(9):788–9.
2007. Ludwig DS, Willett WC. Three daily servings of reduced-fat milk: an evidence-based recommendation? *JAMA Pediatr.* 2013;167(9):788–9.
2008. Tate PL, Bibb R, Larcom LL. Milk stimulates growth of prostate cancer cells in culture. *Nutr Cancer.* 2011;63(8):1361–6.
2009. Ganmaa D, Li XM, Qin LQ, Wang PY, Takeda M, Sato A. The experience of Japan as a clue to the etiology of testicular and prostatic cancers. *Med Hypotheses.* 2003;60(5):724–30.
2010. Ganmaa D, Li XM, Wang J, Qin LQ, Wang PY, Sato A. Incidence and mortality of testicular and prostatic cancers in relation to world dietary practices. *Int J Cancer.* 2002;98(2):262–7.
2011. Epstein SS. Unlabeled milk from cows treated with biosynthetic growth hormones: a case of regulatory abdication. *Int J Health Serv.* 1996;26(1):173–85.
2012. Tate PL, Bibb R, Larcom LL. Milk stimulates growth of prostate cancer cells in culture. *Nutr Cancer.* 2011;63(8):1361–6.
2013. Qin LQ, Xu JY, Wang PY, Kaneko T, Hoshi K, Sato A. Milk consumption is a risk factor for prostate cancer: meta-analysis of case-control studies. *Nutr Cancer.* 2004;48(1):22–7.
2014. Qin LQ, Xu JY, Wang PY, Tong J, Hoshi K. Milk consumption is a risk factor for prostate cancer in Western countries: evidence from cohort studies. *Asia Pac J Clin Nutr.* 2007;16(3):467–76.
2015. Jin S, Je Y. Dairy consumption and total cancer and cancer-specific mortality: a meta-analysis of prospective cohort studies. *Adv Nutr.* 2022;13(4):1063–82.
2016. Mishra S, Baruah K, Malik VS, Ding EL. Dairy intake and risk of hip fracture in prospective cohort studies: non-linear algorithmic dose-response analysis in 486 950 adults. *J Nutr Sci.* 2023;12:e96.
2017. Feskanich D, Bischoff-Ferrari HA, Frazier AL, Willett WC. Milk consumption during teenage years and risk of hip fractures in older adults. *JAMA Pediatr.* 2014;168(1):54–60.
2018. Batey LA, Welt CK, Rohr F, et al. Skeletal health in adult patients with classic galactosemia. *Osteoporos Int.* 2013;24(2):501–9.
2019. Michaëlsson K, Wolk A, Langenskiöld S, et al. Milk intake and risk of mortality and fractures in women and men: cohort studies. *BMJ.* 2014;349:g6015.
2020. Cui X, Wang L, Zuo P, et al. D-galactose-caused life shortening in Drosophila melanogaster and Musca domestica is associated with oxidative stress. *Biogerontology.* 2004;5(5):317–25.
2021. Cui X, Zuo P, Zhang Q, et al. Chronic systemic D-galactose exposure induces memory loss, neurodegeneration, and oxidative damage in mice: protective effects of R-alpha-lipoic acid. *J Neurosci Res.* 2006;84(3):647–54.
2022. Michaëlsson K, Wolk A, Langenskiöld S, et al. Milk intake and risk of mortality and fractures in women and men: cohort studies. *BMJ.* 2014;349:g6015.
2023. Michaëlsson K, Wolk A, Langenskiöld S, et al. Milk intake and risk of mortality and fractures in women and men: cohort studies. *BMJ.* 2014;349:g6015.
2024. Michaëlsson K, Wolk A, Langenskiöld S, et al. Milk intake and risk of mortality and fractures in women and men: cohort studies. *BMJ.* 2014;349:g6015.
2025. Michaëlsson K, Wolk A, Langenskiöld S, et al. Milk intake and risk of mortality and fractures in women and men: cohort studies. *BMJ.* 2014;349:g6015.
2026. Schooling CM. Milk and mortality. *BMJ.* 2014;349:g6205.
2027. Ding M, Li J, Qi L, et al. Associations of dairy intake with risk of mortality in women and men: three prospective cohort studies. *BMJ.* 2019;367:l6204.
2028. Naghshi S, Sadeghi O, Larijani B, Esmaillzadeh A. High vs. low-fat dairy and milk differently affects the risk of all-cause, CVD, and cancer death: a systematic review and dose-response meta-analysis of prospective cohort studies. *Crit Rev Food Sci Nutr.* 2022;62(13):3598–612.
2029. Cancer stat facts: prostate cancer. Surveillance, Epidemiology, and End Results Program

(SEER), National Cancer Institute. https://seer.cancer.gov/statfacts/html/prost.html. Accessed February 12, 2025.
2030. Richman EL, Stampfer MJ, Paciorek A, Broering JM, Carroll PR, Chan JM. Intakes of meat, fish, poultry, and eggs and risk of prostate cancer progression. *Am J Clin Nutr.* 2010;91(3): 712–21.
2031. Richman EL, Stampfer MJ, Paciorek A, Broering JM, Carroll PR, Chan JM. Intakes of meat, fish, poultry, and eggs and risk of prostate cancer progression. *Am J Clin Nutr.* 2010;91(3): 712–21.
2032. Richman EL, Stampfer MJ, Paciorek A, Broering JM, Carroll PR, Chan JM. Intakes of meat, fish, poultry, and eggs and risk of prostate cancer progression. *Am J Clin Nutr.* 2010;91(3): 712–21.
2033. Johansson M, Van Guelpen B, Vollset SE, et al. One-carbon metabolism and prostate cancer risk: prospective investigation of seven circulating B vitamins and metabolites. *Cancer Epidemiol Biomarkers Prev.* 2009;18(5):1538–43.
2034. Richman EL, Stampfer MJ, Paciorek A, Broering JM, Carroll PR, Chan JM. Intakes of meat, fish, poultry, and eggs and risk of prostate cancer progression. *Am J Clin Nutr.* 2010;91(3): 712–21.
2035. Richman EL, Kenfield SA, Stampfer MJ, et al. Choline intake and risk of lethal prostate cancer: incidence and survival. *Am J Clin Nutr.* 2012;96(4):855–63.
2036. Richman EL, Kenfield SA, Stampfer MJ, Giovannucci EL, Chan JM. Egg, red meat, and poultry intake and risk of lethal prostate cancer in the prostate-specific antigen-era: incidence and survival. *Cancer Prev Res* (Phila). 2011;4(12):2110–21.
2037. Tang WH, Wang Z, Levison BS, et al. Intestinal microbial metabolism of phosphatidylcholine and cardiovascular risk. *N Engl J Med.* 2013;368(17):1575–84.
2038. Koeth RA, Wang Z, Levison BS, et al. Intestinal microbiota metabolism of L-carnitine, a nutrient in red meat, promotes atherosclerosis. *Nat Med.* 2013;19:576–85.
2039. Tang WH, Wang Z, Levison BS, et al. Intestinal microbial metabolism of phosphatidylcholine and cardiovascular risk. *N Engl J Med.* 2013;368(17):1575–84.
2040. Choline: there's something fishy about this vitamin. *Harv Health Lett.* 2004;30(1):3.
2041. Mitch Kanter, Ph.D., email communication, January 6, 2010.
2042. Hubbard JD, Inkeles S, Barnard RJ. Nathan Pritikin's heart. *N Engl J Med.* 1985;313(1):52.
2043. Ornish D, Weidner G, Fair WR, et al. Intensive lifestyle changes may affect the progression of prostate cancer. *J Urol.* 2005;174(3):1065–9.
2044. Ornish D, Weidner G, Fair WR, et al. Intensive lifestyle changes may affect the progression of prostate cancer. *J Urol.* 2005;174(3):1065–9.
2045. Barnard RJ, Gonzalez JH, Liva ME, Ngo TH. Effects of a low-fat, high-fiber diet and exercise program on breast cancer risk factors in vivo and tumor cell growth and apoptosis in vitro. *Nutr Cancer.* 2006;55(1):28–34.
2046. Barnard RJ, Ngo TH, Leung PS, Aronson WJ, Golding LA. A low-fat diet and/or strenuous exercise alters the IGF axis in vivo and reduces prostate tumor cell growth in vitro. *Prostate.* 2003;56(3):201–6.
2047. Barnard RJ, Ngo TH, Leung PS, Aronson WJ, Golding LA. A low-fat diet and/or strenuous exercise alters the IGF axis in vivo and reduces prostate tumor cell growth in vitro. *Prostate.* 2003;56(3):201–6.
2048. Barnard RJ, Ngo TH, Leung PS, Aronson WJ, Golding LA. A low-fat diet and/or strenuous exercise alters the IGF axis in vivo and reduces prostate tumor cell growth in vitro. *Prostate.* 2003;56(3):201–6.
2049. Ornish D, Weidner G, Fair WR, et al. Intensive lifestyle changes may affect the progression of prostate cancer. *J Urol.* 2005;174(3):1065–9.
2050. Ornish D, Weidner G, Fair WR, et al. Intensive lifestyle changes may affect the progression of prostate cancer. *J Urol.* 2005;174(3):1065–9.
2051. Ornish D, Magbanua MJ, Weidner G, et al. Changes in prostate gene expression in men

undergoing an intensive nutrition and lifestyle intervention. *Proc Natl Acad Sci USA*. 2008;105(24):8369–74.
2052. Frattaroli J, Weidner G, Dnistrian AM, et al. Clinical events in prostate cancer lifestyle trial: results from two years of follow-up. *Urology*. 2008;72(6):1319–23.
2053. Frey AU, Sønksen J, Fode M. Neglected side effects after radical prostatectomy: a systematic review. *J Sex Med*. 2014;11(2):374–85.
2054. Carmody JF, Olendzki BC, Merriam PA, Liu Q, Qiao Y, Ma Y. A novel measure of dietary change in a prostate cancer dietary program incorporating mindfulness training. *J Acad Nutr Diet*. 2012;112(11):1822–7.
2055. Blanchard CM, Courneya KS, Stein K. Cancer survivors' adherence to lifestyle behavior recommendations and associations with health-related quality of life: results from the American Cancer Society's SCS-II. *J Clin Oncol*. 2008;26(13):2198–204.
2056. Carmody JF, Olendzki BC, Merriam PA, Liu Q, Qiao Y, Ma Y. A novel measure of dietary change in a prostate cancer dietary program incorporating mindfulness training. *J Acad Nutr Diet*. 2012;112(11):1822–7.
2057. Carmody JF, Olendzki BC, Merriam PA, Liu Q, Qiao Y, Ma Y. A novel measure of dietary change in a prostate cancer dietary program incorporating mindfulness training. *J Acad Nutr Diet*. 2012;112(11):1822–7.
2058. Carmody JF, Olendzki BC, Merriam PA, Liu Q, Qiao Y, Ma Y. A novel measure of dietary change in a prostate cancer dietary program incorporating mindfulness training. *J Acad Nutr Diet*. 2012;112(11):1822–7.
2059. Richman EL, Stampfer MJ, Paciorek A, Broering JM, Carroll PR, Chan JM. Intakes of meat, fish, poultry, and eggs and risk of prostate cancer progression. *Am J Clin Nutr*. 2010;91(3):712–21.
2060. Richman EL, Carroll PR, Chan JM. Vegetable and fruit intake after diagnosis and risk of prostate cancer progression. *Int J Cancer*. 2012;131(1):201–10.
2061. Allen NE, Appleby PN, Key TJ, et al. Macronutrient intake and risk of urothelial cell carcinoma in the European Prospective Investigation into Cancer and Nutrition. *Int J Cancer*. 2013;132(3):635–44.
2062. Morton MS, Chan PS, Cheng C, et al. Lignans and isoflavonoids in plasma and prostatic fluid in men: samples from Portugal, Hong Kong, and the United Kingdom. *Prostate*. 1997;32(2):122–8.
2063. van Die MD, Bone KM, Williams SG, Pirotta MV. Soy and soy isoflavones in prostate cancer: a systematic review and meta-analysis of randomized controlled trials. *BJU Int*. 2014;113(5b):E119–30.
2064. Morton MS, Chan PS, Cheng C, et al. Lignans and isoflavonoids in plasma and prostatic fluid in men: samples from Portugal, Hong Kong, and the United Kingdom. *Prostate*. 1997;32(2):122–8.
2065. Lin X, Switzer BR, Demark-Wahnefried W. Effect of mammalian lignans on the growth of prostate cancer cell lines. *Anticancer Res*. 2001;21(6A):3995–9.
2066. Demark-Wahnefried W, Price DT, Polascik TJ, et al. Pilot study of dietary fat restriction and flaxseed supplementation in men with prostate cancer before surgery: exploring the effects on hormonal levels, prostate-specific antigen, and histopathologic features. *Urology*. 2001;58(1):47–52.
2067. Leite KR, Camara-Lopes LH, Cury J, Dall'oglio MF, Sañudo A, Srougi M. Prostate cancer detection at rebiopsy after an initial benign diagnosis: results using sextant extended prostate biopsy. *Clinics* (Sao Paulo). 2008;63(3):339–42.
2068. Demark-Wahnefried W, Robertson CN, Walther PJ, Polascik TJ, Paulson DF, Vollmer RT. Pilot study to explore effects of low-fat, flaxseed-supplemented diet on proliferation of benign prostatic epithelium and prostate-specific antigen. *Urology*. 2004;63(5):900–4.
2069. Demark-Wahnefried W, Polascik TJ, George SL, et al. Flaxseed supplementation (not dietary fat restriction) reduces prostate cancer proliferation rates in men presurgery. *Cancer Epidemiol Biomarkers Prev*. 2008;17(12):3577–87.

2070. Wei JT, Calhoun E, Jacobsen SJ. Urologic Diseases in America Project: benign prostatic hyperplasia. *J Urol.* 2008;179(5 Suppl):S75–80.
2071. Burnett AL, Wein AJ. Benign prostatic hyperplasia in primary care: what you need to know. *J Urol.* 2006;175(3 Pt 2):S19–24.
2072. Taub DA, Wei JT. The economics of benign prostatic hyperplasia and lower urinary tract symptoms in the United States. *Curr Urol Rep.* 2006;7(4):272–81.
2073. Metcalfe C, Poon KS. Long-term results of surgical techniques and procedures in men with benign prostatic hyperplasia. *Curr Urol Rep.* 2011;12(4):265–73.
2074. Burnett AL, Wein AJ. Benign prostatic hyperplasia in primary care: what you need to know. *J Urol.* 2006;175(3 Pt 2):S19–24.
2075. Burnett AL, Wein AJ. Benign prostatic hyperplasia in primary care: what you need to know. *J Urol.* 2006;175(3 Pt 2):S19–24.
2076. Gu F. Epidemiological survey of benign prostatic hyperplasia and prostatic cancer in China. *Chin Med J.* 2000;113(4):299–302.
2077. Barnard RJ, Kobayashi N, Aronson WJ. Effect of diet and exercise intervention on the growth of prostate epithelial cells. *Prostate Cancer Prostatic Dis.* 2008;11(4):362–6.
2078. Zhang W, Wang X, Liu Y, et al. Effects of dietary flaxseed lignan extract on symptoms of benign prostatic hyperplasia. *J Med Food.* 2008;11(2):207–14.
2079. Galeone C, Pelucchi C, Talamini R, et al. Onion and garlic intake and the odds of benign prostatic hyperplasia. *Urology.* 2007;70(4):672–6.
2080. Bravi F, Bosetti C, Dal Maso L, et al. Food groups and risk of benign prostatic hyperplasia. *Urology.* 2006;67(1):73–9.
2081. Zhou Z, Wang Z, Chen C, et al. Transurethral prostate vaporization using an oval electrode in 82 cases of benign prostatic hyperplasia. *Chin Med J.* 1998;111(1):52–5.
2082. Matsuo T, Miyata Y, Sakai H. Effect of salt intake reduction on nocturia in patients with excessive salt intake. *Neurourol Urodyn.* 2019;38(3):927–33.
2083. Bradley CS, Erickson BA, Messersmith EE, et al. Evidence for the impact of diet, fluid intake, caffeine, alcohol and tobacco on lower urinary tract symptoms: a systematic review. *J Urol.* 2017;198(5):1010–20.
2084. Xue Z, Lin Y, Jiang Y, Wei N, Bi J. The evaluation of nocturia in patients with lower urinary tract symptoms suggestive of benign prostatic hyperplasia and the analysis of the curative effect after medical or placebo therapy for nocturia: a randomized placebo-controlled study. *BMC Urol.* 2018;18(1):115.
2085. Johnson TM II, Sattin RW, Parmelee P, Fultz NH, Ouslander JG. Evaluating potentially modifiable risk factors for prevalent and incident nocturia in older adults. *J Am Geriatr Soc.* 2005;53(6):1011–6.
2086. Tani M, Hirayama A, Torimoto K, Matsushita C, Yamada A, Fujimoto K. Guidance on water intake effectively improves urinary frequency in patients with nocturia. *Int J Urol.* 2014;21(6):595–600.
2087. Soda T, Masui K, Okuno H, Terai A, Ogawa O, Yoshimura K. Efficacy of nondrug lifestyle measures for the treatment of nocturia. *J Urol.* 2010;184(3):1000–4.
2088. Cho SY, Lee SL, Kim IS, Koo DH, Kim HK, Oh SJ. Short-term effects of systematized behavioral modification program for nocturia: a prospective study. *Neurourol Urodyn.* 2012;31(1):64–8.
2089. Johnson TM. The chicken-or-egg dilemma with nocturia: which matters most, the water or the salt? *J Clin Hypertens.* 2020;22(4):639–41.
2090. Matsuo T, Miyata Y, Sakai H. Daily salt intake is an independent risk factor for pollakiuria and nocturia. *Int J Urol.* 2017;24(5):384–9.
2091. Alwis US, Monaghan TF, Haddad R, et al. Dietary considerations in the evaluation and management of nocturia. *F1000Res.* 2020;9(F1000 Faculty Rev):165.
2092. Matsuo T, Miyata Y, Sakai H. Effect of salt intake reduction on nocturia in patients with excessive salt intake. *Neurourol Urodyn.* 2019;38(3):927–33.

2093. Monaghan TF, Michelson KP, Wu ZD, et al. Sodium restriction improves nocturia in patients at a cardiology clinic. *J Clin Hypertens (Greenwich)*. 2020;22(4):633–8.
2094. Alwis US, Delanghe J, Dossche L, et al. Could evening dietary protein intake play a role in nocturnal polyuria? *J Clin Med*. 2020;9(8):E2532.
2095. Piantanelli L. Cancer and aging: from the kinetics of biological parameters to the kinetics of cancer incidence and mortality. *Ann N Y Acad Sci*. 1988;521:99–109.
2096. Salvioli S, Capri M, Bucci L, et al. Why do centenarians escape or postpone cancer? The role of IGF-1, inflammation and p53. *Cancer Immunol Immunother*. 2009;58(12):1909–17.
2097. Reed JC. Dysregulation of apoptosis in cancer. *J Clin Oncol*. 1999;17(9):2941–53.
2098. Rowlands MA, Gunnell D, Harris R, Vatten LJ, Holly JM, Martin RM. Circulating insulin-like growth factor peptides and prostate cancer risk: a systematic review and meta-analysis. *Int J Cancer*. 2009;124(10):2416–29.
2099. Guevara-Aguirre J, Balasubramanian P, Guevara-Aguirre M, et al. Growth hormone receptor deficiency is associated with a major reduction in pro-aging signaling, cancer, and diabetes in humans. *Sci Transl Med*. 2011;3(70):70ra13.
2100. Allen NE, Appleby PN, Davey GK, Kaaks R, Rinaldi S, Key TJ. The associations of diet with serum insulin-like growth factor I and its main binding proteins in 292 women meat-eaters, vegetarians, and vegans. *Cancer Epidemiol Biomarkers Prev*. 2002;11(11):1441–8.
2101. Soliman S, Aronson WJ, Barnard RJ. Analyzing serum-stimulated prostate cancer cell lines after low-fat, high-fiber diet and exercise intervention. *Evid Based Complement Alternat Med*. 2011;2011:529053.
2102. Ngo TH, Barnard RJ, Tymchuk CN, Cohen P, Aronson WJ. Effect of diet and exercise on serum insulin, IGF-I, and IGFBP-1 levels and growth of LNCaP cells in vitro (United States). *Cancer Causes Control*. 2002;13(10):929–35.
2103. Allen NE, Appleby PN, Davey GK, Key TJ. Hormones and diet: low insulin-like growth factor-I but normal bioavailable androgens in vegan men. *Br J Cancer*. 2000;83(1):95–7.
2104. Allen NE, Appleby PN, Davey GK, Kaaks R, Rinaldi S, Key TJ. The associations of diet with serum insulin-like growth factor I and its main binding proteins in 292 women meat-eaters, vegetarians, and vegans. *Cancer Epidemiol Biomarkers Prev*. 2002;11(11):1441–8.
2105. Pereira TV, Horwitz RI, Ioannidis JPA. Empirical evaluation of very large treatment effects of medical interventions. *JAMA*. 2012;308(16):1676–84.
2106. Lazarou J, Pomeranz BH, Corey PN. Incidence of adverse drug reactions in hospitalized patients: a meta-analysis of prospective studies. *JAMA*. 1998;279(15):1200–5.
2107. Starfield B. Is US health really the best in the world? *JAMA*. 2000;284(4):483–5.
2108. Kavanagh KT, Saman DM, Bartel R, Westerman K. Estimating hospital-related deaths due to medical error: a perspective from patient advocates. *J Patient Saf*. 2017;13(1):1–5.
2109. Cagle SD, Hutcherson BL, Wiley AT. Health care-associated infections: best practices for prevention. *Am Fam Physician*. 2022;105(3):262–70.
2110. Gilbert K, Stafford C, Crosby K, Fleming E, Gaynes R. Does hand hygiene compliance among health care workers change when patients are in contact precaution rooms in ICUs? *Am J Infect Control*. 2010;38(7):515–7.
2111. Gilbert K, Stafford C, Crosby K, Fleming E, Gaynes R. Does hand hygiene compliance among health care workers change when patients are in contact precaution rooms in ICUs? *Am J Infect Control*. 2010;38(7):515–7.
2112. Leape LL, Berwick DM. Five years after To Err Is Human: what have we learned? *JAMA*. 2005;293(19):2384–90.
2113. Starfield B. Is US health really the best in the world? *JAMA*. 2000;284(4):483–5.
2114. Institute of Medicine (US) Committee on Quality of Health Care in America. *To Err is Human: Building a Safer Health System*. Kohn LT, Corrigan JM, Donaldson MS, eds. Washington (DC): National Academies Press (US); 2000.
2115. Weingart SN, Wilson RM, Gibberd RW, Harrison B. Epidemiology of medical error. *BMJ*. 2000;320(7237):774–7.

2116. Millenson ML. The silence. *Health Aff* (Millwood). 2003;22(2):103–12.
2117. Mills DH. Medical insurance feasibility study. A technical summary. *West J Med*. 1978;128(4): 360–5.
2118. Leape LL. Error in medicine. *JAMA*. 1994;272(23):1851–7.
2119. Millenson ML. The silence. *Health Aff* (Millwood). 2003;22(2):103–12.
2120. Institute of Medicine (US) Committee on Quality of Health Care in America. *To Err is Human: Building a Safer Health System*. Kohn LT, Corrigan JM, Donaldson MS, eds. Washington (DC): National Academies Press (US); 2000.
2121. Millenson ML. The silence. *Health Aff* (Millwood). 2003;22(2):103–12.
2122. Lockley SW, Barger LK, Ayas NT, Rothschild JM, Czeisler CA, Landrigan CP. Effects of health care provider work hours and sleep deprivation on safety and performance. *Jt Comm J Qual Patient Saf*. 2007;33(11 Suppl):7–18.
2123. Barger LK, Ayas NT, Cade BE, et al. Impact of extended-duration shifts on medical errors, adverse events, and attentional failures. *PLoS Med*. 2006;3(12):e487.
2124. Millenson ML. The silence. *Health Aff* (Millwood). 2003;22(2):103–12.
2125. Egger GJ, Binns AF, Rossner SR. The emergence of "lifestyle medicine" as a structured approach for management of chronic disease. *Med J Aust*. 2009;190(3):143–5.
2126. Elek SD. Semmelweis commemoration. Semmelweis and the oath of Hippocrates. *Proc R Soc Med*. 1966;59(4):346–52.
2127. Elek SD. Semmelweis commemoration. Semmelweis and the oath of Hippocrates. *Proc R Soc Med*. 1966;59(4):346–52.
2128. Lamm RD. Marginal medicine. *JAMA*. 1998;280(10):931–3.
2129. Elek SD. Semmelweis commemoration. Semmelweis and the oath of Hippocrates. *Proc R Soc Med*. 1966;59(4):346–52.
2130. Elek SD. Semmelweis commemoration. Semmelweis and the oath of Hippocrates. *Proc R Soc Med*. 1966;59(4):346–52.
2131. Carter KC, Abbott S, Siebach JL. Five documents relating to the final illness and death of Ignaz Semmelweis. *Bull Hist Med*. 1995;69(2):255–70.
2132. Elek SD. Semmelweis commemoration. Semmelweis and the oath of Hippocrates. *Proc R Soc Med*. 1966;59(4):346–52.
2133. Elek SD. Semmelweis commemoration. Semmelweis and the oath of Hippocrates. *Proc R Soc Med*. 1966;59(4):346–52.
2134. Elek SD. Semmelweis commemoration. Semmelweis and the oath of Hippocrates. *Proc R Soc Med*. 1966;59(4):346–52.
2135. Malone J, Guleria R, Craven C, et al. Justification of diagnostic medical exposures: some practical issues. Report of an International Atomic Energy Agency Consultation. *Br J Radiol*. 2012;85(1013):523–38.
2136. Pierce DA, Shimizu Y, Preston DL, Vaeth M, Mabuchi K. Studies of the mortality of atomic bomb survivors. Report 12, part I. Cancer: 1950–1990. 1996. *Radiat Res*. 2012;178(2):AV61–87.
2137. Brenner D, Elliston C, Hall E, Berdon WE. Estimated risks of radiation-induced fatal cancer from pediatric CT. *AJR Am J Roentgenol*. 2001;176(2):289–96.
2138. Rogers LF. Taking care of children: check out the parameters used for helical CT. *AJR Am J Roentgenol*. 2001;176(2):287.
2139. Berrington de Gonzingt A, Mahesh M, Kim KP, et al. Projected cancer risks from computed tomographic scans performed in the United States in 2007. *Arch Intern Med*. 2009;169(22): 2071–7.
2140. Institute of Medicine. *Breast cancer and the environment: a life course approach*. Washington, D.C.: The National Academies Press; 2012.
2141. Picano E. Informed consent and communication of risk from radiological and nuclear medicine examinations: how to escape from a communication inferno. *BMJ*. 2004;329(7470): 849–51.

2142. Schmidt CW. CT scans: balancing health risks and medical benefits. *Environ Health Perspect.* 2012;120(3):A118–21.
2143. Pearce MS, Salotti JA, Little MP, et al. Radiation exposure from CT scans in childhood and subsequent risk of leukaemia and brain tumours: a retrospective cohort study. *Lancet.* 2012;380(9840):499–505.
2144. Limaye MR, Severance H. Pandora's boxes: questions unleashed in airport scanner debate. *J Am Osteopath Assoc.* 2011;111(2):87–8, 119.
2145. Friedberg W, Copeland K, Duke FE, O'Brien K, Darden EB. Radiation exposure during air travel: guidance provided by the Federal Aviation Administration for air carrier crews. *Health Phys.* 2000;79(5):591–5.
2146. Yong LC, Petersen MR, Sigurdson AJ, Sampson LA, Ward EM. High dietary antioxidant intakes are associated with decreased chromosome translocation frequency in airline pilots. *Am J Clin Nutr.* 2009;90(5):1402–10.
2147. Podmore ID, Griffiths HR, Herbert KE, Mistry N, Mistry P, Lunec J. Vitamin C exhibits pro-oxidant properties. *Nature.* 1998;392(6676):559.
2148. Yong LC, Petersen MR, Sigurdson AJ, Sampson LA, Ward EM. High dietary antioxidant intakes are associated with decreased chromosome translocation frequency in airline pilots. *Am J Clin Nutr.* 2009;90(5):1402–10.
2149. Yong LC, Petersen MR, Sigurdson AJ, Sampson LA, Ward EM. High dietary antioxidant intakes are associated with decreased chromosome translocation frequency in airline pilots. *Am J Clin Nutr.* 2009;90(5):1402–10.
2150. Sauvaget C, Kasagi F, Waldren CA. Dietary factors and cancer mortality among atomic-bomb survivors. *Mutat Res.* 2004;551(1–2):145–52.
2151. Kordysh EA, Emerit I, Goldsmith JR, et al. Dietary and clastogenic factors in children who immigrated to Israel from regions contaminated by the Chernobyl accident. *Arch Environ Health.* 2001;56(4):320–6.
2152. Langham WH, Bassett H, Harris PS, Carter RE. Distribution and excretion of plutonium administered intravenously to man. Los Alamos: Los Alamos Scientific Laboratory, LAB1151. *Health Physics.* 1980;38:1031–60.
2153. Loscialpo MJ. Nontherapeutic human research experiments on institutionalized mentally retarded children: civil rights and remedies. *23 New Eng J on Crim & Civ Confinement.* 1997;139:143–5.
2154. Assistant to the Secretary of Defense for Nuclear and Chemical and Biological Defense Programs. Report on search for human radiation experiment records 1944–1994. Department of Defense. https://apps.dtic.mil/sti/pdfs/ADA328641.pdf. June 1997. Accessed February 15, 2025.
2155. Kouvaris JR, Kouloulias VE, Vlahos LJ. Amifostine: the first selective-target and broad-spectrum radioprotector. *Oncologist.* 2007;12(6):738–47.
2156. Rao BN, Archana PR, Aithal BK, Rao BSS. Protective effect of zingerone, a dietary compound against radiation induced genetic damage and apoptosis in human lymphocytes. *Eur J Pharmacol.* 2011;657(1–3):59–66.
2157. Arora R, Gupta D, Chawla R, et al. Radioprotection by plant products: present status and future prospects. *Phytother Res.* 2005;19(1):1–22.
2158. Rakha A, Rehman K, Babar Imran M, Shahid M, Jahan N. Mitigation of 131-I induced oxidative stress by supplementation of turmeric and green cardamom in thyroid patients. *Int J Radiat Res.* 2022;20(1):29–36.
2159. Malekirad AA, Ranjbar A, Rahzani K, et al. Oxidative stress in radiology staff. *Environ Toxicol Pharmacol.* 2005;20(1):215–8.
2160. Zeraatpishe A, Oryan S, Bagheri MH, et al. Effects of Melissa officinalis L. on oxidative status and DNA damage in subjects exposed to long-term low-dose ionizing radiation. *Toxicol Ind Health.* 2011;27(3):205–12.
2161. Zhong W, Maradit-Kremers H, St Sauver JL, et al. Age and sex patterns of drug prescribing in a defined American population. *Mayo Clin Proc.* 2013;88(7):697–707.

2162. The use of medicines in the U.S. 2023. The IQVIA Institute. https://www.iqvia.com/insights/the-iqvia-institute/reports-and-publications/reports/the-use-of-medicines-in-the-us-2023. April 2023. Accessed February 17, 2025.
2163. Santo L, Okeyode T. National Ambulatory Medical Care Survey: 2018 national summary tables. U.S Centers for Disease Control, National Center for Health Statistics. https://www.cdc.gov/nchs/data/ahcd/namcs_summary/2018-namcs-web-tables-508.pdf. Accessed February 16, 2025.
2164. Hudson B, Zarifeh A, Young L, Wells JE. Patients' expectations of screening and preventive treatments. *Ann Fam Med.* 2012;10(6):495–502.
2165. Lytsy P, Westerling R. Patient expectations on lipid-lowering drugs. *Patient Educ Couns.* 2007;67(1–2):143–50.
2166. Trewby PN, Reddy AV, Trewby CS, Ashton VJ, Brennan G, Inglis J. Are preventive drugs preventive enough? A study of patients' expectation of benefit from preventive drugs. *Clin Med.* 2002;2(6):527–33.
2167. Trewby PN, Reddy AV, Trewby CS, Ashton VJ, Brennan G, Inglis J. Are preventive drugs preventive enough? A study of patients' expectation of benefit from preventive drugs. *Clin Med.* 2002;2(6):527–33.
2168. Trewby PN, Reddy AV, Trewby CS, Ashton VJ, Brennan G, Inglis J. Are preventive drugs preventive enough? A study of patients' expectation of benefit from preventive drugs. *Clin Med.* 2002;2(6):527–33.
2169. Raittio E, Ashraf J, Farmer J, Nascimento GG, Aldossri M. Reporting of absolute and relative risk measures in oral health and cardiovascular events studies: a systematic review. *Community Dent Oral Epidemiol.* 2023;51(2):283–91.
2170. Esselstyn CB Jr, Gendy G, Doyle J, Golubic M, Roizen MF. A way to reverse CAD? *J Fam Pract.* 2014;63(7):356–64b.
2171. Esselstyn CB Jr, Gendy G, Doyle J, Golubic M, Roizen MF. A way to reverse CAD? *J Fam Pract.* 2014;63(7):356–64b.
2172. Duthie GG, Wood AD. Natural salicylates: foods, functions and disease prevention. *Food Funct.* 2011;2(9):515–20.
2173. Fuster V, Sweeny JM. Aspirin: a historical and contemporary therapeutic overview. *Circulation.* 2011;123(7):768–78.
2174. Pasche B, Wang M, Pennison M, Jimenez H. Prevention and treatment of cancer with aspirin: where do we stand? *Semin Oncol.* 2014;41(3):397–401.
2175. Karnezis T, Shayan R, Fox S, Achen MG, Stacker SA. The connection between lymphangiogenic signalling and prostaglandin biology: a missing link in the metastatic pathway. *Oncotarget.* 2012;3(8):893–906.
2176. Macdonald S. Aspirin use to be banned in under 16 year olds. *BMJ.* 2002;325(7371):988.
2177. Siller-Matula JM. Hemorrhagic complications associated with aspirin: an underestimated hazard in clinical practice? *JAMA.* 2012;307(21):2318–20.
2178. Sutcliffe P, Connock M, Gurung T, et al. Aspirin in primary prevention of cardiovascular disease and cancer: a systematic review of the balance of evidence from reviews of randomized trials. *PLoS ONE.* 2013;8(12):e81970.
2179. Thun MJ, Jacobs EJ, Patrono C. The role of aspirin in cancer prevention. *Nat Rev Clin Oncol.* 2012;9(5):259–67.
2180. McCarty MF. Minimizing the cancer-promotional activity of cox-2 as a central strategy in cancer prevention. Med *Hypotheses.* 2012;78(1):45–57.
2181. Duthie GG, Wood AD. Natural salicylates: foods, functions and disease prevention. *Food Funct.* 2011;2(9):515–20.
2182. Duthie GG, Wood AD. Natural salicylates: foods, functions and disease prevention. *Food Funct.* 2011;2(9):515–20.
2183. Paterson JR, Blacklock C, Campbell G, Wiles D, Lawrence JR. The identification of salicylates as normal constituents of serum: a link between diet and health? *J Clin Pathol.* 1998;51(7):502–5.

2184. Rinelli S, Spadafranca A, Fiorillo G, Cocucci M, Bertoli S, Battezzati A. Circulating salicylic acid and metabolic and inflammatory responses after fruit ingestion. *Plant Foods Hum Nutr.* 2012;67(1):100–4.
2185. Blacklock CJ, Lawrence JR, Wiles D, et al. Salicylic acid in the serum of subjects not taking aspirin. Comparison of salicylic acid concentrations in the serum of vegetarians, non-vegetarians, and patients taking low dose aspirin. *J Clin Pathol.* 2001;54(7):553–5.
2186. Knutsen SF. Lifestyle and the use of health services. *Am J Clin Nutr.* 1994;59(5 Suppl):1171S–75S.
2187. McCarty MF. Dietary nitrate and reductive polyphenols may potentiate the vascular benefit and alleviate the ulcerative risk of low-dose aspirin. *Med Hypotheses.* 2013;80(2):186–90.
2188. Willcox BJ, Willcox DC, Todoriki H, et al. Caloric restriction, the traditional Okinawan diet, and healthy aging: the diet of the world's longest-lived people and its potential impact on morbidity and life span. *Ann N Y Acad Sci.* 2007;1114:434–55.
2189. McCarty MF. Minimizing the cancer-promotional activity of cox-2 as a central strategy in cancer prevention. *Med Hypotheses.* 2012;78(1):45–57.
2190. Paterson JR, Srivastava R, Baxter GJ, Graham AB, Lawrence JR. Salicylic acid content of spices and its implications. *J Agric Food Chem.* 2006;54(8):2891–6.
2191. Paterson JR, Srivastava R, Baxter GJ, Graham AB, Lawrence JR. Salicylic acid content of spices and its implications. *J Agric Food Chem.* 2006;54(8):2891–6.
2192. Pasche B, Wang M, Pennison M, Jimenez H. Prevention and treatment of cancer with aspirin: where do we stand? *Semin Oncol.* 2014;41(3):397–401.
2193. Paterson JR, Srivastava R, Baxter GJ, Graham AB, Lawrence JR. Salicylic acid content of spices and its implications. *J Agric Food Chem.* 2006;54(8):2891–6.
2194. Baxter GJ, Graham AB, Lawrence JR, Wiles D, Paterson JR. Salicylic acid in soups prepared from organically and non-organically grown vegetables. *Eur J Nutr.* 2001;40(6):289–92.
2195. Scheier L. Salicylic acid: one more reason to eat your fruits and vegetables. *J Am Diet Assoc.* 2001;101(12):1406–8.
2196. Duthie GG, Wood AD. Natural salicylates: foods, functions and disease prevention. *Food Funct.* 2011;2(9):515–20.
2197. Gangwani MK, Aziz A, Dahiya DS, Nawras M, Aziz M, Inamdar S. History of colonoscopy and technological advances: a narrative review. *Transl Gastroenterol Hepatol.* 2023;8:18.
2198. McLachlan SA, Clements A, Austoker J. Patients' experiences and reported barriers to colonoscopy in the screening context—a systematic review of the literature. *Patient Educ Couns.* 2012;86(2):137–46.
2199. Lobel EZ, Korelitz BI. Postendoscopy syndrome: "the doctor never talked to me." *J Clin Gastroenterol.* 2001;33(5):353–4.
2200. McLachlan SA, Clements A, Austoker J. Patients' experiences and reported barriers to colonoscopy in the screening context—a systematic review of the literature. *Patient Educ Couns.* 2012;86(2):137–46.
2201. Huffstetler AN, Fraiman J, Brownlee S, Stoto MA, Lin KW. An estimate of severe harms due to screening colonoscopy: a systematic review. *J Am Board Fam Med.* 2023;36(3):493–500.
2202. Manner H, Plum N, Pech O, Ell C, Enderle MD. Colon explosion during argon plasma coagulation. *Gastrointest Endosc.* 2008;67(7):1123–7.
2203. Levy I, Gralnek IM. Complications of diagnostic colonoscopy, upper endoscopy, and enteroscopy. *Best Pract Res Clin Gastroenterol.* 2016;30(5):705–18.
2204. US Preventive Services Task Force, Davidson KW, Barry MJ, et al. Screening for colorectal cancer: US Preventive Services Task Force recommendation statement. *JAMA.* 2021;325(19):1965–77.
2205. van Hees F, Habbema JD, Meester RG, Lansdorp-Vogelaar I, van Ballegooijen M, Zauber AG. Should colorectal cancer screening be considered in elderly persons without previous screening? A cost-effectiveness analysis. *Ann Intern Med.* 2014;160(11):750–9.

2206. Whitlock EP, Lin JS, Liles E, Beil TL, Fu R. Screening for colorectal cancer: a targeted, updated systematic review for the U.S. Preventive Services Task Force. *Ann Intern Med.* 2008;149(9):638–58.
2207. Brenner H, Stock C, Hoffmeister M. Effect of screening sigmoidoscopy and screening colonoscopy on colorectal cancer incidence and mortality: systematic review and meta-analysis of randomised controlled trials and observational studies. *BMJ.* 2014;348:g2467.
2208. Bretthauer M, Wieszczy P, Løberg M, et al. Estimated lifetime gained with cancer screening tests: a meta-analysis of randomized clinical trials. *JAMA Intern Med.* 2023;183(11):1196–203.
2209. Swan H, Siddiqui AA, Myers RE. International colorectal cancer screening programs: population contact strategies, testing methods and screening rates. *Pract Gastroenter.* 2012;36(8):20–9.
2210. Ling BS, Trauth JM, Fine MJ, et al. Informed decision-making and colorectal cancer screening: is it occurring in primary care? *Med Care.* 2008;46(9 Suppl 1):S23–9.
2211. Ling BS, Trauth JM, Fine MJ, et al. Informed decision-making and colorectal cancer screening: is it occurring in primary care? *Med Care.* 2008;46(9 Suppl 1):S23–9.
2212. Brett AS. Flexible sigmoidoscopy for colorectal cancer screening: more evidence, persistent ironies. *JAMA.* 2014;312(6):601–2.
2213. Yabroff KR, Klabunde CN, Yuan G, et al. Are physicians' recommendations for colorectal cancer screening guideline-consistent? *J Gen Intern Med.* 2011;26(2):177–84.
2214. Swan H, Siddiqui AA, Myers RE. International colorectal cancer screening programs: population contact strategies, testing methods and screening rates. *Pract Gastroenter.* 2012;36(8):20–9.
2215. Swan H, Siddiqui AA, Myers RE. International colorectal cancer screening programs: population contact strategies, testing methods and screening rates. *Pract Gastroenter.* 2012;36(8):20–9.
2216. Butterfield S. Changes coming for colon cancer screening. *ACP Internist.* 2014;34(7):10–1.
2217. Rosenthal E. The $2.7 trillion medical bill: colonoscopies explain why U.S. leads the world in health expenditures. *New York Times.* http://www.nytimes.com/2013/06/02/health/colonoscopies-explain-why-us-leads-the-world-in-health-expenditures.html. June 1, 2013. Accessed February 16, 2025.
2218. Whoriskey P, Keating D. How a secretive panel uses data that distorts doctors' pay. *Washington Post.* http://www.washingtonpost.com/business/economy/how-a-secretive-panel-uses-data-that-distorts-doctors-pay/2013/07/20/ee134e3a-eda8-11e2-9008-61e94a7ea20d_story.html. July 20, 2013. Accessed February 16, 2025.
2219. US Government Accountability Office. Medicare: action needed to address higher use of anatomic pathology services by providers who self-refer. GAO-13-445. http://www.gao.gov/products/GAO-13-445. June 24, 2013. Accessed February 16, 2025.
2220. Spirling LI, Daniels IR. Botanical perspectives on health peppermint: more than just an after-dinner mint. *J R Soc Promot Health.* 2001;121(1):62–3.
2221. Amato A, Liotta R, Mulè F. Effects of menthol on circular smooth muscle of human colon: analysis of the mechanism of action. *Eur J Pharmacol.* 2014;740:295–301.
2222. Leicester RJ, Hunt RH. Peppermint oil to reduce colonic spasm during endoscopy. *Lancet.* 1982;2(8305):989.
2223. Asao T, Mochiki E, Suzuki H, et al. An easy method for the intraluminal administration of peppermint oil before colonoscopy and its effectiveness in reducing colonic spasm. *Gastrointest Endosc.* 2001;53(2):172–7.
2224. Shavakhi A, Ardestani SK, Taki M, Goli M, Keshteli AH. Premedication with peppermint oil capsules in colonoscopy: a double blind placebo-controlled randomized trial study. *Acta Gastroenterol Belg.* 2012;75(3):349–53.
2225. Stange KC. Barbara Starfield: passage of the pathfinder of primary care. *Ann Fam Med.* 2011;9(4):292–6.
2226. Starfield B. Is US health really the best in the world? *JAMA.* 2000;284(4):483–5.

2227. Rappoport J. An exclusive interview with Dr. Barbara Starfield: medically caused death in America. Jon Rappoport's Blog. https://web.archive.org/web/20120831043503/https://jonrappoport.wordpress.com/2009/12/09/an-exclusive-interview-with-dr-barbara-starfield-medically-caused-death-in-america/. December 9, 2009. Accessed February 16, 2025.
2228. Millenson ML. The silence. *Health Aff* (Millwood). 2003;22(2):103–12.
2229. Holtzman NA. Chronicle of an unforetold death. *Arch Intern Med*. 2012;172(15):1174–7.
2230. Anand SS, Islam S, Rosengren A, et al. Risk factors for myocardial infarction in women and men: insights from the INTERHEART study. *Eur Heart J*. 2008;29(7):932–40.
2231. Ornish D, Brown SE, Scherwitz LW, et al. Can lifestyle changes reverse coronary heart disease? The Lifestyle Heart Trial. *Lancet*. 1990;336(8708):129–33.
2232. Gould KL, Ornish D, Scherwitz L, et al. Changes in myocardial perfusion abnormalities by positron emission tomography after long-term, intense risk factor modification. *JAMA*. 1995;274(11):894–901.
2233. Mozaffarian D, Willet WC, Hu FB. The authors reply. *N Engl J Med*. 2011;365(11):1059.
2234. Flynn MM, Schiff AR. Economical healthy diets (2012): including lean animal protein costs more than using extra virgin olive oil. *J Hunger Environ Nutr*. 2015;10(4):467–82.
2235. Bernstein AM, Bloom DE, Rosner BA, Franz M, Willett WC. Relation of food cost to healthfulness of diet among US women. *Am J Clin Nutr*. 2010;92(5):1197–203.
2236. Atwater WO. Foods: nutritive value and cost. *U.S. Department of Agriculture Farmers' Bulletin*. 1894;23:1–30.
2237. Connell CL, Zoellner JM, Yadrick MK, Chekuri SC, Crook LB, Bogle ML. Energy density, nutrient adequacy, and cost per serving can provide insight into food choices in the lower Mississippi Delta. *J Nutr Educ Behav*. 2012;44(2):148–53.
2238. Lo YT, Chang YH, Wahlqvist ML, Huang HB, Lee MS. Spending on vegetable and fruit consumption could reduce all-cause mortality among older adults. *Nutr J*. 2012;11:113.
2239. U.S. Department of Agriculture, U.S. Department of Health and Human Services. *Dietary Guidelines for Americans, 2010*. Washington, D.C.: U.S. Government Printing Office; 2010.
2240. Dietary Guidelines Advisory Committee. *The Report of the Dietary Guidelines Advisory Committee on Dietary Guidelines for Americans, 2010*. Washington, D.C.: U.S. Government Printing Office; 2010.
2241. U.S. Department of Agriculture, U.S. Department of Health and Human Services. *Dietary Guidelines for Americans, 2005*. Washington, D.C.: U.S. Government Printing Office; 2005.
2242. U.S. Department of Agriculture, U.S. Department of Health and Human Services. *Dietary Guidelines for Americans, 2010*. Washington, D.C.: U.S. Government Printing Office; 2010.
2243. U.S. Department of Agriculture, U.S. Department of Health and Human Services. *Dietary Guidelines for Americans, 2010*. Washington, D.C.: U.S. Government Printing Office; 2010.
2244. World Cancer Research Fund, American Institute for Cancer Research. *Food, Nutrition, Physical Activity, and the Prevention of Cancer: a Global Perspective*. Washington, D.C.: AICR; 2007.
2245. Pork Information Gateway. Quick facts—the pork industry at a glance. https://web.archive.org/web/20140327091217/http://www.porkgateway.org/FileLibrary/PIGLibrary/References/NPB%20Quick%20%20Facts%20book.pdf. Accessed February 18, 2025.
2246. Green D. *McDonald's Corporation v. Steel & Morris*, EWHC QB 366 (1997).
2247. United States Department of Agriculture Action Plan. https://www.usda.gov/sites/default/files/documents/usda-tribal-consultation-action-plan.pdf. April 26, 2021. Accessed February 18, 2025.
2248. U.S. Department of Agriculture, U.S. Department of Health and Human Services. *Dietary Guidelines for Americans, 2010*. Washington, D.C.: U.S. Government Printing Office; 2010.
2249. U.S. Department of Agriculture. Our agency. https://www.usda.gov/about-usda/general-information/our-agency#:~:text=We%20have%20a%20vision%20to,through%20conservation%2C%20restored%20forests%2C%20improved. Accessed February 18, 2025.
2250. U.S. Department of Agriculture. Greening Headquarters update. https://web.archive

.org/web/20160330215828/http://3.bp.blogspot.com/-tAFA0tF2hAQ/UBBwlgXK1HI/AAAAAAAAK_E/EZ7yg6hYSv0/s1600/usda.JPG. July 23, 2012. Accessed February 18, 2025.
2251. USDA Retracts Meatless Monday Recommendation. https://web.archive.org/web/20151120235940/http://www.meatlessmonday.com/articles/usda-misses-mark-on-meatless-monday/. July 26, 2012. Accessed February 18, 2025.
2252. Herman J. 2010. Saving U.S. dietary advice from conflicts of interest. *Food and Drug Law Journal.* 65(20):285–316.
2253. Institute of Medicine. *Dietary Reference Intakes for Energy, Carbohydrate, Fiber, Fat, Fatty Acids, Cholesterol, Protein, and Amino Acids.* Washington, D.C.: National Academies Press, 2003.
2254. Institute of Medicine. *Dietary Reference Intakes for Energy, Carbohydrate, Fiber, Fat, Fatty Acids, Cholesterol, Protein, and Amino Acids.* Washington, D.C.: National Academies Press; 2003.
2255. U.S. Department of Agriculture. Fat and fatty acid content of selected foods containing trans-fatty acids. ARS Nutrient Data Laboratory. http://www.ars.usda.gov/SP2UserFiles/Place/12354500/Data/Classics/trans_fa.pdf. Accessed February 18, 2025.
2256. Institute of Medicine. *Dietary Reference Intakes for Energy, Carbohydrate, Fiber, Fat, Fatty Acids, Cholesterol, Protein, and Amino Acids.* Washington, D.C.: National Academies Press; 2003.
2257. Fox M. Report recommends limiting trans-fats in diet. *Reuters.* July 10, 2002.
2258. Krebs-Smith SM, Guenther PM, Subar AF, Kirkpatrick SI, Dodd KW. Americans do not meet federal dietary recommendations. *J Nutr.* 2010;140(10):1832–8.
2259. Krebs-Smith SM, Guenther PM, Subar AF, Kirkpatrick SI, Dodd KW. Americans do not meet federal dietary recommendations. *J Nutr.* 2010;140(10):1832–8.
2260. Krebs-Smith SM, Guenther PM, Subar AF, Kirkpatrick SI, Dodd KW. Americans do not meet federal dietary recommendations. *J Nutr.* 2010;140(10):1832–8.
2261. Stuckler D, McKee M, Ebrahim S, Basu S. Manufacturing epidemics: the role of global producers in increased consumption of unhealthy commodities including processed foods, alcohol, and tobacco. *PLoS Med.* 2012;9(6):e1001235.
2262. Brownell KD. Thinking forward: the quicksand of appeasing the food industry. *PLoS Med.* 2012;9(7):e1001254.
2263. Freedhoff Y, Hébert PC. Partnerships between health organizations and the food industry risk derailing public health nutrition. *CMAJ.* 2011;183(3):291–2.
2264. Neuman W. Save the Children breaks with soda tax effort. *New York Times.* http://www.nytimes.com/2010/12/15/business/15soda.html. December 14, 2010. Accessed February 18, 2025.
2265. Murray CJ, Atkinson C, Bhalla K, et al. The state of US health, 1990–2010: burden of diseases, injuries, and risk factors. *JAMA.* 2013;310(6):591–608.
2266. Neal B. Fat chance for physical activity. *Popul Health Metr.* 2013;11(1):9.
2267. Gilroy DJ, Kauffman KW, Hall RA, Huang X, Chu FS. Assessing potential health risks from microcystin toxins in blue-green algae dietary supplements. *Environ Health Perspect.* 2000;108(5):435–9.
2268. Parker-Pope T. Michael Pollan offers 64 ways to eat food. *New York Times.* January 8, 2010.
2269. Arnold D. British India and the "beriberi problem," 1798–1942. *Med Hist.* 2010;54(3):295–314.
2270. Freeman BB, Reimers K. Tomato consumption and health: emerging benefits. *Am J Lifestyle Med.* 2010; 5(2):182–91.
2271. Denke MA. Effects of cocoa butter on serum lipids in humans: historical highlights. *Am J Clin Nutr.* 1994;60(6 Suppl):1014S–6S.
2272. Feingold Association of the United States. Regulations re 36 colorants covering 80 countries. https://web.archive.org/web/20150824080642/http://www.feingold.org/Research/PDFstudies/List-of-Colorants.pdf. Accessed February 18, 2025.
2273. Galloway D. DIY bacon fat candle. http://lifehacker.com/5929854/diy-bacon-fat-candle. July 28, 2012. Accessed February 18, 2025.

2274. Orlich MJ, Singh PN, Sabaté J, et al. Vegetarian dietary patterns and mortality in Adventist Health Study 2. *JAMA Intern Med.* 2013;173(13):1230–8.
2275. Willcox BJ, Willcox DC, Todoriki H, et al. Caloric restriction, the traditional Okinawan diet, and healthy aging: the diet of the world's longest-lived people and its potential impact on morbidity and life span. *Ann NY Acad Sci.* 2007;1114:434–55.
2276. Kaiser Permanente. The plant-based diet: a healthier way to eat. https://web.archive.org/web/20150219024134/http://mydoctor.kaiserpermanente.org/ncal/Images/New%20Plant%20Based%20Booklet%201214_tcm28-781815.pdf. 2013. Accessed February 18, 2025.
2277. Campbell TC, Parpia B, Chen J. Diet, lifestyle, and the etiology of coronary artery disease: the Cornell China study. *Am J Cardiol.* 1998;82(10B):18T–21T.
2278. Schane RE, Glantz SA, Ling PM. Social smoking implications for public health, clinical practice, and intervention research. *Am J Prev Med.* 2009;37(2):124–31.
2279. Food industry facts. The Food Industry Association. https://www.fmi.org/our-research/food-industry-facts. 2023. Accessed February 18, 2025.
2280. Vohs KD, Heatherton TF. Self-regulatory failure: a resource-depletion approach. *Psychol Sci.* 2000;11(3):249–54.
2281. Kaiser Permanente. The plant-based diet: a healthier way to eat. https://web.archive.org/web/20150219024134/http://mydoctor.kaiserpermanente.org/ncal/Images/New%20Plant%20Based%20Booklet%201214_tcm28-781815.pdf. 2013. Accessed February 18, 2025.
2282. Barnard N, Scialli AR, Bertron P, Hurlick D, Edmondset K. Acceptability of a therapeutic low-fat, vegan diet in premenopausal women. *J Nutr Educ.* 2000;32(6):314–9.
2283. Miller KB, Hurst WJ, Payne MJ, et al. Impact of alkalization on the antioxidant and flavanol content of commercial cocoa powders. *J Agric Food Chem.* 2008;56(18):8527–33.
2284. Kon SK, Klein A. The value of whole potato in human nutrition. *Biochem J.* 1928;22(1):258–60.
2285. Cheah IK, Halliwell B. Ergothioneine; antioxidant potential, physiological function and role in disease. *Biochim Biophys Acta.* 2012;1822(5):784–93.
2286. United States Supreme Court. *Nix v. Hedden*, 149 U.S. 304 (1893).
2287. Arkansas Code of 1987 annotated. Vol 1. https://archive.org/details/govlawarcode012008. Accessed February 18, 2025.
2288. 2025 Dietary Guidelines Advisory Committee. *Scientific Report of the 2025 Dietary Guidelines Advisory Committee: Advisory Report to the Secretary of Health and Human Services and Secretary of Agriculture.* U.S. Department of Health and Human Services. https://doi.org/10.52570/DGAC2025. 2024. Accessed February 18, 2025.
2289. World Cancer Research Fund, American Institute for Cancer Research. *Food, Nutrition, Physical Activity, and the Prevention of Cancer: a Global Perspective.* Washington, D.C.: AICR; 2007.
2290. U.S. Department of Agriculture, Agricultural Research Service. Tofu, raw, firm, prepared with calcium sulfate. FoodData Central. https://fdc.nal.usda.gov/food-details/172475/nutrients. April 1, 2019. Accessed February 18, 2025.
2291. Choi YM, Yoon H, Lee S, et al. Isoflavones, anthocyanins, phenolic content, and antioxidant activities of black soybeans (Glycine max (l.) merrill) as affected by seed weight. *Sci Rep.* 2020;10(1):19960.
2292. Lee M, Sorn SR, Park Y, Park HK. Anthocyanin rich-black soybean testa improved visceral fat and plasma lipid profiles in overweight/obese Korean adults: a randomized controlled trial. *J Med Food.* 2016;19(11):995–1003.
2293. Fields of gold. *Nature.* 2013;497(7447):5–6.
2294. Bøhn T, Cuhra M, Traavik T, Sanden M, Fagan J, Primicerio R. Compositional differences in soybeans on the market: glyphosate accumulates in Roundup Ready GM soybeans. *Food Chem.* 2014;153:207–15.
2295. Aris A, Leblanc S. Maternal and fetal exposure to pesticides associated to genetically modified foods in Eastern Townships of Quebec, Canada. *Reprod Toxicol.* 2011;31(4):528–33.

2296. Bøhn T, Cuhra M, Traavik T, Sanden M, Fagan J, Primicerio R. Compositional differences in soybeans on the market: glyphosate accumulates in Roundup Ready GM soybeans. *Food Chem.* 2014;153:207–15.
2297. Marc J, Mulner-Lorillon O, Boulben S, Hureau D, Durand G, Bellé R. Pesticide Roundup provokes cell division dysfunction at the level of CDK1/cyclin B activation. *Chem Res Toxicol.* 2002;15(3):326–31.
2298. Walsh LP, McCormick C, Martin C, Stocco DM. Roundup inhibits steroidogenesis by disrupting steroidogenic acute regulatory (StAR) protein expression. *Environ Health Perspect.* 2000;108(8):769–76.
2299. Vaughan E. Men! Save your testicles (and humanity): avoid Roundup® and GMO/GE Roundup Ready® foods. https://web.archive.org/web/20140714134611/http://www.drvaughan.com/2013/07/men-save-your-testicles-and-humanity.html. July 29, 2013. Accessed February 18, 2025.
2300. Romano RM, Romano MA, Bernardi MM, Furtado PV, Oliveira CA. Prepubertal exposure to commercial formulation of the herbicide glyphosate alters testosterone levels and testicular morphology. *Arch Toxicol.* 2010;84(4):309–17.
2301. Richard S, Moslemi S, Sipahutar H, Benachour N, Seralini GE. Differential effects of glyphosate and Roundup on human placental cells and aromatase. *Environ Health Perspect.* 2005;113(6):716–20.
2302. De Roos AJ, Blair A, Rusiecki JA, et al. Cancer incidence among glyphosate-exposed pesticide applicators in the Agricultural Health Study. *Environ Health Perspect.* 2005;113(1):49–54.
2303. De Roos AJ, Zahm SH, Cantor KP, et al. Integrative assessment of multiple pesticides as risk factors for non-Hodgkin's lymphoma among men. *Occup Environ Med.* 2003;60(9):E11.
2304. Garry VF, Harkins ME, Erickson LL, Long-Simpson LK, Holland SE, Burroughs BL. Birth defects, season of conception, and sex of children born to pesticide applicators living in the Red River Valley of Minnesota, USA. *Environ Health Perspect.* 2002;110 Suppl 3:441–9.
2305. Thongprakaisang S, Thiantanawat A, Rangkadilok N, Suriyo T, Satayavivad J. Glyphosate induces human breast cancer cells growth via estrogen receptors. *Food Chem Toxicol.* 2013;59:129–36.
2306. IARC Working Group on the Evaluation of Carcinogenic Risks to Humans. *Some Organophosphate Insecticides and Herbicides.* International Agency for Research on Cancer; 2017.
2307. Butler D, Reichhardt T. Long-term effect of GM crops serves up food for thought. *Nature.* 1999;398(6729):651–6.
2308. How GMOs are regulated in the United States. U.S Food and Drug Administration. https://www.fda.gov/food/agricultural-biotechnology/how-gmos-are-regulated-united-states. March 5, 2024. Accessed February 17, 2025.
2309. Smyth S. International considerations of food biotechnology regulatory frameworks. https://web.archive.org/web/20211129201949/http://regulation.upf.edu/exeter-12-papers/Paper%20260%20-%20Smyth%202012%20-%20International%20Considerations%20of%20Food%20Biotechnology%20Regulatory%20Frameworks.pdf. June 29, 2012. Accessed February 17, 2025.
2310. Kramkowska M, Grzelak T, Czyżewska K. Benefits and risks associated with genetically modified food products. *Ann Agric Environ Med.* 2013;20(3):413–9.
2311. Murooka Y, Yamshita M. Traditional healthful fermented products of Japan. *J Ind Microbiol Biotechnol.* 2008;35(8):791–8.
2312. World Cancer Research Fund, American Institute for Cancer Research. *Food, Nutrition, Physical Activity, and the Prevention of Cancer: a Global Perspective.* Washington, D.C.: AICR; 2007.
2313. Parkin DM. 7. Cancers attributable to dietary factors in the UK in 2010. IV. Salt. *Br J Cancer.* 2011;105 Suppl 2:S31–3.
2314. Lee YY, Derakhshan MH. Environmental and lifestyle risk factors of gastric cancer. *Arch Iran Med.* 2013;16(6):358–65.

2315. González CA, Jakszyn P, Pera G, et al. Meat intake and risk of stomach and esophageal adenocarcinoma within the European Prospective Investigation into Cancer and Nutrition (EPIC). *J Natl Cancer Inst.* 2006;98(5):345–54.
2316. Key TJ, Appleby PN, Crowe FL, Bradbury KE, Schmidt JA, Travis RC. Cancer in British vegetarians: updated analyses of 4998 incident cancers in a cohort of 32,491 meat eaters, 8612 fish eaters, 18,298 vegetarians, and 2246 vegans. *Am J Clin Nutr.* 2014;100 Suppl 1:378S–85S.
2317. D'Elia L, Rossi G, Ippolito R, Cappuccio FP, Strazzullo P. Habitual salt intake and risk of gastric cancer: a meta-analysis of prospective studies. *Clin Nutr.* 2012;31(4):489–98.
2318. Yoo JY, Cho HJ, Moon S, et al. Pickled vegetable and salted fish intake and the risk of gastric cancer: two prospective cohort studies and a meta-analysis. *Cancers* (Basel). 2020;12(4):996.
2319. Joossens JV, Hill MJ, Elliott P, et al. Dietary salt, nitrate and stomach cancer mortality in 24 countries. European Cancer Prevention (ECP) and the INTERSALT Cooperative Research Group. *Int J Epidemiol.* 1996;25(3):494–504.
2320. D'Elia L, Rossi G, Ippolito R, Cappuccio FP, Strazzullo P. Habitual salt intake and risk of gastric cancer: a meta-analysis of prospective studies. *Clin Nutr.* 2012;31(4):489–98.
2321. Ko KP, Park SK, Yang JJ, et al. Intake of soy products and other foods and gastric cancer risk: a prospective study. *J Epidemiol.* 2013;23(5):337–43.
2322. D'Elia L, Rossi G, Ippolito R, Cappuccio FP, Strazzullo P. Habitual salt intake and risk of gastric cancer: a meta-analysis of prospective studies. *Clin Nutr.* 2012;31(4):489–98.
2323. Turati F, Pelucchi C, Guercio V, La Vecchia C, Galeone C. Allium vegetable intake and gastric cancer: a case-control study and meta-analysis. *Mol Nutr Food Res.* 2015;59(1):171–9.
2324. He J, Gu D, Wu X, et al. Effect of soybean protein on blood pressure: a randomized, controlled trial. *Ann Intern Med.* 2005;143(1):1–9.
2325. Rivas M, Garay RP, Escanero JF, Cia P, Cia P, Alda JO. Soy milk lowers blood pressure in men and women with mild to moderate essential hypertension. *J Nutr.* 2002;132(7):1900–2.
2326. Kanda A, Hoshiyama Y, Kawaguchi T. Association of lifestyle parameters with the prevention of hypertension in elderly Japanese men and women: a four-year follow-up of normotensive subjects. *Asia Pac J Public Health.* 1999;11(2):77–81.
2327. Ito K. Review of the health benefits of habitual consumption of miso soup: focus on the effects on sympathetic nerve activity, blood pressure, and heart rate. *Environ Health Prev Med.* 2020;25(1):45.
2328. Kondo H, Tomari HS, Yamakawa S, et al. Long-term intake of miso soup decreases nighttime blood pressure in subjects with high-normal blood pressure or stage I hypertension. *Hypertens Res.* 2019;42(11):1757–67.
2329. Du DD, Yoshinaga M, Sonoda M, Kawakubo K, Uehara Y. Blood pressure reduction by Japanese traditional Miso is associated with increased diuresis and natriuresis through dopamine system in Dahl salt-sensitive rats. *Clin Exp Hypertens.* 2014;36(5):359–66.
2330. AskUSDA. Why are green peas and green (string) beans not in the Beans and Peas Vegetable Subgroup? U.S. Department of Agriculture. https://ask.usda.gov/s/article/Why-are-green-peas-and-green-string-beans-not-in-the-Beans-and-Peas-Vegetable-Subgroup. Accessed February 17, 2025.
2331. Jenkins DJ, Wolever TM, Taylor RH, et al. Slow release dietary carbohydrate improves second meal tolerance. *Am J Clin Nutr.* 1982;35(6):1339–46.
2332. Ropert A, Cherbut C, Rozé C, et al. Colonic fermentation and proximal gastric tone in humans. *Gastroenterology.* 1996;111(2):289–96.
2333. Mollard RC, Wong CL, Luhovyy BL, Anderson GH. First and second meal effects of pulses on blood glucose, appetite, and food intake at a later meal. *Appl Physiol Nutr Metab.* 2011;36(5):634–42.
2334. Yashin YI, Nemzer BV, Ryzhnev VY, Yashin AY, Chernousova NI, Fedina PA. Creation of a databank for content of antioxidants in food products by an amperometric method. *Molecules.* 2010;15(10):7450–66.

2335. Zanovec M, O'Neil CE, Nicklas TA. Comparison of nutrient density and nutrient-to-cost between cooked and canned beans. *Food Nutr Sci.* 2011;2(2):66–73.
2336. Zanovec M, O'Neil CE, Nicklas TA. Comparison of nutrient density and nutrient-to-cost between cooked and canned beans. *Food Nutr Sci.* 2011;2(2):66–73.
2337. *Rachael Ray Show.* Buffalo ranch roasted chickpeas. https://www.rachaelrayshow.com/recipes/buffalo-ranch-roasted-chickpeas-recipe. March 23, 2020. Accessed February 19, 2025.
2338. Bazzano LA, Thompson AM, Tees MT, Nguyen CH, Winham DM. Non-soy legume consumption lowers cholesterol levels: a meta-analysis of randomized controlled trials. *Nutr Metab Cardiovasc Dis.* 2011;21(2):94–103.
2339. Anderson JW, Bush HM. Soy protein effects on serum lipoproteins: a quality assessment and meta-analysis of randomized, controlled studies. *J Am Coll Nutr.* 2011;30(2):79–91.
2340. Winham DM, Hutchins AM, Johnston CS. Pinto bean consumption reduces biomarkers for heart disease risk. *J Am Coll Nutr.* 2007;26(3):243–9.
2341. Fuhrman J. Fudgy black bean brownies. *The Dr. Oz Show.* https://web.archive.org/web/20150217165247/http://www.doctoroz.com/recipe/fudgy-black-bean-brownies. November 12, 2014. Accessed February 18, 2025.
2342. Darmadi-Blackberry I, Wahlqvist ML, Kouris-Blazos A, et al. Legumes: the most important dietary predictor of survival in older people of different ethnicities. *Asia Pac J Clin Nutr.* 2004;13(2):217–20.
2343. Darmadi-Blackberry I, Wahlqvist ML, Kouris-Blazos A, et al. Legumes: the most important dietary predictor of survival in older people of different ethnicities. *Asia Pac J Clin Nutr.* 2004;13(2):217–20.
2344. Desrochers N, Brauer PM. Legume promotion in counselling: an e-mail survey of dietitians. *Can J Diet Pract Res.* 2001;62(4):193–8.
2345. Winham DM, Hutchins AM. Perceptions of flatulence from bean consumption among adults in 3 feeding studies. *Nutr J.* 2011;10:128.
2346. Levitt MD, Lasser RB, Schwartz JS, Bond JH. Studies of a flatulent patient. *N Engl J Med.* 1976;295(5):260–2.
2347. Levitt MD, Furne J, Olsson S. The relation of passage of gas and abdominal bloating to colonic gas production. *Ann Intern Med.* 1996;124(4):422–4.
2348. Price KR, Lewis J, Wyatt GM, Fenwick GR. Flatulence—causes, relation to diet and remedies. *Nahrung.* 1988;32(6):609–26.
2349. Matthews SB, Waud JP, Roberts AG, Campbell AK. Systemic lactose intolerance: a new perspective on an old problem. *Postgrad Med J.* 2005;81(953):167–73.
2350. Levitt MD, Lasser RB, Schwartz JS, Bond JH. Studies of a flatulent patient. *N Engl J Med.* 1976;295(5):260–2.
2351. Steggerda FR, Dimmick JF. Effects of bean diets on concentration of carbon dioxide in flatus. *Am J Clin Nutr.* 1966;19(2):120–4.
2352. McEligot AJ, Gilpin EA, Rock CL, et al. High dietary fiber consumption is not associated with gastrointestinal discomfort in a diet intervention trial. *J Am Diet Assoc.* 2002;102(4):549–51.
2353. Jood S, Mehta U, Singh R, Bhat CM. Effect of processing on flatus producing factors in legumes. *J Agric Food Chem.* 1985;3:268–71.
2354. Savitri A, Bhavanishankar TN, Desikachar HSR. Effect of spices on in vitro gas production by Clostridium perfringens. *Food Microbiol.* 1986;3:195–9.
2355. Di Stefano M, Miceli E, Gotti S, Missanelli A, Mazzocchi S, Corazza GR. The effect of oral alpha-galactosidase on intestinal gas production and gas-related symptoms. *Dig Dis Sci.* 2007;52(1):78–83.
2356. How you can limit your gas production. 12 tips for dealing with flatulence. *Harv Health Lett.* 2007;32(12):3.
2357. Magee EA, Richardson CJ, Hughes R, Cummings JH. Contribution of dietary protein to

sulfide production in the large intestine: an in vitro and a controlled feeding study in humans. *Am J Clin Nutr.* 2000;72(6):1488–94.
2358. Gorbach SL. Bismuth therapy in gastrointestinal diseases. *Gastroenterology.* 1990;99(3): 863–75.
2359. Suarez FL, Springfield J, Levitt MD. Identification of gases responsible for the odour of human flatus and evaluation of a device purported to reduce this odour. *Gut.* 1998;43(1): 100–4.
2360. Bouchier IA. Flatulence. *Practitioner.* 1980;224(1342):373–7.
2361. Fardy J, Sullivan S. Gastrointestinal gas. *CMAJ.* 1988;139(12):1137–42.
2362. McCullough ML, Peterson JJ, Patel R, Jacques PF, Shah R, Dwyer JT. Flavonoid intake and cardiovascular disease mortality in a prospective cohort of US adults. *Am J Clin Nutr.* 2012;95(2):454–64.
2363. Hernandez-Marin E, Galano A, Martínez A. Cis carotenoids: colorful molecules and free radical quenchers. *J Phys Chem B.* 2013;117(15):4050–61.
2364. U.S. Department of Agriculture. Oxygen Radical Absorbance Capacity (ORAC) of Selected Foods—2007. http://www.orac-info-portal.de/download/ORAC_R2.pdf. November 2007. Accessed February 18, 2025.
2365. Carlsen MH, Halvorsen BL, Holte K, et al. The total antioxidant content of more than 3100 foods, beverages, spices, herbs and supplements used worldwide. *Nutr J.* 2010;9:3.
2366. Carlsen MH, Halvorsen BL, Holte K, et al. The total antioxidant content of more than 3100 foods, beverages, spices, herbs and supplements used worldwide. *Nutr J.* 2010;9:3.
2367. Carlsen MH, Halvorsen BL, Holte K, et al. The total antioxidant content of more than 3100 foods, beverages, spices, herbs and supplements used worldwide. *Nutr J.* 2010;9:3.
2368. Dinstel RR, Cascio J, Koukel S. The antioxidant level of Alaska's wild berries: high, higher and highest. *Int J Circumpolar Health.* 2013;72.
2369. Carlsen MH, Halvorsen BL, Holte K, et al. The total antioxidant content of more than 3100 foods, beverages, spices, herbs and supplements used worldwide. *Nutr J.* 2010;9:3.
2370. Petta S, Marchesini G, Caracausi L, et al. Industrial, not fruit fructose intake is associated with the severity of liver fibrosis in genotype 1 chronic hepatitis C patients. *J Hepatol.* 2013;59(6):1169–76.
2371. Madero M, Arriaga JC, Jalal D, et al. The effect of two energy-restricted diets, a low-fructose diet versus a moderate natural fructose diet, on weight loss and metabolic syndrome parameters: a randomized controlled trial. *Metab Clin Exp.* 2011;60(11):1551–9.
2372. U.S. Department of Agriculture Economic Research Service. U.S. sugar production. http://www.ers.usda.gov/topics/crops/sugar-sweeteners/background.aspx. November 14, 2014. Accessed February 18, 2025.
2373. Petta S, Marchesini G, Caracausi L, et al. Industrial, not fruit fructose intake is associated with the severity of liver fibrosis in genotype 1 chronic hepatitis C patients. *J Hepatol.* 2013;59(6):1169–76.
2374. Törrönen R, Kolehmainen M, Sarkkinen E, Mykkänen H, Niskanen L. Postprandial glucose, insulin, and free fatty acid responses to sucrose consumed with blackcurrants and lingonberries in healthy women. *Am J Clin Nutr.* 2012;96(3):527–33.
2375. Törrönen R, Kolehmainen M, Sarkkinen E, Mykkänen H, Niskanen L. Postprandial glucose, insulin, and free fatty acid responses to sucrose consumed with blackcurrants and lingonberries in healthy women. *Am J Clin Nutr.* 2012;96(3):527–33.
2376. Törrönen R, Kolehmainen M, Sarkkinen E, Poutanen K, Mykkänen H, Niskanen L. Berries reduce postprandial insulin responses to wheat and rye breads in healthy women. *J Nutr.* 2013;143(4):430–6.
2377. Törrönen R, Kolehmainen M, Sarkkinen E, Mykkänen H, Niskanen L. Postprandial glucose, insulin, and free fatty acid responses to sucrose consumed with blackcurrants and lingonberries in healthy women. *Am J Clin Nutr.* 2012;96(3):527–33.
2378. Manzano S, Williamson G. Polyphenols and phenolic acids from strawberry and apple de-

crease glucose uptake and transport by human intestinal Caco-2 cells. *Mol Nutr Food Res.* 2010;54(12):1773–80.

2379. Sievenpiper JL, Chiavaroli L, de Souza RJ, et al. "Catalytic" doses of fructose may benefit glycaemic control without harming cardiometabolic risk factors: a small meta-analysis of randomised controlled feeding trials. *Br J Nutr.* 2012;108(3):418–23.

2380. Christensen AS, Viggers L, Hasselström K, Gregersen S. Effect of fruit restriction on glycemic control in patients with type 2 diabetes—a randomized trial. *Nutr J.* 2013;12:29.

2381. Meyer BJ, van der Merwe M, du Plessis DG, de Bruin EJ, Meyer AC. Some physiological effects of a mainly fruit diet in man. *S Afr Med J.* 1971;45(8):191–5.

2382. Meyer BJ, de Bruin EJ, du Plessis DG, van der Merwe M, Meyer AC. Some biochemical effects of a mainly fruit diet in man. *S Afr Med J.* 1971;45(10):253–61.

2383. Jenkins DJ, Kendall CW, Popovich DG, et al. Effect of a very-high-fiber vegetable, fruit, and nut diet on serum lipids and colonic function. *Metab Clin Exp.* 2001;50(4):494–503.

2384. Jenkins DJ, Kendall CW, Popovich DG, et al. Effect of a very-high-fiber vegetable, fruit, and nut diet on serum lipids and colonic function. *Metab Clin Exp.* 2001;50(4):494–503.

2385. Ou B, Bosak KN, Brickner PR, Iezzoni DG, Seymour EM. Processed tart cherry products—comparative phytochemical content, in vitro antioxidant capacity and in vitro antiinflammatory activity. *J Food Sci.* 2012;77(5):H105–12.

2386. Mullen W, Stewart AJ, Lean ME, Gardner P, Duthie GG, Crozier A. Effect of freezing and storage on the phenolics, ellagitannins, flavonoids, and antioxidant capacity of red raspberries. *J Agric Food Chem.* 2002;50(18):5197–201.

2387. Marques KK, Renfroe MH, Brevard PB, Lee RE, Gloeckner JW. Differences in antioxidant levels of fresh, frozen and freeze-dried strawberries and strawberry jam. *Int J Food Sci Nutr.* 2010;61(8):759–69.

2388. Blau LW. Cherry diet control for gout and arthritis. *Tex Rep Biol Med.* 1950;8(3):309–11.

2389. Overman T. Pegloticase: a new treatment for gout. *Cleveland Clinic Pharmacotherapy Update.* 2011;14(2):1–3.

2390. Finkelstein Y, Aks SE, Hutson JR, et al. Colchicine poisoning: the dark side of an ancient drug. *Clin Toxicol* (Phila). 2010;48(5):407–14.

2391. Fritsch PO, Sidoroff A. Drug-induced Stevens-Johnson syndrome/toxic epidermal necrolysis. *Am J Clin Dermatol.* 2000;1(6):349–60.

2392. Zhang Y, Chen C, Choi H, et al. Purine-rich foods intake and recurrent gout attacks. *Ann Rheum Dis.* 2012;71(9):1448–53.

2393. Kelley DS, Rasooly R, Jacob RA, Kader AA, Mackey BE. Consumption of Bing sweet cherries lowers circulating concentrations of inflammation markers in healthy men and women. *J Nutr.* 2006;136(4):981–6.

2394. Zielinsky P, Busato S. Prenatal effects of maternal consumption of polyphenol-rich foods in late pregnancy upon fetal ductus arteriosus. *Birth Defects Res C.* 2013;99(4):256–74.

2395. Howatson G, Bell PG, Tallent J, Middleton B, McHugh MP, Ellis J. Effect of tart cherry juice (Prunus cerasus) on melatonin levels and enhanced sleep quality. *Eur J Nutr.* 2012;51(8):909–16.

2396. Huang X, Mazza G. Application of LC and LC-MS to the analysis of melatonin and serotonin in edible plants. *Crit Rev Food Sci Nutr.* 2011;51(4):269–84.

2397. Carlsen MH, Halvorsen BL, Holte K, et al. The total antioxidant content of more than 3100 foods, beverages, spices, herbs and supplements used worldwide. *Nutr J.* 2010;9:3.

2398. Beatty S, Murray IJ, Henson DB, Carden D, Koh H, Boulton ME. Macular pigment and risk for age-related macular degeneration in subjects from a Northern European population. *Invest Ophthalmol Vis Sci.* 2001;42(2):439–46.

2399. Cheng CY, Chung WY, Szeto YT, Benzie IF. Fasting plasma zeaxanthin response to Fructus barbarum L. (wolfberry; Kei Tze) in a food-based human supplementation trial. *Br J Nutr.* 2005;93(1):123–30.

2400. Bucheli P, Vidal K, Shen L, et al. Goji berry effects on macular characteristics and plasma antioxidant levels. *Optom Vis Sci.* 2011;88(2):257–62.

2401. Nakaishi H, Matsumoto H, Tominaga S, Hirayama M. Effects of black currant anthocyanoside intake on dark adaptation and VDT work-induced transient refractive alteration in healthy humans. *Altern Med Rev.* 2000;5(6):553–62.

2402. Wu X, Beecher GR, Holden JM, Haytowitz DB, Gebhardt SE, Prior RL. Concentrations of anthocyanins in common foods in the United States and estimation of normal consumption. *J Agric Food Chem.* 2006;54(11):4069–75.

2403. Muth ER, Laurent JM, Jasper P. The effect of bilberry nutritional supplementation on night visual acuity and contrast sensitivity. *Altern Med Rev.* 2000;5(2):164–73.

2404. Rababah TM, Al-Mahasneh MA, Kilani I, et al. Effect of jam processing and storage on total phenolics, antioxidant activity, and anthocyanins of different fruits. *J Sci Food Agric.* 2011;91(6):1096–102.

2405. Marques KK, Renfroe MH, Brevard PB, Lee RE, Gloeckner JW. Differences in antioxidant levels of fresh, frozen and freeze-dried strawberries and strawberry jam. *Int J Food Sci Nutr.* 2010;61(8):759–69.

2406. Vivian J. Foraging for edible wild plants: a field guide to wild berries. Mother Earth News. https://web.archive.org/web/20140606233803/http://www.motherearthnews.com/organic-gardening/edible-wild-plants.aspx. October/November 1999. Accessed February 18, 2025.

2407. Horton R. GBD 2010: understanding disease, injury, and risk. *Lancet.* 2012;380(9859):2053–4.

2408. GBD 2021 US Burden of Disease Collaborators. The burden of diseases, injuries, and risk factors by state in the USA, 1990–2021: a systematic analysis for the Global Burden of Disease Study 2021. *Lancet.* 2024;404(10469):2314–40.

2409. Institute for Health Metrics and Evaluation (IHME). Diet low in fruits. University of Washington. https://www.healthdata.org/research-analysis/diseases-injuries-risks/factsheets/2021-diet-low-fruits-level-3-risk. Accessed February 17, 2025.

2410. Arranz S, Silván JM, Saura-Calixto F. Nonextractable polyphenols, usually ignored, are the major part of dietary polyphenols: a study on the Spanish diet. *Mol Nutr Food Res.* 2010;54(11):1646–58.

2411. Mullen W, Marks SC, Crozier A. Evaluation of phenolic compounds in commercial fruit juices and fruit drinks. *J Agric Food Chem.* 2007;55(8):3148–57.

2412. Muraki I, Imamura F, Manson JE, et al. Fruit consumption and risk of type 2 diabetes: results from three prospective longitudinal cohort studies. *BMJ.* 2013;347:f5001.

2413. Li N, Shi J, Wang K. Profile and antioxidant activity of phenolic extracts from 10 crabapples (Malus wild species). *J Agric Food Chem.* 2014;62(3):574–81.

2414. Vogel RA. Brachial artery ultrasound: a noninvasive tool in the assessment of triglyceride-rich lipoproteins. *Clin Cardiol.* 1999;22(6 Suppl):II34–9.

2415. Rueda-Clausen CF, Silva FA, Lindarte MA, et al. Olive, soybean and palm oils intake have a similar acute detrimental effect over the endothelial function in healthy young subjects. *Nutr Metab Cardiovasc Dis.* 2007;17(1):50–7.

2416. Casas-Agustench P, López-Uriarte P, Ros E, Bulló M, Salas-Salvadó J. Nuts, hypertension and endothelial function. *Nutr Metab Cardiovasc Dis.* 2011;21 Suppl 1:S21–33.

2417. Vogel RA, Corretti MC, Plotnick GD. The postprandial effect of components of the Mediterranean diet on endothelial function. *J Am Coll Cardiol.* 2000;36(5):1455–60.

2418. Brannan RG, Peters T, Talcott ST. Phytochemical analysis of ten varieties of pawpaw (Asimina triloba [l.] dunal) fruit pulp. *Food Chem.* 2015;168:656–61.

2419. Levine RA, Richards KM, Tran K, Luo R, Thomas AL, Smith RE. Determination of neurotoxic acetogenins in pawpaw (Asimina triloba) fruit by LC-HRMS. *J Agric Food Chem.* 2015;63(4):1053–6.

2420. Majrashi TA, Zulfiqar F, Chittiboyina AG, Ali Z, Khan IA. Isoquinoline alkaloids from Asimina triloba. *Nat Prod Res.* 2019;33(19):2823–9.

2421. McLaughlin JL. Paw paw and cancer: annonaceous acetogenins from discovery to commercial products. *J Nat Prod.* 2008;71(7):1311–21.

2422. Adainoo B. North American pawpaw (Asimina triloba L.) fruit: a critical review of bioactive compounds and their bioactivities. *Trends Food Sci*. 2024;149:104530.
2423. Potts LF, Luzzio FA, Smith SC, Hetman M, Champy P, Litvan I. Annonacin in Asimina triloba fruit: implication for neurotoxicity. *Neurotoxicology*. 2012;33(1):53–8.
2424. Park HK, Ilango SD, Litvan I. Environmental risk factors for progressive supranuclear palsy. *J Mov Disord*. 2021;14(2):103–13.
2425. Park HK, Ilango SD, Litvan I. Environmental risk factors for progressive supranuclear palsy. *J Mov Disord*. 2021;14(2):103–13.
2426. Lannuzel A, Ruberg M, Michel PP. Atypical parkinsonism in the Caribbean island of Guadeloupe: etiological role of the mitochondrial complex I inhibitor annonacin. *Mov Disord*. 2008;23(15):2122–8.
2427. Tran K, Ryan S, McDonald M, Thomas AL, Maia JGS, Smith RE. Annonacin and squamocin contents of pawpaw (Asimina triloba) and marolo (Annona crassiflora) fruits and atemoya (A. squamosa × A. cherimola) seeds. *Biol Trace Elem Res*. 2021;199(6):2320–9.
2428. Cleret de Langavant L, Roze E, Petit A, et al. Annonaceae consumption worsens disease severity and cognitive deficits in degenerative parkinsonism. *Mov Disord*. 2022;37(12):2355–66.
2429. Höllerhage M, Rösler TW, Berjas M, et al. Neurotoxicity of dietary supplements from annonaceae species. *Int J Toxicol*. 2015;34(6):543–50.
2430. Cleret de Langavant L, Roze E, Petit A, et al. Annonaceae consumption worsens disease severity and cognitive deficits in degenerative parkinsonism. *Mov Disord*. 2022;37(12):2355–66.
2431. Lannuzel A, Höglinger GU, Champy P, Michel PP, Hirsch EC, Ruberg M. Is atypical parkinsonism in the Caribbean caused by the consumption of Annonacae? *J Neural Transm Suppl*. 2006;(70):153–7.
2432. Tran K, Ryan S, McDonald M, Thomas AL, Maia JGS, Smith RE. Annonacin and squamocin contents of pawpaw (Asimina triloba) and marolo (Annona crassiflora) fruits and atemoya (A. squamosa × A. cherimola) seeds. *Biol Trace Elem Res*. 2021;199(6):2320–9.
2433. Pomper KW, Lowe JD, Crabtree SB, Keller W. Identification of annonaceous acetogenins in the ripe fruit of the North American pawpaw (Asimina triloba). *J Agric Food Chem*. 2009;57(18):8339–43.
2434. Potts LF, Luzzio FA, Smith SC, Hetman M, Champy P, Litvan I. Annonacin in Asimina triloba fruit: implication for neurotoxicity. *Neurotoxicology*. 2012;33(1):53–8.
2435. McLaughlin JL. Paw paw and cancer: annonaceous acetogenins from discovery to commercial products. *J Nat Prod*. 2008;71(7):1311–21.
2436. Adainoo B. North American pawpaw (Asimina triloba L.) fruit: a critical review of bioactive compounds and their bioactivities. *Trends Food Sci*. 2024;149:104530.
2437. Kaas B, Hillis AE, Pantelyat A. Progressive supranuclear palsy and pawpaw. *Neurol Clin Pract*. 2020;10(2):e17–8.
2438. Park HK, Ilango SD, Litvan I. Environmental risk factors for progressive supranuclear palsy. *J Mov Disord*. 2021;14(2):103–13.
2439. Carlsen MH, Halvorsen BL, Holte K, et al. The total antioxidant content of more than 3100 foods, beverages, spices, herbs and supplements used worldwide. *Nutr J*. 2010;9:3.
2440. Cormio L, De Siati M, Lorusso F, et al. Oral L-citrulline supplementation improves erection hardness in men with mild erectile dysfunction. *Urology*. 2011;77(1):119–22.
2441. Rimando AM, Perkins-Veazie PM. Determination of citrulline in watermelon rind. *J Chromatogr A*. 2005;1078(1–2):196–200.
2442. Pfizer Annual Meeting of Shareholders 2014 Financial Report. https://web.archive.org/web/20160322095143/http://www.pfizer.com/system/files/presentation/2014_Pfizer_Financial_Report.pdf. Accessed February 18, 2025.
2443. Johnson G. Watermelon board approves officers, budget, marketing plan. The Packer. https://web.archive.org/web/20150421102900/http://www.thepacker.com/news/watermelon

-board-approves-officers-budget-marketing-plan. February 24, 2015. Accessed February 18, 2025.
2444. Chai SC, Hooshmand S, Saadat RL, Payton ME, Brummel-Smith K, Arjmandi BH. Daily apple versus dried plum: impact on cardiovascular disease risk factors in postmenopausal women. *J Acad Nutr Diet.* 2012;112(8):1158–68.
2445. Magee E. A nutritional component to inflammatory bowel disease: the contribution of meat to fecal sulfide excretion. *Nutrition.* 1999;15(3):244–6.
2446. Ananthakrishnan AN, Khalili H, Konijeti GG, et al. A prospective study of long-term intake of dietary fiber and risk of Crohn's disease and ulcerative colitis. *Gastroenterology.* 2013;145(5):970–7.
2447. Lin HH, Tsai PS, Fang SC, Liu JF. Effect of kiwifruit consumption on sleep quality in adults with sleep problems. *Asia Pac J Clin Nutr.* 2011;20(2):169–74.
2448. U.S. Food and Drug Administration. FDA announces discontinued marketing of GI drug, Zelnorm, for safety reasons. https://web.archive.org/web/20120203095844/http://www.fda.gov/NewsEvents/Newsroom/PressAnnouncements/2007/ucm108879.htm. March 30, 2007. Accessed February 18, 2025.
2449. Skinner MA. Gold kiwifruit for immune support and reducing symptoms of cold and influenza. *J Food Drug Anal.* 2012;20:261–4.
2450. Hunter DC, Skinner MA, Wolber FM, et al. Consumption of gold kiwifruit reduces severity and duration of selected upper respiratory tract infection symptoms and increases plasma vitamin C concentration in healthy older adults. *Br J Nutr.* 2012;108(7):1235–45.
2451. Orhan F, Karakas T, Cakir M, Aksoy A, Baki A, Gedik Y. Prevalence of immunoglobulin E–mediated food allergy in 6–9-year-old urban schoolchildren in the eastern Black Sea region of Turkey. *Clin Exp Allergy.* 2009;39(7):1027–35.
2452. Rancé F, Grandmottet X, Grandjean H. Prevalence and main characteristics of schoolchildren diagnosed with food allergies in France. *Clin Exp Allergy.* 2005;35(2):167–72.
2453. Szeto YT, To TL, Pak SC, Kalle W. A study of DNA protective effect of orange juice supplementation. *Appl Physiol Nutr Metab.* 2013;38(5):533–6.
2454. Slyskova J, Lorenzo Y, Karlsen A, et al. Both genetic and dietary factors underlie individual differences in DNA damage levels and DNA repair capacity. *DNA Repair (Amst).* 2014;16:66–73.
2455. Szeto YT, Chu WK, Benzie IF. Antioxidants in fruits and vegetables: a study of cellular availability and direct effects on human DNA. *Biosci Biotechnol Biochem.* 2006;70(10):2551–5.
2456. Szeto YT, To TL, Pak SC, Kalle W. A study of DNA protective effect of orange juice supplementation. *Appl Physiol Nutr Metab.* 2013;38(5):533–6.
2457. Song JK, Bae JM. Citrus fruit intake and breast cancer risk: a quantitative systematic review. *J Breast Cancer.* 2013;16(1):72–6.
2458. Miller JA, Lang JE, Ley M, et al. Human breast tissue disposition and bioactivity of limonene in women with early-stage breast cancer. *Cancer Prev Res* (Phila). 2013;6(6):577–84.
2459. Lorenzo Y, Azqueta A, Luna L, Bonilla F, Domínguez G, Collins AR. The carotenoid beta-cryptoxanthin stimulates the repair of DNA oxidation damage in addition to acting as an antioxidant in human cells. *Carcinogenesis.* 2009;30(2):308–14.
2460. Hakim IA, Harris RB, Ritenbaugh C. Citrus peel use is associated with reduced risk of squamous cell carcinoma of the skin. *Nutr Cancer.* 2000;37(2):161–8.
2461. Astley SB, Elliott RM, Archer DB, Southon S. Evidence that dietary supplementation with carotenoids and carotenoid-rich foods modulates the DNA damage: repair balance in human lymphocytes. *Br J Nutr.* 2004;91(1):63–72.
2462. Feskanich D, Willett WC, Hunter DJ, Colditz GA. Dietary intakes of vitamins A, C, and E and risk of melanoma in two cohorts of women. *Br J Cancer.* 2003;88(9):1381–7.
2463. Owira PM, Ojewole JA. The grapefruit: an old wine in a new glass? Metabolic and cardiovascular perspectives. *Cardiovasc J Afr.* 2010;21(5):280–5.
2464. Fuhr U, Klittich K, Staib AH. Inhibitory effect of grapefruit juice and its bitter princi-

pal, naringenin, on CYP1A2 dependent metabolism of caffeine in man. *Br J Clin Pharmacol.* 1993;35(4):431–6.
2465. Ratain MJ, Cohen EE. The value meal: how to save $1,700 per month or more on lapatinib. *J Clin Oncol.* 2007;25(23):3397–8.
2466. Aziz S, Asokumaran T, Intan G. Penetrating ocular injury by durian fruit. *Med J Malaysia.* 2009;64(3):244–5.
2467. Winokur J. *The Traveling Curmudgeon.* Seattle: Sasquatch Books; 2003.
2468. Lenzi M, Fimognari C, Hrelia P. Sulforaphane as a promising molecule for fighting cancer. *Cancer Treat Res.* 2014;159:207–23.
2469. Tarozzi A, Angeloni C, Malaguti M, Morroni F, Hrelia S, Hrelia P. Sulforaphane as a potential protective phytochemical against neurodegenerative diseases. *Oxid Med Cell Longev.* 2013;2013:415078.
2470. Liu H, Smith AJ, Lott MC, et al. Sulforaphane can protect lens cells against oxidative stress: implications for cataract prevention. *Invest Ophthalmol Vis Sci.* 2013;54(8):5236–48.
2471. Heber D, Li Z, Garcia-Lloret M, et al. Sulforaphane-rich broccoli sprout extract attenuates nasal allergic response to diesel exhaust particles. *Food Funct.* 2014;5(1):35–41.
2472. Bahadoran Z, Mirmiran P, Azizi F. Potential efficacy of broccoli sprouts as a unique supplement for management of type 2 diabetes and its complications. *J Med Food.* 2013;16(5):375–82.
2473. Matusheski NV, Juvik JA, Jeffery EH. Heating decreases epithiospecifier protein activity and increases sulforaphane formation in broccoli. *Phytochemistry.* 2004;65(9):1273–81.
2474. Singh K, Connors SL, Macklin EA, et al. Sulforaphane treatment of autism spectrum disorder (ASD). *Proc Natl Acad Sci USA.* 2014;111(43):15550–5.
2475. Vermeulen M, Klöpping-Ketelaars IW, van den Berg R, Vaes WH. Bioavailability and kinetics of sulforaphane in humans after consumption of cooked versus raw broccoli. *J Agric Food Chem.* 2008;56(22):10505–9.
2476. Ferrarini L, Pellegrini N, Mazzeo T, et al. Anti-proliferative activity and chemoprotective effects towards DNA oxidative damage of fresh and cooked Brassicaceae. *Br J Nutr.* 2012;107(9):1324–32.
2477. Collins PJ, Horowitz M, Chatterton BE. Proximal, distal and total stomach emptying of a digestible solid meal in normal subjects. *Br J Radiol.* 1988;61(721):12–8.
2478. Pardini A, Tamasi G, De Rocco F, et al. Kinetics of glucosinolate hydrolysis by myrosinase in Brassicaceae tissues: a high-performance liquid chromatography approach. *Food Chem.* 2021;355:129634.
2479. Dosz EB, Jeffery EH. Modifying the processing and handling of frozen broccoli for increased sulforaphane formation. *J Food Sci.* 2013;78(9):H1459–63.
2480. Olsen H, Grimmer S, Aaby K, Saha S, Borge GI. Antiproliferative effects of fresh and thermal processed green and red cultivars of curly kale (Brassica oleracea L. convar. acephala var. sabellica). *J Agric Food Chem.* 2012;60(30):7375–83.
2481. Dosz EB, Jeffery EH. Commercially produced frozen broccoli lacks the ability to form sulforaphane. *Journal of Functional Foods.* 2013;(5)2:987–90.
2482. Ghawi SK, Methven L, Niranjan K. The potential to intensify sulforaphane formation in cooked broccoli (Brassica oleracea var. italica) using mustard seeds (Sinapis alba). *Food Chem.* 2013;138(2–3):1734–41.
2483. Dosz EB, Jeffery EH. Modifying the processing and handling of frozen broccoli for increased sulforaphane formation. *J Food Sci.* 2013;78(9):H1459–63.
2484. Economic Research Service. Red cabbage—average retail price, 2022. U.S. Department of Agriculture. https://www.ers.usda.gov/data-products/fruit-and-vegetable-prices. Accessed February 18, 2025.
2485. U.S. Department of Agriculture. Oxygen Radical Absorbance Capacity (ORAC) of Selected Foods—2007. http://www.orac-info-portal.de/download/ORAC_R2.pdf. November 2007. Accessed February 18, 2025.
2486. Economic Research Service. Red cabbage—average retail price, 2022. U.S. Department of

Agriculture. https://www.ers.usda.gov/data-products/fruit-and-vegetable-prices. Accessed February 18, 2025.

2487. Gu Y, Guo Q, Zhang L, Chen Z, Han Y, Gu Z. Physiological and biochemical metabolism of germinating broccoli seeds and sprouts. *J Agric Food Chem.* 2012;60(1):209–13.

2488. Clarke JD, Hsu A, Riedl K, et al. Bioavailability and inter-conversion of sulforaphane and erucin in human subjects consuming broccoli sprouts or broccoli supplement in a cross-over study design. *Pharmacol Res.* 2011;64(5):456–63.

2489. Shapiro TA, Fahey JW, Dinkova-Kostova AT, et al. Safety, tolerance, and metabolism of broccoli sprout glucosinolates and isothiocyanates: a clinical phase I study. *Nutr Cancer.* 2006;55(1):53–62.

2490. Sestili P, Paolillo M, Lenzi M, et al. Sulforaphane induces DNA single strand breaks in cultured human cells. *Mutat Res.* 2010;689(1–2):65–73.

2491. Kwak CS, Moon SC, Lee MS. Antioxidant, antimutagenic, and antitumor effects of pine needles (Pinus densiflora). *Nutr Cancer.* 2006;56(2):162–71.

2492. Grivetti LE, Corlett JL, Gordon BM, Lockett GT. Food in American history: part 10. Greens: part 1. Vegetable greens in a historical context. *Nutr Today.* 2008;42(2):88–94.

2493. Krebs-Smith SM, Guenther PM, Subar AF, Kirkpatrick SI, Dodd KW. Americans do not meet federal dietary recommendations. *J Nutr.* 2010;140(10):1832–8.

2494. Walker FB. Myocardial infarction after diet-induced warfarin resistance. *Arch Intern Med.* 1984;144(10):2089–90.

2495. Tamakoshi A, Tamakoshi K, Lin Y, Yagyu K, Kikuchi S. Healthy lifestyle and preventable death: findings from the Japan Collaborative Cohort (JACC) Study. *Prev Med.* 2009;48(5):486–92.

2496. Hung HC, Joshipura KJ, Jiang R, et al. Fruit and vegetable intake and risk of major chronic disease. *J Natl Cancer Inst.* 2004;96(21):1577–84.

2497. Joshipura KJ, Hu FB, Manson JE, et al. The effect of fruit and vegetable intake on risk for coronary heart disease. *Ann Intern Med.* 2001;134(12):1106–14.

2498. Joshipura KJ, Ascherio A, Manson JE, et al. Fruit and vegetable intake in relation to risk of ischemic stroke. *JAMA.* 1999;282(13):1233–9.

2499. Patent publication number EP 1069819 B1. Method for selective increase of the anticarcinogenic glucosinolates in brassica species. https://patents.google.com/patent/EP1069819B1. July 24, 2002. Accessed February 18, 2025.

2500. Archetti M, Döring TF, Hagen SB, et al. Unravelling the evolution of autumn colours: an interdisciplinary approach. *Trends Ecol Evol (Amst).* 2009;24(3):166–73.

2501. Benaron DA, Cheong WF, Stevenson DK. Tissue optics. *Science.* 1997;276(5321):2002–3.

2502. Pietrzak M, Halicka HD, Wieczorek Z, Wieczorek J, Darzynkiewicz Z. Attenuation of acridine mutagen ICR-191—DNA interactions and DNA damage by the mutagen interceptor chlorophyllin. *Biophys Chem.* 2008;135(1–3):69–75.

2503. Jubert C, Mata J, Bench G, et al. Effects of chlorophyll and chlorophyllin on low-dose aflatoxin B(1) pharmacokinetics in human volunteers. *Cancer Prev Res* (Phila). 2009;2(12):1015–22.

2504. Bachem A. Reed CI. The penetration of light through human skin. *Am J Physiol.* 1931;97:86–91.

2505. Benaron DA, Cheong WF, Stevenson DK. Tissue optics. *Science.* 1997;276(5321):2002–3.

2506. Xu C, Zhang J, Mihai DM, Washington I. Light-harvesting chlorophyll pigments enable mammalian mitochondria to capture photonic energy and produce ATP. *J Cell Sci.* 2014;127(Pt 2):388–99.

2507. Qu J, Ma L, Zhang J, Jockusch S, Washington I. Dietary chlorophyll metabolites catalyze the photoreduction of plasma ubiquinone. *Photochem Photobiol.* 2013;89(2):310–3.

2508. Ahmad K, Manongi NJ, Rajapandian R, et al. Effectiveness of coenzyme Q10 supplementation in statin-induced myopathy: a systematic review. *Cureus.* 2024;16(8):e68316.

2509. Olsen H, Grimmer S, Aaby K, Saha S, Borge GI. Antiproliferative effects of fresh and thermal processed green and red cultivars of curly kale (Brassica oleracea L. convar. acephala var. sabellica). *J Agric Food Chem.* 2012;60(30):7375–83.

2510. De Nicola GR, Bagatta M, Pagnotta E, et al. Comparison of bioactive phytochemical content and release of isothiocyanates in selected brassica sprouts. *Food Chem.* 2013;141(1):297–303.

2511. Capaldi ED, Privitera GJ. Decreasing dislike for sour and bitter in children and adults. *Appetite.* 2008;50(1):139–45.

2512. Capaldi ED, Privitera GJ. Decreasing dislike for sour and bitter in children and adults. *Appetite.* 2008;50(1):139–45.

2513. Sharafi M, Hayes JE, Duffy VB. Masking vegetable bitterness to improve palatability depends on vegetable type and taste phenotype. *Chemosens Percept.* 2013;6(1):8–19.

2514. Ottaviani JI, Ensunsa JL, Fong RY, et al. Impact of polyphenol oxidase on the bioavailability of flavan-3-ols in fruit smoothies: a controlled, single blinded, cross-over study. *Food Funct.* 2023;14(18):8217–28.

2515. Brown MJ, Ferruzzi MG, Nguyen ML, et al. Carotenoid bioavailability is higher from salads ingested with full-fat than with fat-reduced salad dressings as measured with electrochemical detection. *Am J Clin Nutr.* 2004;80(2):396–403.

2516. Unlu NZ, Bohn T, Clinton SK, Schwartz SJ. Carotenoid absorption from salad and salsa by humans is enhanced by the addition of avocado or avocado oil. *J Nutr.* 2005;135(3):431–6.

2517. Roodenburg AJ, Leenen R, van het Hof KH, Weststrate JA, Tijburg LB. Amount of fat in the diet affects bioavailability of lutein esters but not of alpha-carotene, beta-carotene, and vitamin E in humans. *Am J Clin Nutr.* 2000;71(5):1187–93.

2518. Bongoni R, Verkerk R, Steenbekkers B, Dekker M, Stieger M. Evaluation of different cooking conditions on broccoli (Brassica oleracea var. italica) to improve the nutritional value and consumer acceptance. *Plant Foods Hum Nutr.* 2014;69(3):228–34.

2519. Johnston CS, Steplewska I, Long CA, Harris LN, Ryals RH. Examination of the antiglycemic properties of vinegar in healthy adults. *Ann Nutr Metab.* 2010;56(1):74–9.

2520. Johnston CS, Gaas CA. Vinegar: medicinal uses and antiglycemic effect. *MedGenMed.* 2006;8(2):61.

2521. White AM, Johnston CS. Vinegar ingestion at bedtime moderates waking glucose concentrations in adults with well-controlled type 2 diabetes. *Diabetes Care.* 2007;30(11):2814–5.

2522. Johnston CS, White AM, Kent SM. Preliminary evidence that regular vinegar ingestion favorably influences hemoglobin A1c values in individuals with type 2 diabetes mellitus. *Diabetes Res Clin Pract.* 2009;84(2):e15–7.

2523. Chung CH. Corrosive oesophageal injury following vinegar ingestion. *Hong Kong Med J.* 2002;8(5):365–6.

2524. Lhotta K, Höfle G, Gasser R, Finkenstedt G. Hypokalemia, hyperreninemia and osteoporosis in a patient ingesting large amounts of cider vinegar. *Nephron.* 1998;80(2):242–3.

2525. Wu D, Kimura F, Takashima A, et al. Intake of vinegar beverage is associated with restoration of ovulatory function in women with polycystic ovary syndrome. *Tohoku J Exp Med.* 2013;230(1):17–23.

2526. Sakakibara S, Murakami R, Takahashi M, et al. Vinegar intake enhances flow-mediated vasodilatation via upregulation of endothelial nitric oxide synthase activity. *Biosci Biotechnol Biochem.* 2010;74(5):1055–61.

2527. Kajimoto O, Ohshima Y, Tayama K, Hirata H, Nishimura A, Tsukamoto Y. Hypotensive effects of drinks containing vinegar on high normal blood pressure and mild hypertensive subjects. *J Nutr Food.* 2003;6:51–68.

2528. Takano-Lee M, Edman JD, Mullens BA, Clark JM. Home remedies to control head lice: assessment of home remedies to control the human head louse, Pediculus humanus capitis (Anoplura: Pediculidae). *J Pediatr Nurs.* 2004;19(6):393–8.

2529. Kondo T, Kishi M, Fushimi T, Ugajin S, Kaga T. Vinegar intake reduces body weight, body fat mass, and serum triglyceride levels in obese Japanese subjects. *Biosci Biotechnol Biochem.* 2009;73(8):1837–43.

2530. Bergquist SA, Gertsson UE, Knuthsen P, Olsson ME. Flavonoids in baby spinach (Spinacia oleracea L.): changes during plant growth and storage. *J Agric Food Chem.* 2005;53(24):9459–64.

2531. Xiao Z, Lester GE, Luo Y, Wang Q. Assessment of vitamin and carotenoid concentrations of emerging food products: edible microgreens. *J Agric Food Chem.* 2012;60(31):7644–51.

2532. Dechet AM, Herman KM, Chen Parker C, et al. Outbreaks caused by sprouts, United States, 1998–2010: lessons learned and solutions needed. *Foodborne Pathog Dis.* 2014;11(8):635–44.

2533. Singh M, Brar J. Egg safety in the realm of preharvest food safety. *Microbiol Spectr.* 2016;4(4).

2534. Murray CJ, Atkinson C, Bhalla K, et al. The state of US health, 1990–2010: burden of diseases, injuries, and risk factors. *JAMA.* 2013;310(6):591–608.

2535. Institute for Health Metrics and Evaluation (IHME). GBD 2021 results. University of Washington. https://vizhub.healthdata.org/gbd-results/. Accessed December 13, 2024.

2536. O'Hara JK. The $11 trillion reward: how simple dietary changes can save lives and money, and how we get there. https://www.ucsusa.org/resources/11-trillion-dollar-reward#:~:text=According%20to%20a%202013%20UCS,from%20heart%20disease%20each%20year. August 2013. Accessed February 20, 2025.

2537. Murakami A, Ohnishi K. Target molecules of food phytochemicals: food science bound for the next dimension. *Food Funct.* 2012;3(5):462–76.

2538. Watzl B, Bub A, Brandstetter BR, Rechkemmer G. Modulation of human T-lymphocyte functions by the consumption of carotenoid-rich vegetables. *Br J Nutr.* 1999;82(5):383–9.

2539. Willcox JK, Catignani GL, Lazarus S. Tomatoes and cardiovascular health. *Crit Rev Food Sci Nutr.* 2003;43(1):1–18.

2540. Dutta-Roy AK, Crosbie L, Gordon MJ. Effects of tomato extract on human platelet aggregation in vitro. *Platelets.* 2001;12(4):218–27.

2541. O'Kennedy N, Crosbie L, Whelan S, et al. Effects of tomato extract on platelet function: a double-blinded crossover study in healthy humans. *Am J Clin Nutr.* 2006;84(3):561–9.

2542. O'Kennedy N, Crosbie L, van Lieshout M, Broom JI, Webb DJ, Duttaroy AK. Effects of antiplatelet components of tomato extract on platelet function in vitro and ex vivo: a time-course cannulation study in healthy humans. *Am J Clin Nutr.* 2006;84(3):570–9.

2543. Fuentes E, Forero-Doria O, Carrasco G, et al. Effect of tomato industrial processing on phenolic profile and antiplatelet activity. *Molecules.* 2013;18(9):11526–36.

2544. Nurk E, Refsum H, Drevon CA, et al. Cognitive performance among the elderly in relation to the intake of plant foods. The Hordaland Health Study. *Br J Nutr.* 2010;104(8):1190–201.

2545. Putnam J, Allshouse J, Kantor LS. U.S. per capita food supply trends: more calories, refined carbohydrates, and fats. *FoodReview.* 2002;25:2–15.

2546. Bhupathiraju SN, Tucker KL. Greater variety in fruit and vegetable intake is associated with lower inflammation in Puerto Rican adults. *Am J Clin Nutr.* 2011;93(1):37–46.

2547. Cooper AJ, Sharp SJ, Lentjes MA, et al. A prospective study of the association between quantity and variety of fruit and vegetable intake and incident type 2 diabetes. *Diabetes Care.* 2012;35(6):1293–300.

2548. Lichtenstein AH, Appel LJ, Brands M, et al. Diet and lifestyle recommendations revision 2006: a scientific statement from the American Heart Association Nutrition Committee. *Circulation.* 2006;114(1):82–96.

2549. Büchner FL, Bueno-de-Mesquita HB, Ros MM, et al. Variety in fruit and vegetable consumption and the risk of lung cancer in the European prospective investigation into cancer and nutrition. *Cancer Epidemiol Biomarkers Prev.* 2010;19(9):2278–86.

2550. Dias JS. Nutritional quality and health benefits of vegetables: a review. *Food and Nutrition Sciences.* 2012;3(10):1354–74.

2551. Sillanpää S, Salminen JP, Eeva T. Breeding success and lutein availability in great tit (Parus major). *Acta Oecologica.* 2009;35(6):805–10.
2552. Whitehead RD, Coetzee V, Ozakinci G, Perrett DI. Cross-cultural effects of fruit and vegetable consumption on skin color. *Am J Public Health.* 2012;102(2):212–3.
2553. Stephen ID, Law Smith MJ, Stirrat MR, Perrett DI. Facial skin coloration affects perceived health of human faces. *Int J Primatol.* 2009;30(6):845–57.
2554. Whitehead RD, Re D, Xiao D, Ozakinci G, Perrett DI. You are what you eat: within-subject increases in fruit and vegetable consumption confer beneficial skin-color changes. *PLoS ONE.* 2012;7(3):e32988.
2555. Whitehead RD, Ozakinci G, Stephen ID, Perrett DI. Appealing to vanity: could potential appearance improvement motivate fruit and vegetable consumption? *Am J Public Health.* 2012;102(2):207–11.
2556. Nagata C, Nakamura K, Wada K, et al. Association of dietary fat, vegetables and antioxidant micronutrients with skin ageing in Japanese women. *Br J Nutr.* 2010;103(10):1493–8.
2557. Greens to be gorgeous: Why eating your five fruit and veg a day makes you sexy. *Daily Mail.* http://www.dailymail.co.uk/health/article-1228348/Eating-fruit-veg-makes-attractive-opposite-sex.html. November 17, 2009. Accessed February 20, 2025.
2558. Paul BD, Snyder SH. The unusual amino acid L-ergothioneine is a physiologic cytoprotectant. *Cell Death Differ.* 2010;17(7):1134–40.
2559. Paul BD, Snyder SH. The unusual amino acid L-ergothioneine is a physiologic cytoprotectant. *Cell Death Differ.* 2010;17(7):1134–40.
2560. Berk L, Castle WB. Observations on the etiologic relationship of achylia gastrica to pernicious anemia; activity of vitamin B12 as food, extrinsic factor. *N Engl J Med.* 1948;239(24):911–3.
2561. Ey J, Schömig E, Taubert D. Dietary sources and antioxidant effects of ergothioneine. *J Agric Food Chem.* 2007;55(16):6466–74.
2562. Nguyen TH, Nagasaka R, Ohshima T. Effects of extraction solvents, cooking procedures and storage conditions on the contents of ergothioneine and phenolic compounds and antioxidative capacity of the cultivated mushroom Flammulina velutipes. *Int J Food Sci Tech.* 2012;47(6):1193–205.
2563. Schulzová V, Hajslová J, Peroutka R, Gry J, Andersson HC. Influence of storage and household processing on the agaritine content of the cultivated Agaricus mushroom. *Food Addit Contam.* 2002;19(9):853–62.
2564. Gry J. Mushrooms traded as food. Vol II sec 2. http://norden.diva-portal.org/smash/get/diva2:733528/FULLTEXT01.pdf. July 18, 2012. Accessed February 20, 2025.
2565. Mitchell SC. Food idiosyncrasies: beetroot and asparagus. *Drug Metab Dispos.* 2001;29(4 Pt 2):539–43.
2566. Donado-Pestana CM, Mastrodi Salgado J, de Oliveira Rios A, dos Santos PR, Jablonski A. Stability of carotenoids, total phenolics and in vitro antioxidant capacity in the thermal processing of orange-fleshed sweet potato (Ipomoea batatas Lam) cultivars grown in Brazil. *Plant Foods Hum Nutr.* 2012;67(3):262–70.
2567. Padda MS, Picha DH. Phenolic composition and antioxidant capacity of different heat-processed forms of sweetpotato cv. "Beauregard." *Int J Food Sci Tech.* 2008;43(8):1404–9.
2568. Bovell-Benjamin AC. Sweet potato: a review of its past, present, and future role in human nutrition. *Adv Food Nutr Res.* 2007;52:1–59.
2569. Center for Science in the Public Interest. 10 best foods. https://web.archive.org/web/20160301011207/http://www.nutritionaction.com/free-downloads/what-to-eat-10-best-foods/. Accessed February 20, 2025.
2570. Wilson CD, Pace RD, Bromfield E, Jones G, Lu JY. Consumer acceptance of vegetarian sweet potato products intended for space missions. *Life Support Biosph Sci.* 1998;5(3):339–46.
2571. Drewnowski A. New metrics of affordable nutrition: which vegetables provide most nutrients for least cost? *J Acad Nutr Diet.* 2013;113(9):1182–7.
2572. Ameny MA, Wilson PW. Relationship between hunter color values and b-carotene con-

tents in white-fleshed African sweet potatoes (Ipomoea batatas Lam). *J Sci Food Agric.* 1997;73:301–6.

2573. Kaspar KL, Park JS, Brown CR, Mathison BD, Navarre DA, Chew BP. Pigmented potato consumption alters oxidative stress and inflammatory damage in men. *J Nutr.* 2011;141(1):108–11.

2574. Vinson JA, Demkosky CA, Navarre DA, Smyda MA. High-antioxidant potatoes: acute in vivo antioxidant source and hypotensive agent in humans after supplementation to hypertensive subjects. *J Agric Food Chem.* 2012;60(27):6749–54.

2575. Carlsen MH, Halvorsen BL, Holte K, et al. The total antioxidant content of more than 3100 foods, beverages, spices, herbs and supplements used worldwide. *Nutr J.* 2010;9:3.

2576. Vinson JA, Demkosky CA, Navarre DA, Smyda MA. High-antioxidant potatoes: acute in vivo antioxidant source and hypotensive agent in humans after supplementation to hypertensive subjects. *J Agric Food Chem.* 2012;60(27):6749–54.

2577. Lim S, Xu J, Kim J, et al. Role of anthocyanin-enriched purple-fleshed sweet potato p40 in colorectal cancer prevention. *Mol Nutr Food Res.* 2013;57(11):1908–17.

2578. Olsen A, Ritz C, Kramer L, Møller P. Serving styles of raw snack vegetables. What do children want? *Appetite.* 2012;59(2):556–62.

2579. Roberto CA, Baik J, Harris JL, Brownell KD. Influence of licensed characters on children's taste and snack preferences. *Pediatrics.* 2010;126(1):88–93.

2580. Kros W, Paulis WD, van der Wouden JC. Increasing vegetable intake in Mexican-American youth: design and analysis issues. *J Am Diet Assoc.* 2011;111(11):1657.

2581. Fisher JO, Mennella JA, Hughes SO, Liu Y, Mendoza PM, Patrick H. Offering "dip" promotes intake of a moderately-liked raw vegetable among preschoolers with genetic sensitivity to bitterness. *J Acad Nutr Diet.* 2012;112(2):235–45.

2582. Isoldi KK, Dalton S, Rodriguez DP, Nestle M. Classroom "cupcake" celebrations: observations of foods offered and consumed. *J Nutr Educ Behav.* 2012;44(1):71–5.

2583. Spill MK, Birch LL, Roe LS, Rolls BJ. Hiding vegetables to reduce energy density: an effective strategy to increase children's vegetable intake and reduce energy intake. *Am J Clin Nutr.* 2011;94(3):735–41.

2584. Blatt AD, Roe LS, Rolls BJ. Hidden vegetables: an effective strategy to reduce energy intake and increase vegetable intake in adults. *Am J Clin Nutr.* 2011;93(4):756–63.

2585. Vereecken C, Rovner A, Maes L. Associations of parenting styles, parental feeding practices and child characteristics with young children's fruit and vegetable consumption. *Appetite.* 2010;55(3):589–96.

2586. World Cancer Research Fund, American Institute for Cancer Research. *Food, Nutrition, Physical Activity, and the Prevention of Cancer: a Global Perspective.* Washington, D.C.: AICR; 2007.

2587. Annema N, Heyworth JS, McNaughton SA, Iacopetta B, Fritschi L. Fruit and vegetable consumption and the risk of proximal colon, distal colon, and rectal cancers in a case-control study in Western Australia. *J Am Diet Assoc.* 2011;111(10):1479–90.

2588. Boivin D, Lamy S, Lord-Dufour S, et al. Antiproliferative and antioxidant activities of common vegetables: a comparative study. *Food Chem.* 2009;112:374–80.

2589. Boivin D, Lamy S, Lord-Dufour S, et al. Antiproliferative and antioxidant activities of common vegetables: a comparative study. *Food Chem.* 2009;112:374–80.

2590. Boivin D, Lamy S, Lord-Dufour S, et al. Antiproliferative and antioxidant activities of common vegetables: a comparative study. *Food Chem.* 2009;112:374–80.

2591. Boivin D, Lamy S, Lord-Dufour S, et al. Antiproliferative and antioxidant activities of common vegetables: a comparative study. *Food Chem.* 2009;112:374–80.

2592. Boivin D, Lamy S, Lord-Dufour S, et al. Antiproliferative and antioxidant activities of common vegetables: a comparative study. *Food Chem.* 2009;112:374–80.

2593. Abdull Razis AF, Noor NM. Cruciferous vegetables: dietary phytochemicals for cancer prevention. *Asian Pac J Cancer Prev.* 2013;14(3):1565–70.

2594. Nicastro HL, Ross SA, Milner JA. Garlic and onions: their cancer prevention properties. *Cancer Prev Res* (Phila). 2015;8(3):181–9.

2595. Oude Griep LM, Geleijnse JM, Kromhout D, Ocké MC, Verschuren WM. Raw and processed fruit and vegetable consumption and 10-year coronary heart disease incidence in a population-based cohort study in the Netherlands. *PLoS ONE.* 2010;5(10):e13609.
2596. Gliszczyńska-Swigło A, Ciska E, Pawlak-Lemańska K, Chmielewski J, Borkowski T, Tyrakowska B. Changes in the content of health-promoting compounds and antioxidant activity of broccoli after domestic processing. *Food Addit Contam.* 2006;23(11):1088–98.
2597. Ghavami A, Coward WA, Bluck LJ. The effect of food preparation on the bioavailability of carotenoids from carrots using intrinsic labelling. *Br J Nutr.* 2012;107(9):1350–66.
2598. Garcia AL, Koebnick C, Dagnelie PC, et al. Long-term strict raw food diet is associated with favourable plasma beta-carotene and low plasma lycopene concentrations in Germans. *Br J Nutr.* 2008;99(6):1293–300.
2599. Bohm V, Bitsch R. Intestinal absorption of lycopene from different matrices and interactions to other carotenoids, the lipid status, and the antioxidant capacity of human plasma. *Eur J Nutr.* 1999;38:118–25.
2600. Kahlon TS, Chiu MM, Chapman MH. Steam cooking significantly improves in vitro bile acid binding of collard greens, kale, mustard greens, broccoli, green bell pepper and cabbage. *Nutr Res.* 2008;28:351–7.
2601. Javitt NB, Budai K, Miller DG, Cahan AC, Raju U, Levitz M. Breast-gut connection: origin of chenodeoxycholic acid in breast cyst fluid. *Lancet.* 1994;343(8898):633–5.
2602. Stott-Miller M, Neuhouser ML, Stanford JL. Consumption of deep-fried foods and risk of prostate cancer. *Prostate.* 2013;73(9):960–9.
2603. Chen MJ, Hsu HT, Lin CL, Ju WY. A statistical regression model for the estimation of acrylamide concentrations in French fries for excess lifetime cancer risk assessment. *Food Chem Toxicol.* 2012;50(10):3867–76.
2604. Lineback DR, Coughlin JR, Stadler RH. Acrylamide in foods: a review of the science and future considerations. *Annu Rev Food Sci Technol.* 2012;3:15–35.
2605. Jiménez-Monreal AM, García-Diz L, Martínez-Tomé M, Mariscal M, Murcia MA. Influence of cooking methods on antioxidant activity of vegetables. *J Food Sci.* 2009;74(3): H97–103.
2606. Jiménez-Monreal AM, García-Diz L, Martínez-Tomé M, Mariscal M, Murcia MA. Influence of cooking methods on antioxidant activity of vegetables. *J Food Sci.* 2009;74(3):H97–103.
2607. Jiménez-Monreal AM, García-Diz L, Martínez-Tomé M, Mariscal M, Murcia MA. Influence of cooking methods on antioxidant activity of vegetables. *J Food Sci.* 2009;74(3):H97–103.
2608. Barański M, Srednicka-Tober D, Volakakis N, et al. Higher antioxidant and lower cadmium concentrations and lower incidence of pesticide residues in organically grown crops: a systematic literature review and meta-analyses. *Br J Nutr.* 2014;112(5):794–811.
2609. Krol WJ. Removal of trace pesticide residues from produce. Connecticut Agricultural Experiment Station. https://portal.ct.gov/caes/fact-sheets/analytical-chemistry/removal-of-trace-pesticide-residues-from-produce. June 28, 2012. Accessed February 20, 2025.
2610. Krieger RI, Brutsche-Keiper P, Crosby HR, Krieger AD. Reduction of pesticide residues of fruit using water only or Plus Fit Fruit and Vegetable Wash. *Bull Environ Contam Toxicol.* 2003;70(2):213–8.
2611. Krol WJ, Arsenault TL, Pylypiw HM, Incorvia Mattina MJ. Reduction of pesticide residues on produce by rinsing. *J Agric Food Chem.* 2000;48(10):4666–70.
2612. Wang Z, Huang J, Chen J, Li F. Effectiveness of dishwashing liquids in removing chlorothalonil and chlorpyrifos residues from cherry tomatoes. *Chemosphere.* 2013;92(8):1022–8.
2613. Zohair A. Behaviour of some organophosphorus and organochlorine pesticides in potatoes during soaking in different solutions. *Food Chem Toxicol.* 2001;39(7):751–5.
2614. Zhang ZY, Liu XJ, Hong XY. Effects of home preparation on pesticide residues in cabbage. *Food Control.* 2007;18(12):1484–7.
2615. Zohair A. Behaviour of some organophosphorus and organochlorine pesticides in potatoes during soaking in different solutions. *Food Chem Toxicol.* 2001;39(7):751–5.

2616. Organic food sales in the United States from 2005 to 2023. Statista. https://www.statista.com/statistics/196952/organic-food-sales-in-the-us-since-2000/. Accessed February 19, 2025.
2617. Understanding the USDA Organic label. U.S. Department of Agriculture. https://www.usda.gov/about-usda/news/blog/understanding-usda-organic-label. July 22, 2016. Accessed February 19, 2025.
2618. Monette M. The science of pesticide-free potato chips. *CMAJ.* 2012;184(14):E741–2.
2619. Smith-Spangler C, Brandeau ML, Hunter GE, et al. Are organic foods safer or healthier than conventional alternatives?: a systematic review. *Ann Intern Med.* 2012;157(5):348–66.
2620. Barański M, Srednicka-Tober D, Volakakis N, et al. Higher antioxidant and lower cadmium concentrations and lower incidence of pesticide residues in organically grown crops: a systematic literature review and meta-analyses. *Br J Nutr.* 2014;112(5):794–811.
2621. Forman J, Silverstein J. Organic foods: health and environmental advantages and disadvantages. *Pediatrics.* 2012;130(5):e1406–15.
2622. Barański M, Srednicka-Tober D, Volakakis N, et al. Higher antioxidant and lower cadmium concentrations and lower incidence of pesticide residues in organically grown crops: a systematic literature review and meta-analyses. *Br J Nutr.* 2014;112(5):794–811.
2623. Lindén A, Andersson K, Oskarsson A. Cadmium in organic and conventional pig production. *Arch Environ Contam Toxicol.* 2001;40(3):425–31.
2624. Lee WCJ, Shimizu M, Kniffin KM, Wansink B. You taste what you see: do organic labels bias taste perceptions? *Food Qual Prefer.* 2013;29(1):33–9.
2625. Williams PR, Hammitt JK. Perceived risks of conventional and organic produce: pesticides, pathogens, and natural toxins. *Risk Anal.* 2001;21(2):319–30.
2626. Hammitt JK. Risk perceptions and food choice: an exploratory analysis of organic- versus conventional-produce buyers. *Risk Anal.* 1990;10(3):367–74.
2627. Reiss R, Johnston J, Tucker K, Desesso JM, Keen CL. Estimation of cancer risks and benefits associated with a potential increased consumption of fruits and vegetables. *Food Chem Toxicol.* 2012;50(12):4421–7.
2628. Winter CK. Pesticide residues in imported, organic, and "suspect" fruits and vegetables. *J Agric Food Chem.* 2012;60(18):4425–9.
2629. Singh KK, Mridula D, Rehal J, Barnwal P. Flaxseed: a potential source of food, feed and fiber. *Crit Rev Food Sci Nutr.* 2011;51(3):210–22.
2630. Hyvärinen HK, Pihlava JM, Hiidenhovi JA, Hietaniemi V, Korhonen HJ, Ryhänen EL. Effect of processing and storage on the stability of flaxseed lignan added to bakery products. *J Agric Food Chem.* 2006;54(1):48–53.
2631. Cunnane SC, Hamadeh MJ, Liede AC, Thompson LU, Wolever TM, Jenkins DJ. Nutritional attributes of traditional flaxseed in healthy young adults. *Am J Clin Nutr.* 1995;61(1):62–8.
2632. Davidi A, Reynolds J, Njike VY, Ma Y, Doughty K, Katz DL. The effect of the addition of daily fruit and nut bars to diet on weight, and cardiac risk profile, in overweight adults. *J Hum Nutr Diet.* 2011;24(6):543–51.
2633. Chai SC, Hooshmand S, Saadat RL, Payton ME, Brummel-Smith K, Arjmandi BH. Daily apple versus dried plum: impact on cardiovascular disease risk factors in postmenopausal women. *J Acad Nutr Diet.* 2012;112(8):1158–68.
2634. Peterson JM, Montgomery S, Haddad E, Kearney L, Tonstad S. Effect of consumption of dried California mission figs on lipid concentrations. *Ann Nutr Metab.* 2011;58(3):232–8.
2635. Chai SC, Hooshmand S, Saadat RL, Payton ME, Brummel-Smith K, Arjmandi BH. Daily apple versus dried plum: impact on cardiovascular disease risk factors in postmenopausal women. *J Acad Nutr Diet.* 2012;112(8):1158–68.
2636. Puglisi MJ, Vaishnav U, Shrestha S, et al. Raisins and additional walking have distinct effects on plasma lipids and inflammatory cytokines. *Lipids Health Dis.* 2008;7:14.
2637. Chai SC, Hooshmand S, Saadat RL, Arjmandi BH. Daily apple consumption promotes cardiovascular health in postmenopausal women. *The FASEB Journal.* 2011;25:971.10.
2638. Keast DR, O'Neil CE, Jones JM. Dried fruit consumption is associated with improved diet

quality and reduced obesity in US adults: National Health and Nutrition Examination Survey, 1999–2004. *Nutr Res.* 2011;31(6):460–7.
2639. Edel AL, Rodriguez-Leyva D, Maddaford TG, et al. Dietary flaxseed independently lowers circulating cholesterol and lowers it beyond the effects of cholesterol-lowering medications alone in patients with peripheral artery disease. *J Nutr.* 2015;145(4):749–57.
2640. Fraser GE, Shavlik DJ. Ten years of life: is it a matter of choice? *Arch Intern Med.* 2001;161(13):1645–52.
2641. Carlsen MH, Halvorsen BL, Holte K, et al. The total antioxidant content of more than 3100 foods, beverages, spices, herbs and supplements used worldwide. *Nutr J.* 2010;9(1):3.
2642. Ros E, Mataix J. Fatty acid composition of nuts—implications for cardiovascular health. *Br J Nutr.* 2006;96 Suppl 2:S29–35.
2643. Xiao Y, Huang W, Peng C, et al. Effect of nut consumption on vascular endothelial function: a systematic review and meta-analysis of randomized controlled trials. *Clin Nutr.* 2018;37(3):831–9.
2644. Yang J, Liu RH, Halim L. Antioxidant and antiproliferative activities of common edible nut seeds. *Food Sci Tech.* 2009;42(1):1–8.
2645. Bao Y, Han J, Hu FB, et al. Association of nut consumption with total and cause-specific mortality. *N Engl J Med.* 2013;369(21):2001–11.
2646. Luu HN, Blot WJ, Xiang YB, et al. Prospective evaluation of the association of nut/peanut consumption with total and cause-specific mortality. *JAMA Intern Med.* 2015;175(5):755–66.
2647. Fernández-Montero A, Bes-Rastrollo M, Barrio-López MT, et al. Nut consumption and 5-y all-cause mortality in a Mediterranean cohort: the SUN project. *Nutrition.* 2014;30(9):1022–7.
2648. Estruch R, Ros E, Salas-Salvadó J, et al. Primary prevention of cardiovascular disease with a Mediterranean diet. *N Engl J Med.* 2013;368(14):1279–90.
2649. Supplement to: Estruch R, Ros E, Salas-Salvadó J, et al. Primary prevention of cardiovascular disease with a Mediterranean diet. *N Engl J Med.* 2013;368:1279–90.
2650. Estruch R, Ros E, Salas-Salvadó J, et al. Retraction and republication: primary prevention of cardiovascular disease with a Mediterranean diet. *N Engl J Med.* 2013;368:1279–90. *N Engl J Med.* 2018;378(25):2441–2.
2651. Stroke facts. U.S. Center for Disease Control and Prevention. https://www.cdc.gov/stroke/data-research/facts-stats/index.html. October 24, 2024. Accessed February 26, 2025.
2652. Guasch-Ferré M, Bulló M, Martínez-González MA, et al. Frequency of nut consumption and mortality risk in the PREDIMED nutrition intervention trial. *BMC Med.* 2013;11:164.
2653. Guasch-Ferré M, Hu FB, Martínez-González MA, et al. Olive oil intake and risk of cardiovascular disease and mortality in the PREDIMED Study. *BMC Med.* 2014;12:78.
2654. Keys A. Olive oil and coronary heart disease. *Lancet.* 1987;1(8539):983–4.
2655. Guasch-Ferré M, Bulló M, Martínez-González MA, et al. Frequency of nut consumption and mortality risk in the PREDIMED nutrition intervention trial. *BMC Med.* 2013;11:164.
2656. Toner CD. Communicating clinical research to reduce cancer risk through diet: walnuts as a case example. *Nutr Res Pract.* 2014;8(4):347–51.
2657. Natoli S, McCoy P. A review of the evidence: nuts and body weight. *Asia Pac J Clin Nutr.* 2007;16(4):588–97.
2658. Martínez-González MA, Bes-Rastrollo M. Nut consumption, weight gain and obesity: epidemiological evidence. *Nutr Metab Cardiovasc Dis.* 2011;21 Suppl 1:S40–5.
2659. Wang X, Li Z, Liu Y, Lv X, Yang W. Effects of pistachios on body weight in Chinese subjects with metabolic syndrome. *Nutr J.* 2012;11:20.
2660. Painter, J. The pistachio principle: calorie reduction without calorie restriction. *Weight Management Matters.* 2008;6:8.
2661. Murakami K, Sasaki S, Takahashi Y, et al. Hardness (difficulty of chewing) of the habitual

diet in relation to body mass index and waist circumference in free-living Japanese women aged 18–22 y. *Am J Clin Nutr.* 2007;86(1):206–13.
2662. McKiernan F, Lokko P, Kuevi A, et al. Effects of peanut processing on body weight and fasting plasma lipids. *Br J Nutr.* 2010;104(3):418–26.
2663. Brennan AM, Sweeney LL, Liu X, Mantzoros CS. Walnut consumption increases satiation but has no effect on insulin resistance or the metabolic profile over a 4-day period. *Obesity (Silver Spring).* 2010;18(6):1176–82.
2664. Mattes RD, Kris-Etherton PM, Foster GD. Impact of peanuts and tree nuts on body weight and healthy weight loss in adults. *J Nutr.* 2008;138(9):1741S–5S.
2665. Tapsell L, Batterham M, Tan SY, Warensjö E. The effect of a calorie controlled diet containing walnuts on substrate oxidation during 8-hours in a room calorimeter. *J Am Coll Nutr.* 2009;28(5):611–7.
2666. Mark KP, Arenella K, Girard A, Herbenick D, Fu J, Coleman E. Erectile dysfunction prevalence in the United States: report from the 2021 National Survey of Sexual Wellbeing. *J Sex Med.* 2024;21(4):296–303.
2667. Chiurlia E, D'Amico R, Ratti C, Granata AR, Romagnoli R, Modena MG. Subclinical coronary artery atherosclerosis in patients with erectile dysfunction. *J Am Coll Cardiol.* 2005;46(8):1503–6.
2668. Montorsi P, Ravagnani PM, Galli S, et al. The artery size hypothesis: a macrovascular link between erectile dysfunction and coronary artery disease. *Am J Cardiol.* 2005;96(12B):19M–23M.
2669. Montorsi P, Montorsi F, Schulman CC. Is erectile dysfunction the "tip of the iceberg" of a systemic vascular disorder? *Eur Urol.* 2003;44(3):352–4.
2670. Montorsi F, Briganti A, Salonia A, et al. Erectile dysfunction prevalence, time of onset and association with risk factors in 300 consecutive patients with acute chest pain and angiographically documented coronary artery disease. *Eur Urol.* 2003;44(3):360–4.
2671. Montorsi P, Ravagnani PM, Galli S, et al. The artery size hypothesis: a macrovascular link between erectile dysfunction and coronary artery disease. *Am J Cardiol.* 2005;96(12B):19M–23M.
2672. Meldrum DR, Gambone JC, Morris MA, Meldrum DA, Esposito K, Ignarro LJ. The link between erectile and cardiovascular health: the canary in the coal mine. *Am J Cardiol.* 2011;108(4):599–606.
2673. Corona G, Fagioli G, Mannucci E, et al. Penile doppler ultrasound in patients with erectile dysfunction (ED): role of peak systolic velocity measured in the flaccid state in predicting arteriogenic ED and silent coronary artery disease. *J Sex Med.* 2008;5(11):2623–34.
2674. Schwartz BG, Kloner RA. How to save a life during a clinic visit for erectile dysfunction by modifying cardiovascular risk factors. *Int J Impot Res.* 2009;21(6):327–35.
2675. Inman BA, Sauver JL, Jacobson DJ, et al. A population-based, longitudinal study of erectile dysfunction and future coronary artery disease. *Mayo Clin Proc.* 2009;84(2):108–13.
2676. Jackson G. Erectile dysfunction and coronary disease: evaluating the link. *Maturitas.* 2012;72(3):263–4.
2677. Fung MM, Bettencourt R, Barrett-Connor E. Heart disease risk factors predict erectile dysfunction 25 years later: the Rancho Bernardo Study. *J Am Coll Cardiol.* 2004;43(8):1405–11.
2678. Gupta BP, Murad MH, Clifton MM, Prokop L, Nehra A, Kopecky SL. The effect of lifestyle modification and cardiovascular risk factor reduction on erectile dysfunction: a systematic review and meta-analysis. *Arch Intern Med.* 2011;171(20):1797–803.
2679. Jackson G. Problem solved: erectile dysfunction (ED) = early death (ED). *Int J Clin Pract.* 2010;64(7):831–2.
2680. Aldemir M, Okulu E, Neşelioğlu S, Erel O, Kayıgil O. Pistachio diet improves erectile function parameters and serum lipid profiles in patients with erectile dysfunction. *Int J Impot Res.* 2011;23(1):32–8.

2681. Esposito K, Ciotola M, Maiorino MI, et al. Hyperlipidemia and sexual function in premenopausal women. *J Sex Med.* 2009;6(6):1696–703.
2682. Baer HJ, Glynn RJ, Hu FB, et al. Risk factors for mortality in the Nurses' Health Study: a competing risks analysis. *Am J Epidemiol.* 2011;173(3):319–29.
2683. Ros E, Hu FB. Consumption of plant seeds and cardiovascular health: epidemiological and clinical trial evidence. *Circulation.* 2013;128(5):553–65
2684. Hawkins AT, Wise PE, Chan T, et al. Diverticulitis: an update from the age old paradigm. *Curr Probl Surg.* 2020;57(10):100862.
2685. Korzenik JR. Case closed? Diverticulitis: epidemiology and fiber. *J Clin Gastroenterol.* 2006;40 Suppl 3:S112–6.
2686. Hawkins AT, Wise PE, Chan T, et al. Diverticulitis: an update from the age old paradigm. *Curr Probl Surg.* 2020;57(10):100862.
2687. Painter NS, Burkitt DP. Diverticular disease of the colon, a 20th century problem. *Clin Gastroenterol.* 1975;4(1):3–21.
2688. Korzenik JR. Case closed? Diverticulitis: epidemiology and fiber. *J Clin Gastroenterol.* 2006;40 Suppl 3:S112–6.
2689. Painter NS, Burkitt DP. Diverticular disease of the colon: a deficiency disease of Western civilization. *Br Med J.* 1971;2(5759):450–4.
2690. Painter NS, Burkitt DP. Diverticular disease of the colon, a 20th century problem. *Clin Gastroenterol.* 1975;4(1):3–21.
2691. Painter NS, Burkitt DP. Diverticular disease of the colon: a deficiency disease of Western civilization. *Br Med J.* 1971;2(5759):450–4.
2692. Burkitt DP. Dietary fibre and "pressure diseases." *J R Coll Physicians Lond.* 1975;9(2):138–46.
2693. Painter NS, Burkitt DP. Diverticular disease of the colon, a 20th century problem. *Clin Gastroenterol.* 1975;4(1):3–21.
2694. Tuohy KM, Gougoulias C, Shen Q, Walton G, Fava F, Ramnani P. Studying the human gut microbiota in the trans-omics era—focus on metagenomics and metabonomics. *Curr Pharm Des.* 2009;15(13):1415–27.
2695. Burkitt DP. Dietary fibre and "pressure diseases." *J R Coll Physicians Lond.* 1975;9(2):138–46.
2696. Burkitt DP, Walker AR, Painter NS. Dietary fiber and disease. *JAMA.* 1974;229(8):1068–1074.
2697. Hawkins AT, Wise PE, Chan T, et al. Diverticulitis: an update from the age old paradigm. *Curr Probl Surg.* 2020;57(10):100862.
2698. Korzenik JR. Case closed? Diverticulitis: epidemiology and fiber. *J Clin Gastroenterol.* 2006;40 Suppl 3:S112–6.
2699. Tarleton S, DiBaise JK. Low-residue diet in diverticular disease: putting an end to a myth. *Nutr Clin Pract.* 2011;26(2):137–42.
2700. Schechter S, Mulvey J, Eisenstat TE. Management of uncomplicated acute diverticulitis: results of a survey. *Dis Colon Rectum.* 1999;42(4):470–5; discussion 475–6.
2701. Hawkins AT, Wise PE, Chan T, et al. Diverticulitis: an update from the age old paradigm. *Curr Probl Surg.* 2020;57(10):100862.
2702. Strate LL, Liu YL, Syngal S, Aldoori WH, Giovannucci EL. Nut, corn, and popcorn consumption and the incidence of diverticular disease. *JAMA.* 2008;300(8):907–14.
2703. Prasad S, Ewigman B. Let them eat nuts—this snack is safe for diverticulosis patients. *J Fam Pract.* 2009;58(2):82–4.
2704. Godman H. The dos and don'ts of managing diverticular disease. *Harvard Health.* https://www.health.harvard.edu/diseases-and-conditions/the-dos-and-donts-of-managing-diverticular-disease. January 1, 2022. Accessed February 26, 2025.
2705. Zeratsky K. Diverticulitis: can certain foods trigger an attack? Mayo Clinic. https://www.mayoclinic.org/healthy-lifestyle/nutrition-and-healthy-eating/expert-answers/diverticulitis-diet/faq-20058293#. July 9, 2024. Accessed February 26, 2025.
2706. Diverticular disease: greatest myths and facts. Cleveland Clinic. https://health.clevelandclinic

.org/diverticular-disease-greatest-myths-and-facts. January 9, 2020. Accessed February 26, 2025.
2707. Pérez-Jiménez J. Dietary fiber: still alive. *Food Chem.* 2024;439:138076.
2708. Srinivasan K. Antioxidant potential of spices and their active constituents. *Crit Rev Food Sci Nutr.* 2014;54(3):352–72.
2709. Carlsen MH, Halvorsen BL, Holte K, et al. The total antioxidant content of more than 3100 foods, beverages, spices, herbs and supplements used worldwide. *Nutr J.* 2010;9:3.
2710. Tapsell LC, Hemphill I, Cobiac L, et al. Health benefits of herbs and spices: the past, the present, the future. *Med J Aust.* 2006;185(4 Suppl):S4–24.
2711. Shishodia S, Sethi G, Aggarwal BB. Curcumin: getting back to the roots. *Ann NY Acad Sci.* 2005;1056:206–17.
2712. Agarwal KA, Tripathi CD, Agarwal BB, Saluja S. Efficacy of turmeric (curcumin) in pain and postoperative fatigue after laparoscopic cholecystectomy: a double-blind, randomized placebo-controlled study. *Surg Endosc.* 2011;25(12):3805–10.
2713. Chandran B, Goel A. A randomized, pilot study to assess the efficacy and safety of curcumin in patients with active rheumatoid arthritis. *Phytother Res.* 2012;26(11):1719–25.
2714. Kuptniratsaikul V, Dajpratham P, Taechaarpornkul W, et al. Efficacy and safety of Curcuma domestica extracts compared with ibuprofen in patients with knee osteoarthritis: a multicenter study. *Clin Interv Aging.* 2014;9:451–8.
2715. Khajehdehi P, Zanjaninejad B, Aflaki E, et al. Oral supplementation of turmeric decreases proteinuria, hematuria, and systolic blood pressure in patients suffering from relapsing or refractory lupus nephritis: a randomized and placebo-controlled study. *J Ren Nutr.* 2012;22(1):50–7.
2716. Vecchi Brumatti L, Marcuzzi A, Tricarico PM, Zanin V, Girardelli M, Bianco AM. Curcumin and inflammatory bowel disease: potential and limits of innovative treatments. *Molecules.* 2014;19(12):21127–53.
2717. Lang A, Salomon N, Wu JC, et al. Curcumin in combination with mesalamine induces remission in patients with mild-to-moderate ulcerative colitis in a randomized controlled trial. *Clin Gastroenterol Hepatol.* 2015;13(8):1444–49.e1.
2718. Peng Z, Li D, Wu N, et al. Safety and efficacy of curcumin in the treatment of ulcerative colitis: an updated systematic review and meta-analysis of randomized controlled trials. *Explore (NY).* 2025;21(1):103083.
2719. Percival SS, Vanden Heuvel JP, Nieves CJ, Montero C, Migliaccio AJ, Meadors J. Bioavailability of herbs and spices in humans as determined by ex vivo inflammatory suppression and DNA strand breaks. *J Am Coll Nutr.* 2012;31(4):288–94.
2720. Gupta SC, Sung B, Kim JH, Prasad S, Li S, Aggarwal BB. Multitargeting by turmeric, the golden spice: from kitchen to clinic. *Mol Nutr Food Res.* 2013;57(9):1510–28.
2721. Siruguri V, Bhat RV. Assessing intake of spices by pattern of spice use, frequency of consumption and portion size of spices consumed from routinely prepared dishes in southern India. *Nutr J.* 2015;14:7.
2722. Gilani AH, Rahman AU. Trends in ethnopharmacology. *J Ethnopharmacol.* 2005;100(1–2):43–9.
2723. Newman DJ, Cragg GM. Natural products as sources of new drugs over the last 25 years. *J Nat Prod.* 2007;70(3):461–77.
2724. Atal CK, Dubey RK, Singh J. Biochemical basis of enhanced drug bioavailability by piperine: evidence that piperine is a potent inhibitor of drug metabolism. *J Pharmacol Exp Ther.* 1985;232(1):258–62.
2725. Shoba G, Joy D, Joseph T, Majeed M, Rajendran R, Srinivas PS. Influence of piperine on the pharmacokinetics of curcumin in animals and human volunteers. *Planta Med.* 1998;64(4):353–6.
2726. Anand P, Kunnumakkara AB, Newman RA, Aggarwal BB. Bioavailability of curcumin: problems and promises. *Mol Pharm.* 2007;4(6):807–18.

2727. Anand P, Kunnumakkara AB, Newman RA, Aggarwal BB. Bioavailability of curcumin: problems and promises. *Mol Pharm.* 2007;4(6):807–18.
2728. Jacobson MS. Cholesterol oxides in Indian ghee: possible cause of unexplained high risk of atherosclerosis in Indian immigrant populations. *Lancet.* 1987;2(8560):656–8.
2729. Percival SS, Vanden Heuvel JP, Nieves CJ, Montero C, Migliaccio AJ, Meadors J. Bioavailability of herbs and spices in humans as determined by ex vivo inflammatory suppression and DNA strand breaks. *J Am Coll Nutr.* 2012;31(4):288–94.
2730. Arjmandi BH, Khalil DA, Lucas EA, et al. Soy protein may alleviate osteoarthritis symptoms. *Phytomedicine.* 2004;11(7–8):567–75.
2731. Agarwal KA, Tripathi CD, Agarwal BB, Saluja S. Efficacy of turmeric (curcumin) in pain and postoperative fatigue after laparoscopic cholecystectomy: a double-blind, randomized placebo-controlled study. *Surg Endosc.* 2011;25(12):3805–10.
2732. Aggarwal BB, Yuan W, Li S, Gupta SC. Curcumin-free turmeric exhibits anti-inflammatory and anticancer activities: identification of novel components of turmeric. *Mol Nutr Food Res.* 2013;57(9):1529–42.
2733. Kim JH, Gupta SC, Park B, Yadav VR, Aggarwal BB. Turmeric (Curcuma longa) inhibits inflammatory nuclear factor (NF)-κB and NF-κB-regulated gene products and induces death receptors leading to suppressed proliferation, induced chemosensitization, and suppressed osteoclastogenesis. *Mol Nutr Food Res.* 2012;56(3):454–65.
2734. Aggarwal BB, Yuan W, Li S, Gupta SC. Curcumin-free turmeric exhibits anti-inflammatory and anticancer activities: identification of novel components of turmeric. *Mol Nutr Food Res.* 2013;57(9):1529–42.
2735. Bengmark S, Mesa MD, Gil A. Plant-derived health: the effects of turmeric and curcuminoids. *Nutr Hosp.* 2009;24(3):273–81.
2736. Cao J, Jia L, Zhou HM, Liu Y, Zhong LF. Mitochondrial and nuclear DNA damage induced by curcumin in human hepatoma G2 cells. *Toxicol Sci.* 2006;91(2):476–83.
2737. Halegoua-DeMarzio D, Navarro V, Ahmad J, et al. Liver injury associated with turmeric—a growing problem: ten cases from the Drug Induced Liver Injury Network [DILIN]. *Am J Med.* 2023;136(2):200–6.
2738. Dostal AM, Samavat H, Bedell S, et al. The safety of green tea extract supplementation in postmenopausal women at risk for breast cancer: results of the Minnesota Green Tea Trial. *Food Chem Toxicol.* 2015;83:26–35.
2739. Molani-Gol R, Dehghani A, Rafraf M. Effects of curcumin/turmeric supplementation on the liver enzymes, lipid profiles, glycemic index, and anthropometric indices in non-alcoholic fatty liver patients: an umbrella meta-analysis. *Phytother Res.* 2024;38(2):539–55.
2740. Forsyth JE, Nurunnahar S, Islam SS, et al. Turmeric means "yellow" in Bengali: lead chromate pigments added to turmeric threaten public health across Bangladesh. *Environ Res.* 2019;179(Pt A):108722.
2741. Cowell W, Ireland T, Vorhees D, Heiger-Bernays W. Ground turmeric as a source of lead exposure in the United States. *Public Health Rep.* 2017;132(3):289–93.
2742. Forsyth JE, Baker M, Nurunnahar S, et al. Food safety policy enforcement and associated actions reduce lead chromate adulteration in turmeric across Bangladesh. *Environ Res.* 2023;232:116328.
2743. Forsyth JE, Mistree D, Nash E, Angrish M, Luby SP. Evidence of turmeric adulteration with lead chromate across South Asia. *Sci Total Environ.* 2024;949:175003.
2744. Turmeric and curcumin supplements and spices. https://www.consumerlab.com/reviews/turmeric-curcumin-supplements-spice-review/turmeric/. June 15, 2023. Updated February 18, 2025. Accessed February 22, 2025.
2745. Rasyid A, Lelo A. The effect of curcumin and placebo on human gall-bladder function: an ultrasound study. *Aliment Pharmacol Ther.* 1999;13(2):245–9.
2746. Rasyid A, Rahman AR, Jaalam K, Lelo A. Effect of different curcumin dosages on human gall bladder. *Asia Pac J Clin Nutr.* 2002;11(4):314–8.

2747. Asher GN, Spelman K. Clinical utility of curcumin extract. *Altern Ther Health Med.* 2013;19(2):20–2.
2748. Goel A, Kunnumakkara AB, Aggarwal BB. Curcumin as "curecumin": from kitchen to clinic. *Biochem Pharmacol.* 2008;75(4):787–809.
2749. Ghosh Das S, Savage GP. Total and soluble oxalate content of some Indian spices. *Plant Foods Hum Nutr.* 2012;67(2):186–90.
2750. Asher GN, Spelman K. Clinical utility of curcumin extract. *Altern Ther Health Med.* 2013;19(2):20–2.
2751. Ahmad A, Husain A, Mujeeb M, et al. A review on therapeutic potential of Nigella sativa: a miracle herb. *Asian Pac J Trop Biomed.* 2013;3(5):337–52.
2752. Sharma NK, Ahirwar D, Jhade D, Gupta S. Medicinal and phamacological potential of Nigella sativa: a review. *Ethnobotanical Review.* 2009;13:946–55.
2753. Agricultural Research Service, United States Department of Agriculture. Sweet sunnah, whole black seeds nigella sativa. FoodData Central. https://fdc.nal.usda.gov/fdc-app.html#/food-details/468991/nutrients. April 1, 2019. Accessed May 8, 2021.
2754. Sahebkar A, Beccuti G, Simental-Mendía LE, Nobili V, Bo S. Nigella sativa (black seed) effects on plasma lipid concentrations in humans: a systematic review and meta-analysis of randomized placebo-controlled trials. *Pharmacol Res.* 2016;106:37–50.
2755. Sahebkar A, Soranna D, Liu X, et al. A systematic review and meta-analysis of randomized controlled trials investigating the effects of supplementation with Nigella sativa (black seed) on blood pressure. *J Hypertens.* 2016;34(11):2127–35.
2756. Daryabeygi-Khotbehsara R, Golzarand M, Ghaffari MP, Djafarian K. Nigella sativa improves glucose homeostasis and serum lipids in type 2 diabetes: a systematic review and meta-analysis. *Complement Ther Med.* 2017;35:6–13.
2757. Ibrahim RM, Hamdan NS, Mahmud R, et al. A randomised controlled trial on hypolipidemic effects of Nigella Sativa seeds powder in menopausal women. *J Transl Med.* 2014;12:82.
2758. Latiff LA, Parhizkar S, Dollah MA, Hassan ST. Alternative supplement for enhancement of reproductive health and metabolic profile among perimenopausal women: a novel role of Nigella sativa. *Iran J Basic Med Sci.* 2014;17(12):980–5.
2759. Ibrahim RM, Hamdan NS, Mahmud R, et al. A randomised controlled trial on hypolipidemic effects of Nigella Sativa seeds powder in menopausal women. *J Transl Med.* 2014;12:82.
2760. Sahebkar A, Beccuti G, Simental-Mendía LE, Nobili V, Bo S. Nigella sativa (black seed) effects on plasma lipid concentrations in humans: a systematic review and meta-analysis of randomized placebo-controlled trials. *Pharmacol Res.* 2016;106:37–50.
2761. Mousavi SM, Sheikhi A, Varkaneh HK, Zarezadeh M, Rahmani J, Milajerdi A. Effect of Nigella sativa supplementation on obesity indices: a systematic review and meta-analysis of randomized controlled trials. *Complement Ther Med.* 2018;38:48–57.
2762. Montazeri RS, Fatahi S, Sohouli MH, et al. The effect of Nigella sativa on biomarkers of inflammation and oxidative stress: a systematic review and meta-analysis of randomized controlled trials. *J Food Biochem.* 2021;45(4):e13625.
2763. He T, Xu X. The influence of Nigella sativa for asthma control: a meta-analysis. *Am J Emerg Med.* 2020;38(3):589–93.
2764. Khabbazi A, Javadivala Z, Seyedsadjadi N, Malek Mahdavi A. A systematic review of the potential effects of *Nigella sativa* on rheumatoid arthritis. *Planta Med.* 2020;86(7):457–69.
2765. Tajmiri S, Abbasalizad Farhangi M, Dehghan P. *Nigella Sativa* treatment and serum concentrations of thyroid hormones, transforming growth factor β (TGF-β) and interleukin 23 (IL-23) in patients with Hashimoto's thyroiditis. *Eur J Integr Med.* 2016;8(4):576–80.
2766. Ardakani Movaghati MR, Yousefi M, Saghebi SA, Sadeghi Vazin M, Iraji A, Mosavat SH. Efficacy of black seed *(Nigella sativa* L.) on kidney stone dissolution: a randomized, double-blind, placebo-controlled, clinical trial. *Phytother Res.* 2019;33(5):1404–12.

2767. Korzeniewski K, Nitsch-Osuch A, Guzek A, Juszczak D. High altitude pulmonary edema in mountain climbers. *Respir Physiol Neurobiol.* 2015;209:33–8.
2768. Greenwald AJ, Allen TH, Bancroft RW. Abdominal gas volume at altitude and at ground level. *J Appl Physiol.* 1969;26(2):177–81.
2769. Auerbach P, Miller YE. High altitude flatus expulsion (HAFE). *West J Med.* 1981;134(2):173–4.
2770. Swaminathan A, Sridhara SRC, Sinha S, et al. Nitrites derived from *Foeniculum vulgare* (fennel) seeds promotes vascular functions. *J Food Sci.* 2012;77(12):H273–9.
2771. Türkyilmaz Z, Karabulut R, Sönmez K, Can Başaklar A. A striking and frequent cause of premature thelarche in children: *Foeniculum vulgare. J Pediatr Surg.* 2008;43(11):2109–11.
2772. Ghasemi V, Kheirkhah M, Neisani Samani L, Vahedi M. The effect of herbal tea containing fennel seed on breast milk sufficiency signs and growth parameters of Iranian infants. *Shiraz E-Med J.* 2014;15(4):e22262.
2773. Lee HW, Ang L, Lee MS, Alimoradi Z, Kim E. Fennel for reducing pain in primary dysmenorrhea: a systematic review and meta-analysis of randomized controlled trials. *Nutrients.* 2020;12(11):E3438.
2774. Javidnia K, Dastgheib L, Mohammadi Samani S, Nasiri A. Antihirsutism activity of Fennel (fruits of *Foeniculum vulgare*) extract—a double-blind placebo controlled study. *Phytomedicine.* 2003;10(6–7):455–8.
2775. Khan TM, Wu DBC, Dolzhenko AV. Effectiveness of fenugreek as a galactagogue: a network meta-analysis. *Phytother Res.* 2018;32(3):402–12.
2776. Bumrungpert A, Somboonpanyakul P, Pavadhgul P, Thaninthranon S. Effects of fenugreek, ginger, and turmeric supplementation on human milk volume and nutrient content in breastfeeding mothers: a randomized double-blind controlled trial. *Breastfeed Med.* 2018;13(10):645–50.
2777. Younesy S, Amiraliakbari S, Esmaeili S, Alavimajd H, Nouraei S. Effects of fenugreek seed on the severity and systemic symptoms of dysmenorrhea. *J Reprod Infertil.* 2014;15(1):41–8.
2778. Ashihara H. *De novo* biosynthesis of trigonelline in fenugreek (*Trigonella foenum-graecum*) seedlings. *Nat Prod Commun.* 2016;11(8):1093–6.
2779. Khanna A, John F, Das S, et al. Efficacy of a novel extract of fenugreek seeds in alleviating vasomotor symptoms and depression in perimenopausal women: a randomized, double-blinded, placebo-controlled study. *J Food Biochem.* 2020;44(12):e13507.
2780. Steels E, Steele ML, Harold M, Coulson S. Efficacy of a proprietary *Trigonella foenum-graecum* L. de-husked seed extract in reducing menopausal symptoms in otherwise healthy women: a double-blind, randomized, placebo-controlled study. *Phytother Res.* 2017;31(9):1316–22.
2781. Hakimi S, Charandabi SMA, Shadbad MRS, et al. Effect of Fenugreek seed on early menopausal symptoms. *Pharm Sci.* 2005;(2):83–90.
2782. Rao A, Steels E, Beccaria G, Inder WJ, Vitetta L. Influence of a specialized *Trigonella foenum-graecum* seed extract (libifem), on testosterone, estradiol and sexual function in healthy menstruating women, a randomised placebo controlled study. *Phytother Res.* 2015;29(8):1123–30.
2783. Steels E, Steele ML, Harold M, Coulson S. Efficacy of a proprietary *Trigonella foenum-graecum* L. de-husked seed extract in reducing menopausal symptoms in otherwise healthy women: a double-blind, randomized, placebo-controlled study. *Phytother Res.* 2017;31(9):1316–22.
2784. Safary M, Hakimi S, Mobaraki-Asl N, Amiri P, Tvassoli H, Delazar A. Comparison of the effects of fenugreek vaginal cream and ultra low-dose estrogen on atrophic vaginitis. *Curr Drug Deliv.* 2020;17(9):815–22.
2785. Park HJ, Lee KS, Lee EK, Park NC. Efficacy and safety of a mixed extract of *Trigonella foenum-graecum* seed and *Lespedeza cuneata* in the treatment of testosterone deficiency syndrome: a randomized, double-blind, placebo-controlled clinical trial. *World J Mens Health.* 2018;36(3):230–8.

2786. Idris S, Mishra A, Khushtar M. Recent therapeutic interventions of fenugreek seed: a mechanistic approach. *Drug Res (Stuttg)*. 2021;71(4):180–92.
2787. Khodamoradi K, Khosropanah MH, Ayati Z, et al. The effects of fenugreek on cardiometabolic risk factors in adults: a systematic review and meta-analysis. *Complement Ther Med*. 2020;52:102416.
2788. Askarpour M, Alami F, Campbell MS, Venkatakrishnan K, Hadi A, Ghaedi E. Effect of fenugreek supplementation on blood lipids and body weight: a systematic review and meta-analysis of randomized controlled trials. *J Ethnopharmacol*. 2020;253:112538.
2789. Mansoori A, Hosseini S, Zilaee M, Hormoznejad R, Fathi M. Effect of fenugreek extract supplement on testosterone levels in male: a meta-analysis of clinical trials. *Phytother Res*. 2020;34(7):1550–5.
2790. Rao A, Steels E, Inder WJ, Abraham S, Vitetta L. Testofen, a specialised *Trigonella foenum-graecum* seed extract reduces age-related symptoms of androgen decrease, increases testosterone levels and improves sexual function in healthy aging males in a double-blind randomised clinical study. *The Aging Male*. 2016;19(2):134–42.
2791. Rao A, Steels E, Inder WJ, Abraham S, Vitetta L. Testofen, a specialised *Trigonella foenum-graecum* seed extract reduces age-related symptoms of androgen decrease, increases testosterone levels and improves sexual function in healthy aging males in a double-blind randomised clinical study. *Aging Male*. 2016;19(2):134–42.
2792. Poole C, Bushey B, Foster C, et al. The effects of a commercially available botanical supplement on strength, body composition, power output, and hormonal profiles in resistance-trained males. *J Int Soc Sports Nutr*. 2010;7:34.
2793. Askarpour M, Alami F, Campbell MS, Venkatakrishnan K, Hadi A, Ghaedi E. Effect of fenugreek supplementation on blood lipids and body weight: a systematic review and meta-analysis of randomized controlled trials. *J Ethnopharmacol*. 2020;253:112538.
2794. Khodamoradi K, Khosropanah MH, Ayati Z, et al. The effects of fenugreek on cardiometabolic risk factors in adults: a systematic review and meta-analysis. *Complement Ther Med*. 2020;52:102416.
2795. Mebazaa R, Rega B, Camel V. Analysis of human male armpit sweat after fenugreek ingestion: characterisation of odour active compounds by gas chromatography coupled to mass spectrometry and olfactometry. *Food Chem*. 2011;128(1):227–35.
2796. Marsh TL, Arriola PE. The science of salsa: antimicrobial properties of salsa components to learn scientific methodology. *J Microbiol Biol Educ*. 2009;10(1):3–8.
2797. Mauer L, El-Sohemy A. Prevalence of cilantro (Coriandrum sativum) disliking among different ethnocultural groups. *Flavour*. 2012;1:8.
2798. Eriksson N, Wu S, Do CB, et al. A genetic variant near olfactory receptor genes influences cilantro preference. *Flavour*. 2012;1:22.
2799. Knaapila A, Hwang LD, Lysenko A, et al. Genetic analysis of chemosensory traits in human twins. *Chem Senses*. 2012;37(9):869–81.
2800. Eriksson N, Wu S, Do CB, et al. A genetic variant near olfactory receptor genes influences cilantro preference. *Flavour*. 2012;1:22.
2801. Sahib NG, Anwar F, Gilani AH, Hamid AA, Saari N, Alkharfy KM. Coriander (Coriandrum sativum L.): a potential source of high-value components for functional foods and nutraceuticals—a review. *Phytother Res*. 2013;27(10):1439–56.
2802. Rajeshwari CU, Siri S, Andallu B. Antioxidant and antiarthritic potential of coriander (Coriandrum sativum L.) leaves. *e-SPEN J*. 2012;7(6):e223–8.
2803. Geppetti P, Fusco BM, Marabini S, Maggi CA, Fanciullacci M, Sicuteri F. Secretion, pain and sneezing induced by the application of capsaicin to the nasal mucosa in man. *Br J Pharmacol*. 1988;93(3):509–14.
2804. Nesbitt AD, Goadsby PJ. Cluster headache. *BMJ*. 2012;344:e2407.
2805. Fusco BM, Marabini S, Maggi CA, Fiore G, Geppetti P. Preventative effect of repeated nasal applications of capsaicin in cluster headache. *Pain*. 1994;59(3):321–5.

2806. Nozu T, Kudaira M. Altered rectal sensory response induced by balloon distention in patients with functional abdominal pain syndrome. *Biopsychosoc Med.* 2009;3:13.
2807. Bortolotti M, Porta S. Effect of red pepper on symptoms of irritable bowel syndrome: preliminary study. *Dig Dis Sci.* 2011;56(11):3288–95.
2808. Bortolotti M, Coccia G, Grossi G. Red pepper and functional dyspepsia. *N Engl J Med.* 2002;346(12):947–8.
2809. Hennessy S, Leonard CE, Newcomb C, Kimmel SE, Bilker WB. Cisapride and ventricular arrhythmia. *Br J Clin Pharmacol.* 2008;66(3):375–85.
2810. Mustafa T, Srivastava KC. Ginger (Zingiber officinale) in migraine headache. *J Ethnopharmacol.* 1990;29(3):267–73.
2811. Gottlieb MS. Discovering AIDS. *Epidemiology.* 1998;9(4):365–7.
2812. Ghofrani HA, Osterloh IH, Grimminger F. Sildenafil: from angina to erectile dysfunction to pulmonary hypertension and beyond. *Nat Rev Drug Discov.* 2006;5(8):689–702.
2813. Vandenbroucke JP. In defense of case reports and case series. *Ann Intern Med.* 2001;134(4):330–4.
2814. Maghbooli M, Golipour F, Moghimi Esfandabadi A, Yousefi M. Comparison between the efficacy of ginger and sumatriptan in the ablative treatment of the common migraine. *Phytother Res.* 2014;28(3):412–5.
2815. Desai HG, Kalro RH, Choksi AP. Effect of ginger & garlic on DNA content of gastric aspirate. *Indian J Med Res.* 1990;92:139–41.
2816. Wasson S, Jayam VK. Coronary vasospasm and myocardial infarction induced by oral sumatriptan. *Clin Neuropharmacol.* 2004;27(4):198–200.
2817. Laine K, Raasakka T, Mäntynen J, Saukko P. Fatal cardiac arrhythmia after oral sumatriptan. *Headache.* 1999;39(7):511–2.
2818. Maghbooli M, Golipour F, Moghimi Esfandabadi A, Yousefi M. Comparison between the efficacy of ginger and sumatriptan in the ablative treatment of the common migraine. *Phytother Res.* 2014;28(3):412–5.
2819. Coco AS. Primary dysmenorrhea. *Am Fam Physician.* 1999;60(2):489–96.
2820. Kashefi F, Khajehei M, Tabatabaeichehr M, Alavinia M, Asili J. Comparison of the effect of ginger and zinc sulfate on primary dysmenorrhea: a placebo-controlled randomized trial. *Pain Manag Nurs.* 2014;15(4):826–33.
2821. Rahnama P, Montazeri A, Huseini HF, Kianbakht S, Naseri M. Effect of Zingiber officinale R. rhizomes (ginger) on pain relief in primary dysmenorrhea: a placebo randomized trial. *BMC Complement Altern Med.* 2012;12:92.
2822. Ozgoli G, Goli M, Moattar F. Comparison of effects of ginger, mefenamic acid, and ibuprofen on pain in women with primary dysmenorrhea. *J Altern Complement Med.* 2009;15(2):129–32.
2823. Kashefi F, Khajehei M, Alavinia M, Golmakani E, Asili J. Effect of ginger (Zingiber officinale) on heavy menstrual bleeding: a placebo-controlled, randomized clinical trial. *Phytother Res.* 2015;29(1):114–9.
2824. Khayat S, Kheirkhah M, Behboodi Moghadam Z, Fanaei H, Kasaeian A, Javadimehr M. Effect of treatment with ginger on the severity of premenstrual syndrome symptoms. *ISRN Obstet Gynecol.* 2014;2014:792708.
2825. Mowrey DB, Clayson DE. Motion sickness, ginger, and psychophysics. *Lancet.* 1982;1(8273):655–7.
2826. Palatty PL, Haniadka R, Valder B, Arora R, Baliga MS. Ginger in the prevention of nausea and vomiting: a review. *Crit Rev Food Sci Nutr.* 2013;53(7):659–69.
2827. Ding M, Leach M, Bradley H. The effectiveness and safety of ginger for pregnancy-induced nausea and vomiting: a systematic review. *Women Birth.* 2013;26(1):e26–30.
2828. Carlsen MH, Halvorsen BL, Holte K, et al. The total antioxidant content of more than 3100 foods, beverages, spices, herbs and supplements used worldwide. *Nutr J.* 2010;9:3.
2829. American Thyroid Association Taskforce on Radioiodine Safety, Sisson JC, Freitas

J, et al. Radiation safety in the treatment of patients with thyroid diseases by radioiodine 131I: practice recommendations of the American Thyroid Association. *Thyroid.* 2011;21(4):335–46.
2830. Metso S, Auvinen A, Huhtala H, Salmi J, Oksala H, Jaatinen P. Increased cancer incidence after radioiodine treatment for hyperthyroidism. *Cancer.* 2007;109(10):1972–9.
2831. Arami S, Ahmadi A, Haeri SA. The radioprotective effects of Origanum vulgare extract against genotoxicity induced by (131)I in human blood lymphocyte. *Cancer Biother Radiopharm.* 2013;28(3):201–6.
2832. Berrington D, Lall N. Anticancer activity of certain herbs and spices on the cervical epithelial carcinoma (HeLa) cell line. *Evid Based Complement Alternat Med.* 2012;2012:564927.
2833. Gunawardena D, Shanmugam K, Low M, et al. Determination of anti-inflammatory activities of standardised preparations of plant-and mushroom-based foods. *Eur J Nutr.* 2014;53(1):335–43.
2834. Al Dhaheri Y, Attoub S, Arafat K, et al. Anti-metastatic and anti-tumor growth effects of Origanum majorana on highly metastatic human breast cancer cells: inhibition of NFκB signaling and reduction of nitric oxide production. *PLoS ONE.* 2013;8(7):e68808.
2835. Haj-Husein I, Tukan S, Alkazaleh F. The effect of marjoram (Origanum majorana) tea on the hormonal profile of women with polycystic ovary syndrome: a randomised controlled pilot study. *J Hum Nutr Diet.* 2016;29(1):105–11.
2836. Shirvani H, Bazgir B, Shamsoddini A, et al. Oregano (Origanum vulgare) consumption reduces oxidative stress and markers of muscle damage after combat readiness tests in soldiers. *Nutrients.* 2022;15(1):137.
2837. Nikaein F, Babajafari S, Mazloomi SM, Zibaeenezhad M, Zargaran A. The effects of Satureja hortensis l. dried leaves on serum sugar, lipid profiles, hs-CRP, and blood pressure in metabolic syndrome patients: a double-blind randomized clinical trial. *Iran Red Crescent Med J.* 2016;19(1).
2838. Ference BA, Ginsberg HN, Graham I, et al. Low-density lipoproteins cause atherosclerotic cardiovascular disease. 1. Evidence from genetic, epidemiologic, and clinical studies. A consensus statement from the European Atherosclerosis Society Consensus Panel. *Eur Heart J.* 2017;38(32):2459–72.
2839. Carlsen MH, Halvorsen BL, Holte K, et al. The total antioxidant content of more than 3100 foods, beverages, spices, herbs and supplements used worldwide. *Nutr J.* 2010;9:3.
2840. Carlsen MH, Halvorsen BL, Holte K, et al. The total antioxidant content of more than 3100 foods, beverages, spices, herbs and supplements used worldwide. *Nutr J.* 2010;9:3.
2841. Baliga MS, Dsouza JJ. Amla (Emblica officinalis Gaertn), a wonder berry in the treatment and prevention of cancer. *Eur J Cancer Prev.* 2011;20(3):225–39.
2842. Carlsen MH, Halvorsen BL, Holte K, et al. The total antioxidant content of more than 3100 foods, beverages, spices, herbs and supplements used worldwide. *Nutr J.* 2010;9:3.
2843. Darvin ME, Patzelt A, Knorr F, Blume-Peytavi U, Sterry W, Lademann J. One-year study on the variation of carotenoid antioxidant substances in living human skin: influence of dietary supplementation and stress factors. *J Biomed Opt.* 2008;13(4):044028.
2844. Mohanty P, Hamouda W, Garg R, Aljada A, Ghanim H, Dandona P. Glucose challenge stimulates reactive oxygen species (ROS) generation by leucocytes. *J Clin Endocrinol Metab.* 2000;85(8):2970–3.
2845. Ghanim H, Mohanty P, Pathak R, Chaudhuri A, Sia CL, Dandona P. Orange juice or fructose intake does not induce oxidative and inflammatory response. *Diabetes Care.* 2007;30(6):1406–11.
2846. Prior RL, Gu L, Wu X, et al. Plasma antioxidant capacity changes following a meal as a measure of the ability of a food to alter in vivo antioxidant status. *J Am Coll Nutr.* 2007;26(2):170–81.
2847. Carlsen MH, Halvorsen BL, Holte K, et al. The total antioxidant content of more than 3100 foods, beverages, spices, herbs and supplements used worldwide. *Nutr J.* 2010;9:3.

2848. Saper RB, Kales SN, Paquin J, et al. Heavy metal content of Ayurvedic herbal medicine products. *JAMA*. 2004;292(23):2868–73.
2849. Martena MJ, van der Wielen JC, Rietjens IM, Klerx WN, de Groot HN, Konings EJ. Monitoring of mercury, arsenic, and lead in traditional Asian herbal preparations on the Dutch market and estimation of associated risks. *Food Addit Contam Part A*. 2010;27(2):190–205.
2850. Rao MM, Kumarmeena A, Galib null. Detection of toxic heavy metals and pesticide residue in herbal plants which are commonly used in the herbal formulations. *Environ Monit Assess*. 2011;181(1–4):267–71.
2851. Skulas-Ray AC, Kris-Etherton PM, Teeter DL, Chen CYO, Vanden Heuvel JP, West SG. A high antioxidant spice blend attenuates postprandial insulin and triglyceride responses and increases some plasma measures of antioxidant activity in healthy, overweight men. *J Nutr*. 2011;141(8):1451–7.
2852. Tomita LY, Roteli-Martins CM, Villa LL, Franco EL, Cardoso MA, BRINCA Study Team. Associations of dietary dark-green and deep-yellow vegetables and fruits with cervical intraepithelial neoplasia: modification by smoking. *Br J Nutr*. 2011;105(6):928–37.
2853. Fritschi G, Prescott WR Jr. Morphine levels in urine subsequent to poppy seed consumption. *Forensic Sci Int*. 1985;27(2):111–7.
2854. Hahn A, Michalak H, Begemann K, et al. Severe health impairment of a 6-week-old infant related to the ingestion of boiled poppy seeds. *Clin Toxicol*. 2008;46:607.
2855. Sproll C, Perz RC, Lachenmeier DW. Optimized LC/MS/MS analysis of morphine and codeine in poppy seed and evaluation of their fate during food processing as a basis for risk analysis. *J Agric Food Chem*. 2006;54(15):5292–8.
2856. European Food Safety Authority. Scientific opinion on the risks for public health related to the presence of opium alkaloids in poppy seeds. *EFSA J*. 2011;9(11):2405.
2857. Lachenmeier DW, Sproll C, Musshoff F. Poppy seed foods and opiate drug testing—where are we today? *Ther Drug Monit*. 2010;32(1):11–8.
2858. Sproll C, Perz RC, Lachenmeier DW. Optimized LC/MS/MS analysis of morphine and codeine in poppy seed and evaluation of their fate during food processing as a basis for risk analysis. *J Agric Food Chem*. 2006;54(15):5292–8.
2859. Lachenmeier DW, Sproll C, Musshoff F. Poppy seed foods and opiate drug testing—where are we today? *Ther Drug Monit*. 2010;32(1):11–8.
2860. H.R.6512—*Stephen Hacala Poppy Seed Safety Act 2023*. www.congress.gov/bill/118th-congress/house-bill/6512/text. November 29, 2023. Accessed February 26, 2025.
2861. Idle JR. Christmas gingerbread (Lebkuchen) and Christmas cheer—review of the potential role of mood elevating amphetamine-like compounds formed in vivo and in furno. *Prague Med Rep*. 2005;106(1):27–38.
2862. Payne RB. Nutmeg intoxication. *N Engl J Med*. 1963;269:36–8.
2863. Cushny AR. Nutmeg poisoning. *Proc R Soc Med*. 1908;1(Ther Pharmacol Sect):39–44.
2864. Williams EY, West F. The use of nutmeg as a psychotropic drug. Report of two cases. *J Natl Med Assoc*. 1968;60(4):289–90.
2865. Williams EY, West F. The use of nutmeg as a psychotropic drug. Report of two cases. *J Natl Med Assoc*. 1968;60(4):289–90.
2866. Scholefield JH. Nutmeg—an unusual overdose. *Arch Emerg Med*. 1986;3(2):154–5.
2867. Davis PA, Yokoyama W. Cinnamon intake lowers fasting blood glucose: meta-analysis. *J Med Food*. 2011;14(9):884–9.
2868. Solomon TPJ, Blannin AK. Effects of short-term cinnamon ingestion on in vivo glucose tolerance. *Diabetes Obes Metab*. 2007;9(6):895–901.
2869. Solomon TPJ, Blannin AK. Changes in glucose tolerance and insulin sensitivity following 2 weeks of daily cinnamon ingestion in healthy humans. *Eur J Appl Physiol*. 2009;105(6):969–76.
2870. Fotland TØ, Paulsen JE, Sanner T, Alexander J, Husøy T. Risk assessment of coumarin using

the bench mark dose (BMD) approach: children in Norway which regularly eat oatmeal porridge with cinnamon may exceed the TDI for coumarin with several folds. *Food Chem Toxicol.* 2012;50(3–4):903–12.

2871. Wickenberg J, Lindstedt S, Berntorp K, Nilsson J, Hlebowicz J. Ceylon cinnamon does not affect postprandial plasma glucose or insulin in subjects with impaired glucose tolerance. *Br J Nutr.* 2012;107(12):1845–9.

2872. Davis PA, Yokoyama W. Cinnamon intake lowers fasting blood glucose: meta-analysis. *J Med Food.* 2011;14(9):884–9.

2873. World Cancer Research Fund, American Institute for Cancer Research. *Food, Nutrition, Physical Activity, and the Prevention of Cancer: a Global Perspective.* Washington, D.C.: AICR; 2007.

2874. 100% whole grains infographic. American Heart Association. https://www.heart.org/en/healthy-living/healthy-eating/eat-smart/nutrition-basics/whole-grains-infographic. Accessed February 20, 2025.

2875. Shan Z, Li Y, Baden MY, et al. Association between healthy eating patterns and risk of cardiovascular disease. *JAMA Intern Med.* 2020;180(8):1090–100.

2876. Wu H, Flint AJ, Qi Q, et al. Association between dietary whole grain intake and risk of mortality: two large prospective studies in US men and women. *JAMA Intern Med.* 2015;175(3):373–84.

2877. Tang G, Wang D, Long J, Yang F, Si L. Meta-analysis of the association between whole grain intake and coronary heart disease risk. *Am J Cardiol.* 2015;115(5):625–9.

2878. Aune D, Norat T, Romundstad P, Vatten LJ. Whole grain and refined grain consumption and the risk of type 2 diabetes: a systematic review and dose-response meta-analysis of cohort studies. *Eur J Epidemiol.* 2013;28(11):845–58.

2879. Cho SS, Qi L, Fahey GC, Klurfeld DM. Consumption of cereal fiber, mixtures of whole grains and bran, and whole grains and risk reduction in type 2 diabetes, obesity, and cardiovascular disease. *Am J Clin Nutr.* 2013;98(2):594–619.

2880. Institute for Health Metrics and Evaluation (IHME). GBD 2021 cause and risk summary: diet low in whole grains—level 3 risk. University of Washington. https://www.healthdata.org/research-analysis/diseases-injuries-risks/factsheets/2021-diet-low-whole-grains-level-3-risk. Accessed December 7, 2024.

2881. Lefevre M, Jonnalagadda S. Effect of whole grains on markers of subclinical inflammation. *Nutr Rev.* 2012;70(7):387–96.

2882. Montonen J, Boeing H, Fritsche A, et al. Consumption of red meat and whole-grain bread in relation to biomarkers of obesity, inflammation, glucose metabolism and oxidative stress. *Eur J Nutr.* 2013;52(1):337–45.

2883. Goletzke J, Buyken AE, Joslowski G, et al. Increased intake of carbohydrates from sources with a higher glycemic index and lower consumption of whole grains during puberty are prospectively associated with higher IL-6 concentrations in younger adulthood among healthy individuals. *J Nutr.* 2014;144(10):1586–93.

2884. Sofi F, Ghiselli L, Cesari F, et al. Effects of short-term consumption of bread obtained by an old Italian grain variety on lipid, inflammatory, and hemorheological variables: an intervention study. *J Med Food.* 2010;13(3):615–20.

2885. Vitaglione P, Mennella I, Ferracane R, et al. Whole-grain wheat consumption reduces inflammation in a randomized controlled trial on overweight and obese subjects with unhealthy dietary and lifestyle behaviors: role of polyphenols bound to cereal dietary fiber. *Am J Clin Nutr.* 2015;101(2):251–61.

2886. Esposito K, Nappo F, Giugliano F, et al. Meal modulation of circulating interleukin 18 and adiponectin concentrations in healthy subjects and in patients with type 2 diabetes mellitus. *Am J Clin Nutr.* 2003;78(6):1135–40.

2887. Masters RC, Liese AD, Haffner SM, Wagenknecht LE, Hanley AJ. Whole and refined grain intakes are related to inflammatory protein concentrations in human plasma. *J Nutr.* 2010;140(3):587–94.

2888. Vitaglione P, Mennella I, Ferracane R, et al. Whole-grain wheat consumption reduces inflammation in a randomized controlled trial on overweight and obese subjects with unhealthy dietary and lifestyle behaviors: role of polyphenols bound to cereal dietary fiber. *Am J Clin Nutr.* 2015;101(2):251–61.

2889. Qi L, van Dam RM, Liu S, Franz M, Mantzoros C, Hu FB. Whole-grain, bran, and cereal fiber intakes and markers of systemic inflammation in diabetic women. *Diabetes Care.* 2006;29(2):207–11.

2890. Sofi F, Ghiselli L, Cesari F, et al. Effects of short-term consumption of bread obtained by an old Italian grain variety on lipid, inflammatory, and hemorheological variables: an intervention study. *J Med Food.* 2010;13(3):615–20.

2891. Esposito K, Giugliano D. Whole-grain intake cools down inflammation. *Am J Clin Nutr.* 2006;83(6):1440–1.

2892. Jacobs DR Jr, Andersen LF, Blomhoff R. Whole-grain consumption is associated with a reduced risk of noncardiovascular, noncancer death attributed to inflammatory diseases in the Iowa Women's Health Study. *Am J Clin Nutr.* 2007;85(6):1606–14.

2893. Rubio-Tapia A, Ludvigsson JF, Brantner TL, Murray JA, Everhart JE. The prevalence of celiac disease in the United States. *Am J Gastroenterol.* 2012;107(10):1538–44.

2894. Cooper BT, Holmes GK, Ferguson R, Thompson RA, Allan RN, Cooke WT. Gluten-sensitive diarrhea without evidence of celiac disease. *Gastroenterology.* 1980;79(5 Pt 1):801–6.

2895. Falchuk ZM. Gluten-sensitive diarrhea without enteropathy: fact or fancy? *Gastroenterology.* 1980;79(5 Pt 1):953–5.

2896. Aziz I, Hadjivassiliou M, Sanders DS. Does gluten sensitivity in the absence of coeliac disease exist? *BMJ.* 2012;345:e7907.

2897. Mansueto P, Seidita A, D'Alcamo A, Carroccio A. Non-celiac gluten sensitivity: literature review. *J Am Coll Nutr.* 2014;33(1):39–54.

2898. Genuis SJ. Sensitivity-related illness: the escalating pandemic of allergy, food intolerance and chemical sensitivity. *Sci Total Environ.* 2010;408(24):6047–61.

2899. Di Sabatino A, Corazza GR. Nonceliac gluten sensitivity: sense or sensibility? *Ann Intern Med.* 2012;156(4):309–11.

2900. McCarter DF. Non-celiac gluten sensitivity: important diagnosis or dietary fad? *Am Fam Physician.* 2014;89(2):82–3.

2901. Ferch CC, Chey WD. Irritable bowel syndrome and gluten sensitivity without celiac disease: separating the wheat from the chaff. *Gastroenterology.* 2012;142(3):664–6.

2902. Carroccio A, Mansueto P, Iacono G, et al. Non-celiac wheat sensitivity diagnosed by double-blind placebo-controlled challenge: exploring a new clinical entity. *Am J Gastroenterol.* 2012;107(12):1898–906.

2903. Carroccio A, Mansueto P, Iacono G, et al. Non-celiac wheat sensitivity diagnosed by double-blind placebo-controlled challenge: exploring a new clinical entity. *Am J Gastroenterol.* 2012;107(12):1898–906.

2904. Biesiekierski JR, Peters SL, Newnham ED, Rosella O, Muir JG, Gibson PR. No effects of gluten in patients with self-reported non-celiac gluten sensitivity after dietary reduction of fermentable, poorly absorbed, short-chain carbohydrates. *Gastroenterology.* 2013;145(2):320–8.e1–3.

2905. Peters SL, Biesiekierski JR, Yelland GW, Muir JG, Gibson PR. Randomised clinical trial: gluten may cause depression in subjects with non-coeliac gluten sensitivity—an exploratory clinical study. *Aliment Pharmacol Ther.* 2014;39(10):1104–12.

2906. Aziz I, Hadjivassiliou M, Sanders DS. Editorial: noncoeliac gluten sensitivity—a disease of the mind or gut? *Aliment Pharmacol Ther.* 2014;40(1):113–4.

2907. Picarelli A, Borghini R, Isonne C, Di Tola M. Reactivity to dietary gluten: new insights into differential diagnosis among gluten-related gastrointestinal disorders. *Pol Arch Med Wewn.* 2013;123(12):708–12.

2908. Rubio-Tapia A, Ludvigsson JF, Brantner TL, Murray JA, Everhart JE. The prevalence of celiac disease in the United States. *Am J Gastroenterol.* 2012;107(10):1538–44.
2909. Riddle MS, Murray JA, Porter CK. The incidence and risk of celiac disease in a healthy US adult population. *Am J Gastroenterol.* 2012;107(8):1248–55.
2910. Volta U, Bardella MT, Calabrò A, Troncone R, Corazza GR. An Italian prospective multicenter survey on patients suspected of having non-celiac gluten sensitivity. *BMC Med.* 2014;12:85.
2911. Holmes G. Non coeliac gluten sensitivity. *Gastroenterol Hepatol Bed Bench.* 2013;6(3):115–9.
2912. Gaesser GA, Angadi SS. Gluten-free diet: imprudent dietary advice for the general population? *J Acad Nutr Diet.* 2012;112(9):1330–3.
2913. De Palma G, Nadal I, Collado MC, Sanz Y. Effects of a gluten-free diet on gut microbiota and immune function in healthy adult human subjects. *Br J Nutr.* 2009;102(8):1154–60.
2914. Gaesser GA, Angadi SS. Gluten-free diet: imprudent dietary advice for the general population? *J Acad Nutr Diet.* 2012;112(9):1330–3.
2915. Horiguchi N, Horiguchi H, Suzuki Y. Effect of wheat gluten hydrolysate on the immune system in healthy human subjects. *Biosci Biotechnol Biochem.* 2005;69(12):2445–9.
2916. Di Sabatino A, Corazza GR. Nonceliac gluten sensitivity: sense or sensibility? *Ann Intern Med.* 2012;156(4):309–11.
2917. Koerner TB, Cleroux C, Poirier C, et al. Gluten contamination of naturally gluten-free flours and starches used by Canadians with celiac disease. *Food Addit Contam Part A.* 2013;30(12):2017–21.
2918. McCarter DF. Non-celiac gluten sensitivity: important diagnosis or dietary fad? *Am Fam Physician.* 2014;89(2):82–3.
2919. Tavakkoli A, Lewis SK, Tennyson CA, Lebwohl B, Green PH. Characteristics of patients who avoid wheat and/or gluten in the absence of celiac disease. *Dig Dis Sci.* 2014;59(6):1255–61.
2920. Pietzak M. Celiac disease, wheat allergy, and gluten sensitivity: when gluten free is not a fad. *JPEN J Parenter Enteral Nutr.* 2012;36(1 Suppl):68S–75S.
2921. Goufo P, Trindade H. Rice antioxidants: phenolic acids, flavonoids, anthocyanins, proanthocyanidins, tocopherols, tocotrienols, γ-oryzanol, and phytic acid. *Food Sci Nutr.* 2014;2(2):75–104.
2922. Choi SP, Kang MY, Koh HJ, Nam SH, Friedman M. Antiallergic activities of pigmented rice bran extracts in cell assays. *J Food Sci.* 2007;72(9):S719–26.
2923. Pintha K, Yodkeeree S, Limtrakul P. Proanthocyanidin in red rice inhibits MDA-MB-231 breast cancer cell invasion via the expression control of invasive proteins. *Biol Pharm Bull.* 2015;38(4):571–81.
2924. Suttiarporn P, Chumpolsri W, Mahatheeranont S, Luangkamin S, Teepsawang S, Leardkamolkarn V. Structures of phytosterols and triterpenoids with potential anti-cancer activity in bran of black non-glutinous rice. *Nutrients.* 2015;7(3):1672–87.
2925. Egilman D, Mailloux C, Valentin C. Popcorn-worker lung caused by corporate and regulatory negligence: an avoidable tragedy. *Int J Occup Environ Health.* 2007;13(1):85–98.
2926. Egilman DS, Schilling JH. Bronchiolitis obliterans and consumer exposure to butter-flavored microwave popcorn: a case series. *Int J Occup Environ Health.* 2012;18(1):29–42.
2927. Su LJ, Chiang TC, O'Connor SN. Arsenic in brown rice: do the benefits outweigh the risks? *Front Nutr.* 2023;10:1209574.
2928. Schmidt CW. Arsenical association: inorganic arsenic may accumulate in the meat of treated chickens. *Environ Health Perspect.* 2013;121(7):A226.
2929. Rajkowska-Myśliwiec M, Ciemniak A, Karp G. Arsenic in rice and rice-based products with regard to consumer health. *Foods.* 2024;13(19):3153.
2930. International Agency for Research on Cancer. *IARC Monographs on the Evaluation of Carcinogenic Risks to Humans, Volume 100 C, Arsenic, Metals, Fibres, and Dusts: This Publication Represents the Views and Expert Opinions of an IARC Working Group on the Evaluation of Carcinogenic Risks to Humans, Which Met in Lyon, 17-24 March 2009.* IARC; 2012.

2931. Arsenic in rice and rice products risk assessment report. U.S. Food and Drug Administration. http://www.fda.gov/Food/FoodScienceResearch/RiskSafetyAssessment/default.htm. May 13, 2014. Updated March 2016. Accessed February 20, 2025.
2932. Rajkowska-Myśliwiec M, Ciemniak A, Karp G. Arsenic in rice and rice-based products with regard to consumer health. *Foods.* 2024;13(19):3153.
2933. Nelson K, Stojanovska L, Vasiljevic T, Mathai M. Germinated grains: a superior whole grain functional food? *Can J Physiol Pharmacol.* 2013;91(6):429–41.
2934. Hovey AL, Jones GP, Devereux HM, Walker KZ. Whole cereal and legume seeds increase faecal short chain fatty acids compared to ground seeds. *Asia Pac J Clin Nutr.* 2003;12(4):477–82.
2935. Stephen AM, Cummings JH. The microbial contribution to human faecal mass. *J Med Microbiol.* 1980;13(1):45–56.
2936. Fechner A, Fenske K, Jahreis G. Effects of legume kernel fibres and citrus fibre on putative risk factors for colorectal cancer: a randomised, double-blind, crossover human intervention trial. *Nutr J.* 2013;12:101.
2937. Hovey AL, Jones GP, Devereux HM, Walker KZ. Whole cereal and legume seeds increase faecal short chain fatty acids compared to ground seeds. *Asia Pac J Clin Nutr.* 2003;12(4):477–82.
2938. Tan J, McKenzie C, Potamitis M, Thorburn AN, Mackay CR, Macia L. The role of short-chain fatty acids in health and disease. *Adv Immunol.* 2014;121:91–119.
2939. Molteberg EL, Solheim R, Dimberg LH, Frølich W. Variation in oat groats due to variety, storage and heat treatment. II: sensory quality. *J Cereal Sci.* 1996;24(3):273–82.
2940. Cerio R, Dohil M, Downie J, et al. Mechanism of action and clinical benefits of colloidal oatmeal for dermatologic practice. *J Drugs Dermatol.* 2010;9(9):1116–20.
2941. Boisnic S, Branchet-Gumila MC, Coutanceau C. Inhibitory effect of oatmeal extract oligomer on vasoactive intestinal peptide-induced inflammation in surviving human skin. *Int J Tissue React.* 2003;25(2):41–6.
2942. Alexandrescu DT, Vaillant JG, Dasanu CA. Effect of treatment with a colloidal oatmeal lotion on the acneform eruption induced by epidermal growth factor receptor and multiple tyrosine-kinase inhibitors. *Clin Exp Dermatol.* 2007;32(1):71–4.
2943. Wild R, Fager K, Flefleh C, et al. Cetuximab preclinical antitumor activity (monotherapy and combination based) is not predicted by relative total or activated epidermal growth factor receptor tumor expression levels. *Mol Cancer Ther.* 2006;5(1):104–13.
2944. Guo W, Nie L, Wu D, et al. Avenanthramides inhibit proliferation of human colon cancer cell lines in vitro. *Nutr Cancer.* 2010;62(8):1007–16.
2945. Clemens R, van Klinken BJW. Oats, more than just a whole grain: an introduction. *Br J Nutr.* 2014;112 Suppl 2:S1–3.
2946. Eidson M, Saenz B. Average portion sizes of pasta from Italian casual dining restaurants in Tarrant County. https://web.archive.org/web/20150105091129/http://www.srs.tcu.edu/previous_posters/Nutritional_Sciences/2010/148-Eidson-Gorman.pdf. 2010. Accessed February 20, 2025.
2947. Popkin BM, Armstrong LE, Bray GM, Caballero B, Frei B, Willett WC. A new proposed guidance system for beverage consumption in the United States. *Am J Clin Nutr.* 2006;83(3):529–42.
2948. Rush EC. Water: neglected, unappreciated and under researched. *Eur J Clin Nutr.* 2013;67(5):492–5.
2949. Rush EC. Water: neglected, unappreciated and under researched. *Eur J Clin Nutr.* 2013;67(5):492–5.
2950. Jéquier E, Constant F. Water as an essential nutrient: the physiological basis of hydration. *Eur J Clin Nutr.* 2010;64(2):115–23.
2951. Vivanti AP. Origins for the estimations of water requirements in adults. *Eur J Clin Nutr.* 2012;66(12):1282–9.

2952. Adolph EF. The regulation of the water content of the human organism. *J Physiol* (Lond). 1921;55(1–2):114–32.
2953. Walsh NP, Fortes MB, Purslow C, Esmaeelpour M. Author response: is whole body hydration an important consideration in dry eye? *Invest Ophthalmol Vis Sci.* 2013;54(3):1713–4.
2954. Goodman AB, Blanck HM, Sherry B, Park S, Nebeling L, Yaroch AL. Behaviors and attitudes associated with low drinking water intake among US adults, Food Attitudes and Behaviors Survey, 2007. *Prev Chronic Dis.* 2013;10:E51.
2955. Negoianu D, Goldfarb S. Just add water. *J Am Soc Nephrol.* 2008;19(6):1041–3.
2956. Michaud DS, Spiegelman D, Clinton SK, et al. Fluid intake and the risk of bladder cancer in men. *N Engl J Med.* 1999;340(18):1390–7.
2957. Chan J, Knutsen SF, Blix GG, Lee JW, Fraser GE. Water, other fluids, and fatal coronary heart disease: the Adventist Health Study. *Am J Epidemiol.* 2002;155(9):827–33.
2958. Guest S, Essick GK, Mehrabyan A, Dessirier JM, McGlone F. Effect of hydration on the tactile and thermal sensitivity of the lip. *Physiol Behav.* 2014;123:127–35.
2959. Benelam B, Wyness L. Hydration and health: a review. *Nutr Bull.* 2010;35:3–25.
2960. Vivanti AP. Origins for the estimations of water requirements in adults. *Eur J Clin Nutr.* 2012;66(12):1282–9.
2961. Benelam B, Wyness L. Hydration and health: a review. *Nutr Bull.* 2010;35:3–25.
2962. Killer SC, Blannin AK, Jeukendrup AE. No evidence of dehydration with moderate daily coffee intake: a counterbalanced cross-over study in a free-living population. *PLoS ONE.* 2014;9(1):e84154.
2963. Ruxton CH, Hart VA. Black tea is not significantly different from water in the maintenance of normal hydration in human subjects: results from a randomised controlled trial. *Br J Nutr.* 2011;106(4):588–95.
2964. Benelam B, Wyness L. Hydration and health: a review. *Nutr Bull.* 2010;35:3–25.
2965. Saleh MA, Abdel-Rahman FH, Woodard BB, et al. Chemical, microbial and physical evaluation of commercial bottled waters in greater Houston area of Texas. *J Environ Sci Health A Tox Hazard Subst Environ Eng.* 2008;43(4):335–47.
2966. Li H, Zhu L, Ma M, Wu H, An L, Yang Z. Occurrence of microplastics in commercially sold bottled water. *Sci Total Environ.* 2023;867:161553.
2967. Valtin H. "Drink at least eight glasses of water a day." Really? Is there scientific evidence for "8 x 8"? *Am J Physiol Regul Integr Comp Physiol.* 2002;283(5):R993–1004.
2968. Kempton MJ, Ettinger U, Foster R, et al. Dehydration affects brain structure and function in healthy adolescents. *Hum Brain Mapp.* 2011;32(1):71–9.
2969. Stookey JD, Brass B, Holliday A, Arieff A. What is the cell hydration status of healthy children in the USA? Preliminary data on urine osmolality and water intake. *Public Health Nutr.* 2012;15(11):2148–56.
2970. Edmonds CJ, Burford D. Should children drink more water?: the effects of drinking water on cognition in children. *Appetite.* 2009;52(3):776–9.
2971. Pross N, Demazières A, Girard N, et al. Influence of progressive fluid restriction on mood and physiological markers of dehydration in women. *Br J Nutr.* 2013;109(2):313–21.
2972. Péronnet F, Mignault D, du Souich P, et al. Pharmacokinetic analysis of absorption, distribution and disappearance of ingested water labeled with D_2O in humans. *Eur J Appl Physiol.* 2012;112(6):2213–22.
2973. Bateman DN. Effects of meal temperature and volume on the emptying of liquid from the human stomach. *J Physiol* (Lond). 1982;331:461–7.
2974. Armstrong LE, Ganio MS, Klau JF, Johnson EC, Casa DJ, Maresh CM. Novel hydration assessment techniques employing thirst and a water intake challenge in healthy men. *Appl Physiol Nutr Metab.* 2014;39(2):138–44.
2975. Cuomo R, Grasso R, Sarnelli G, et al. Effects of carbonated water on functional dyspepsia and constipation. *Eur J Gastroenterol Hepatol.* 2002;14(9):991–9.

2976. Duregon E, Bernier M, de Cabo R. A glance back at the journal of gerontology—coffee, dietary interventions and life span. *J Geront A Biol Sci Med Sci.* 2020;75(11):2029–30.
2977. Li Q, Liu Y, Sun X, et al. Caffeinated and decaffeinated coffee consumption and risk of all-cause mortality: a dose–response meta-analysis of cohort studies. *J Hum Nut Diet.* 2019;32(3):279–87.
2978. Spiegelhalter D. Using speed of ageing and "microlives" to communicate the effects of lifetime habits and environment. *BMJ.* 2012;345:e8223.
2979. Poole R, Kennedy OJ, Roderick P, Fallowfield JA, Hayes PC, Parkes J. Coffee consumption and health: umbrella review of meta-analyses of multiple health outcomes. *BMJ.* 2017;359:j5024.
2980. Loftfield E, Cornelis MC, Caporaso N, Yu K, Sinha R, Freedman N. Association of coffee drinking with mortality by genetic variation in caffeine metabolism: findings from the UK Biobank. *JAMA Intern Med.* 2018;178(8):1086.
2981. Shimamoto T, Yamamichi N, Kodashima S, et al. No association of coffee consumption with gastric ulcer, duodenal ulcer, reflux esophagitis, and non-erosive reflux disease: a cross-sectional study of 8,013 healthy subjects in Japan. *PLoS ONE.* 2013;8(6):e65996.
2982. Wendl B, Pfeiffer A, Pehl C, Schmidt T, Kaess H. Effect of decaffeination of coffee or tea on gastro-oesophageal reflux. *Aliment Pharmacol Ther.* 1994;8(3):283–7.
2983. Li M, Wang M, Guo W, Wang J, Sun X. The effect of caffeine on intraocular pressure: a systematic review and meta-analysis. *Graefes Arch Clin Exp Ophthalmol.* 2011;249(3):435–42.
2984. Kang JH, Willett WC, Rosner BA, Hankinson SE, Pasquale LR. Caffeine consumption and the risk of primary open-angle glaucoma: a prospective cohort study. *Invest Ophthalmol Vis Sci.* 2008;49(5):1924–31.
2985. Bonilha L, Li LM. Heavy coffee drinking and epilepsy. *Seizure.* 2004;13(4):284–5.
2986. Lloret-Linares C, Lafuente-Lafuente C, Chassany O, et al. Does a single cup of coffee at dinner alter the sleep? A controlled cross-over randomised trial in real-life conditions. *Nutrition & Dietetics.* 2012;69(4):250–5.
2987. Urgert R, Katan MB. The cholesterol-raising factor from coffee beans. *Annu Rev Nutr.* 1997;17:305–24.
2988. Corrêa TAF, Rogero MM, Mioto BM, et al. Paper-filtered coffee increases cholesterol and inflammation biomarkers independent of roasting degree: a clinical trial. *Nutrition.* 2013;29(7–8):977–81.
2989. Bhave PD, Hoffmayer K. Caffeine and atrial fibrillation: friends or foes? *Heart.* 2013;99(19):1377–8.
2990. Patanè S, Marte F, La Rosa FC, La Rocca R. Atrial fibrillation associated with chocolate intake abuse and chronic salbutamol inhalation abuse. *Int J Cardiol.* 2010;145(2):e74–6.
2991. Krittanawong C, Tunhasiriwet A, Wang Z, et al. Is caffeine or coffee consumption a risk for new-onset atrial fibrillation? A systematic review and meta-analysis. *Eur J Prev Cardiol.* 2021;28(12):e13–5.
2992. Cao Y, Liu X, Xue Z, et al. Association of coffee consumption with atrial fibrillation risk: an updated dose-response meta-analysis of prospective studies. *Front Cardiovasc Med.* 2022;9:894664.
2993. Poole R, Kennedy OJ, Roderick P, Fallowfield JA, Hayes PC, Parkes J. Coffee consumption and health: umbrella review of meta-analyses of multiple health outcomes. *BMJ.* 2017;359:j5024.
2994. Son H, Song HJ, Seo HJ, Lee H, Choi SM, Lee S. The safety and effectiveness of self-administered coffee enema: a systematic review of case reports. *Medicine.* 2020;99(36):e21998.
2995. Glade MJ. Caffeine—not just a stimulant. *Nutrition.* 2010;26(10):932–8.
2996. Bhave PD, Hoffmayer K. Caffeine and atrial fibrillation: friends or foes? *Heart.* 2013;99(19):1377–8.

2997. Sepkowitz KA. Energy drinks and caffeine-related adverse effects. *JAMA*. 2013;309(3): 243–4.
2998. Dirks-Naylor AJ. The benefits of coffee on skeletal muscle. *Life Sci*. 2015;143:182–6.
2999. Juliano LM, Griffiths RR. A critical review of caffeine withdrawal: empirical validation of symptoms and signs, incidence, severity, and associated features. *Psychopharmacology* (Berl). 2004;176(1):1–29.
3000. O'Keefe JH, Bhatti SK, Patil HR, DiNicolantonio JJ, Lucan SC, Lavie CJ. Effects of habitual coffee consumption on cardiometabolic disease, cardiovascular health, and all-cause mortality. *J Am Coll Cardiol*. 2013;62(12):1043–51.
3001. Tzellos TG, Sardeli C, Lallas A, Papazisis G, Chourdakis M, Kouvelas D. Efficacy, safety and tolerability of green tea catechins in the treatment of external anogenital warts: a systematic review and meta-analysis. *J Eur Acad Dermatol Venereol*. 2011;25(3):345–53.
3002. Dunne EF, Friedman A, Datta SD, Markowitz LE, Workowski KA. Updates on human papillomavirus and genital warts and counseling messages from the 2010 Sexually Transmitted Diseases Treatment Guidelines. *Clin Infect Dis*. 2011;53 Suppl 3:S143–52.
3003. Tjeerdsma F, Jonkman MF, Spoo JR. Temporary arrest of basal cell carcinoma formation in a patient with basal cell naevus syndrome (BCNS) since treatment with a gel containing various plant extracts. *J Eur Acad Dermatol Venereol*. 2011;25(2):244–5.
3004. Trudel D, Labbé DP, Bairati I, Fradet V, Bazinet L, Têtu B. Green tea for ovarian cancer prevention and treatment: a systematic review of the in vitro, in vivo and epidemiological studies. *Gynecol Oncol*. 2012;126(3):491–8.
3005. Butler LM, Wu AH. Green and black tea in relation to gynecologic cancers. *Mol Nutr Food Res*. 2011;55(6):931–40.
3006. Onakpoya I, Spencer E, Heneghan C, Thompson M. The effect of green tea on blood pressure and lipid profile: a systematic review and meta-analysis of randomized clinical trials. *Nutr Metab Cardiovasc Dis*. 2014;24(8):823–36.
3007. Liu G, Mi XN, Zheng XX, Xu YL, Lu J, Huang XH. Effects of tea intake on blood pressure: a meta-analysis of randomised controlled trials. *Br J Nutr*. 2014;112(7):1043–54.
3008. Maruyama K, Iso H, Sasaki S, Fukino Y. The association between concentrations of green tea and blood glucose levels. *J Clin Biochem Nutr*. 2009;44(1):41–5.
3009. Maki KC, Reeves MS, Farmer M, et al. Green tea catechin consumption enhances exercise-induced abdominal fat loss in overweight and obese adults. *J Nutr*. 2009;139(2):264–70.
3010. Arab L, Khan F, Lam H. Epidemiologic evidence of a relationship between tea, coffee, or caffeine consumption and cognitive decline. *Adv Nutr*. 2013;4(1):115–22.
3011. Arab L, Liu W, Elashoff D. Green and black tea consumption and risk of stroke: a meta-analysis. *Stroke*. 2009;40(5):1786–92.
3012. Yang WS, Wang WY, Fan WY, Deng Q, Wang X. Tea consumption and risk of type 2 diabetes: a dose-response meta-analysis of cohort studies. *Br J Nutr*. 2014;111(8):1329–39.
3013. Koyama Y, Kuriyama S, Aida J, et al. Association between green tea consumption and tooth loss: cross-sectional results from the Ohsaki Cohort 2006 Study. *Prev Med*. 2010;50(4): 173–9.
3014. Watanabe I, Kuriyama S, Kakizaki M, et al. Green tea and death from pneumonia in Japan: the Ohsaki cohort study. *Am J Clin Nutr*. 2009;90(3):672–9.
3015. Maeda-Yamamoto M, Ema K, Monobe M, et al. The efficacy of early treatment of seasonal allergic rhinitis with benifuuki green tea containing O-methylated catechin before pollen exposure: an open randomized study. *Allergol Int*. 2009;58(3):437–44.
3016. Masuda S, Maeda-Yamamoto M, Usui F, Fujisawa T. 'Benifuuki' green tea containing O-methylated catechin reduces symptoms of Japanese cedar pollinosis: a randomized, double-blind, placebo-controlled trial. *Allergol Int*. 2014;63(2):211–7.
3017. Millet D. The origins of EEG. Seventh Annual Meeting of the International Society for the History of the Neurosciences (ISHN). https://web.archive.org/web/20110716085043/http://www.bri.ucla.edu/nha/ishn/ab24-2002.htm. June 3, 2002. Accessed February 20, 2025.

3018. Nobre AC, Rao A, Owen GN. L-theanine, a natural constituent in tea, and its effect on mental state. *Asia Pac J Clin Nutr.* 2008;17 Suppl 1:167–8.
3019. Wang ZM, Zhou B, Wang YS, et al. Black and green tea consumption and the risk of coronary artery disease: a meta-analysis. *Am J Clin Nutr.* 2011;93(3):506–15.
3020. Rusak G, Komes D, Likić S, Horžić D, Kovač M. Phenolic content and antioxidative capacity of green and white tea extracts depending on extraction conditions and the solvent used. *Food Chem.* 2008;110(4):852–8.
3021. Green RJ, Murphy AS, Schulz B, Watkins BA, Ferruzzi MG. Common tea formulations modulate in vitro digestive recovery of green tea catechins. *Mol Nutr Food Res.* 2007;51(9):1152–62.
3022. Santana-Rios G, Orner GA, Amantana A, Provost C, Wu SY, Dashwood RH. Potent antimutagenic activity of white tea in comparison with green tea in the Salmonella assay. *Mutat Res.* 2001;495(1–2):61–74.
3023. Yang DJ, Hwang LS, Lin JT. Effects of different steeping methods and storage on caffeine, catechins and gallic acid in bag tea infusions. *J Chromatogr A.* 2007;1156(1–2):312–20.
3024. Venditti E, Bacchetti T, Tiano L, Carloni P, Greci L, Damiani E. Hot vs. cold water steeping of different teas: do they affect antioxidant activity? *Food Chem.* 2010;119(4):1597–1604.
3025. Karak T, Bhagat R. Trace elements in tea leaves, made tea and tea infusion: a review. *Food Res Int.* 2010;43(9):2234–52.
3026. Shen FM, Chen HW. Element composition of tea leaves and tea infusions and its impact on health. *Bull Environ Contam Toxicol.* 2008;80(3):300–4.
3027. Kochman J, Jakubczyk K, Antoniewicz J, Mruk H, Janda K. Health benefits and chemical composition of matcha green tea: a review. *Molecules.* 2020;26(1):85.
3028. Crozier TWM, Stalmach A, Lean MEJ, Crozier A. Espresso coffees, caffeine and chlorogenic acid intake: potential health implications. *Food Funct.* 2012;3(1):30–3.
3029. Kole AS, Jones HD, Christensen R, Gladstein J. A case of kombucha tea toxicity. *J Intensive Care Med.* 2009;24(3):205–7.
3030. Goenka P, Sarawgi A, Karun V, Nigam AG, Dutta S, Marwah N. Camellia sinensis (tea): implications and role in preventing dental decay. *Pharmacogn Rev.* 2013;7(14):152–6.
3031. Kakumanu N, Rao SD. Images in clinical medicine. Skeletal fluorosis due to excessive tea drinking. *N Engl J Med.* 2013;368(12):1140.
3032. Malinowska E, Inkielewicz I, Czarnowski W, Szefer P. Assessment of fluoride concentration and daily intake by human from tea and herbal infusions. *Food Chem Toxicol.* 2008;46(3):1055–61.
3033. Malinowska E, Inkielewicz I, Czarnowski W, Szefer P. Assessment of fluoride concentration and daily intake by human from tea and herbal infusions. *Food Chem Toxicol.* 2008;46(3):1055–61.
3034. Quock RL, Gao JX, Chan JT. Tea fluoride concentration and the pediatric patient. *Food Chem.* 2012;130:615–7.
3035. Carlsen MH, Halvorsen BL, Holte K, et al. The total antioxidant content of more than 3100 foods, beverages, spices, herbs and supplements used worldwide. *Nutr J.* 2010;9:3.
3036. Chu CH, Pang KKL, Lo ECM. Dietary behavior and knowledge of dental erosion among Chinese adults. *BMC Oral Health.* 2010;10:13.
3037. Attin T, Siegel S, Buchalla W, Lennon AM, Hannig C, Becker K. Brushing abrasion of softened and remineralised dentin: an in situ study. *Caries Res.* 2004;38(1):62–6.
3038. Bassiouny MA, Yang J. Influence of drinking patterns of carbonated beverages on dental erosion. *Gen Dent.* 2005;53(3):205–10.
3039. Phillips KM, Carlsen MH, Blomhoff R. Total antioxidant content of alternatives to refined sugar. *J Am Diet Assoc.* 2009;109(1):64–71.
3040. Matsui M, Matsui K, Kawasaki Y, et al. Evaluation of the genotoxicity of stevioside and steviol using six in vitro and one in vivo mutagenicity assays. *Mutagenesis.* 1996;11(6):573–9.

3041. Koyama E, Kitazawa K, Ohori Y, et al. In vitro metabolism of the glycosidic sweeteners, stevia mixture and enzymatically modified stevia in human intestinal microflora. *Food Chem Toxicol.* 2003;41(3):359–74.
3042. Joint FAO/WHO Expert Committee on Food Additives. Evaluation of certain food additives. *World Health Organ Tech Rep Ser.* 2009;(952):1–208.
3043. Tey SL, Salleh NB, Henry CJ, Forde CG. Effects of non-nutritive (artificial vs natural) sweeteners on 24-h glucose profiles. *Eur J Clin Nutr.* 2017;71(9):1129–32.
3044. Nutrition facts—original 20 fl oz. Coca-Cola. https://us.coca-cola.com/products/coca-cola/original. Accessed February 20, 2025.
3045. Tey SL, Salleh NB, Henry J, Forde CG. Effects of aspartame-, monk fruit-, stevia- and sucrose-sweetened beverages on postprandial glucose, insulin and energy intake. *Int J Obes (Lond).* 2017;41(3):450–7.
3046. Pepino MY, Tiemann CD, Patterson BW, Wice BM, Klein S. Sucralose affects glycemic and hormonal responses to an oral glucose load. *Diabetes Care.* 2013;36(9):2530–5.
3047. Witkowski M, Nemet I, Alamri H, et al. The artificial sweetener erythritol and cardiovascular event risk. *Nat Med.* 2023;29(3):710–8.
3048. Witkowski M, Wilcox J, Province V, et al. Ingestion of the non-nutritive sweetener erythritol, but not glucose, enhances platelet reactivity and thrombosis potential in healthy volunteers-brief report. *Arterioscler Thromb Vasc Biol.* 2024;44(9):2136–41.
3049. Witkowski M, Nemet I, Li XS, et al. Xylitol is prothrombotic and associated with cardiovascular risk. *Eur Heart J.* 2024;45(27):2439–52.
3050. Yang Q. Gain weight by "going diet?" Artificial sweeteners and the neurobiology of sugar cravings: neuroscience 2010. *Yale J Biol Med.* 2010;83(2):101–8.
3051. Yang Q. Gain weight by "going diet?" Artificial sweeteners and the neurobiology of sugar cravings: neuroscience 2010. *Yale J Biol Med.* 2010;83(2):101–8.
3052. Porikos KP, Booth G, Van Itallie TB. Effect of covert nutritive dilution on the spontaneous food intake of obese individuals: a pilot study. *Am J Clin Nutr.* 1977;30(10):1638–44.
3053. Mattes R. Effects of aspartame and sucrose on hunger and energy intake in humans. *Physiol Behav.* 1990;47(6):1037–44.
3054. Yang Q. Gain weight by "going diet?" Artificial sweeteners and the neurobiology of sugar cravings: neuroscience 2010. *Yale J Biol Med.* 2010;83(2):101–8.
3055. Emmerich SD, Fryar CD, Stierman B, Ogden CL. Obesity and severe obesity prevalence in adults: United States, August 2021–August 2023. *NCHS Data Brief.* 2024;(508):10.15620/cdc/159281.
3056. Laskowski ER. The role of exercise in the treatment of obesity. *PMR.* 2012;4(11):840–4.
3057. Emmerich SD, Fryar CD, Stierman B, Ogden CL. Obesity and severe obesity prevalence in adults: United States, August 2021–August 2023. *NCHS Data Brief.* 2024;(508):10.15620/cdc/159281.
3058. May AL, Freedman D, Sherry B, Blanck HM, Centers for Disease Control and Prevention (CDC). Obesity—United States, 1999–2010. *MMWR Suppl.* 2013;62(3):120–128.
3059. Emmerich SD, Fryar CD, Stierman B, Gu Q, Afful J, Ogden CL. Trends in obesity-related measures among US children, adolescents, and adults. *JAMA.* Published online February 13, 2025:e2427676.
3060. Laskowski ER. The role of exercise in the treatment of obesity. *PMR.* 2012;4(11):840–4.
3061. Olshansky SJ, Passaro DJ, Hershow RC, et al. A potential decline in life expectancy in the United States in the 21st century. *N Engl J Med.* 2005;352(11):1138–45.
3062. Freedhoff Y, Hébert PC. Partnerships between health organizations and the food industry risk derailing public health nutrition. *CMAJ.* 2011;183(3):291–2.
3063. Westerterp KR, Speakman JR. Physical activity energy expenditure has not declined since the 1980s and matches energy expenditures of wild mammals. *Int J Obes* (Lond). 2008;32(8):1256–63.

3064. Dwyer-Lindgren L, Freedman G, Engell RE, et al. Prevalence of physical activity and obesity in US counties, 2001–2011: a road map for action. *Popul Health Metr.* 2013;11:7.
3065. Laskowski ER. The role of exercise in the treatment of obesity. *PMR.* 2012;4(11):840–4.
3066. Swinburn B, Sacks G, Ravussin E. Increased food energy supply is more than sufficient to explain the US epidemic of obesity. *Am J Clin Nutr.* 2009;90(6):1453–6.
3067. Matthews J, International Food Information Council Foundation. Food & Health Survey: Consumer Attitudes Toward Food Safety, Nutrition & Health. https://web.archive.org/web/20140630011645/http://www.foodinsight.org/2011_Food_Health_Survey_Consumer_Attitudes_Toward_Food_Safety_Nutrition_Health. August 31, 2011. Accessed February 20, 2025.
3068. U.S. Department of Agriculture, Agricultural Research Service. Chicken, broilers or fryers, leg, meat only, cooked, stewed. FoodData Central. https://fdc.nal.usda.gov/food-details/172381/nutrients. April 1, 2019. Accessed February 20, 2025.
3069. Archer E, Hand GA, Blair SN. Correction: Validity of U.S. Nutritional Surveillance: National Health and Nutrition Examination Survey Caloric Energy Intake Data, 1971–2010. *PLoS One.* 2013;8(10):10.1371/annotation/c313df3a-52bd-4cbe-af14–6676480d1a43. Erratum for: *PLoS One.* 2013;8(10):e76632.
3070. Blair SN. Physical inactivity: the biggest public health problem of the 21st century. *Br J Sports Med.* 2009;43(1):1–2.
3071. Institute for Health Metrics and Evaluation (IHME). GBD 2021 results. University of Washington. https://vizhub.healthdata.org/gbd-results/. Accessed December 13, 2024.
3072. Institute for Health Metrics and Evaluation (IHME). GBD 2021 cause and risk summary: low physical activity—level 2 risk. University of Washington. https://www.healthdata.org/research-analysis/diseases-injuries-risks/factsheets/2021-low-physical-activity-level-2-risk. Accessed December 7, 2024.
3073. Institute for Health Metrics and Evaluation (IHME). GBD 2021 cause and risk summary: dietary risks—level 2 risk. University of Washington. https://www.healthdata.org/research-analysis/diseases-injuries-risks/factsheets/2021-dietary-risks-level-2-risk. Accessed December 7, 2024.
3074. Wang YC, McPherson K, Marsh T, Gortmaker SL, Brown M. Health and economic burden of the projected obesity trends in the USA and the UK. *Lancet.* 2011;378(9793):815–25.
3075. Dunstan DW, Barr ELM, Healy GN, et al. Television viewing time and mortality: the Australian Diabetes, Obesity and Lifestyle Study (AusDiab). *Circulation.* 2010;121(3):384–91.
3076. Stamatakis E, Hamer M, Dunstan DW. Screen-based entertainment time, all-cause mortality, and cardiovascular events: population-based study with ongoing mortality and hospital events follow-up. *J Am Coll Cardiol.* 2011;57(3):292–9.
3077. Chaput JP, Klingenberg L, Sjödin A. Do all sedentary activities lead to weight gain: sleep does not. *Curr Opin Clin Nutr Metab Care.* 2010;13(6):601–7.
3078. Patel AV, Bernstein L, Deka A, et al. Leisure time spent sitting in relation to total mortality in a prospective cohort of US adults. *Am J Epidemiol.* 2010;172(4):419–29.
3079. Van Uffelen JG, Wong J, Chau JY, et al. Occupational sitting and health risks: a systematic review. *Am J Prev Med.* 2010;39(4):379–88.
3080. Patel AV, Bernstein L, Deka A, et al. Leisure time spent sitting in relation to total mortality in a prospective cohort of US adults. *Am J Epidemiol.* 2010;172(4):419–29.
3081. Mosley M. Calorie burner: how much better is standing up than sitting? *BBC News Magazine.* http://www.bbc.com/news/magazine-24532996. October 16, 2013. Accessed February 20, 2025.
3082. Fock KM, Khoo J. Diet and exercise in management of obesity and overweight. *J Gastroenterol Hepatol.* 2013;28 Suppl 4:59–63.
3083. Thosar SS, Johnson BD, Johnston JD, Wallace JP. Sitting and endothelial dysfunction: the role of shear stress. *Med Sci Monit.* 2012;18(12):RA173–80.
3084. Koepp GA, Manohar CU, McCrady-Spitzer SK, et al. Treadmill desks: a 1-year prospective trial. *Obesity* (Silver Spring). 2013;21(4):705–11.

3085. Healy GN, Dunstan DW, Salmon J, et al. Breaks in sedentary time: beneficial associations with metabolic risk. *Diabetes Care.* 2008;31(4):661–6.
3086. Peddie MC, Bone JL, Rehrer NJ, Skeaff CM, Gray AR, Perry TL. Breaking prolonged sitting reduces postprandial glycemia in healthy, normal-weight adults: a randomized crossover trial. *Am J Clin Nutr.* 2013;98(2):358–66.
3087. Esen AM, Barutcu I, Acar M, et al. Effect of smoking on endothelial function and wall thickness of brachial artery. *Circ J.* 2004;68(12):1123–6.
3088. Alexopoulos N, Vlachopoulos C, Aznaouridis K, et al. The acute effect of green tea consumption on endothelial function in healthy individuals. *Eur J Cardiovasc Prev Rehabil.* 2008;15(3):300–5.
3089. Akazawa N, Choi Y, Miyaki A, et al. Curcumin ingestion and exercise training improve vascular endothelial function in postmenopausal women. *Nutr Res.* 2012;32(10):795–9.
3090. Sugawara J, Akazawa N, Miyaki A, et al. Effect of endurance exercise training and curcumin intake on central arterial hemodynamics in postmenopausal women: pilot study. *Am J Hypertens.* 2012;25(6):651–6.
3091. McHugh M. The health benefits of cherries and potential applications in sports. *Scand J Med Sci Sports.* 2011;21(5):615–6.
3092. Aptekmann NP, Cesar TB. Orange juice improved lipid profile and blood lactate of overweight middle-aged women subjected to aerobic training. *Maturitas.* 2010;67(4):343–7.
3093. McAnulty LS, Nieman DC, Dumke CL, et al. Effect of blueberry ingestion on natural killer cell counts, oxidative stress, and inflammation prior to and after 2.5 h of running. *Appl Physiol Nutr Metab.* 2011;36(6):976–84.
3094. Connolly DA, McHugh MP, Padilla-Zakour OI, Carlson L, Sayers SP. Efficacy of a tart cherry juice blend in preventing the symptoms of muscle damage. *Br J Sports Med.* 2006;40(8):679–83.
3095. Kuehl KS, Perrier ET, Elliot DL, Chesnutt JC. Efficacy of tart cherry juice in reducing muscle pain during running: a randomized controlled trial. *J Int Soc Sports Nutr.* 2010;7:17.
3096. Howatson G, McHugh MP, Hill JA, et al. Influence of tart cherry juice on indices of recovery following marathon running. *Scand J Med Sci Sports.* 2010;20(6):843–52.
3097. Tarazona-Díaz MP, Alacid F, Carrasco M, Martínez I, Aguayo E. Watermelon juice: potential functional drink for sore muscle relief in athletes. *J Agric Food Chem.* 2013;61(31):7522–8.
3098. Mastaloudis A, Yu TW, O'Donnell RP, Frei B, Dashwood RH, Traber MG. Endurance exercise results in DNA damage as detected by the comet assay. *Free Radic Biol Med.* 2004;36(8):966–75.
3099. Tsai K, Hsu TG, Hsu KM, et al. Oxidative DNA damage in human peripheral leukocytes induced by massive aerobic exercise. *Free Radic Biol Med.* 2001;31(11):1465–72.
3100. Fogarty MC, Hughes CM, Burke G, et al. Exercise-induced lipid peroxidation: implications for deoxyribonucleic acid damage and systemic free radical generation. *Environ Mol Mutagen.* 2011;52(1):35–42.
3101. Childs A, Jacobs C, Kaminski T, Halliwell B, Leeuwenburgh C. Supplementation with vitamin C and N-acetyl-cysteine increases oxidative stress in humans after an acute muscle injury induced by eccentric exercise. *Free Radic Biol Med.* 2001;31(6):745–53.
3102. Fogarty MC, Hughes CM, Burke G, Brown JC, Davison GW. Acute and chronic watercress supplementation attenuates exercise-induced peripheral mononuclear cell DNA damage and lipid peroxidation. *Br J Nutr.* 2013;109(2):293–301.
3103. Trapp D, Knez W, Sinclair W. Could a vegetarian diet reduce exercise-induced oxidative stress? A review of the literature. *J Sports Sci.* 2010;28(12):1261–8.
3104. U.S. Department of Health and Human Services. *Physical Activity Guidelines for Americans,* 2nd edition. Washington, DC: U.S. Department of Health and Human Services; 2018.
3105. U.S. Surgeon General. Physical activity and health—a report of the Surgeon General. https://web.archive.org/web/20090607065311/http://www.cdc.gov/nccdphp/sgr/pdf/sgrfull.pdf. November 17, 1999. Accessed February 20, 2025.

3106. Pate RR, Pratt M, Blair SN, et al. Physical activity and public health. A recommendation from the Centers for Disease Control and Prevention and the American College of Sports Medicine. *JAMA*. 1995;273(5):402–7.
3107. U.S. Department of Health and Human Services. *Physical Activity Guidelines for Americans, 2nd edition*. Washington, DC: U.S. Department of Health and Human Services; 2018.
3108. Samitz G, Egger M, Zwahlen M. Domains of physical activity and all-cause mortality: systematic review and dose-response meta-analysis of cohort studies. *Int J Epidemiol*. 2011;40(5):1382–400.
3109. Woodcock J, Franco OH, Orsini N, Roberts I. Non-vigorous physical activity and all-cause mortality: systematic review and meta-analysis of cohort studies. *Int J Epidemiol*. 2011;40(1):121–38.
3110. Samitz G, Egger M, Zwahlen M. Domains of physical activity and all-cause mortality: systematic review and dose-response meta-analysis of cohort studies. *Int J Epidemiol*. 2011;40(5):1382–400.
3111. Samitz G, Egger M, Zwahlen M. Domains of physical activity and all-cause mortality: systematic review and dose-response meta-analysis of cohort studies. *Int J Epidemiol*. 2011;40(5):1382–400.
3112. Pes GM, Dore MP, Errigo A, Poulain M. Analysis of physical activity among free-living nonagenarians from a Sardinian longevous population. *J Aging Phys Act*. 2018;26(2):254–8.
3113. Saint-Maurice PF, Troiano RP, Bassett DR, et al. Association of daily step count and step intensity with mortality among US adults. *JAMA*. 2020;323(12):1151–60.
3114. Aguiar EJ, Ducharme SW, Thomas DM. Is 4400 steps per day the new 10 000 steps per day? *JAMA Intern Med*. 2019;179(11):1601.
3115. Abbasi J. For mortality, busting the myth of 10 000 steps per day. *JAMA*. 2019;322(6):492–3.
3116. Arem H, Moore SC, Patel A, et al. Leisure time physical activity and mortality: a detailed pooled analysis of the dose-response relationship. *JAMA Intern Med*. 2015;175(6):959–67.
3117. U.S. Centers for Disease Control and Prevention (CDC). Adult participation in aerobic and muscle-strengthening physical activities—United States, 2011. *MMWR Morb Mortal Wkly Rep*. 2013;62(17):326–30.
3118. Shimizu N, Iwamoto M, Nakano Y, et al. Long-term electrocardiographic follow-up from childhood of an adult patient with Brugada syndrome associated with sick sinus syndrome. *Circ J*. 2009;73(3):575–9.
3119. Lacunza J, San Román I, Moreno S, García-Molina E, Gimeno J, Valdés M. Heat stroke, an unusual trigger of Brugada electrocardiogram. *Am J Emerg Med*. 2009;27(5):634.e1–3.
3120. Smith J, Hannah A, Birnie DH. Effect of temperature on the Brugada ECG. *Heart*. 2003;89(3):272.
3121. Dillehay TD, Rossen J, Ugent D, et al. Early Holocene coca chewing in northern Peru. *Antiquity*. 2010;84(326):939–53.
3122. Iozzo P, Guiducci L, Guzzardi MA, Pagotto U. Brain PET imaging in obesity and food addiction: current evidence and hypothesis. *Obes Facts*. 2012;5(2):155–64.
3123. Volkow ND, Wang GJ, Fowler JS, Tomasi D, Baler R. Food and drug reward: overlapping circuits in human obesity and addiction. *Curr Top Behav Neurosci*. 2012;11:1–24.
3124. Volkow ND, Wang GJ, Tomasi D, Baler RD. Obesity and addiction: neurobiological overlaps. *Obes Rev*. 2013;14(1):2–18.
3125. Frank S, Linder K, Kullmann S, et al. Fat intake modulates cerebral blood flow in homeostatic and gustatory brain areas in humans. *Am J Clin Nutr*. 2012;95(6):1342–9.
3126. Smeets PA, de Graaf C, Stafleu A, van Osch MJ, van der Grond J. Functional MRI of human hypothalamic responses following glucose ingestion. *Neuroimage*. 2005;24(2):363–8.
3127. Burger KS, Stice E. Frequent ice cream consumption is associated with reduced striatal response to receipt of an ice cream–based milkshake. *Am J Clin Nutr*. 2012;95(4):810–7.
3128. Burger KS, Stice E. Frequent ice cream consumption is associated with reduced striatal response to receipt of an ice cream–based milkshake. *Am J Clin Nutr*. 2012;95(4):810–7.

3129. Albayrak Ö, Wölfle SM, Hebebrand J. Does food addiction exist? A phenomenological discussion based on the psychiatric classification of substance-related disorders and addiction. *Obes Facts.* 2012;5(2):165–79.
3130. Lisle DJ, Goldhamer A. *The Pleasure Trap: Mastering the Hidden Force That Undermines Health & Happiness.* Summertown, TN: Book Publishing Company; 2007.
3131. Grosshans M, Loeber S, Kiefer F. Implications from addiction research toward the understanding and treatment of obesity. *Addict Biol.* 2011;16(2):189–98.
3132. Drewnowski A, Krahn DD, Demitrack MA, Nairn K, Gosnell BA. Taste responses and preferences for sweet high-fat foods: evidence for opioid involvement. *Physiol Behav.* 1992;51(2):371–9.
3133. Wang GJ, Volkow ND, Thanos PK, Fowler JS. Imaging of brain dopamine pathways: implications for understanding obesity. *J Addict Med.* 2009;3(1):8–18.
3134. Garavan H, Pankiewicz J, Bloom A, et al. Cue-induced cocaine craving: neuroanatomical specificity for drug users and drug stimuli. *Am J Psychiatry.* 2000;157(11):1789–98.
3135. Martin-Sölch C, Magyar S, Künig G, Missimer J, Schultz W, Leenders KL. Changes in brain activation associated with reward processing in smokers and nonsmokers. A positron emission tomography study. *Exp Brain Res.* 2001;139(3):278–86.
3136. Kelly J. Heal thyself. *University of Chicago Magazine.* http://mag.uchicago.edu/science-medicine/heal-thyself. Jan–Feb 2015. Accessed February 20, 2025.
3137. Farmer B, Larson BT, Fulgoni VL III, Rainville AJ, Liepa GU. A vegetarian dietary pattern as a nutrient-dense approach to weight management: an analysis of the National Health and Nutrition Examination Survey 1999–2004. *J Am Diet Assoc.* 2011;111(6):819–27.
3138. Clarys P, Deliens T, Huybrechts I, et al. Comparison of nutritional quality of the vegan, vegetarian, semi-vegetarian, pesco-vegetarian and omnivorous diet. *Nutrients.* 2014;6(3):1318–32.
3139. Pawlak R, Parrott SJ, Raj S, Cullum-Dugan D, Lucus D. How prevalent is vitamin B(12) deficiency among vegetarians? *Nutr Rev.* 2013;71(2):110–7.
3140. Mądry E, Lisowska A, Grebowiec P, Walkowiak J. The impact of vegan diet on B-12 status in healthy omnivores: five-year prospective study. *Acta Sci Pol Technol Aliment.* 2012;11(2):209–13.
3141. Brocadello F, Levedianos G, Piccione F, Manara R, Pesenti FF. Irreversible subacute sclerotic combined degeneration of the spinal cord in a vegan subject. *Nutrition.* 2007;23(7–8):622–4.
3142. Kuo SC, Yeh CB, Yeh YWY, Tzeng NS. Schizophrenia-like psychotic episode precipitated by cobalamin deficiency. *Gen Hosp Psychiatry.* 2009;31(6):586–8.
3143. Milea D, Cassoux N, LeHoang P. Blindness in a strict vegan. *N Engl J Med.* 2000;342(12):897–8.
3144. Haler D. Death after vegan diet. *Lancet.* 1968;2(7560):170.
3145. Roschitz B, Plecko B, Huemer M, Biebl A, Foerster H, Sperl W. Nutritional infantile vitamin B12 deficiency: pathobiochemical considerations in seven patients. *Arch Dis Child Fetal Neonatal Ed.* 2005;90(3):F281–2.
3146. Donaldson MS. Metabolic vitamin B12 status on a mostly raw vegan diet with follow-up using tablets, nutritional yeast, or probiotic supplements. *Ann Nutr Metab.* 2000;44(5–6):229–34.
3147. Institute of Medicine. *Dietary Reference Intakes for Thiamin, Riboflavin, Niacin, Vitamin B6, Folate, Vitamin B12, Pantothenic Acid, Biotin, and Choline.* Washington, D.C.: National Academy Press; 1998.
3148. Eussen SJ, de Groot LC, Clarke R, et al. Oral cyanocobalamin supplementation in older people with vitamin B12 deficiency: a dose-finding trial. *Arch Intern Med.* 2005;165(10):1167–72.
3149. Hill MH, Flatley JE, Barker ME, et al. A vitamin B-12 supplement of 500 μg/d for eight weeks does not normalize urinary methylmalonic acid or other biomarkers of vitamin B-12 status in elderly people with moderately poor vitamin B-12 status. *J Nutr.* 2013;143(2):142–7.
3150. Bor MV, von Castel-Roberts KM, Kauwell GPA, et al. Daily intake of 4 to 7 μg dietary vitamin B-12 is associated with steady concentrations of vitamin B-12-related biomarkers in a healthy young population. *Am J Clin Nutr.* 2010;91(3):571–7.

3151. Bischoff-Ferrari HA. Optimal serum 25-hydroxyvitamin D levels for multiple health outcomes. *Adv Exp Med Biol.* 2014;810:500–25.
3152. Mulligan GB, Licata A. Taking vitamin D with the largest meal improves absorption and results in higher serum levels of 25-hydroxyvitamin D. *J Bone Miner Res.* 2010;25(4):928–30.
3153. Harris SS. Vitamin D and African Americans. *J Nutr.* 2006;136(4):1126–9.
3154. Holick MF, Matsuoka LY, Wortsman J. Age, vitamin D, and solar ultraviolet. *Lancet.* 1989;2(8671):1104–5.
3155. Wacker M, Holick MF. Sunlight and vitamin D: a global perspective for health. *Dermatoendocrinol.* 2013;5(1):51–108.
3156. Wacker M, Holick MF. Sunlight and vitamin D: a global perspective for health. *Dermatoendocrinol.* 2013;5(1):51–108.
3157. Langdahl JH, Schierbeck LL, Bang UC, Jensen JEB. Changes in serum 25-hydroxyvitamin D and cholecalciferol after one whole-body exposure in a commercial tanning bed: a randomized study. *Endocrine.* 2012;42(2):430–5.
3158. O'Sullivan NA, Tait CP. Tanning bed and nail lamp use and the risk of cutaneous malignancy: a review of the literature. *Australas J Dermatol.* 2014;55(2):99–106.
3159. Levine JA, Sorace M, Spencer J, Siegel DM. The indoor UV tanning industry: a review of skin cancer risk, health benefit claims, and regulation. *J Am Acad Dermatol.* 2005;53(6):1038–44.
3160. Moan J, Grigalavicius M, Dahlback A, Baturaite Z, Juzeniene A. Ultraviolet-radiation and health: optimal time for sun exposure. *Adv Exp Med Biol.* 2014;810:423–8.
3161. Dasgupta PK, Liu Y, Dyke JV. Iodine nutrition: iodine content of iodized salt in the United States. *Environ Sci Technol.* 2008;42(4):1315–23.
3162. Institute for Health Metrics and Evaluation (IHME). GBD 2021 results. University of Washington. https://vizhub.healthdata.org/gbd-results/. Accessed December 13, 2024.
3163. Leung AM, Braverman LE, Pearce EN. History of U.S. iodine fortification and supplementation. *Nutrients.* 2012;4(11):1740–6.
3164. Teas J, Pino S, Critchley A, Braverman LE. Variability of iodine content in common commercially available edible seaweeds. *Thyroid.* 2004;14(10):836–41.
3165. Rose M, Lewis J, Langford N, et al. Arsenic in seaweed forms, concentration and dietary exposure. *Food Chem Toxicol.* 2007;45(7):1263–7.
3166. Teas J, Pino S, Critchley A, Braverman LE. Variability of iodine content in common commercially available edible seaweeds. *Thyroid.* 2004;14(10):836–41.
3167. Di Matola T, Zeppa P, Gasperi M, Vitale M. Thyroid dysfunction following a kelp-containing marketed diet. *BMJ Case Rep.* 2014;bcr2014206330.
3168. Greger M. Do Eden beans have too much iodine? http://nutritionfacts.org/2012/07/05/do-eden-beans-have-too-much-iodine/. July 5, 2012. Accessed February 20, 2025.
3169. Tonstad S, Nathan E, Oda K, Fraser G. Vegan diets and hypothyroidism. *Nutrients.* 2013;5(11):4642–52.
3170. Leung AM, LaMar A, He X, Braverman LE, Pearce EN. Iodine status and thyroid function of Boston-area vegetarians and vegans. *J Clin Endocrinol Metab.* 2011;96(8):E1303–7.
3171. Shaikh MG, Anderson JM, Hall SK, Jackson MA. Transient neonatal hypothyroidism due to a maternal vegan diet. *J Pediatr Endocrinol Metab.* 2003;16(1):111–3.
3172. Becker DV, Braverman LE, Delange F, et al. Iodine supplementation for pregnancy and lactation—United States and Canada: recommendations of the American Thyroid Association. *Thyroid.* 2006;16(10):949–51.
3173. Vannice G, Rasmussen H. Position of the Academy of Nutrition and Dietetics: dietary fatty acids for healthy adults. *J Acad Nutr Diet.* 2014;114(1):136–53.
3174. Harris WS. Achieving optimal n-3 fatty acid status: the vegetarian's challenge . . . or not. *Am J Clin Nutr.* 2014;100 Suppl 1:449S–52S.
3175. Sarter B, Kelsey KS, Schwartz TA, Harris WS. Blood docosahexaenoic acid and eicosapentaenoic acid in vegans: associations with age and gender and effects of an algal-derived omega-3 fatty acid supplement. *Clin Nutr.* 2015;34(2):212–8.

3176. Bourdon JA, Bazinet TM, Arnason TT, Kimpe LE, Blais JM, White PA. Polychlorinated biphenyls (PCBs) contamination and aryl hydrocarbon receptor (AhR) agonist activity of omega-3 polyunsaturated fatty acid supplements: implications for daily intake of dioxins and PCBs. *Food Chem Toxicol.* 2010;48(11):3093–7.

3177. Yokoo EM, Valente JG, Grattan L, Schmidt SL, Platt I, Silbergeld EK. Low level methylmercury exposure affects neuropsychological function in adults. *Environ Health.* 2003;2(1):8.

3178. Chang JW, Pai MC, Chen HL, Guo HR, Su HJ, Lee CC. Cognitive function and blood methylmercury in adults living near a deserted chloralkali factory. *Environ Res.* 2008;108(3):334–9.

3179. Masley SC, Masley LV, Gualtierei T. Effect of mercury levels and seafood intake on cognitive function in middle-aged adults. *Integr Med.* 2012;11(3)32–40.

3180. Arterburn LM, Oken HA, Hoffman JP, et al. Bioequivalence of docosahexaenoic acid from different algal oils in capsules and in a DHA-fortified food. *Lipids.* 2007;42(11):1011–24.

3181. Greene J, Ashburn SM, Razzouk L, Smith DA. Fish oils, coronary heart disease, and the environment. *Am J Public Health.* 2013;103(9):1568–76.

3182. Lane K, Derbyshire E, Li W, Brennan C. Bioavailability and potential uses of vegetarian sources of omega-3 fatty acids: a review of the literature. *Crit Rev Food Sci Nutr.* 2014;54(5):572–9.

3183. Witte AV, Kerti L, Hermannstädter HM, et al. Long-chain omega-3 fatty acids improve brain function and structure in older adults. *Cereb Cortex.* 2014;24(11):3059–68.

3184. Farmer B, Larson BT, Fulgoni VL, Rainville AJ, Liepa GU. A vegetarian dietary pattern as a nutrient-dense approach to weight management: an analysis of the National Health and Nutrition Examination Survey 1999–2004. *J Am Diet Assoc.* 2011;111(6):819–27.

3185. Food Surveys Research Group. Usual nutrient intake from food and beverages, by gender and age, What We Eat in America, NHANES 2017-March 2020 prepandemic. USDA, Agricultural Research Service. www.ars.usda.gov/nea/bhnrc/fsrg. 2023. Accessed February 20, 2025.

3186. Davis B, Melina V. *Becoming Vegan: The Complete Guide to Adopting a Plant-Based Diet (Comprehensive Edition).* Summertown, TN: Book Publishing Company; 2014.

3187. Craig WJ, Mangels AR. Position of the American Dietetic Association: vegetarian diets. *J Am Diet Assoc.* 2009;109(7):1266–82.

3188. Spock B. Good nutrition for kids. *Good Medicine.* 1998;7(2).

Index

Page references in *italics* indicate figures and tables.

abdominal fat, 155, 167–68, *168*, 339, 374
açaí berries, 187–88, 340
ACE inhibitors, 113, 118
acid reflux, 125, 138–41, 447
acid-inducing diet, 199–200, 202, 204–6, *205*
advanced glycation end products (AGEs), 70–71
Africa, 21–22, 234, 473
  Alzheimer's disease in, 65, 66
  colorectal cancer in, 129
  diverticulosis in, 405
  heart disease in, 21, 28, 274
  hypertension in, 103, 114
  Kenya, 103–4
  Nigeria, 65, 66
  Uganda, 21, 129
African Americans, 65, 189, 244–45, 278
AGEs. *See* advanced glycation end products
aging, 20–21, 79–80, 161, 206, 224
  blood flow and, 63–64
  cellular, 8–9
  free radical theory of, 58
  genetics and, 7
  oxidative stress cause for, 60
  sirtuins and, 70–71
AHA. *See* American Heart Association
AICR. *See* American Institute for Cancer Research
AIDS, 77, 197–98
air pollution, 43, 44, 45–47
alcohol consumption, 24, 84, 444
  breast cancer risk with, 232–33
  digestive cancer risk and, 135, 138
  liver disease with, 170, 171, 172–73, 181

alfalfa sprouts, 375–76
alkalinity, 199, 202, 204–5, *205*
allergies
  asthma and, 46, 47
  cancer risk and, 91
  to kiwifruit, 356
  seasonal, 91, 449
  treating and preventing, 86, 91–92, 360, 449
  to wheat, 434, 435
allium vegetables. *See* garlic; onions
Alzheimer's disease, 62–75, 265
  AGEs and, 70–71
  animal-based foods and, 66, 73
  annual deaths from, *11*, 53
  atherosclerosis causing, 53–54, 63–65
  diet and prevention of, 65–69, 73–75, 414
  exercise and, 72
  genetics compared to diet in, 65–67
American Heart Association (AHA), 4–5, 13, 379
  blood pressure guidelines and recommendations, 103, 113, 115
  on coronary artery calcium tests, 28
  on omega-3 fish oil supplementation, 22–23
  on primordial prevention, 4
  "Simple 7" recommendations, 4, 7
  sodium intake guidelines, 106, 109, 111, 331
American Institute for Cancer Research (AICR), 210, 231, 309, 328, 385
Americans, 4–5, 6–7, 308. *See also* standard American diet
  blood pressure of, 103, 113
  heart disease in, 2, 19, 20, 21–22
  life expectancy of, 3

amino acids, 199, 219, 381–82
amla, 425–26
amyloid, 54, 64–65, 265
anemia, 133, 134–35, 185, 188
aneurysms, 102
angina, xiii, 20, 30
animal fat, 22, 30, 66, 153, 159, 174, 267, 291, 401
animal protein, 73, 197, 198–99, 203–5, 232, 278, 283–84
animal viruses, 77, 136, 190–92, 194
animal-based foods, 6. *See also* beef; cooked meat; fish; pork; poultry; processed meat
  acid reflux with, 139–40
  AGEs and, 70–71
  aging and, 8
  antibiotics in, 100, 190
  antioxidant lack in, 61
  BMI with, 149
  calories in, *157*, 159–60
  cancers associated with, 42–44, 129–30, 132–34, 139–40, 190–92, 236–40, 332, 389
  disease risk from, 44–45, 48, 65–67, 132–34, 153–54, *153*, 158–59, 244–45, 283
  fiber deficiency with, 54–55
  flatulence and, 337–38
  food poisoning in, 92–99, 207, 375
  industry pressure for, 32
  inflammation with, 30, 199, 201, 214–15
  iron excess with, 129
  kidney problems with, 197–202
  mental health and, 214–16
  pregnancy risk with, 43
  weight gain and, 110, 160, 163
antacids, 140
antibiotics, 94, 96, 99, 100, 190, 247
anticancer agents, 41–42, 83, 130
antidepressants. *See* prescription drugs
antioxidants, 68–69
  in apple peels, 243, 341
  of berries, 83, 341–42, 345–47
  in beverages, 119, 450, 452
  as brain food, 68–69
  depression protection with, 224–25
  in food over supplements, 50, 187, 290–91, 364
  foods high in, 60–62, 119, 180, 363

  in greens, 368, 369–70
  in herbs and spices, 41, 61, 188, 407–8, 423–27, 429
  inflammation reduction with, 62, 461
  measuring, 425
  nitric oxide and, 121
  oxidative stress and, 60–61
  pigments as, 82, 180
  smoking and, 40
  stroke risk and, 58–62
  in vitamin C, 210–11
apolipoprotein E4 (ApoE4), 66–67
apples, 71, 82, 140, 349
  antioxidants in peels of, 243, 341
  cancer reduction with, 243
  dried, 395
arachidonic acid, 214–16
Aricept. *See* donepezil
arsenic, 254–55, 437–38, 476
arteries, 20, 21, 22, 24, 28–30
arthritis
  childhood obesity and, 149
  food poisoning and, 97
  gout, 149, 175, 204, 263, 345, 419
  osteoarthritis, 408, 411
  rheumatoid arthritis, 408, 415
artificial flavorings, 437
artificial sweeteners, 221–22, 453–55
asbestos, 136, 137
Asian populations, 316
  cancer in, 13, 49, 127–28, 250–51, 278, 296
  diabetes in, 158
  enlarged prostate in, 280
  heart disease in, 21, 28
aspartame, 222, 453, 454
aspirin, 215, 294–97, 345, 378, 409
asthma, *11*, 36–37, 45, 47–51, 86
atherosclerosis, 20–21, 22, 24, 25, 104
  as Alzheimer's cause, 63–65
  erectile dysfunction with, 403
  LDL cholesterol and, 24
atherosclerotic plaque, 20, 22, 24, 28, 30, 53–55, 63–64
athletes, 83, 90–91, 104, 105, 116, 123, 147, 460, 465
Atkins corporation, 100–101
autism, 360
autoimmune diseases, 97, 432–35
avocados, 135, 154, 348, 372
Ayurveda, 425, 426

INDEX | 637

B cells, 79
B vitamins. *See* folate; vitamin B12
babies, 86
bacon, 43–44, *71*, 102, 209–10, 238, 261, 309, 315, 425
bananas, 56–57, 342, 348, 351, 371
Barnard, Neal, 34, 319
Barrett's esophagus, 139
beans, 15, 382, 476
  cancer prevention with, 127–28, 129, 130
  canned, 335, 476
  flatulence with, 337–38
  for hypertension, 117
  life extension with, 337
  prebiotics in, 87
  recipes for, 327–28, 335–36
  stroke prevention and, 55
  toxin defense with, 82
  types and daily serving for, 323–24, *324*
  weight loss link to, 154–55
beef, 94–95, 204–5, *205*, 215
beetroot, 121–23
bell peppers/capsicum, 259, 267, 386, 390
benign prostatic hyperplasia (BPH), 279–81
berries, 324
  anti-inflammatory influence of, 62, 460
  antioxidant power of, 83, 341–42, 345–47
  blood sugar and, 343
  clinical trials on, 346
  colorectal cancer reversal with, 131–32
  disease prevention with, 266, 340–41
  frozen compared to fresh, 344
  immune boost with, 83–84, 340
  memory ability and, 68
  types and daily serving for, 340
  vision improvement with, 345, 346
beta-carotene, 82, 187
beverages, *324*, 325
  beneficial, 119–20, 135, 442–55
  recipes for, 179–80, 446, 453–54
bicarbonate of soda, 202
blackberries, 342
Blackburn, Elizabeth, 9
bladder infections. *See* urinary tract infections
blood cancers, 183–85
  animal viruses and, 190–92
  annual deaths from, *11*, 185
  categories of, 184–85
  children and, 183–84
  plant-based foods for, 186–89, 194

blood donation, 134, 176
blood flow, 53–54, 57
blood pressure, high, 5, 102–4
  beetroot for, 121–23
  clinical trials on, 107, 112, 118–20, 339
  DASH diet for, 113–16
  deaths due to, *11,* 102
  drugs for, 112–13, 114, 120, 121
  fiber and reduction of, 55
  nitrates treatment for, 120–23
  plant-based diet treatment of, 102–4, 108, 113–24, 332, 384
  risks of, 102–4
  sodium and, 106–11, 331–33
  soya as defense to, 331–33
  on standard diet, 103–4, 115–16
  whole grains treating, 112–13
blood pressure, normal, 4, 103, 107, 332
blood sugar, 4, 144–46
  drugs lowering, 161–62
  fats raising, 146–47
  plant-based diet management of, 80, 155, 157, 163–66, 343, 429
  vinegar for, 373
blood thinners, 294, 301
blueberries
  antioxidant power of, 83–84, 224, 341, 342
  memory ability and, 68
  Parkinson's risk and, 266
body mass index (BMI), 149, 163, 167–68, *168*, 415, 458
bone density, 130, 271–72
bottled water, 443, 445
bowel movement, 54, 128–29, 142, 264, 344, 405. *See also* constipation
BPH. *See* benign prostatic hyperplasia
brain diseases, *11*, 53–54, 408. *See also* Alzheimer's disease; stroke
breast cancer, 39, 40, 227–29
  alcohol and risk of, 232–33
  annual deaths from, *11*
  antihypertensive drugs and risk of, 112–13
  detection of, 227
  exercise and prevention of, 237
  fiber-rich diet and prevention of, 241–43
  flaxseeds and reduction of, 246–48, 394
  genetics and, 249–50
  mammograms and, 229–31
  meat consumption and risk of, 192, 237–40, 244

breast cancer (*continued*)
  melatonin and risk of, 233–34, 236
  plant-based diet for, 6, 130, 131, 180, 240–51, 275, 356, 385–86
  soya and, 248–50, 330, 339
  stem cell suppression in, 245–46
broccoli, 156, 157, 325, 359–61, 378
  cancer prevention with, 39–40, 244–46
  DNA damage prevention with, 359–60
  immune boost with, 81–82
  liver detox with, 46–47
  supplements, 364
broccoli sprouts, 14, 46–47, 246, 359, 363–64
bronchitis, 36, 38, 44
brussels sprouts, 385, 386
Burkitt, Denis, 129
butter. *See* dairy

C. diff. See Clostridium difficile
cabbage, 39, 186, 188, 205–6, 363
caffeine, 446–48. *See also* coffee; tea
calcium, 130, 160, 203–4, 308, 310, 328, 414
calcium-channel blockers, 113, 118
calories, 111, 155, 156–57, *157*, 160, 163, 401–2
cancer, 5, 10
  allergies and risk of, 91
  alliums for fighting, 332, 387, 388
  animal-based foods and, 42–44, 129–30, 132–34, 139–40, 190–92, 236–40, 332, 389
  in Asian populations, 13, 49, 127–28, 250–51, 278, 296
  aspirin and risk of, 294–96
  broccoli for prevention of, 39–40, 244–46
  clinical trials on, 41, 130, 142, 189, 248
  diagnostic radiation and, 289–92
  eggs and risk for, 239, 273–74, 278, 283–84
  exercise and, 274–76, 283, 458
  fiber for reducing risk of, 54, 128–29, 241–43
  genetics and, 13–15, 125, 132, 249–50
  growth hormones and, 232, 271, 282
  herbs and spices for, 41–42, 126–28, 137–38, 188–89, 386, 387, 388, 408, 424–27
  Ornish's studies on, 14, 274, 276, 277

plant-based foods for, 6, 39–40, 82–83, 126–28, 130, 142–43, 227–28, 231, 240–51, 275–79, 328, 359–60, 361, 380, 385–87
poultry-related, 136–37, 139, 190, 237, 273, 278
smoking-related, 29, 36, 37, 51, 135, 136, 137, 138, 261
tea protecting against, 449, 450
water benefits for, 443–44
cannabis. *See* marijuana
cannibalistic feed, 76, 266–67
capsicum. *See* bell peppers
Captopril, 120
carbohydrate consumption, 146–47, 219–20
carbohydrate-fiber ratio, 438–40, *439*
carcinogen blockers, 41, 332, 368–69
carcinogens, 38–39, 42–43, 47, 209, 210
cardamom, 84
carotenoids, 187, 224, 371, 372, 380
carrots, 377, 378, 383, 386, 388, 390
cauliflower, 39, 338, 359, 360, 362, 378
cayenne pepper, 419–20
CDC. *See* Centers for Disease Control and Prevention
celery, 387, 390
celery juice, 210
celiac disease, 432–35
Centers for Disease Control and Prevention (CDC), 257
  on alcohol consumption, 172
  on chemical pollutants, 253
  on diabetes rates, 145, 168
  on food poisoning, 92, 94, 98
  on heart attack prevention, 207
  on hypertension management, 113–14
  on infection-related deaths, 77
  on leukemia diagnoses, 185
  lifestyle behaviors for health by, 7
cesarean section, 86
cheese. *See* dairy
chemopreventive agents, 41
chemotherapy, 14, 42, 127, 137, 186, 187, 235, 440–41
cherries, tart, 345
chest pain. *See* angina
chia seeds, 354, 398, 399, 476
chicken. *See* poultry
children, 93
  asthma in, 36–37, 47–48
  dehydration in, 445

INDEX | 639

diabetes in, 148–50
fiber intake for, 55
incense exposure and, 49
leukemia in, 184, 448
obesity and prediabetes in, 148–50, 313, 457
PAHs and development of, 43
plant-based diet for, 148–50, 291, 384–85
toxins passed to, 253–54
China-Cornell-Oxford Project, 21
Chinese medicine, 109
chlorella, 437
chlorophyll, 58, 340, 368–70
cholesterol, blood, 4, 293. *See also* LDL cholesterol
   coffee and, 447
   diseases linked to high, 20, 22, 24–26, 54, 55, 63–67, 75, 174–75, 197
   kale's influence on, 40
   plant-based diet and, 21–22, 25, 28–31
   pregnancy and, 24
   sexual dysfunction with high, 404
choline, 273–74
chronic obstructive pulmonary disease (COPD), 11, 36, 44–45, 51
cinnamon, 61, 218, 338, 407, 424, 429
circadian body clock, 234–35
cirrhosis. *See* liver disease
citrus zest, 356
clinical trials, 86, 179. *See also* Global Burden of Disease Study; NIH-AARP study
   on Alzheimer's, 69, 72–73
   on animal protein, 199, 201, 203
   on autism, 360
   on berries, 346
   on beverages, 446, 449
   on black cumin, 415
   on blood pressure, 107, 112, 119–20, 339
   on blood sugar, 164, 373
   on cancer, 41, 130, 142, 189, 248
   on diabetes, 105–6, 155, 158, 373
   on fenugreek, 416, 417
   on fish oil, 23
   on flaxseeds, 117–18, 247
   on ginger, 421
   on gluten, 433
   on heart disease, 23
   on kidneys, 199, 201
   on liver disease, 181–82, 413

   on mental health, 194, 216–17, 220, 221, 223, 224
   on migraine headaches, 421
   on nuts and seeds, 399–401
   on PCOS, 424
   on probiotics, 86–87
   on turmeric and curcumin, 41, 189, 292, 408, 412, 413
   on weight loss, 157, 158, 179
Clostridium difficile (C. diff), 98–99
cloves, 188, 218, 424–25
Coca-Cola, 32, 33, 188, 206, 222, 310, 312–13, 453, 457
cocoa powder, 314, 344, 345
coenzyme Q10 (CoQ10), 369–70
coffee, 442, 444, 446–48
   cholesterol levels and, 447
   liver protection with, 178, 181–82
   longevity with, 446
   Parkinson's and, 258
   suicide risk and, 221
collard greens, 186, 211, 245, 325, 336, 359, 366, 371
colon cancer. *See* colorectal cancer
colonoscopy, 126, 170, 293, 297–300
colorectal cancer, 126–35
   annual deaths from, 11, 125
   diagnosis and prevention of, 126–28, 129–32, 297–301
   diet as cause of and cure for, 7, 113, 129–35, 210, 232, 243, 385
   in India, 296
   in Japan compared with U.S., 13
   stool size and, 128–29
   turmeric and, 126–28, 137
complexion, 380–81
constipation, 128–29, 264–65
cooked meat, 43–44, 70–71, 190–91, 237–40, 244–45, 389
cooked vegetables, 360–62, 370–72, 388–90
cooking methods, 388–90
COPD. *See* chronic obstructive pulmonary disease
CoQ10. *See* coenzyme Q10
coriander 122, 407, 418–19
COVID-19 pandemic, 19
   deaths from, 77, 78
   plant-based diet and, 87–88
   life expectancy impacted by, 3
   "long COVID" syndrome, 88
cranberries, 68–69, 179–80, 340, 342

cruciferous vegetables, 39–40, 323, *324*,
    359–65. *See also* broccoli; kale
  cancer protection and reversal with, 39–40,
    46, 186, 187, 244, 245–46, 278,
    359–60
  immune system defense with, 81–82
  raw benefits in cooked, 360–62
  recipes for, 362–64
  stem cell suppression with, 246
  types and daily servings of, 325, 359
CT scans, 289–90
curcumin, 408–14, 460
  cancer prevention and treatment with, 41–42,
    126–28, 137–38, 188–89
  supplement compared with whole food, 409,
    411–13

Daily Dozen, 306, 321, 323–26, *324*
dairy, 109, 262–63, 310, 442, 476
  acid load and, 199, *205*
  asthma and, 48
  blood pressure and, 115, 116
  cancer and bone fractures with, 263, 270–73
  flatulence with, 337–38
  Parkinson's link to, 262–63
  pollutants and pathogens in, 82, 93, 95, 192,
    255, 256, 262–63
  saturated and trans fats in, 154, 166
DART trial, 23
DASH diet, 113–16
dates, 180, 344, 348, 349–50
DDT, 253–54, 255, 256, 262, 263, 264,
    390
death
  from air pollution, 45
  from Alzheimer's, *11*, 53, 62
  from cancer, 10, *11*, 35–36, 37, 125, 129, 138,
    181, 185, 227
  from COVID-19, 77, 78
  from diabetes, *11*, 145
  dietary factors in, 1, 3, 10, 102, 104, 201,
    210, 348, 377
  from food poisoning, 93
  from heart disease, 1, 4, *11*, 20–22, 23, 102
  from high blood pressure, *11*, 102
  from kidney disease, *11*, 197
  leading causes of, 1, 2, 5, 10, *11*, 197
  from liver disease, *11*, 170–71, 172
  from medical error and medical care, 285–87,
    300
  from Parkinson's disease, *11*, 252
  from prescription drugs, 285
  responsibility for, 469–70
  screen time and risk of, 458
  from suicide, *11*, 212
"decision fatigue," 316–17
dementia, 54, 63, 64, 65–66, 73
depression. *See* mental health; suicide
desserts, 325–26, 336–37, 344, 411
detoxification. *See* toxins
diabetes, type 1, 145–46, 147, 148
diabetes, type 2, 54, 87, 144–45.
    See also prediabetes
  annual deaths from, *11*
  in Asia, 158
  calories for, 162
  causes of, 146–48
  exercise and, 168–69, 458
  fruit juice and risk of, 349
  genetics and, 146, 156, 169
  heart disease risk with, 157
  medication risks, 161
  neuropathy treatment in, 165–67
  obesity and, 144, 145, 148–49, 150–53
  omnivores and, 153–54, *153*, 158
  pesticides in food link to, 159
  plant-based diet with, 144, 146, 152–60,
    163–67, 360, 429–30
  processed foods and, 5–6
  statins and risk of, 26–27
  symptoms of, 145
  therapies for, 160–67, 429
diagnostic medical radiation. *See* radiation
diet. *See also* plant-based diet; standard
    American diet; vegan diet;
    vegetarian diet
  addictions in, 466–68
  big picture importance in, 313–17
  cancer cause and prevention with, 5–7, 125,
    129–34, 135–37, 139–41, 227–28,
    237–50, 296
  child development and, 149, 478
  death risk and, 1, 3, 10, 102, 104, 201, 210,
    348, 377
  as disease cause and cure, xiii–xiv, xv, 1–6,
    10–13, 21–22, 25, 26–34, 36–38,
    259–66, 293, 340
  evidence-based, 11, 320–22, 469
  inflammation reduction with, 45, 62, 88, 92,
    118, 345, 379, 384, 440, 460
  for mental health, 215–21, 224–25, 434
  physicians advising on, 33
  quality of, 6, 9
  willpower and habits with, 316–19

dietary guidelines, 113–16, 442. *See also* Daily Dozen
government-based, 7, 32, 109, 111, 308–13, 327–28
from Kaiser Permanente, 12–13, 316, 317–18
digestive cancers, *11*, 125. *See also* colorectal cancer; pancreatic cancer
dioxins, 82, 190, 254, 255, 256–57, 263, 264
diuretics, 114, 333
diverticulosis, 142, 405–6
DNA, 8, 14, 70
DNA damage, 59–60, 249–50, 412, 453
  chlorophyll preventing, 368–70
  exercise and, 461
  foods preventing, 39, 41, 290–92, 359, 368–69, 382
  foods repairing, 80, 182, 356
  free radicals and, 243, 381–82
  herbs and spices preventing, 409, 410, 423, 450
  incense and, 49
  meat and, 43–44, 238–39
  pesticides and, 265
  tobacco use and, 36, 39, 41
  viruses and, 191, 192
doctors. *See* physicians
donepezil (Aricept), 69
dopamine, 218, 466–68
drug addiction, 466–68
drug overdose, 171
durian fruit, 357

E. coli, 93, 94, 95, 96
eczema, 47, 86
edamame, 327, 333, 334
Edison, Thomas, 2, 13
egg industry, 32, 33, 93, 274, 346
eggs
  acid load and, 204–5, *205*
  antioxidant lack in, 61
  arachidonic acid in, 215
  asthma attacks and, 48
  cancer risk and, 239, 273–74, 278, 283
  flax as substitute for, 329, 397
  LDL cholesterol and, 25
  pollutants in, 255, 256, 267
  Salmonella with, 93, 95, 375
  sensitivity to, 433–34
emphysema, 36, 44, 45, 258
empowerment, xi, xv, xvii, 7, 12, 14, 15, 469

endothelial function, 459–60
endotoxins, 29–30
EPIC study, 136–37, 190, 200–201
EPIC-PANACEA, 160, 162–63
epigenetics, 13–14
Epstein-Barr virus, 90
erectile dysfunction, 114, 120, 169, 270, 354, 403–4
ergothioneine, 323, 381–82
erythritol, 453
esophageal cancer, *11*, 14, 125, 138–43
esophageal varices, 170
Esselstyn, Caldwell, Jr., 28, 293–94
essential tremor, 259–62
estrogen, 143, 233, 237, 417
  fennel and, 416
  lignans and, 247, 396
  receptors, 241, 243, 245, 248–49, 330
  relieving excess, 240–43
  soya and, 248–50, 339, 396
exercise, 267, *324*, 325, 457–58
  benefits of, 457–58
  breast cancer prevention with, 237
  cancer treatment with, 274–76, 283
  cellular aging and, 10
  for depression, 223
  diabetes treatment with, 168–69, 458
  as health factor, 4, 7, 9
  heart disease reversal and, xiii–xiv, 458
  immune boost with, 88–91
  memory improvement with, 72
  moderation in, 88–89
  oxidative stress in, 461–62
  plant-based diet with, 460–62
  types and duration of, 456, 458–60, 462–63

fast food, 174, 217, 351, 435
fat. *See also* animal fat; cholesterol, blood; omega-3 fats; saturated fat; trans fat
  body, 6, 103, 146, 152, 167–68, 241, 264
  enzyme for burning, 160
  in nuts, 400
  in poultry, 162–63
  turmeric with, 410
  types of, 154
fat consumption
  addiction to, 467
  carbohydrate compared to, 146–47

fat consumption (*continued*)
  diseases linked to, 24–25, 67–68, 139–40, 146–47, 173–74, 181
  greens pairing with, 371–72
  pancreatic cancer and, 135–36
fat soluble nutrients, 346, 371, 447
FDA. *See* Food and Drug Administration, U.S.
fecal contamination, 92, 94–95, 97
fenugreek, 407, 417–18
fiber. *See also* carbohydrate-fiber ratio
  breast cancer risk and, 241–43
  colorectal cancer protection and, 128–29
  deficiency risks, 54–56, 143, 241–43, 405–6
  diverticulitis and, 405–6
  foods high in, 55–56, 88, 241, 327, 339
  hiatal hernias and, 141–42
  prebiotics in, 87
  stroke risk reduction with, 54–56
  from supplements versus foods, 242
fish, 87, 116, 149, 153, 156, *157*
  acid load and, 203, 204, 205
  arachidonic acid in, 215
  farm-raised risks, 159, 256
  kidney stones and, 203
  iodine in, 475
  pollutants and pathogens in, 43, 71, 82, 175, 191, 240, 255–57, 264, 476–77
  salted, 332
  from supplements versus foods, 476
  in traditional Asian diets, 158
fish oil, 22–23, 217, 255, 476
flatulence, 337–39
flavor conditioning, 370–71
flaxseeds, 323, *324*, 325, 394–97, 476
  blood pressure treatment with, 117–18
  cancer reduction with, 246–48, 278–79, 280–81
  suggestions for using, 329, 375, 394–97, 426
fluoride, 451–52
FOIA. *See* Freedom of Information Act
folate, 225, 327, 339
food addictions, 466–68
food additives, 206–8
Food and Drug Administration, U.S. (FDA), 93, 336
  aducanumab approved by, 75
  antidepressant trial data, 225–26
  on arsenic in rice, 437–38
  on aspartame, 222
  on dioxins, 257
  food additive safety and, 207–8

  on pawpaws, 353
  PPI safety alert issued by, 140
  retail-meat survey by, 94
  on statin safety labeling, 26
food industry, 457. *See also* meat industry
  food safety and, 93, 95–96, 207–8
  information suppression in, 109, 274
  profits and claims by, 33–34, 94, 98, 312–13, 319–20
  standard diet influenced by, 311–13, 466
food poisoning, 92–93
  with alfalfa sprouts, 375–76
  eggs and, 93, 95, 375
  in meat and poultry, 94–99, 176, 207
  by superbugs, 98–99
  UTIs and, 96–97
food pollutants, 159, 253–57, 262–64, 266–67, 476–77
food safety, 94–96, 98, 207, 208, 413
foods, 102, 367. *See also* animal-based foods; fried food; frozen food
  in acid-inducing diet, 204–5, *205*
  allergies to, 356, 434, 435
  calories per portion of, 156–57, *157*
  cost of healthy, 307–8
  for disease prevention, 178–82, 195, 359–60
  DNA damage prevention with, 39, 41, 290–92, 359, 368–69, 382
  epigenetic influence of, 14
  fiber-rich, 55–56, 88, 241, 327, 339
  heavy metals in, 254–55, 264, 267, 291, 413
  immune system boost with, 90–91, 100–101
  over drugs, 10, 12–13, 14, 51, 112–13, 118, 120, 132, 220, 280, 293–97
  over supplements, 50, 60, 187–88, 202, 225, 250, 379, 411–13, 473
  pollutants in, 159, 253–57, 262–64, 266–67, 476–77
  for radiation protection, 290–91
  rating system for, 308–10, *309*
forest bathing, 84–86
free radicals, 58, 59, 68, 109, 120–21, 224
Freedom of Information Act (FOIA), 225–26, 274
fried food, 42–44, 71, 238, 239, 244, 261, 389
frozen food, 344, 361
fruit-and-nut bars, 395
fruits, *324*. *See also* berries
  alkalinity with, 204–5, *205*
  in beverages, 446
  citrus, benefits of, 57, 356

diet lacking in, 102, 348
DNA repair with, 356
lung disease and, 44, 45
phytonutrients in, 57, 82
recipes for, 344, 345
suggestions for, 348, 350–51, 354–55
variety of, benefit of eating, 378–81, 385–86
wash for, 390–91
whole over juicing, 314, 349

galactose, 263, 272
gallbladder, 414
garlic, 83, 281, 292, 338, 386, 387, 388
gastric bypass surgery, 162
genetics, 2. *See also* epigenetics
 aging and, 7
 Alzheimer's and, 65–67
 cancer and, 13–15, 125, 132, 249–50
 coriander and, 418
 diabetes and, 146, 156, 169
 diet and lifestyle over, 13–15, 66, 276–77
gerontotoxins, 70–71
ginger, 291–92, 338, 355, 407, 421–23
Global Burden of Disease Study, 102, 348, 377
gluten, 432–35
GMOs, 329–31
goji berries, 292, 325, 340, 345–46
grapefruit, 348, 356, 357, 371
grapes, 68, 127, 179, 233, 340
GRAS ("generally recognized as safe"), 208
Graves' disease, 97
green beans, 387, 390
green tea, 14, 119, 218, 250–51, 378, 412–13, 442, 448–52
greens, 15, *324*, 366–76
 alkalinity of, 204, *205*
 anti-inflammatory influence of, 62
 antioxidant power of, 366, 368, 369–70
 blood cancer benefit from, 186–87, 194
 cooking suggestions for, 370–73
 nitrates in, 121, 122, *122*
 phytonutrients in, 372, 375
 potassium in, 57
 in salads, 374–75
 types and daily servings of, 366
growth hormones, 232, 271, 282–83

habits, 316–19
HCAs. *See* heterocyclic amines
headaches, 419–20, 421
healing process, 28–29
health care system, xiii–xvii, 11–12, 299

heart attack
 aspirin and risk of, 294–96
 atherosclerosis leading to, 20–21
 foods preventing, 312, 367
 mainstream prevention of, 3–4
heart disease, 206, 263, 447–48.
  See also stroke
 berries and prevention of, 340
 death from, 1, 4, *11*, 20–22, 23, 102
 diabetics and, 146, 157, 160–61
 exercise and, xiii–xiv, 458–59
 global occurrences of, 21–22, 28
 kidney damage link to, 196
 LDL cholesterol influence on, 24–26
 meat consumption and, 132–33
 Ornish's studies on, xiv, 12, 28, 30, 72, 305
 plant-based diet for, xiii–xiv, 10, 21–22, 25, 28–31, 131, 305–6, 431, 469
 potassium and, 56
 processed foods and, 6
 sodium intake and, 106–7
 water benefits for, 443, 444
 whole grains treating, 113
 women and, 301
heavy metals. *See also* mercury
 in foods, 254–55, 264, 267, 291, 413
 in supplements, 413, 426
 women and, 253
heme iron. *See* iron
hemoglobin A1c, 163–64
hemorrhagic strokes, 54
hemorrhoids, 128, 142, 214
hepatitis, viral, 175–77, 181
herbs and spices, 296, *324*
 antioxidant power of, 40, 61, 188, 341, 407–8, 423, 424–27, 429
 for brain and mood health, 69, 219, 220
 for cancer, 41–42, 126–28, 137–38, 188–89, 386, 387, 388, 408, 424–27
 cautions with, 427–30
 DNA damage prevention with, 409, 410, 423, 450
 for inflammation reduction, 408, 410, 412, 413, 415, 418, 423–24
 with pregnancy, 414, 422, 423
 recommendations for, 407–8, 414–27
hernia. *See* hiatal hernia
hesperidin, 57
heterocyclic amines (HCAs), 43, 190, 237–39, 244, 273, 389
hexachlorobenzene, 159, 255
hiatal hernia, 128, 141–42

hibiscus tea, 117, 119–20, 442, 452
Hodgkin's lymphoma, 185
horseradish, 359, 362, 407
hot dogs, 71, 102, 209
Huntington's disease, 263, 265
hypertension. *See* blood pressure, high

iatrogenic cause. *See* medical error
IBS. *See* irritable bowel syndrome
IgA, 89
IGF-1, 232, 282–84
immune system
  berries for, 83–84, 340
  depression and, 213
  exercise and diet boosting, 88–91
  function of, 79–80
  infection prevention and, 78–80
  plant-based diet boosting, 80–84, 87–88, 90–91
incense, 48–50
India, 126, 127
indigestion, 420
infectious diseases, 11. *See also* COVID-19 pandemic
  hand hygiene to prevent, 78
  immune system and, 79–80
  meat industry and, 77
  prevention of, 79–80, 86–91, 285–86
inflammation
  of arteries, 29–30
  berries reducing, 62, 460
  diet for reduction of, 45, 62, 88, 91, 118, 345, 379, 384, 440, 460
  greens reducing, 62
  herbs and spices for, 408, 410, 412, 413, 415, 418, 423–24
  with meat consumption, 30, 199, 201, 214
  mushrooms reducing, 90–91
  saturated fat causing, 154
  tart cherry and, 345
  whole grains and, 432
influenza, 77, 78, 89, 213
insulin, 144–48, 152–57, 164–65, 169
insulin resistance, 80, 146–48, 153, 154, 161
intestines, 81, 92, 94, 125, 127, 128, 131, 133, 134
iodine, 475–76
iron, 129, 132–35, 310
irritable bowel syndrome (IBS), 355, 420, 433, 434, 435
ischemic stroke, 54

Journal of the American Medical Association, 22–23, 24, 32, 286, 298, 300
juice, fruit and vegetable, 57, 121–22, 123, 210
  Alzheimer's risk and, 68–69
  whole food compared to, 180, 233, 314, 349, 356

Kaiser Permanente, 12, 221, 316, 317
kale, 40, 80–81, 186, 211, 278, 363, 370
kelp, 476
Kempner, Walter, 108
kidney disease, 102, 263
  animal-based food link to, 197, 200–201
  annual deaths from, 11, 197
  diet causing, 195–99, 206–7
  foods for prevention of, 195–96, 209
  heart disease from, 196
  phosphorus excess and, 206–7
  tobacco and hot dog link to, 209
kidney function, 195–96, 197–201
kidney stones, 131, 202–5, 414, 416, 443
kiwifruit, 117, 355–56
kombucha, 451
Komen, Susan G., 312

lactovegetarian diet, 114
lavender, 221
LDL cholesterol, 155, 451
  Alzheimer's link to, 65
  foods to lower, 31, 40, 157, 201, 329, 344, 355, 395, 415, 418, 424
  heart disease risk and, 24–26
  levels for health, 25–26
  statins and, 27–28
legumes. *See* beans
lentils, 324, 326, 327, 328, 334, 335, 336
lettuce, 122, 386–87
leukemia. *See* blood cancers
life expectancy, 3
lifestyle behaviors, xiv–xv, 7, 9, 295–96
  of Americans, 3, 5, 7, 308
  over genetics, 13–14, 65–67, 276–77
lifestyle-based diseases, 5, 11–12
lignans, 246–47, 278–79, 323
liver cancer, 136, 171, 174, 175, 179, 181
liver disease. *See also* hepatitis, viral
  alcohol-related, 170, 171, 172–73, 181
  berries and, 340
  death from, 11, 170–71, 172
  fast food and, 174, 175

foods for prevention of, 178–82
nonalcoholic fatty, 173–75, 182
obesity as cause for, 174
pork link to, 176–77
from statins, 26
types of, 171
weight-loss supplements and, 177–78
liver function, 171, 244
lung cancer, *11*, 29, 35–36, 37–44, 45, 49, 51, 126, 137
lung disease, 5, *11*, 35–36, 51. *See also* asthma; chronic obstructive pulmonary disease
lycopene, 82, 224, 314, 341, 372, 380, 388–89
lymphoma, *11*, 184–85, 186, 187, 190–91, 192, 360

mad cow disease, 76, 77, 265, 266
magnesium, 160, 308, 473, 477
mammograms, 228–31
mangos, 351
MAO. *See* monoamine oxidase
marijuana, 38–39
Mayo Clinic, 3, 78, 94, 187, 406
McDonald's, 29, 32, 33, 71, 110, 139, 174, 175, 310
McGovern Committee, 32
meat consumption. *See* animal-based foods
meat fumes, 42–44
meat industry
 cannibalistic feed in, 76, 266–67
 infectious diseases and, 77
 power of, 32–33, 76–77, 94–96, 311
 on *Salmonella*, 94–96
meat industry workers, 136, 137, 176, 191
meat substitutes, 43–44, 200–201, 238, 333
meat-to-vegetable ratio, 130
medical error, 285–87
medical establishment, 2, 32–33, 183–84
medical literature, xv, xvii, 468
medical training, xv, 1–2, 12, 169
Mediterranean diet, 67, 174, 217, 259, 401
MeIQx, 190
melatonin, 233–34, 236
memory ability, 68, 72
men, 254, 264, 266, 329–30, 443–44. *See also* erectile dysfunction; prostate cancer
menstruation, 134, 219, 247, 319, 417, 421–22
mental health. *See also* suicide
 antioxidants and, 224–25
 artificial sweeteners and, 221–22

clinical trials on, 194, 216–17, 220, 221, 223, 224
diet and, 214–22, 224–25, 434
drug side effects, 218, 220, 226
exercise for, 223
free radicals and, 224
green tea and, 218
major depression, 212, 215, 216–17, 221, 223
onions and, 218
physical health link to, 213–14
prescription drugs for, 218, 220, 223, 225–26
saffron for, 220
tests for, 214
mercury, 95, 143, 255–56, 264, 267, 392, 477
metastasis, 40, 138, 239, 248, 249, 359
MGUS, 188–89
microgreens, 375
migration studies, 13, 21, 65, 405
milk. *See* dairy
milk substitutes, 115, 249, 271, 314, 328, 332
mint, 180, 292, 299–300, 371, 407, 423, 426, 442, 446, 453
miso, 327, 328, 331–33
mitochondria, 58, 59, 154, 160, 381–82
molasses, 453
money
 corruption of, xvi, 31–34
 food safety and, 94, 97–99, 207, 208
 junk food industry and, 33
 prescription drugs and, 167
 supplement industry and, 177, 178
monoamine oxidase (MAO), 218
monounsaturated fat, 154, 155
Monsanto, 263, 329, 367
muscle damage, 26
mushrooms, 90–91, 204, 233, 250–51, 377, 378, 381–83
mustard greens and seeds, 336, 359, 361–62, 366, 367, 411
myeloma, *11*, 184–86, 188–89, 194

natural killer cells, 79, 83–84, 85, 86, 131, 434
nausea, 420, 422
neuropathy, 145, 165–67
neurotoxins, 261, 262, 265, 352–53
Nigerian paradox, 66
nightshades, 258–59
NIH-AARP study, 133, 135–36, 190, 209–10, 221–22
nitrates, 121–22, 123, 209–11, 295, 416
nitric oxide (NO), 120–22, 295, 416
nitrites, 44, 209–11

nitroglycerin, 29, 120
nitrosamines, 43, 209–10
NO. *See* nitric oxide
nocturia, 281–82
non-Hodgkin's lymphoma. *See* blood cancers
Novick, Jeff, 111, 318
nutmeg, 218, 407, 428–29
nutrition, xv–xvi
  diseases due to, 5, 307
  literature on, xvi, 468–69
  medical school training in, xv, 1–2, 12, 169
  in plant-based diet, 155, 308, 310, 366, 375
  reference book for, 477–78
  in standard American diet, 6, 54–55, 56, 348
nutritional yeast, 90–91, 333
NutritionFacts.org, ix, xvi, 144, 169, 318, 320, 336, 438, 469, 477
nuts and seeds, 154, 314, 331
  blended, 398–99
  for cholesterol control, 31
  clinical trials on, 398–99
  fat in, 402–3
  mental health with, 219–20
  sexual function with, 403–4
  types and daily servings of, 324, *324*, 398
  weight loss with, 401–3

oatmeal, 178–79, 314, 328, 440–41
obesity, 162–63, 431, 457
  anti-obesity drugs, 157
  diabetes and, 144, 145, 148–49, 150–53
  in children, 148–49, 313, 457, 458
  liver disease due to, 174
  pollutants and, 159
  processed foods and, 6
oils, 350–51
olives and olive oil, 146, 350–51, 400–401
omega-3 fats, 22–23, 217, 246, 395, 399, 476–77
omnivores, 116, 129, 153–54, *153*, 158, 215
The Omnivore's Dilemma (Pollan), 313
onions, 179, 218, 281, 332, 341, 377, 388, 407–8
online resources, ix, xvi, 27, 60, 149, 318, 320, 336, 438, 469, 477
oregano and marjoram, 61, 218, 407, 423–24
organic food, 15, 131, 243, 270, 271, 296, 326, 330, 390–93
organochlorines, 262, 263, 264

Ornish, Dean, 9, 10, 72–75, 157
  cancer studies by, 14, 274, 276, 277
  heart disease studies by, xiv, 12, 28, 30, 72, 305
osteoarthritis, 408, 411
osteoporosis, 130, 271
over-the-counter drugs, 141, 171, 294–97
overweight. *See* obesity; weight gain
oxidative stress, 60, 109, 461–62

PAHs. *See* polycyclic aromatic hydrocarbons
pain relief, 165–67, 419–22, 460
pandemic. *See* COVID-19 pandemic
pancreas, 144, 145–47
pancreatic cancer, *11*, 125, 135–38, 386
Parkinson's disease, 252–56
  berries and prevention of, 264–66
  coffee for, 258
  constipation link to, 264–65
  dairy consumption and, 262–63
  death from, *11*, 252
  essential tremor, 259–62
  plant-based diet and, 263–66
  pollutants and risk of, 253–56, 259–62, 263–64, 266–67
  risk reduction tips for, 267
  tobacco and, 257–59
PCBs, 159, 253, 255, 256, 257, 262, 263, 476
PCOS. *See* polycystic ovary syndrome
peanut butter, 325, 384
peas, 334
pepper, black, 292, 338, 383, 410, 412
persistent lipophilic organic pollutants (PLOPs), 267
pesco-vegetarian diet, 149, *153*
pesticides, 235, 253, 296
  cancer risk with, 391–92
  diabetes risk and, 159
  GMOs and, 329–31
  Parkinson's risk and, 253, 254–56, 262–63, 264, 265–66
  reducing, 390–91
pets, 192–93
pharmaceutical industry, xv, 12
Philip Morris, 33, 37
phosphate salts, 207
phosphorus, 206–8
physicians, 1–2, 12, 33, 298–99. *See also* health care system; medical establishment
phytates, 128, 129–31
phytoestrogens, 246, 248–49, 278, 339, 396

phytonutrients, 127. *See also* carotenoids
  in fruits, 57, 82, 180
  in greens, 372, 375
  in tea, 119, 448, 450
  toxin defense with, 82
  tumor growth blocked by, 127, 131
  unique profiles of, 378–80
pickled foods, 332
pigment phytonutrients, 378
  greens and, 368
  mental health with, 224
  power of, 82, 126, 179–80, 341, 436
pineal gland, 234, 236
pistachios, 372, 398, 401–2, 403–4
plant-based diet, 6, 8, 9, 34. *See also* vegan diet; vegetarian diet
  acid reflux prevention with, 139–40
  Alzheimer's prevention with, 65–69, 73–75, 414
  angina and, 30
  antioxidant power of, 60–62
  aspirin-like benefits with, 296–97
  asthma improvement with, 48, 50–51
  blood cancer risk with, 186–88, 194
  blood pressure treatment with, 102–4, 108, 113–24, 332, 384
  blood sugar control with, 157, 163–65, 343, 429
  breast cancer prevention and treatment with, 6, 130, 131, 180, 240–51, 275, 356, 385–86
  cancer prevention and treatment with, 6, 39–40, 82–83, 126–28, 130, 141–43, 227–28, 231, 240–51, 275–79, 328, 359–60, 361, 380, 385–87
  for children, 478
  cholesterol control with, 21–22, 25, 28–31
  COPD prevention and management with, 44–45
  daily checklist for, 323–26, *324*
  definition and outline of, 315–16, 323–26
  diabetes risk and treatment with, 144, 146, 152–60, 163–67, 360, 429–30
  disease prevention and treatment with, 5–6, 8–10, 293, 296–97, 309–10
  dopamine levels with, 468
  with exercise, 460–62
  heart disease treatment with, xiii–xiv, 10, 21–22, 25, 28–31, 131, 305–6, 431, 469
  immune system strength with, 80–84, 87–88, 90–91
  iron sufficiency in, 133–34
  kidney function with, 195–96, 209
  mental health with, 214–22, 224–25, 434
  neuropathy treatment with, 165–68
  nutrition from, 155, 308, 310, 366, 375
  Parkinson's risk and, 262–64
  prostate cancer and, 14, 274–77, 283–84
  radiation protection with, 290–92
  toxin reduction with, 82, 255–56, 263–64, 360
  variety benefits in, 61–62, 378–80, 386
  weight regulation with, 149, 153–60
PLOPs. *See* persistent lipophilic organic pollutants
PMS. *See* premenstrual syndrome
pneumonia, 78, 80, 83, 89, 140
Pollan, Michael, 313
pollutants. *See* food pollutants; toxins
polycyclic aromatic hydrocarbons (PAHs), 43
polycystic ovary syndrome (PCOS), 374, 424
polyps, 127, 130, 131–32, 170, 297
popcorn, 406, 431, 437
poppy seeds, 427–28
pork, 92, 94, 97–98, 176–77, 204, *205*, 215
potassium, 56–57, 160, 308, 327, 328
potatoes, 306, 341, 384
poultry, 71, 77, 382
  acid load with, 204, *205*
  cancer risk with, 136–37, 139, 190, 237, 273, 278
  fat content in, 162–63
  food poisoning with, 94–99, 175, 207
  sodium levels in, 110
  toxins in, 256–57
  UTIs link to, 96–97
  workers and cancer risk, 136, 191
prebiotics, 87, 334, 338, 434
prediabetes, 148–50, 155, 158, 164, 168
PREDIMED trial, 399–401
pregnancy, 86–87
  animal-based food risk in, 43
  blood cholesterol and, 24
  coffee consumption during, 448
  hepatitis E and, 177
  herbs and spices with, 345, 414, 422–23
  incense use during, 49
  iodine with, 476
  pollutants in, 253–54, 255
premenstrual syndrome (PMS), 219

prescription drugs, 357
 benefits of, 292–94
 for blood sugar, 161, 164–65
 death from, 285
 for depression, 218, 220, 223, 225–26
 food treatment compared to, 10, 12–13, 51, 112–13, 118, 120, 132, 202, 220, 280, 292–97
 market in U.S. for, 2–3
 side effects of, 10, 26–27, 30, 110, 111, 120, 130, 161, 195, 218, 220, 226, 280–81, 285, 355, 367, 421
Pritikin, Nathan, xiii–xiv, 28, 274, 280
probiotics, 86–87, 331
processed foods, 466
 definition of, 313–15
 diseases linked to, 5–6, 55, 68
 phosphate caution with, 207
 sodium levels in, 106–7, 109, 111
 trans fats in, 25
 ultra-processed foods, 200–201
 whole grains compared to, 438–40
processed meat, 102, 200, 201, 209–11, 255, 264, 309
profits, 12, 97, 100, 110, 207, 226, 299, 312, 320, 466
pro-oxidant, 45, 133, 180, 384
prostate, enlarged, 279–81
prostate cancer
 annual deaths from, *11*
 cell growth regulation and, 131, 275, 360
 dairy and eggs, 270–74, 278
 diet and risk of, 270–74, 180
 flaxseed and, 278–79, 396
 plant-based diet and reversal of, 14, 274–77, 283–84
 screening for, 268–70
 surgery for, 280
protein. *See also* animal protein
 animal to plant ratio for, 277
 in beans, 327
 kidney function and, 197–99
 malformation of, 265
Prozac, 220, 221, 226
PSA levels, 268–70, 276, 277, 279

radiation, 289–92, 422
radishes, 359, 362, 386
ranolazine (Ranexa), 30
raspberries, 340, 342, 344
raw food, 117, 360, 382, 388–89, 411

recipes
 for beans, 328–29, 335–36
 for beverages, 179–80, 446, 453–54
 cancer-fighting salad, 386–87
 for cruciferous vegetables, 362–64
 for desserts, 336–37, 344
 easy and cheap, 318, 372
 for flaxseeds, 396–97
 for fruit, 344, 345
 for ginger, 422–23
 for greens, 371–73
 miso soup, 331
 mushroom, 382–83
 for nuts and seeds, 398–99
 online sources for, 318
 pesto, 436–37
 salad, 374–75, 386–87
 for spice mixes, 112, 426–27
 tempeh, 328–29
 for turmeric, 410–11
 whole grain, 436–37, 441
rectal cancer. *See* colorectal cancer
registered dietitian, 33
respiratory disease, 44, 49, 50
resting heart rate, 104–6
rhinoconjunctivitis, 47
rice, 113, 313–14
rocket, *122*, 186, 211, 359, 366
Roundup, 329–30

Sacks, Frank, 114–15
SAD. *See* standard American diet
saffron, 69, 220, 225, 407, 414
salads, 374–75, 386–87
salicylic acid, 294–97
salmon, 159
Salmonella, 92–97, 375, 376
salt. *See* sodium
salt industry, 109
salt water, 391
saturated fat, 154–56, 242, 310–11
sauces, 398–99, 436–37
seaweeds, 475–76
secondhand smoke, 37, 42, 48, 210, 258
seizures, 178, 447
Semmelweis, Ignaz Philipp, 287–89
serotonin, 218, 219–20
side effects
 of antacids, 140–41
 of blood pressure drugs, 112–13, 114, 120
 of diabetes medications, 161
 of mental health drugs, 218, 220, 226

of prescription drugs, 10, 26–27, 30, 110, 111, 120, 130, 161, 195, 218, 220, 226, 280–81, 285, 355, 367, 421
"Simple 7" factors, 4, 7
sirtuins, 70–71
sitting, 458–60
sleep, 58, 235, 236, 449
smoking, 8, 313, 466
  cancers from, 29, 36, 37, 51, 135, 136, 137, 138, 209, 261
  COPD from, 44–45
  cruciferous vegetables and, 39, 40, 46
  as health factor, 4, 7, 8, 460
  Parkinson's and, 257–59
  smoking cessation, 8, 27, 33–34, 173, 181, 316, 337, 427
smoothies, 321, 371, 411, 426, 451
sodium, 308, 475
  blood pressure and, 106–11, 117, 331–33
  cancer risk with excess, 332
  in canned beans, 335
  intake guidelines, 106, 109, 111, 331
soft drinks, 102, 110, 158, 174, 194, 201, 222, 312–13, 343, 454–55. *See also* Coca-Cola
sorbitol, 453
soya, 199, 336
  blood pressure and, 331–33
  breast cancer and, 248–50, 330, 339
  calcium in, 328
  GMOs in, 329–31
  miso, 327, 328, 331–33
  tempeh, 43–44, 324, 327, 328
  tofu, 198, 324, 327, 328, 332, 338, 411
  unprocessed, 328–29
soya milk, 115, 249, 328, 332, 396, 411
spices. *See* herbs and spices
spinach, 92, 366, 369, 375, 386
Spock, Benjamin, 478
sprouted food, 46–47, 334, 363–64, 375–76
Spurlock, Morgan, 174
Stadtman, Earl, 58
standard American diet (SAD), 3
  blood pressure with, 103–4, 116
  brain and mood health with, 65–67, 219–20
  cancer with, 129, 239–40, 275
  diseases from, 20, 48, 65–67, 197, 204, 239, 403
  food industry's part in, 312–15, 466
  nutrition lack in, 6, 312–13, 425–26
  sodium in, 109

transition from, 317–19, 333–34
typical fare in, 48, 377, 387, 425–26
Starfield, Barbara, 300–301
statin drugs, 4, 10, 26–28, 31, 65, 197, 202, 293, 370, 395, 415
stem cells, 245–46
stevia, 453
stool. *See* bowel movement
strawberries, 68, 142–43, 156, *157*, 266, 340, 342, 344, 347
stress. *See* mental health
stroke, 54–62, 263
  antioxidants reducing risk of, 58–62
  deaths from, *11*, 54
  dietary prevention for, 6, 54–57, 367, 400, 431
  sleep duration and risk of, 58
sugars, 308, 337–38, 342–44, 371, 466–68
suicide, *11*, 212, 215, 221, 235
sulforaphane, 46, 186, 245–47, 323, 360–64
sulfur additives, 355
Super Size Me, 174
superbugs, 98–99
superoxide, 59–60, 109, 340
supplements
  caution with, 177–78, 413, 414, 426, 473–78
  foods over, 50, 60, 187, 202, 225, 242, 250, 264, 290–91, 364, 379, 409, 411–13, 473, 476
  recommendations for, 473–78
surgery, 161–62, 238, 246, 248, 270, 276–77, 287, 408, 422, 423
sweet potatoes, 57, 383–84
sweeteners, 453–55
swine flu, 77

tea, 448–52. *See also* green tea; hibiscus tea
  cancer protection with, 449, 450
  fluoride in, 451
  leaves, 424, 426, 446, 451
  phytonutrients in, 119, 448, 450
  types and servings of, 442, 448
telomeres, 8–10, 72
tempeh, 43–44, 324, 327, 328. *See also* soya
textured vegetable protein (TVP), 201, 281
thyroid function, 475–76
tobacco. *See* smoking
tobacco industry, 33, 109, 257–58, 270, 312, 466
tofu, 198, 324, 327, 328, 332, 338, 411. *See also* soya

tomatoes, 32, 224, 225, 258, 259, 314, 324, 378–79, 387. *See also* lycopene
toxins. *See also* heavy metals; pesticides
  in bodies, 253–54
  fiber intake and, 143
  in food, 159
  monounsaturated fats eliminating, 154
  phytonutrients defense against, 82
  plant-based foods reducing, 82, 255–56, 263–64, 360
  in saturated fat, 155
  in supplements, 413
  trans fat, 22, 25, 113, 166–67, 207–8, 310–11
tryptophan, 219–20
tumor. *See* cancer; polyps
turmeric, 292, 407, 408–14. *See also* curcumin
  cancer-fighting properties of, 41–42, 126–28, 137, 189, 194
  cautions with, 414
  clinical trials on, 41, 189, 292, 408, 412, 413
  flatulence reduction with, 338
  suggestions for consumption of, 112, 325, 407, 410
  supplement compared to whole food of, 411–13
  synergistic foods for, 411
TVP. *See* textured vegetable protein

uric acid, 175, 198, 199, 203, 204–5, 263, 419
urinary tract infections, 95–97
U.S. Department of Agriculture (USDA), 6, 95–96, 188, 257, 307, 309, 310–11, 391

V8 juice, 122
vaccinations, 80, 175, 181, 182, 255
varicose veins, 128, 142, 170, 214
vascular disorder, 63–65
vegan diet, 200–201, 316
  angina and, 30
  blood pressure on, 116
  BMI and, 149
  bowel movements with, 129
  diabetes occurrence with, 153, *153*, 154, 158, 165
  nutrition in, 159, 242–43
  pollutants with, 263
  prostate cancer and, 277, 278
vegetables
  cancer-fighting, 385–87
  meal options for, 383–84, 393
  strategies for kids eating, 384–85
  types and daily servings of, 377
  variety in diet benefit, 378–80, 385–87
  wash for, 390–91
vegetarian diet, 134, 140, 203, 239, 241, 267, 311, 316
  blood cancer incidence with, 186
  blood pressure with, 114–15
  BMI and, 149–50
  bowel movement with, 129
  dementia occurrence with, 66, 73
  diabetes occurrence with, *153*, 158, 159–60
  fat burning enzyme in, 160
  meat-eating transition to, 5–6
  urine alkalinity with, 199–200
vinegar, 373–74, 391
vision, 145, 161, 167, 345, 346, 365
vitamin A, 160, 187, 388, 473
vitamin B12, 73, 382, 473, 474, 478
vitamin C, 128, 160, 242, 375, 388, 389, 405, 461, 473
  antioxidant power of, 108, 187, 210, 290
  iron absorption with, 135
  plant-based diet and, 8
  supplement form of, 290, 379
vitamin D, 234, 370, 473, 474–75
vitamin E, 50, 160, 187, 425, 473
vitamin K, 367, 371, 375

Waist-to-Height Ratio (WHtR), 167–68, *168*
walnuts, 325, 371, 372, 374–75, 398, 399–401, 402, 404, 476
warfarin, 367
water, 442, 443–46, 450–51, 455
watermelon, 117, 324, 348, 354, 379
weight, body, 4, 6, 116. *See also* body mass index; obesity
weight gain, 160, 162–63, 454–55
weight loss, 168
  bean consumption link to, 154–55
  clinical trials on, 157, 158, 179
  nuts and, 401–3
  oatmeal and, 179
  with plant-based diet, 149, 154–60, 164
  supplements for, 177–78
  vinegar for, 374
weight stigma, 150–52
wheat sensitivity, 433–35
wheatgrass juice, 365
white blood cells, 79, 80, 81, 83, 86, 90, 184–85

whole grains, 129, 296, *324*, 326, 431–41
  blood pressure health with, 112–13
  inflammation and, 432
  liver health with, 178–79
  processed compared to, 436–37
  suggestions for, 436–38
  types and daily servings of, 325, 431
willpower, 317–19
wine, 117, 172, 233, 261, 355
Winfrey, Oprah, 76, 100, 187
women, 158, 219, 247, 270–71, 444. *See also* breast cancer; menstruation
  fat intake study with, 67–68
  heart disease and, 301
  iron deficiency in, 134–35
  kidney disease study on, 197
  nuts benefit for, 404
  pollutants in bodies of, 253–55
World Health Organization, 4, 49, 78, 99–100, 173, 210, 212, 257, 426, 444, 453, 476

x-rays, 289–90, 292
xylitol, 453

Yersinia, 97–98

zoonosis, 96, 176

About the Author

A founding member and fellow of the American College of Lifestyle Medicine, Michael Greger, M.D., FACLM, is a physician, a *New York Times* bestselling author, and an internationally recognized speaker on nutrition, food safety, and public health issues. He has lectured at the Conference on World Affairs and testified before Congress and was invited as an expert witness in the defense of Oprah Winfrey in the infamous "meat defamation" trial. In 2017, Dr. Greger was honored with the ACLM Lifestyle Medicine Trailblazer Award. He is a graduate of Cornell University's School of Agriculture and Life Sciences and the Tufts University School of Medicine. His books *How Not to Die*, *The How Not to Die Cookbook*, *How Not to Diet*, and *How Not to Age* became instant *New York Times* bestsellers. Dr. Greger is the founder of the science-based nonprofit health and research organization NutritionFacts.org, which provides free updates on the latest in nutrition research via videos, blogs, podcasts, and infographics and is strictly noncommercial, without any sponsors, ads, brand partnerships, or paid subscriptions. All proceeds he receives from his books, DVDs, and speaking engagements are donated to charity.